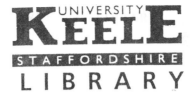

LIBRARY

Please return by the last date shown

10. JUN. 1994		

PROSTAGLANDINS

CURRENT ENDOCRINOLOGY: BASIC AND CLINICAL ASPECTS
Louis V. Avioli, *Series Editor-in-Chief*

TITLES IN **CURRENT ENDOCRINOLOGY**

ENDOCRINE CONTROL OF GROWTH
William H. Daughaday, *Editor-in-Chief*

GLUCAGON
Roger H. Unger and Lelio Orci, *Editors-in-Chief*

PROLACTIN
Robert B. Jaffe, *Editor-in-Chief*

ENDOCRINE ASPECTS OF AGING
Stanley G. Korenman, *Editor-in-Chief*

PROSTAGLANDINS
James B. Lee, *Editor-in-Chief*

CLINICAL REPRODUCTIVE NEUROENDOCRINOLOGY
Judith L. Vaitukaitis, *Editor-in-Chief*

PROSTAGLANDINS

Edited by
James B. Lee, M.D.

Professor of Medicine
State University of New York
Erie County Medical Center
Buffalo, New York

ELSEVIER · NEW YORK
New York · Amsterdam · Oxford

Elsevier North Holland, Inc.
52 Vanderbilt Avenue, New York, New York 10017

Sole distributors outside the United States and Canada:
Elsevier Science Publishers B.V.
P.O. Box 211, 1000 AE Amsterdam, The Netherlands

Library of Congress Cataloging in Publication Data

Main entry under title:

Prostaglandins.

(Current endocrinology)

Bibliography: p.
Includes index.
1. Prostaglandins. I. Lee, James B., 1930–   . II. Series.
[DNLM: 1. Prostaglandins — Physiology. QU 90 P9662 1981]
QP801.P68P7223   612'.405   81-12613
ISBN 0-444-00645-1   AACR2

Manufactured in the United States of America

CONTENTS

PROSTACYCLIN, PROSTAGLANDINS, THROMBOXANES, AND PLATELET FUNCTION

Ryszard J. Gryglewski

PROSTAGLANDINS AND SKELETAL METABOLISM

Lawrence G. Raisz

FOREWORD

Although endocrinology textbooks satisfy a fundamental educational need and are routinely used as reference standards, an information gap often exists between the current state of the art and the published contents. Refinements in laboratory methods and assay techniques, the ever increasing awareness of metabolic and endocrine correlates that were once unapparent, and the dramatic discoveries in molecular biology and genetics make it extremely difficult to present an up-to-date volume at time of publication. The endocrinology textbook may effectively serve the academic community only for 3–5 years.

Despite the constant change in the state of the art, new discoveries defining relationships between endocrinology and molecular biology, physiology, genetics, biochemistry, biophysics, and immunology do not proceed at comparable rates. In fact, certain areas of endocrinology have been dormant for years.

In an attempt to offer timely reviews, a number of well-established authorities were offered the challenge of editing small editions that characterize the state-of-the-art in *specific* areas of endocrinology. This format relieves the editor (or editors) from the nearly impossible task of producing a "current textbook" of endocrinology and facilitates the process of rapid and timely revision. Moreover, a specific endocrine discipline review can be revised if and when necessary without revising an entire textbook.

Endocrine Control of Growth, edited by W. Daughaday, was the first review in this series, *Current Endocrinology: Basic and Clinical Aspects*. This has been followed by individual texts on *Glucagon* and *Prolactin*, edited by R. Unger and L. Orci, and R. Jaffe, respectively. This series presents those current aspects of endocrinology of interest to the basic scientist, clinician, house officer, trainee, and medical student alike. These initial volumes will be followed by others on *Thyroid, Posterior Pituitary, Clinical Reproductive Neuroendocrinology, Androgens-Hirsutism, Molecular Action of Hormones, The Adrenal, Hormonal Control of Skeletal Remodeling, Gastrointestinal Hormones,* and *Endocrine Aspects of Aging*. We are confident that this complete series and its revised editions, when appropriate, will serve the academic community well.

Louis V. Avioli, M.D.

PREFACE

Since the original discovery of biological activity ultimately attributable to prostaglandins by the independent observations of Kurzrok and Lieb, U. S. von Euler, and M. W. Goldblatt in the early 1930s, a voluminous literature has appeared to the extent of thousands of articles each year. Although the prostaglandins have the most diverse and potent biological activities of any of the known autocoids, a precise physiological or pathological role has not been defined in all the organ systems in which they have been studied.

Because the literature on prostaglandins is so vast and filled with numerous conflicting and at times irreconcilable observations, basic science investigators and clinicians, involved as well as uninvolved in prostaglandin research, have often found it difficult to perceive a rational continuum underlying many of the observations with these ubiquitous and fascinating compounds. Although this book makes no claim to provide a thread of rationale on this subject, it is intended to bring together as concisely and, hopefully, as lucidly as possible, the current state of the art in a modestly comprehensive fashion. The bibliographies are arbitrarily selective and extensive but not exhaustive. There is some unavoidable overlap among the various chapters, particularly with regard to synthesis and metabolism, the cardiovascular and renal systems, and the immune and inflammatory responses that hopefully will be regarded as a positive factor, enabling the reader to profit from several different points of view.

The editor wishes to express his thanks and deep appreciation to the numerous authorities who have contributed so much time and effort in surveying their respective fields of interest in prostaglandin research. The editor also wishes to thank Ms. Diane Drobnis of Elsevier North Holland for her patience and valuable assistance during the preparation of the manuscripts. Lastly, the editor is indebted to Audrey, James, Jr., John, David, and Steven for forbearance and support.

James B. Lee, M.D.

CONTRIBUTORS

AHMAD A. ATTALLAH, Ph.D.
Research Assistant Professor of Medicine, State University of New York, Department of Medicine, Erie County Medical Center, Buffalo, New York

HAROLD R. BEHRMAN, Ph.D.
Associate Professor of Obstetrics/Gynecology and Pharmacology, Yale University School of Medicine, Departments of Obstetrics, Gynecology, and Pharmacology, New Haven, Connecticut

MARC BYGDEMAN, M.D.
Professor, Department of Obstetrics and Gynecology, World Health Organization, Research and Training Centre on Human Reproduction, Karolinska Institutet, Stockholm, Sweden

THOMAS M. FITZPATRICK, Ph.D.
Research Associate, Department of Physiology and Biophysics, Georgetown University Schools of Medicine and Dentistry, Washington, D.C.

A. GILLESPIE, M.D.
Department of Obstetrics and Gynecology, University of Adelaide, Queen Victoria Hospital, Adelaide, South Australia, Australia

RYSZARD J. GRYGLEWSKI, M.D.
Chairman and Professor, Department of Pharmacology, Copernicus Academy of
Medicine, Cracow, Poland

ALAN K. HALL, Ph.D.
Post Doctoral Fellow, Departments of Obstetrics, Gynecology, and Pharmacology, Yale
University School of Medicine, New Haven, Connecticut

PETER A. KOT, M.D.
Professor, Department of Physiology and Biophysics, Georgetown University Schools
of Medicine and Dentistry, Washington, D.C.

JAMES B. LEE, M.D.
Professor of Medicine, Department of Medicine, State University of New York, Erie
County Medical Center, Buffalo, New York

CHARLES W. PARKER, M.D.
Professor of Medicine, Microbiology, and Immunology, Investigator, Howard Hughes
Medical Institute and Department of Medicine, Washington University School of
Medicine, St. Louis, Missouri

LAWRENCE G. RAISZ, M.D.
Professor of Medicine, Head, Endocrinology and Metabolism, Department of Medicine,
University of Connecticut Health Center, Farmington, Connecticut

ANDRÉ ROBERT, M.D., Ph.D.
Distinguished Research Scientist, Department of Experimental Biology, The Upjohn
Company, Kalamazoo, Michigan

MARY J. RUWART, Ph.D.
Research Scientist, Department of Experimental Biology, The Upjohn Company,
Kalamazoo, Michigan

WILLIAM F. STENSON, M.D.
Assistant Professor of Medicine, Chief, Division of Gastroenterology, Jewish Hospital of
St. Louis, Washington University School of Medicine, St. Louis, Missouri

ROBERT B. ZURIER, M.D.
Professor of Medicine, Chief, Rheumatology Section, University of Pennsylvania School
of Medicine, Philadelphia, Pennsylvania

PROSTAGLANDINS

ALAN K. HALL, Ph.D.

HAROLD R. BEHRMAN, Ph.D.

PROSTAGLANDINS: BIOSYNTHESIS, METABOLISM, AND MECHANISM OF CELLULAR ACTION

INTRODUCTION

Prostaglandins, prostacyclins, and thromboxanes comprise groups of polyunsaturated, hydroxylated long chain fatty acids that can evoke a wide spectrum of biological actions at extremely low concentrations in a variety of tissues. Since their discovery in the early 1930s by the Swedish biochemist von Euler, prostaglandins have been subjected to much research and numerous literature reviews. This chapter deals with some of the salient features of the biosynthesis and metabolism of prostaglandin, prostacyclin, and thromboxane, and embraces a number of possible mechanisms by which these "autocoids" might act within the cell.

Prostaglandins, thromboxanes, and prostacyclins occur naturally in many of the tissues so far examined. Prostaglandins per se have been implicated as playing a functional role in such physiological processes as vasodilation and vasoconstriction [114], regulation of body temperature [160], platelet aggregation [158,219,220], reproduction [58,102,115], inflammation [249], gastrointestinal function [213,258], autonomic neurotransmission [226], and cardiovascular and renal function [136,178,-

From the Reproductive Biology Section, Departments of Obstetrics, Gynecology, and Pharmacology, Yale University School of Medicine, New Haven, Connecticut.

1

253]. Clinical and pharmacological applications of prostaglandins are dealt with extensively in a recent review by Elattar [41].

The bulk of thromboxane research to date has been focused on platelet and cardiovascular function [6,19,145]. However, other studies have recognized the involvement of thromboxanes in uterine function [165], in the inflammation and permeability of granulomal tissue [31], in gastric mucosal tissue function [5], in the control of blood vessel tone [6], and in neurotransmission [91]. In a provocative scenario composed by Horrobin et al. in 1978, thromboxane A_2 (TXA_2) is allocated a central role in the control of a multitude of processes ranging from ultraviolet radiation effects on perfused rat mesentery to the inevitable modulation of calcium flux [101]. Also, for researchers who are anxious to discover other physiological processes affected by TXA_2, it has recently been suggested that enhanced neural TXA_2 formation may be responsible (at least in part) for their anxiety [100]!

Continued study of the products of arachidonic acid metabolism, together with the isolation of an enzyme system localized within vascular endothelium, gave rise to the innovative characterization of prostacyclin (PGI_2, formerly designated PGX) [24,111,217]. Because of its relative novelty, little is known of the effects of PGI_2 apart from its superior inhibitory action on vasoconstriction and platelet aggregation [24,175, 257].

In view of the formidable evidence for an involvement of prostaglandins, thromboxanes, and prostacyclins in the processes outlined above, it is not surprising that a good deal of attention has polarized around the mechanism(s) by which these substances are made, released, and degraded.

BIOSYNTHESIS

Origins and Release of Precursors

Prostaglandins are not stored within the cell to any great extent [134,198], thus any stimulation of their release requires the a priori mobilization of substrate precursor(s) such as free fatty acid (FFA). The major fraction of cellular FFA occurs tightly sequestered in the esterified form as cholesteryl esters (CEs), triglycerides (TGs), or phospholipids (PLs) (Fig. 1). It is the general consensus that a cardinal rate-limiting phase in prostaglandin (and presumably thromboxane) formation is precursor availability [133,134]. Polyunsaturated fatty acids (PUFAs) like arachidonic acid ($C_{20:4\omega6}$) (Fig. 1) are the principal substrates for prostaglandin (PG) and thromboxane formation. Release of PUFAs is facilitated by the hydrolytic action of a class of membrane-associated enzymes referred to as phospholipases. These phospholipases are classified in accordance with the site on a PL molecule where they catalyze a hydrolytic cleavage. Thus phospholipase A_1 specifically removes the fatty acid moiety (deacylation) from the carbon-1 position. Exquisite coverage of phospho-

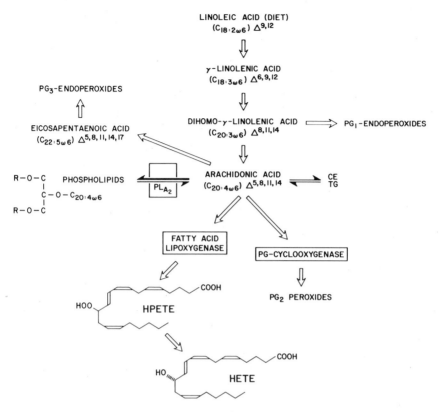

FIGURE 1. Cellular origin and metabolism of arachidonic acid. Linoleic acid (EFA) is obtained from dietary intake. PGE_1 and $PGF_{1\alpha}$ (monenoic PGs) are a relatively rare occurrence, since $C_{20:4\omega6}$ is a major precursor FFA.

lipase involvement with prostaglandin biosynthesis has recently been reviewed.

Typically, phospholipase A_2 (phosphatide-2-acyl-hydrolase, E.C. 3.1.1.4) catalyzes the selective deacylation of arachidonic acid [127] (Fig. 1). Indeed, it has been shown that as much as 95% of cellular arachidonic acid is bound and esterified in the phosphatide fraction, at least in the platelet [16,19]. Also, phosphatidylcholine (lecithin) is known to lose its arachidonate moiety during PG formation in spleen slices. The importance of phospholipase activation assumes significance in view of the finding that naturally occurring "nascent" free arachidonic acid is a distant cellular rarity. Indeed, even when free arachidonic acid is mobilized by esterase enzymes, its inherent hydrophobicity causes a large portion of it to be mopped up by the plethora of avid lipophilic binding sites on serum albumin [52,76,230].

Several of the phospholipases studied thus far appear to be calcium dependent [55], a finding that is supported by the stimulatory effect of carboxylic acid ionophores A23187 and X537A [188] on prostaglandin and thromboxane biosynthesis. In platelets, such proaggregatory agents as collagen and thrombin are known to stimulate release of arachidonate from phospholipids.

Metabolism of Arachidonic Acid

The liberation of free arachidonic acid is soon followed by the evolution of prostaglandin endoperoxides and the subsequent formation of prostaglandins, thromboxanes, and prostacyclins, along with the multitude of other arachidonic acid metabolites depending on the system under investigation. Arachidonic acid is degraded by the so-called arachidonic acid cascade [205] which is comprised of two distinct pathways (Fig. 1). Arachidonic acid ($C_{20:4\omega6}$) is hydroxylated in one pathway by fatty acid lipoxygenase (mainly in blood platelets), which results in the evolution of such hydroxy acids as hydroxyeicosatetraenoic acid (HETE) [186]. Alternatively, arachidonic acid (or other FFAs, Fig. 1) can interact with prostaglandin endoperoxide synthetase (E.C.1.14.99.1) (also referred to as fatty acid cyclooxygenase), a membrane-bound multienzyme complex that specifically catalyzes the incorporation of molecular oxygen into PUFA [134], thereby generating 15-hydroxyprostaglandin endoperoxides (PGG$_2$ and PGH$_2$ if substrate is $C_{20:4\omega6}$) [83]; in addition, under certain conditions, light is emitted because of the presence of singlet oxygen [154].

Prostaglandin synthetase has been studied in a variety of organs; in 1974 Miyamoto et al. [167] solubilized the complex from bovine vesicular gland and found that it was composed of two well-defined fractions. Fraction 1 (the cyclooxygenase) was found to be dependent on L-tryptophan and hemoglobin for maximal activity, whereas the second fraction (isomerase) exhibited an exclusive glutathione requirement. The importance of cofactors in prostaglandin biosynthesis is illustrated by the observation that the presence of reduced glutathione (GSH) and Cu^{2+} is associated with the predominant formation of F-type prostaglandins [133,149]. Ascorbic acid, by virtue of its redox property, favors production of E-type prostaglandins at least in tracheal tissue [203]; gold salts are inhibitory [235].

A number of compounds such as catecholamines, hydroquinone, L-tryptophan, and serotonin (5'HT) are documented as essential cofactors for prostaglandin biosynthesis [227,244]; such claims are substantiated by the finding that these compounds will enhance catalytic conversion of arachidonic acid to the PG endoperoxides PGH$_2$ and PGG$_2$ [168,243]. In the case of epinephrine, prostaglandin biosynthesis is thought to be stimulated by the intrinsic affinity of epinephrine for oxygen radicals [40,241]. Other agents like α-tocopherol (vitamin E) will attenuate prostaglandin endoperoxide formation, at least in rat blood [98]. Compounds that can retard or inhibit prostaglandin formation are, for example: aspirin, indomethacin, probenecid, ethacrynic acid [reviewed extensively (51,215)], phenacetin and acetaminophin (paracetomol) [56], feneprofen [96], suprofen, and other substituted arylacetic acids, such as ibuprofen [109].

These substances, particularly aspirin and indomethacin, attack the cyclooxygenase moiety of prostaglandin synthetase [134,206,245]. Antiinflammatory agents such as glucocorticoids act by blocking the catalytic degradation of membrane PL by phospholipase A_2, thus attenuating the flow of activated PUFA into the arachidonic acid cascade (Fig. 1) [29,75]. More recently some interesting work carried out by Flower and Blackwell [50] has demonstrated that antiinflammatory steroids such as dexamethasone are able to induce an endogenous inhibitor of phospholipase A_2, an effect apparently dependent on de novo protein synthesis.

Endoperoxide Degradation

Little is known of the biological actions of endoperoxides PGG_2 and PGH_2 [187,248] except that they are intermediates in the synthesis of prostaglandins and thromboxanes. Recently, however, it was shown that incubation of $[1-^{14}C]PGH_2$ with solubilized rabbit aorta microsomal prostaglandin I synthetase results in the exclusive formation of PGI_2 [184]; this observation is in accordance with the finding that intravenously infused arachidonic acid is rapidly transformed into PGI_2 upon passage through lungs in anesthetized dogs [177]. Gorman and colleagues [61] have reported that PGH_2 can inhibit basal and hormone-stimulated adenylate cyclase activity in adipocyte ghosts; PGG_2 can apparently attenuate the stimulatory effect of PGE_1 on cyclic AMP formation in platelets [15,24]. On the other hand, cyclic AMP has been shown to inhibit PGG_2 formation in human platelets [151]. The situation is confusing to say the least, but studies utilizing long-acting (epoxy-methano) analogues of PG endoperoxides may further elucidate their physiological role(s) in platelet function [15,219]. Inhibition of cyclic AMP accumulation by PG endoperoxides may well be a plausible mechanism whereby the endoperoxides induce platelet aggregation.

Some of the presently known products of prostaglandin endoperoxide transformations are depicted in Fig. 2. At least six primary products may be formed from endoperoxide transformations, and these are apparently controlled by specific enzymes. Products of endoperoxide metabolism also vary with the presence of cofactors and molecular oxygen. All the products produced from endoperoxides are rapidly degraded to form thromboxanes, prostaglandins, or prostacyclins.

Prostaglandins

The term "prostaglandins" is of course a misnomer: it was coined by von Euler in 1935 in the belief that this substance emanated from the prostate gland. This contention was found to be incorrect when it was

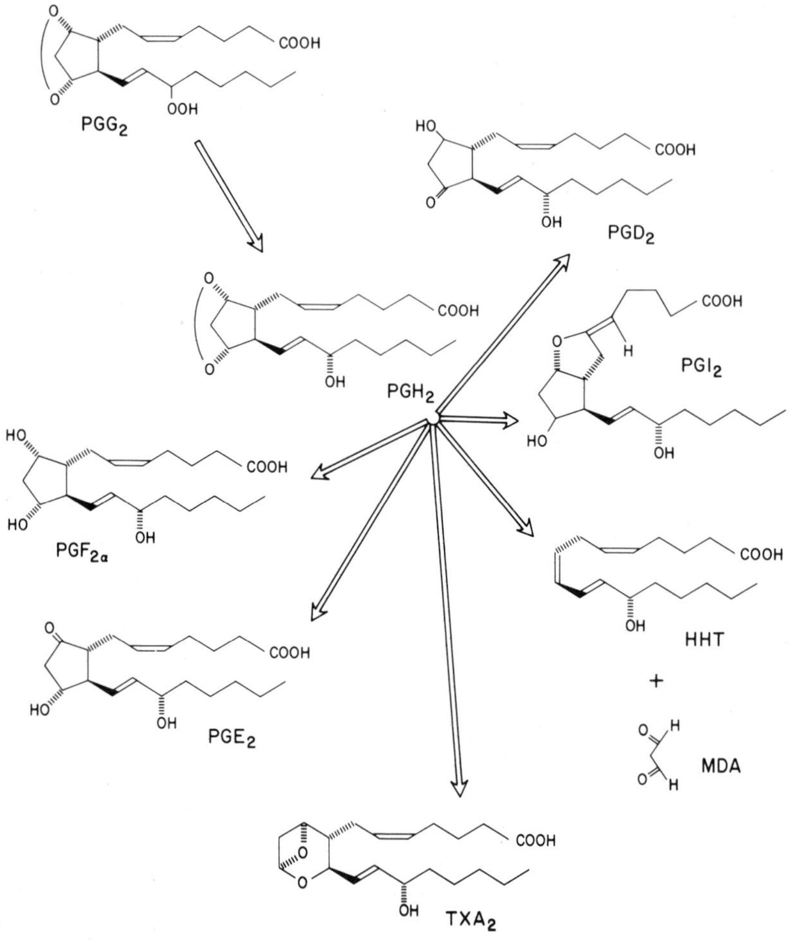

FIGURE 2. Metabolism of prostaglandin endoperoxides.

demonstrated that these pharmacologically active compounds were primarily produced in the seminal vesicles [42]. Some years later, the family of prostaglandins was described and their respective structures determined [14].

The occurrence, synthesis, and biological actions of prostaglandins have been summarized [8,14,114,166,218]. The widespread distribution of the enzymes responsible for prostaglandin biosynthesis is reflected by the observation that they occur in lung, thymus, umbilical cord, uterus, kidney, and heart, and in amniotic and menstrual fluids. The significance of very high concentrations of prostaglandins in human seminal plasma remains a mystery, save for their possible involvement in sperm transport [58,115]. Prostaglandins can even be isolated from a Caribbean coral *(Plexaura hormamalla)*, the predominant prostaglandins being 15-epi-PGA_2 and its diester.

The biosynthesis of prostaglandins from tissues occurs readily in response to a diverse array of pathological stimuli such as the presence of malignant tumors [201,106], fever, trauma, and burns (reviewed by Nakano [178]). Many tissues apparently disgorge prostaglandins at the slightest provocation [20,153]; for example, stretching of uterine tissue will release prostaglandins [198,202]. It certainly appears that the singular most important trigger for prostaglandin liberation may well be perturbation of membrane integrity.

Several well-written accounts deal with the nomenclature [185], biological aspects [8], and organic synthesis [166] of the prostaglandins. Structurally, all prostaglandins are comprised of a cyclopentanone nucleus with two side chains, giving the archetypal "hairpin" prostanoic acid configuration. Primary prostaglandins contain a 15-hydroxyl group and a 13,14-trans double bond. Each type of prostaglandin is currently allocated a group letter, A, B, C, D, E, or F, in accordance with the functionality of the cyclopentanone ring (see Fig. 3). Generally speaking these group letters indicate the degree of prostaglandin lipophilicity, that is, F > E > A > B > 11-deoxy-E [8,9]. A subscript number follows the group letter; this denotes the number of double bonds (degree of unsaturation) in the side chains. Immediately following this subscript number is a further classification index, either α or β, as in $PGF_{2\alpha}$ or $PGF_{2\beta}$: this merely refers to the stereochemistry of the C_9 hydroxyl group (see Fig. 3).

Prostaglandins arise by transformation of prostaglandin endoperoxides (Fig. 2). Endoperoxides were proposed as intermediates in prostaglandin biosynthesis following an elegant series of experiments using $^{18}O_2$ incorporation; it was discovered that the two oxygen atoms that reside in the cyclopentanone ring were derived from the same molecule of oxygen [84,85]. Lands et al. [133] recently reported a kinetic analysis of the mechanism of prostaglandin biosynthesis in soy bean and vesicular tissue; oxygenation of PUFA is apparently modulated by substrate availability, concentration of glutathione, and the presence of an enzyme activator. TXA_2 and HHT are mainly produced by platelets [19,186], along with negligible amounts of prostaglandins. PGE_2 appears to be the major product produced by kidney, whereas blood vessels [72,171], forestomach [193], uterus [46,164], and corpus luteum [142] form mainly PGI_2, as judged by appearance of 6-keto-$PGF_{1\alpha}$. HHT is produced by most tissues but does not appear to have much biological activity. All the products formed from endoperoxide are rapidly metabolized; PGE_2 and $PGF_{2\alpha}$ have a half-life of only a few minutes in the bloodstream.

Thromboxanes

Thromboxanes are formed by the degradation of cyclic prostaglandin endoperoxides (PGG_2 and PGH_2) [37,48,86] (Fig. 2). These unstable non-prostanoate compounds were designated "thromboxane" to indicate

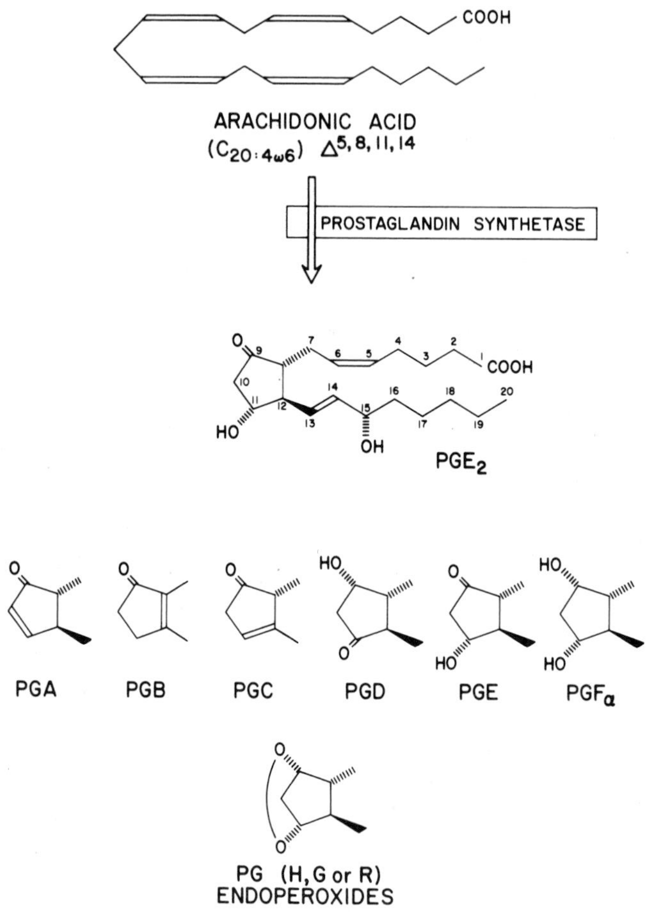

FIGURE 3. Nomenclature of prostaglandins.

their structure and origin. Nomenclature of thromboxanes was discussed in a recent paper [105], and it seems likely that a system similar to that of the primary prostaglandins will be adopted, "thrombanoic acid" being the name describing the basic 20-carbon-substituted tetrahydropyran with the carbon numbering system shown in Fig. 4. Structurally, thromboxane A_2 (TXA$_2$) is best described as an unstable derivative of PGH$_2$ (15-hydroxy-9α,11α-peroxido-prosta-5,13-dienoic acid), which arises from the sequential transformation of PGG$_2$ [15-hydroperoxy-9α,11α-peroxido-prosta-5,13-dienoic acid (Fig. 2)] [86,172]. The appearance of TXA$_2$ in platelets, as a result of arachidonic acid metabolism, is accompanied by formation of malondialdehyde (MDA), a cytotoxic degradation product of the prostaglandin endoperoxide pentanone nucleus, and hydroxylated fatty acids such as 12-hydroxy-8-cis,10-cis-heptadecatrienoic acid (HHT) and hydroxyeicosatetraenoic acid (HETE) [186].

The amount of HHT and HETE or prostaglandins formed in any one system is dependent on the relative activity of prostaglandin cyclooxygenase, and fatty acid lipoxygenase (also the availability of O_2). Platelet thromboxane synthetase has been solubilized (Triton X-100) and is found to be primarily localized within the microsomal fraction of tissue homogenates [87]; activity of this complex is apparently not dependent on cystine or cysteine residues because N-ethylmaleimide (NEM) and dithiothreitol (DTT) do not inhibit formation of the primary metabolite of TXA_2, namely TXB_2 [TXB_2 is trivial name for 8-(1-hydroxy-3-oxopropyl) 9,12-L-dihydroxy-5,10-heptadecadienoic acid or 9α,11,15(S)-trihydroxythromba-5,13-dienoic acid, using nomenclature suggested by Jackson-Roberts et al. in 1978 [105]. It was suggested by Hammarström and Falardeau [87] that 12-L-hydroperoxy-5,8,10,14-eicosatetraenoic acid (HPETE) inhibits TXB_2 biosynthesis; these authors postulate that HPETE might fulfill a role as an endogenous regulator or TXA_2 biosynthesis [44,87].

Substrate specificity studies of thromboxane synthetase reveal that degree of saturation and length of the carbon chain in prostaglandin endoperoxides appear to be the major determinants of substrate activity [181], although it was recently suggested that since TXA_1 and TXA_3 could be formed [134], this specificity may be restricted to endoperoxides and not PUFA. Ho et al. [97] have studied the cofactor requirements of platelet thromboxane synthetase and have demonstrated a requirement for ferriprotoporphyrin IX and L-tryptophan for maximal activity; in contrast to prostaglandin synthetase, the enzyme complex was unaffected by glutathione. The same authors also demonstrated that thromboxane synthetase is rapidly inactivated following TXB_2 formation. Indeed, a similar phenomenon is recognized in the case of prostaglandin cyclooxygenase [135]; it was suggested that this loss of activity might represent a mechanism of hormone-induced desensitization.

As with prostaglandin synthetase [51,215], many agents are capable of retarding the formation of thromboxanes, but few exhibit a selective action, and act by affecting a broad spectrum of enzymes involved in arachidonic acid metabolism. Relatively specific thromboxane synthetase inhibitors are imidazole (a putative buffer substance) (Fig. 5) [170,182] and such nonacidic antiinflammatory compounds as 2-isopropyl-3-nicotinyl-indole (L8027) [180] and dipyridamole (an antithrombotic agent) [6,173]. To confuse matters, sodium-p-benzyl-4-[1-oxo-2(4-chlorobenzyl)-3-phenylpropyl] phenylphosphonate (better known as N-0164) has

FIGURE 4. Carbon numbering system for thrombanoic acid. [After Jackson-Roberts et al. (105)].

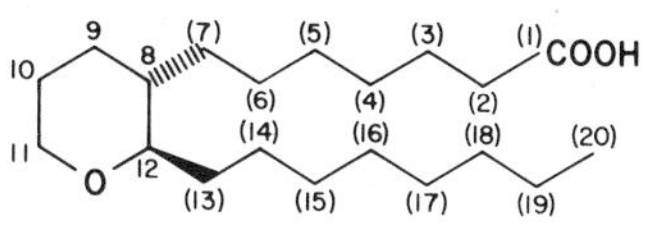

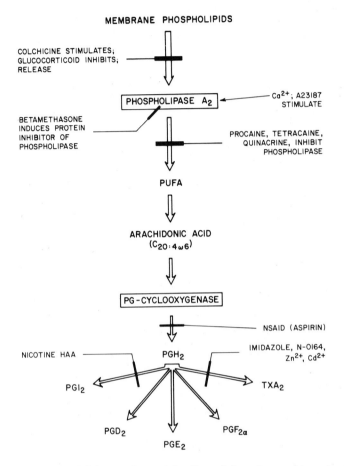

FIGURE 5. Inhibition of prostaglandin and thromboxane biosynthesis.

been cited as both a selective [39,134] and a nonselective [180] inhibitor of thromboxane biosynthesis. In platelets, both cyclic AMP and dibutyryl cyclic AMP exert inhibitory actions on TXA_2 biosynthesis [145,151,162]. Conversely, TXA_2 will lower the platelet concentration of cyclic AMP [63]. Meanwhile, onion and garlic have recently been placed among the more exotic inhibitors of platelet TXA_2 formation [150]. Certain transition metals, particularly Zn^{2+} and Cd^{2+}, also attenuate TXB_2 synthesis in platelets [97]. The divalent cation ionophore A23187 [209] will stimulate platelet and renal prostaglandin and thromboxane formation [123,188], an action that implicates a Ca^{2+}-dependent step in their respective biosyntheses. Pickett et al. [197] suggest that this stimulatory effect of A23187 is directed toward activation of Ca^{2+}-dependent phospholipases [188], which leads to a relatively nonspecific arachidonate mobilization (Figs. 1 and 5).

Prostacyclins

Prostacyclin (PGI$_2$) is the trivial name used to describe 9-deoxy-6,9α-epoxy-Δ^5-PGF$_{1\alpha}$ [111,112]. Being a highly unstable vinyl ether, PGI$_2$ will undergo nonenzymatic "facile hydrolysis" in aqueous solution, particularly at a low pH [32], to form 6-keto-PGF$_{1\alpha}$ (Fig. 6). PGI$_2$ is apparently more stable under basic conditions (1M Tris-buffer, pH 9.5) and low temperatures (0°C).

Prostacyclin formation occurs mainly in the intimal region of arterial tissue [25,171,183], although other studies have revealed that a variety of tissues can produce PGI$_2$, often as a major product of arachidonate metabolism [36,104] in corpus luteum [239], human follicular tissue [142], uterine tissue [46,164,259], bovine seminal vesicles [30], renal tissues [179,239], rat carrageenan-induced granuloma tissue [31], and homogenates of rat stomach [193]. Needleman et al. [179] have suggested that the widespread occurrence of prostacyclin synthetase, as illustrated above, might be attributed to the inclusion of vascular elements in vitro tissue preparations. This apparently justifiable criticism makes interpretation of many tissue slice or homogenate studies somewhat erroneous if not enigmatic. This problem is further compounded by the recent disclosure that the ratio of tissue-reduced or -oxidized pyridine nucleotide (NADPH or NADP$^+$) might predetermine whether PGI$_2$ is released intact or as a metabolite [240,262,263].

It was previously proposed that endothelial tissue "scavenges" PG endoperoxides that are generated by local platelets; the subsequent endothelial evolution and release of PGI$_2$ thus prevents localized thrombus

FIGURE 6. Metabolism of prostacyclin.

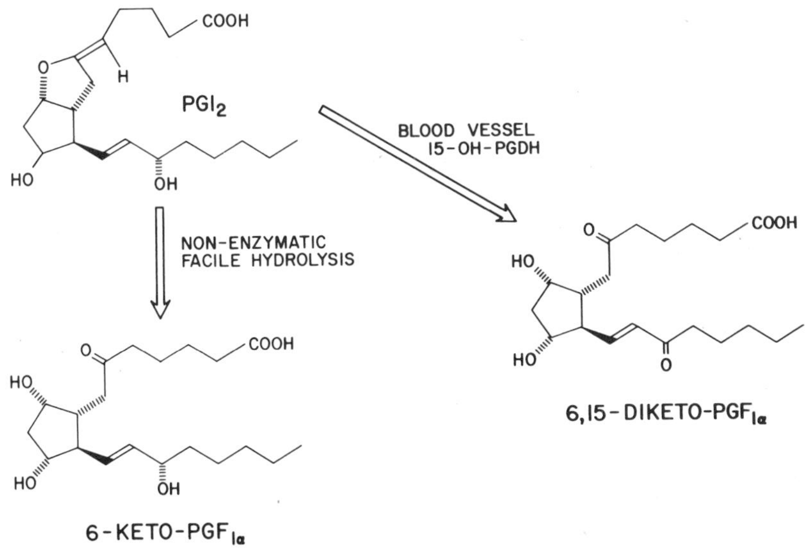

formation via inhibition of platelet aggregation. A very recent paper, however, takes issue with this concept [184]. Hence, PGI_2 has been considered to be the endogenous antithrombotic agent [25,72], an action that is diametrically opposed to that of TXA_2. The suggestion of opposing actions of TXA_2 and PGI_2 vis à vis platelet aggregation and vascular tone has provoked a flurry of interest in the search for specific pharmacological agents capable of selective modulation of the synthesis-metabolism or receptor-binding of PGI_2 and TXA_2 [53,112,180].

There is conclusive evidence that aspirin irreversibly acetylates the catalytic subunit of PG cyclooxygenase [51,215], but there is some disagreement about its use in clinical treatment of cardiovascular disease. Aspirin, particularly in large doses, will abolish the effects of dipyridamole, an agent that acts by potentiation of PGI_2 by phosphodiesterase inhibition [173]. Studies involving culture of porcine endothelial cells indicated that inhibition of PGI_2 biosynthesis by aspirin is dose dependent; low doses of aspirin (100 μM) exert a reversible inhibition, but high doses (1 mM) provide an inhibition of PGI_2 formation that remains some 24 hours after drug removal [59]. The same authors concluded that aspirin administration to infarct patients is potentially dangerous and recommended substitution of sulfinpyrazone for aspirin. A more extensive study of this dilemma was executed by Jaffe and Weksler [108], who showed that endothelial PGI_2 synthetase can recover from aspirin inhibition within 36 hours. The conclusion of this study was that vascular endothelium produces sufficient PGI_2 to counter platelet TXA_2. Apparently, platelet and endothelial cyclooxygenases are equisensitive to aspirin, but recovery of the platelet enzyme from aspirin inhibition is tardy or even incomplete [26,108].

In tobacco consumers, nicotine has been associated with the development of cardiovascular disease [60,255] by virtue of its inhibitory action on PGI_2 biosynthesis. PGI_2 is the main product of arachidonate metabolism in cardiac tissue [36,179], and nicotine will induce a dose-dependent inhibition of $[1-^{14}C]$arachidonate incorporation into $[1-^{14}C]6$-keto-$PGF_{1\alpha}$ in cardiac tissue, which is accompanied by increased release of $[^{14}C]PGE_2$ [255]. Platelet thromboxane synthesis seems to be unaffected by nicotine.

METABOLISM

15-Hydroxy Prostaglandin Dehydrogenase

Primary prostaglandins such as PGE_2, $PGF_{2\alpha}$, or PGA_2 are rapidly inactivated in vivo by passage through the pulmonary circulation [47,198] (PGA_2 can also be degraded by fungi [224]), and this property alone subsequently argues strongly against a function of prostaglandins as circulating hormones (with the possible exception of PGI_2). It has however been suggested that prostaglandins may gain slight protection by macromolecular binding to serum albumin [52,76,230]. The first and most important catabolic step with respect to biological inactivation of primary prostaglandins is the oxidation of the 15-hydroxyl group to a 15-keto moiety, an action catalyzed by the enzyme 15-hydroxyprosta-glandin dehydrogenase (15-OH-PGDH, E.C.1.1.1.141) (Fig. 7). Lee and Levine [137] solubilized 15-OH-PGDH and demonstrated the existence of two types of enzyme that were distinguishable in terms of pyridine nucleotide requirement. Type 1 is NAD$^+$-dependent, whereas type 2 has an exclusive NADP$^+$ requirement. These observations have now been confirmed by affinity chromatography using PGF$_{2\alpha}$-Sepharose [191]. By and large, type 2 15-OH-PGDH plays the cardinal role in pros-taglandin metabolism (reviewed by Hansen in 1976 [89]).

FIGURE 7. Metabolism of prostaglandin E$_2$.

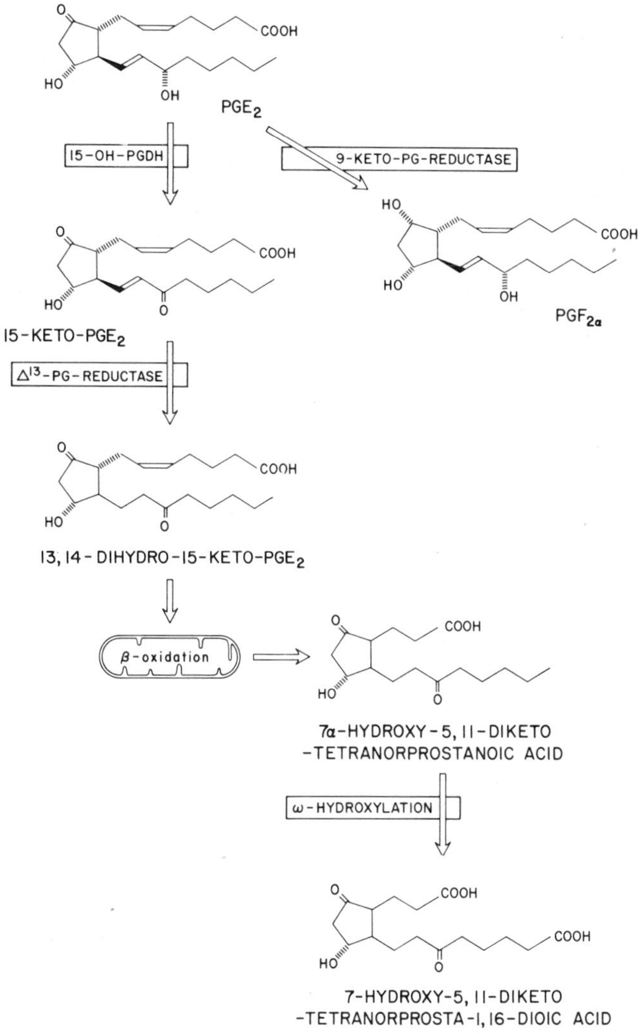

Some studies of 15-OH-PGDH have focused on structural requirements for substrate binding [157], whereas others have documented the
biological distribution of 15-OH-PGDH in tissues (of swine); highest
concentrations of this enzyme are found in lungs, followed by spleen
and then kidney cortex [89]. A recent report has provided convincing
evidence that 15-OH-PGDH is also localized in both mesenteric arteries
and veins [262], the importance of which is discussed below. Additional
work suggests that despite its low activity, 15-OH-PGDH may make a
valid contribution to prostaglandin degradation in brain tissue [247]. It
appears that as in the case of prostaglandin cyclooxygenase [135], 15-
OH-PGDH has a very short biological half-life as demonstrated by the
use of inhibitors of protein synthesis [18].

Recent studies have shown that 15-OH-PGDH displays a characteristic
substrate specificity, in that any modification of the prostanoate structure
in the vicinity of the reaction site (carbon-15) greatly modifies the substrate activity [9,238]. On a scale where $PGF_{2\alpha}$ exhibits 100% substrate
activity, it has been demonstrated that the following prostaglandins may
be classified: $PGE_2 > PGH_2 > PGA_2 >$ 11-deoxy-$PGF_{2\alpha}$ [238]. Apparently,
neither PGG_2, PGD_2, nor PGB_2 is a substrate for 15-OH-PGDH, at least
in the monkey lung.

Dehydrogenation at carbon-15 results in almost complete loss of biological activity with and the subsequent formation of the 15-keto derivative; this is a structural change that activates the 13,14 double bond
as a substrate for 13,14-prostaglandin reductase (Fig. 7). Recently it was
shown that PGI_2 may be a circulating hormone [174]; this observation
is reinforced by the finding that exogenous PGI_2 can traverse the perfused rabbit heart [179] without being metabolized. Indeed, PGI_2 is apparently released from the lungs, an effect potentiated by hyperventilation [74]. A recent communication [262] has suggested that PGI_2 is
metabolized by 15-OH-PGDH in vascular endothelium, the principal
metabolite being 6,15-diketo-$PGF_{1\alpha}$ (Fig. 6). The same authors suggest
that since radiolabeled 6-keto-$PGF_{1\alpha}$ is not degraded by mesenteric arterial and venous homogenates, measurement of this substance on the
assumption that it is the only stable metabolite of PGI_2 may be mislead-
ing.

A growing number of projects now underway utilize TXB_2 as an index
of TXA_2 biosynthesis [65,165,260]; but it is evident from studies involving
the infusion of [^{3}H]TXB_2 in the monkey that TXB_2 may be further metabolized, primarily by a one-step β-oxidation (Fig. 8) [105]. TXB_2 will,
it is thought, act as a substrate for 15-OH-PGDH in sensitized guinea
pig lung, leading to the formation of 15-keto-13,14 dihydro-TXB_2, but
this property is accorded little importance.

The physiologic importance of 15-OH-PGDH has served to focus much
attention on agents that will selectively modify this enzyme's action
[242]. Inhibitors of 15-OH-PGDH are discussed in several reviews [8,
51,89,134,143,155,196]. Hansen's review [89] presents a well-referenced
list of compounds and miscellaneous agents that inhibit 15-OH-PGDH.

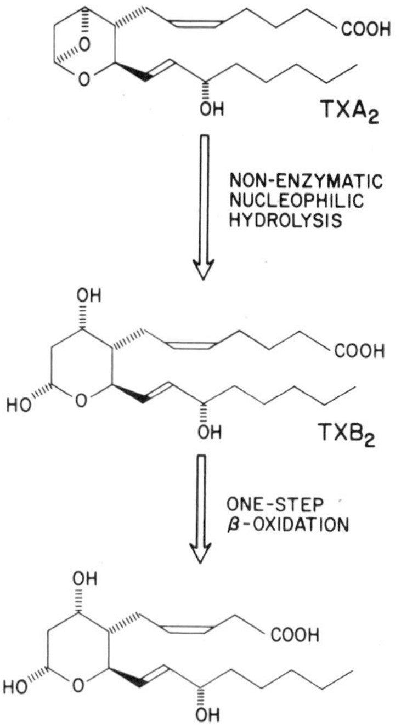

TXA$_2$

NON-ENZYMATIC
NUCLEOPHILIC
HYDROLYSIS

TXB$_2$

ONE-STEP
β-OXIDATION

$7\alpha, 9\alpha, 13$-TRIHYDROXY-THROMBAMONOIC
ACID

FIGURE 8. Metabolism of thromboxane A$_2$.

Interestingly, indomethacin, a known PG synthetase inhibitor will inhibit 15-OH-PGDH [88] and at low concentrations will also inhibit the
action of 13,14-PG reductase and 9-hydroxyprostaglandin dehydrogenase (9-PGDH) [195]. In this context, indomethacin has been documented
as potentiating the effect of dibutyryl cyclic AMP on toad bladder by
phosphodiesterase inhibition [3,49]. Steroid hormones can affect the
activity of 15-OH-PGDH, an action probably directed toward de novo
protein biosynthesis, which is believed to regulate turnover of 15-OH-
PGDH [18]. Certainly, progesterone and estrogen inhibit partially purified term human placental 15-OH-PGDH [223], which incidentally has
a higher Michaelis constant for PGF$_{2\alpha}$ than the monkey lung enzyme
[238]. Lerner and Carminati [140] have delineated fluctuations of PG
metabolism in rat placental, ovarian, lung, and kidney tissue during
pregnancy, a finding that also implies a steroidal influence on metabolism of prostaglandins. Other work has provided a more lucid descrip-
tion of "age-related" changes in the activity not only of 15-OH-PGDH,
but of the whole "multiplicity of enzymes" involved in PG catabolism
(e.g. 13,14-PG reductase and 9-PGDH) [194].

13,14-Prostaglandin Reductase

The next phase in the sequential degradation of most prostaglandins is catalyzed by 13,14-PG reductase (13-PGR), which selectively desaturates the 13,14-trans double bond, an action that requires activation of this bond by a conjugated ketone (Fig. 7). 13-PGR activity was first detected in guinea pig lung homogenates and later in tissues of the swine. The enzyme is specific for 15-keto-prostaglandins, which rapidly undergo saturation at Δ^{13} to form 13,14-dihydro-15-keto-prostaglandins; this action requires reduced pyridine nucleotide (preferentially NADPH) as electron donors (Fig. 7) [138]. The 15-keto and 13,14-dihydro-15-keto PG derivatives so formed are virtually devoid of biological activity.

Essentially, 13-PGR has a cellular distribution similar to that of 15-OH-PGDH, being primarily located in the soluble fraction of tissue homogenates. A study of highly purified (7000-fold) chicken heart 13-PGR [138] revealed that the enzyme has a molecular weight of 70,000, which makes it slightly larger than 15-OH-PGDH (60,000) and PGE 9-keto-reductase (45,000), as determined by Sephadex G-200 chromatography. In contrast to PGE-9-keto-reductase, 13-PGR is not inhibited by the presence of oxidized pyridine nucleotides (NAD^+ or $NADP^+$). There appears to be no evidence that prostacyclins or thromboxanes can interact with 13-PGR. Since blood vessel homogenates (containing 15-OH-PGDH) fail to degrade 6-keto-PGF$_{1\alpha}$ [262], it is possible that the presence of a keto group at carbon-6 negates degradation by both 15-OH-PGDH and possibly by 13-PGR.

Prostaglandin E-9-Keto-(α)-Reductase

Various enzymes exist that are able to transform stable prostaglandins. One such enzyme is prostaglandin E-9-keto-(α)-reductase (9-PGR), which specifically reduces PGE to PGF (Fig. 7). This enzyme is well represented in distribution, occurring in sheep red blood cells [93] guinea pig liver [82], certain tissues of the rat [141], and even in baker's yeast [224]. In the rat, 9-PGR activity was detected using PGF$_{2\alpha}$ antiserum; activity was found to be highest in heart, followed by kidney, brain, and liver, respectively; no activity of 9-PGR was detected in striated muscle, spleen, or ileum [141]. Chicken heart 9-PGR can be separated into two fractions by phosphocellulose chromatography [139]. 9-PGR is one of the enzymes concerned with prostaglandin metabolism that seems to have been neglected.

β- and ω-Oxidation

Following initial deactivation by 15-OH-PGDH and 13-PGR, the prostanoid molecule undergoes β- and ω-oxidation of the side chains. It must be borne in mind, however, that intravenous bolus injections of prostaglandins can lead directly to their β-oxidation. The β-oxidation of prostaglandins was proposed because it was found that [3-^{14}C], [5,6-

[3H2]PGE1, when injected into rats and recovered in the urine, had lost part of the β-carboxylic side chain beyond carbon-3; similar experiments involving injection of [5,6-3H2]PGF1α gave rise to dinor-PGF1α (7α,9α,13-trihydroxyprostadienoic acid) [64,68]. Indeed, it was originally shown that PGF1α, PGF1β, PGE1, and PGB all underwent at least one step of β-oxidation in isolated liver mitochondria, losing a two-carbon unit and forming the corresponding C_{18} homologues [81]. Figure 7 illustrates the metabolic rate of PGE_2 in the rat. The 13,14-dihydro-15-keto derivative undergoes two steps of β-oxidation to form 7α-hydroxy-15,11-diketo-tetranorprostanoic acid (C_{16}) and finally 7-hydroxy-5,11-diketo-tetranor-prosta-1,16-dioic acid by ω-oxidation (hydroxylation of chain containing the 15-keto grouping). $PGF_{2α}$ has a very similar metabolic profile, 5α,7α-dihydroxy-11-ketotetranorprosta-1,16-dioic acid being the major urinary metabolite in the human [66].

MECHANISMS OF CELLULAR ACTION

Introduction

Despite the myriad biological and pharmacological properties of prostaglandins, relatively little is known of the method or methods by which these compounds act. This dilemma is not reflected in the apparent surplus of reviews pertinent to their mechanisms of cellular action [10,90,94,101,113,126,228,266]. It is perhaps the polyfunctional nature of the prostanoate molecule that facilitates a formidably wide spectrum of cellular effects. Its lipophilic side chains give the prostaglandin molecule an intrinsic lipid solubility and membrane permeability [17] that permit flirtation with such glamorous hypotheses as alteration of membrane fluidity [113,128], and the interaction with membrane-associated enzymes such as adenylate cyclase [94,131,246], phospholipases [176], lysosomal hydrolases [254], and phosphodiesterase [7], as well as intracellular enzymes such as 20-α-hydroxysteroid dehydrogenase [12], 3β-Δ5-hydroxysteroid dehydrogenase [78,99], cholesterol ester hydrolase and synthetase [11], and cholesterol side-chain cleavage [78]. This section deals with a few of these actions and investigates some of the more recent hypotheses of cellular action in greater detail.

Receptors

It is a presently accepted premise that the initial phase(s) in the mechanism of action of many hormones is characterized by specific binding of the hormone to a receptor. Receptors may reside in intra-, sub-, or transcellular compartments, but most receptors studied so far appear to be localized on the plasma membrane. Prompted by a striking dose-response relationship between added PGE1 and formation of cyclic AMP by isolated mouse ovaries, Kuehl and Humes [125] were the first researchers to provide fundamental information on prostaglandin receptor in rat lipocytes. Structural requirements for binding of PGE1 to its receptor were later delineated by Oien et al. [189]; in accordance with the major metabolic fate of prostaglandins (i.e. by 15-OH-PGDH [89] and 13,14-PG-isomerase), it was found that removal or substitution of 9-keto or 15-hydroxyl groupings drastically reduced binding.

Following such pioneering work, many other researchers embarked on studies of prostaglandin receptors in a multitude of tissues. Of the primary prostaglandins, PGE_1 receptor has now been investigated in bovine corpus luteum [144,211], bovine thyroid membranes [169], rat thymocytes [71,221], human myometrium [117,222], human, monkey, rat, and hamster uterine tissues [110,252], fallopian tubes [251], rat liver plasma membranes and mitochondria [27,229], fat cells [62,125], human and ovine adrenal glands [35], and platelets [147], to name a few examples. Though mainly restricted to reproductive organs, an equally impressive array of studies have been concerned with $PGF_{2\alpha}$ receptor in, for instance, human [200], rat [264], bovine [212], and equine [119] corpus luteum, in human, monkey, and hamster uterus [118,250,252], and in rat skin [67,146]. The goal of much of the work on the $PGF_{2\alpha}$ receptor has been to understand the mechanism of $PGF_{2\alpha}$-induced luteolysis, which is not yet fully understood.

Following the recent isolation of prostacyclin [171], specific binding of [3H]prostacyclin has now been described for human platelets [225]. Inevitable Scatchard analysis suggests a heterogeneous population of PGI_2 receptors; apparently there are 93 high affinity (K_d 12.1 nM) and 2700 low affinity (K_d 0.9 μM) PGI_2 binding sites per platelet. The authors suggest that patients displaying a history of thrombotic proclivities may exhibit reduced populations of platelet PGI_2 receptors (or perhaps overabundance of endothelial TXA_2 receptor?). Some currently available data, based on the use of a specific prostaglandin endoperoxide antagonist ("trimethoquinol") would, at least indirectly, support the existence of TXA_2 receptors in vascular endothelium [147,148].

A concept central to the study of receptors is the possibility of synthesizing specific ligand antagonists or long-acting analogues of prostaglandins, prostacyclins, and thromboxanes. Much of the impetus in this pursuit has, in the past, been restricted to primary prostaglandins (e.g. PGE_2 or $PGF_{2\alpha}$). A veritable plethora of potent, relatively specific, prostaglandin analogues [9,15,53] and antagonists [103,148] now exist for research and clinical purposes. Future developments are likely to include analogues of PGI_2 and TXA_2; indeed, synthesis of 20-methyl-PGI_2 analogues has already allowed a study of structure-activity relationships of PGI_2 in vitro and in vivo [53]. Desaturation of the 13,14-double bond to give 13,14-dihydro-20-methyl analogue of PGI_2 greatly enhances the antiaggregatory effect in platelets, though sacrificing stability of the molecule. In circular contrast, the same authors show that introduction of a CH_3 grouping at C_{20} did little for biological potency (viz., vasodilation and inhibition of platelet aggregation) but extended the half-life.

The physicochemical properties of PGE_2 and $PGF_{2\alpha}$ receptors have been examined in bovine corpus luteum [212]; phospholipase A treatment reduces binding, as does n-ethylmaleimide [80]. The phospholipase action, it is speculated, may be due to a detergent effect of PUFA. Calcium apparently will alter the receptor affinity for PGE_2 in bovine corpus luteum [211], in rat liver mitochondria [27], and in platelets. In bovine corpus luteum [212] it was postulated that E- and F-type prostaglandins shared a common receptor; more recent investigations have revealed that PGE_2 and $PGF_{2\alpha}$ receptors exist as quite separate entities. From such a data base, one might conclude that most of the actions of prostaglandins are receptor mediated.

Ion Flux; Possible Ionophoretic Action

One of the more attractive theories of prostaglandin action is that which proposes an ionophoretic ability. Apart from Na^+ and K^+ flux in red blood cells [204], most of the evidence in this context is primarily concerned with Ca^{2+} flux. Interrelationships between Ca^{2+} and prostaglandins are by no means clear at present, although it is becoming increasingly evident that prostaglandins may exert many of their actions by alteration of Ca^{2+} metabolism.

An ionophoretic action has already been proposed for PGE_1 [120] and PGE_2 and $PGF_{2\alpha}$ [28,38]. These actions are supported by the ability of prostaglandins to form metastable calcium (and proton) complexes in aqueous phase [2]. The ionophoretic activity of prostaglandins may also be determined by their ability to form micelles in solution at a specific critical concentration [216]. The apparent involvement of Ca^{2+} and prostaglandins is further highlighted by the observation that excessive and inappropriate endogenous prostaglandin production by malignant tumors (breast cancer in particular) is believed to be responsible for the hypercalcemia and bone resorbtion associated with neoplastic carcinoma [121]. Indeed, hypercalcemia and bone resorbtion often linked with breast cancer can in some cases be reversed by indomethacin treatment [201].

PGE_1 and PGE_2 modify the size of the soluble Ca^{2+} pool in red blood cells [208] and in plasma as a whole [13], whereas in other tissues Ca^{2+} will antagonize the inhibitory effect of PGE_2 upon noradrenaline release from the sympathetic nerves of cat spleen [234]. In isolated liver mitochondria, low concentrations of PGE_1 (10^{-7} M) have been shown to provoke efflux of actively accumulated $^{45}Ca^{2+}$, an effect that is pH dependent [27]. The same study also demonstrated that small doses of Ca^{2+} (500 μM) stimulate an extremely transient uptake of $[^3H]PGE_1$ by mitochondria; this effect is, however, nonspecific: it can also be achieved with Sr^{2+} and Mn^{2+}. Such a study nevertheless indicates mitochondrially sequestered Ca^{2+} as an intracellular target for prostaglandins. Mitochondria are of course central to the control of the ionic concentrations in the "milieu interior" [207].

Thromboxane A_2 also appears to be intrinsic to the control of cellular Ca^{2+} flux [101], and there is some direct experimental evidence of Ca^{2+} mobilization by TXA_2 [54]. There exists a possibility that ambient Ca^{2+}

concentration may in turn modulate prostaglandin and thromboxane biosynthesis; it is now well established that the majority of phospholipases exhibit a distinct calcium dependence [188]. A Ca^{2+}-ionophoretic action of $PGF_{2\alpha}$ [28,38] might explain the recent report that this prostaglandin can stimulate phospholipase A_2 activity in brain slice incubations [176].

It has been implied that Ca^{2+} may cause the depolymerization of microtubules, an action probably mediated by calcium-dependent regulatory protein (CDR) [152]. In this context, colchicine has been found to stimulate PGE_1 formation in platelets [220] to attain concentrations that will inhibit platelet aggregation.

In the field of reproductive biology, it has been suggested that a possible mechanism of $PGF_{2\alpha}$-induced luteolysis might involve an Ca^{2+}-ionophoretic [38] and calcium-related [214] action. The small size of the prostaglandin molecule (only 8.5 Å in length), coupled with its characteristic "hairpin" configuration [9,40], appear to make the "ionophoretic theory" feasible, an effect that may reflect the susceptibility of plasma membrane phospholipid matrices to changes in ionic strength.

Effects on Membrane-Associated Enzymes

Some, if not most of the effects exerted by prostaglandins appear to be directed at enzymes localized within the plasma membrane. Such effects may arise from prostaglandin-induced changes in membrane fluidity [128], transmembranal diffusion or mobility of proteins (receptors?), or alterations of phospholipid distribution by enhanced flip-flop [95,124]; or they may simply be due to an allosteric action of the prostaglandin. Johnson and Ramwell [113], who reviewed and studied the actions of PGE_1 and PGE_2 on some membrane enzymes, reported that PGE_1 was more potent than PGE_2 in inhibiting platelet ATPase, an action that was competitively attenuated by 7-oxa-13-prostynoic acid (15 μM). The same authors confirmed and extended the earlier work of Polis et al. [199], who had originally demonstrated a regenerative effect of PGB_1 on oxidative phosphorylation in isolated mitochondria obtained from acceleration-stressed rats. Apparently, PGE_1, PGE_2, and PGB_1 all inhibit ATPase; in an earlier study Fassina and Contessa [45] failed to observe such effects of PGE_1 on ATPase obtained from human erythrocytes. Fassina and Contessa did however show an inhibitory effect of PGE_1 on norepinephrine-stimulated lipolysis and FFA release from rat epididymal fat pad preparations, which was evidently dependent on reduced Ca^{2+} and the complete absence of K^+ from the incubation medium.

Adenylate kinase, an enzyme responsible for maintenance of intracellular ATP levels, is also subject to the modifying influences of prostaglandins [1,113]. PGE_2 (10^{-6} M) apparently increases the affinity of muscle adenylate kinase for ADP and AMP, whereas equimolar PGE_3 has the opposite action. It was suggested, since PGE_3 caused a dose-dependent ADP inhibition of the enzyme only when PGE_2 stimulation was operational, that PGE_3 serves as a modulator of PGE_2 action at this level [1].

Many of the effects of prostaglandins are manifest through changes in the intracellular concentration of cyclic AMP [126,265,266]. The involvement of the adenylate cyclase–cyclic AMP system in the mechanism of action of prostaglandins has long been debated and remains subject to controversy. Kuehl has compiled literature both favoring and opposing interactions between prostaglandins and the cyclic nucleotide system [126]. It was proposed that since 7-oxa-13-prostynoic acid, a relatively specific prostaglandin antagonist [103], could inhibit the stimulatory effect of luteinizing hormone (LH) on ovarian adenylate cyclase, the prostaglandin receptor molecule functioned as an obligatory intermediate between the LH-receptor complex and the catalytic subunit of adenylate cyclase. This hypothesis has been met with a degree of skepticism, since Kuehl later published work demonstrating inhibition of cyclic AMP-dependent protein kinase by 7-oxa-13-prostynoic acid. The rejection of Kuehl's hypothesis was also indicated by the finding that LH and PGE_2 can elicit an additive stimulation of ovarian adenylate cyclase.

Prostaglandins E_1, E_2, A_1, $F_{2\alpha}$, $F_{1\beta}$, $F_{2\alpha}$ [126,156,265], and PGI_2 [57,134] all enhance the formation of cyclic AMP. Studies by Armstrong's group showed that very high concentrations (15 $\mu g/ml$) of PGI_2 are required for stimulation of granulosa cell adenylate cyclase, a system in which PGE_2 exerts superior potency [57]. Stimulatory effects of PGE_1 and PGI_2 on platelet adenylate cyclase are believed to be a component in the mechanism by which these agents counter aggregation [220,259]. To date, little work has been done to investigate the possible actions of thromboxanes on adenylate cyclase, except for the recent study of Gorman et al. [63], who showed that TXA_2 inhibits PGE_1 stimulation of platelet adenylate cyclase [63]. This succinct experimental finding is clearly at variance with the rather elaborate theory proposed by Horrobin et al. [101], which also postulates an action of TXA_2 on cyclic AMP-phosphodiesterase (PDE). Amer and Marquis [7] have studied the effects of prostaglandins on phosphodiesterase; PGE_1 (1.4×10^{-6} M) and $PGF_{2\alpha}$ (2×10^{-4} M) are both inhibitory in membrane-supplemented whole homogenates of human blood platelets.

Generally speaking, F-type prostaglandins are less potent stimulators of adenylate cyclase, and are even inhibitory in some cases, especially in ovarian luteal tissue [69,131,246]. In the case of ovarian adenylate cyclase, it appears that young cells are refractory to the inhibitory effects of $PGF_{2\alpha}$ [10,116]. This question of refractoriness of adenylate cyclase is further complicated by the disclosure that LH can desensitize the enzyme [21]. Age-related changes in cyclase sensitivity may well reflect some intrinsic physical-chemical property of the plasma membrane; old membranes might be less fluid as a result of retarded phospholipid turnover, or adenylate cyclase synthesis may be slowed in aging cell membranes.

It is now a generally accepted premise that most actions of cyclic AMP are opposed by cyclic GMP; little work, however, has been carried out on guanylate cyclase as a possible target enzyme for prostaglandins. Arachidonic acid, in contrast to PGE_1, has a slightly stimulatory effect on platelet cyclic GMP formation [15]. The significance of this finding is puzzling, although it has been suggested that there is a yin-yang mechanism controlling cell exocytosis via transient alterations in microtubule equilibrium. For example, it was proposed that agents that elevate intracellular cyclic AMP diminish release, whereas elevation of cyclic GMP has the opposite effect [254].

Interrelationships between calcium, prostaglandins, thromboxanes, and cyclic nucleotides in the platelet are many and complex [54,220]. Prostaglandin endoperoxide synthesis is inhibited by elevated platelet cyclic AMP levels [151], an effect tentatively attributed to restriction of the availability of arachidonic acid [161]. Conversely, it was recently shown that increased TXA_2 formation lowers the intraplatelet concentration of cyclic AMP in a calcium-dependent mechanism involving blockade of PGI_2-stimulated adenylate cyclase [63]. In addition, it is now known that the inhibitory effect of cyclic AMP on platelet TXA_2 biosynthesis is secondary to the effect of this nucleotide on platelet aggregation [145].

The observed stimulatory effects of ionophores on platelet thromboxane and prostaglandin biosynthesis [188] suggest calcium involvement. Extended studies show that the primary target for ionophore action (A23187, X537A, Nigericin) is probably a membranal phospholipase (A_2), with a high affinity binding site for Ca^{2+} [77], which is mandatory for phospholipid hydrolysis. This calcium binding site is central, and probably modifies the "interfacial recognition site" on the phospholipase A_2. In this context, $PGF_{2\alpha}$ (8×10^{-7} M) has been shown to increase the incorporation of arachidonic acid into choline and ethanolamine-phosphoglycerides in brain slice incubations, implying a $PGF_{2\alpha}$-induced activation of lysosomal phospholipase A_2 [176]. Also pertinent is the finding that phospholipids (phosphoglycerides) and diglyceride kinase activity are present in microtubular structures associated with membranes, at least in chicken embryo, muscle and brain, and HeLa cells [33]. It was proposed that phospholipids (and phospholipase?) functioned to modify the assembly and disassembly of tubulin [33]. Prostaglandins may act at this level [176], and it may be an indirect mechanism involving microtubules and microfilaments (as suggested in the last subsection), possibly mediated by changes in calcium flux initiated by ionophoretic effects of prostaglandins (see "Ion Flux," above).

Interactions with Intracellular Enzymes

Prostaglandins may also exert their many different effects by interacting with a number of intracellular enzyme systems. Both cellular carbohydrate and lipid metabolisms appear to be targets for prostaglandin action. Early investigations showed that PGE_1 and PGB_1 stimulate oxidative phosphorylation [199], an effect presumably mediated by alteration of mitochondrial ion flux [27,207]. More recent work suggests an involvement of thromboxanes with pyruvate and lactate metabolism and in the control of collagen biosynthesis [101]. Studies with isolated rat adipocytes reveal that PGE_1 (2.8×10^{-6} M) depresses cleavage of triacylglycerides and subsequent release of glycerol, and enhances glucose oxidation in a dose-dependent fashion; this antilipolytic action of PGE_1 has been compared to that exerted by insulin [22]. In the same study, in vivo administration of PGE_1 (1 mg/kg body weight, intraperitoneally) in fed male rats, elevated blood glucose by 80% after 30 minutes by increased liver glycogenolysis, an effect accompanied by a concomitant fall in adrenal catecholamine content.

That lipid metabolism is a biochemical focus for prostaglandin action is illustrated by the finding that treatment of pregnant rats for 4 days with $PGF_{2\alpha}$ correlates with histologically detectable cytosolic lipid accumulation in corpus luteum [190]. Moreover, studies on regressing rat corpus luteum reveal elevated intracellular concentrations of triglycerides and lipids [236]. $PGF_{2\alpha}$ (2×10^{-6} M) will stimulate lipoprotein lipase activity in differentiating 3T3-L1 adipocytes [232], an action resulting in the formation of FFA and glycerol, which are usually reesterified to form triacylglycerols in adipocytes.

Other intracellular enzymes affected by $PGF_{2\alpha}$ include cholesterol ester synthetase (sterol acyl transferase, E.C. 3.1.22) and cholesterol ester hydrolase [11], mitochondrial cholesterol side-chain cleavage [78], $\Delta^5,3\beta$-hydroxysteroid dehydrogenase [78,99], 17α-hydroxylase [70], and microsomal 20α-hydroxysteroid dehydrogenase [12,266]. Other prostaglandins also modify the activities of steroidogenic enzymes; PGA_1, PGA_2, PGB_1, PGE_2, and $PGF_{1\alpha}$ will inhibit LH-stimulated testosterone production in isolated testicular interstitial cells [70]. PGE_2 (1 mg/rat) will stimulate a 15-fold increase in the activity of ovarian ornithine decarboxylase [132], an enzyme involved in the biosynthesis of polyamines. PGE_1 and PGE_2 have also been documented as stimulating rat ovarian granulosa cells to produce plasminogen activator—an enzyme intrinsic to ovum escape [237].

Possible Interactions with Cytoskeleton; Microtubules and Microfilaments

At present, evidence for interactions between prostaglandins, prostacyclins, or thromboxanes with cell cytoskeleton components such as microtubules or microfilaments is scarce. However, there is a growing awareness that because prostaglandins exert their major effects on smooth muscle complexes in many tissues, especially blood vessels [73,178], these autocoids may modulate activity of such intracellular contractile elements as microtubules and microfilaments, particularly in blood platelets that possess a well-organized microtubule system [233,256].

Microfilaments and microtubules are primarily but not exclusively involved in the maintenance of cell morphology and intracellular support [23] for such organelles as mitochondria, with which they are often associated [92], and in the intracellular transport of hormones [130]. To construct a coherent hypothesis linking prostaglandins with microtubule function, it is necessary to review the available data. Unfortunately, most of the material appears to be either circumstantial or indirect.

Colchicine, an agent that specifically causes the depolymerization of microtubules, has long been used in the treatment of rheumatoid arthritis and cancer. This and other related alkaloids (e.g. vinblastine) have been shown to stimulate prostaglandin biosynthesis and release in cultured rheumatoid synovial cells. Other more limited studies have documented the binding of [3H]PGE_2 to microtubular protein obtained from brain homogenates [261]. These authors also showed that the ability of tubulin to polymerize in vitro was retarded slightly by E-type prostaglandins; and based on the anticonvulsive action of PGE_2, they postulated an interplay between prostaglandins, PGI_2, TXA_2, and brain microtubules.

FIGURE 9. Interrelationships between microtubules, prostaglandins, and cyclic nucleotide in the luteal cell. $PGF_{2\alpha}$ may provoke Ca^{2+} influx and activate phospholipase A_2; release of PUFA and PGs may then modulate microtubule equilibrium at the level of membrane by interaction with a specific $PGF_{2\alpha}$ receptor ($PGF_{2\alpha R}$).

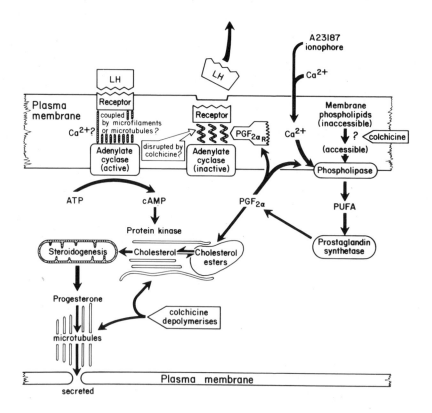

The platelet release reaction, triggered by thrombin, collagen, ADP, or epinephrine [63,220], is apparently associated with a clearly defined transient decrease in the pool of polymerized tubulin [233], which is evident 15 seconds after addition of aggregatory agent and is subject to colchicine blockade [107,145,256]. The antiaggregatory action of colchicine does not involve elevation of platelet cyclic AMP formation, but it does include inhibition of TXB_2 biosynthesis. This may indicate that the locus of activity for colchicine is at the level of phospholipase A_2. Thus the platelet provides a model that illustrates an interplay between prostaglandins, thromboxanes, prostacyclin, and microtubules.

A similar situation might occur in ovarian tissue. Microtubules have also been inferred in the process of internalization and metabolism of low density lipoprotein (LDL), a source of cholesterol, the major substrate for steroidogenesis [192]. It might be speculated that prostaglandins, by initiating a local calcium flux, act at the level of microtubules, thereby inhibiting uptake of LDL and thus inhibiting steroidogenesis by deforming cell surface conformation. There is certainly evidence that both PGE_1 and PGE_2 can induce shape changes in cultured rat ovarian granulosa cells [4].

Prostaglandins may modify mobility of membrane-associated receptor proteins by interacting with microfilaments [210] in that vicinity, an action permitted by the lipophilic nature of the prostaglandins. Zor et al. have recently implied an involvement of microtubules or microfilaments in the coupling of gonadotrophin receptor complexes to the catalytic subunit of ovarian adenylate cyclase.

In summary, some speculative ideas are illustrated in Figure 9, which depicts possible interrelationships between cyclic AMP, prostaglandins, microtubules, and calcium in the luteal cell.

ACKNOWLEDGMENTS

This work was supported by National Institutes of Health grant HD-10718. Alan K. Hall is supported by Ford Foundation grant 770-0534 and acknowledges receipt of a travel grant awarded by the Wellcome Trust. The authors are indebted to Ms. M. Eaton and Ms. S. Losacco for typing the manuscript.

REFERENCES

1. Abdulla, Y. H., and MacFarlane, D. E. (1971) Control of adenylate kinase by PGE_2 and PGE_3. Biochem. Pharmacol. 20, 1726.
2. Advani, A. T., and Pettit, L. D. (1973) The formation constants of the proton and calcium complexes of prostaglandin E_1 and $F_{1\beta}$. Chem. Biol. Interactions. 7, 181.
3. Ahfelt-Rønne, I. (1978) In vitro stimulation of prostaglandin biosynthesis by methylxanthines. Prostaglandins 16(5), 711–724.
4. Albertini, D. F., and Clark, J. I. (1975) Membrane-microtubule interactions. Con A capping induced redistribution of cytoplasmic microtubules and colchicine binding. Proc. Natl. Acad. Sci. (U.S.) 72(12), 4976–4980.
5. Ali, M., Zamecnik, J., Cerskus, A. L., Stoessl, A. J., Barnett, W. H., and McDonald, J. W. D. (1977) Synthesis of thromboxane B_2 and prostaglandins by bovine gastric mucosal microsomes. Prostaglandins 14(5), 819–828.

6. Ally, A. I., Manku, M. S., Horrobin, D. F., Morgan, R. O., Karmazin, M., and Karmali, R. A. (1977) Dipyridamole: A possible potent inhibitor of thromboxane A_2 synthetase in vascular smooth muscle. Prostaglandins 14, 607–609.

7. Amer, M. A., and Marquis, N. R. (1972) In: P. W. Ramwell and B. B. Pharriss (eds.), Prostaglandins in Cellular Biology, Plenum Press, New York, pp. 93.

8. Andersen, N. H., and Ramwell, P. W. (1974) Biological aspects of prostaglandins. Arch. Intern. Med. 133, 30–50.

9. Andersen, N. H., Ramwell, P. W., Leovey, E. M. K., and Johnson, M. (1976) Biological consequences of prostaglandin molecular conformations. In: B. Samuelsson and R. Paoletti (eds.), Advances in Prostaglandin and Thromboxane Research, Vol. 1, Raven Press, New York, pp. 271–289.

10. Behrman, H. R., Grinwich, D. L., and Hichens, M. (1976) Studies on the mechanism of $PGF_{2\alpha}$ and gonadotropin interactions on LH receptor function in corpora lutea during luteolysis. In: B. B. Samuelsson and R. Paoletti (eds.), Advances in Prostaglandin and Thromboxane Research, Vol. 2, Raven Press, New York, pp. 655–656.

11. Behrman, H. R., MacDonald, G., and Greep, R. O. (1971) Regulation of ovarian cholesterol esters; Evidence for the enzymatic sites of prostaglandin-induced loss of corpus luteum function. Lipids 6, 791–796.

12. Behrman, H. R., Yoshinaga, K., and Greep, R. O. (1971) Extraluteal effects of prostaglandins. Ann. NY Acad. Sci. 180, 426–433.

13. Beliel, O. M., Singer, F. R., and Coburn, J. W. (1973) Effects of prostaglandins on plasma calcium. Prostaglandins 3, 237–241.

14. Bergström, S., Carlson, L. A., and Weeks, J. R. (1968) The prostaglandins; A family of biologically active lipids. Pharmacol. Rev. 20, 1–48.

15. Best, L. C., McGuire, M. B., Martin, T. J., Preston, F. E., and Russell, R. G. G. (1979) Effects of epoxymethano analogues of prostaglandin endoperoxides on aggregation, on release of 5'-hydroxytryptamine and on the metabolism of 3'5'-cyclic AMP and cyclic GMP in human platelets. Biochim. Biophys. Acta 583, 344–351.

16. Bills, T. K., and Silver, M. J. (1975) Phosphatidylcholine is the primary source of arachidonic acid utilized by platelet prostaglandin synthetase. Fed. Proc. 34, 79.

17. Bito, L. Z. (1975) Are prostaglandins intracellular, transcellular, or extracellular autocoids? Prostaglandins 9(9), 851–855.

18. Blackwell, G. J., Flower, R. J., and Vane, J. R. (1975) Rapid reduction of prostaglandin 15-hydroxy-prostaglandin dehydrogenase activity in rat tissues after treatment with protein synthesis inhibitors. Br. J. Pharmacol. 55, 233–238.

19. Blackwell, G. J., Duncombe, W. G., Flower, R. J., Parsons, M. F., and Vane, J. R. (1977) The distribution and metabolism of arachidonic acid in rabbit platelets during aggregation and its modification by drugs. Br. J. Pharmacol. 59, 353–366.

20. Block, A. J., Feinberg, H., Herbaczynska-Cedro, K., and Vane, J. R. (1975) Anoxia-induced release of prostaglandins in rabbit isolated hearts. Circ. Res. 36, 34–42.

21. Bockaert, J., Hunzicker, D. M., and Birnbaumer, L. (1976) Hormone-stimulated desensitization of hormone-dependent adenylate cyclase. J. Biol. Chem. 247, 7073–7081.

22. Bohle, E., and May, B. (1967) Metabolic effects of prostaglandin E_1 upon lipid and carbohydrate metabolism. In: P. W. Ramwell and J. E. Shaw (eds.), Prostaglandin Symposium of the Worcester Foundation for Experimental Biology, Interscience, New York, pp. 115–129.

23. Brecher, S. (1975) The occurrence and role of 80–100 A filaments in PtK_1 cells. Exp. Cell Res. 96, 303–310.

24. Bunting, S., Gryglewski, R., Moncada, S., and Vane, J. R. (1976) Arterial walls generate from prostaglandin endoperoxides a substance (PGX) which relaxes strips of mesenteric and coeliac arteries and inhibits platelet aggregation. Prostaglandins 12(6), 897–913.

25. Bunting, S., Moncada, S., and Vane, J. R. (1977) Anti-thrombotic properties of vascular endothelium. Lancet 2, 1075–1076.

26. Burch, J. W., Stanford, N., and Majerus, P. W. (1977) Inhibition of platelet prosta-glandin synthetase by oral aspirin. J. Clin. Invest. 61, 314–319.

27. Carafoli, E., and Crovetti, F. (1973) Interactions between PGE_1 and Ca^{2+} at the level of the mitochondrial membrane. Arch. Biochem. Biophys. 154, 40–46.

28. Carsten, M. E., and Miller, J. D. (1977) Effects of prostaglandin and oxytocin on calcium release from a uterine microsomal fraction; Hypothesis for ionophoretic action of prostaglandins. J. Biol. Chem. 252 (5), 1576–1581.

29. Chang, J. A., Lewis, G. P., and Piper, P. J. (1977) Inhibition by glucocorticoids of prostaglandin release from adipose tissue in vitro. Br. J. Pharmacol. 59, 425–432.

30. Chang, W. C., and Murota, S. I. (1977) Identification of 6-keto-prostaglandin $F_{1\alpha}$ formed from arachidonic acid in bovine seminal vesicles. Biochim. Biophys. Acta 486, 136–144.

31. Chang, W. C., Murota, S. I., and Tsurufujii, S. (1978) Inhibition of thromboxane B_2 and 6-keto-prostaglandin $F_{1\alpha}$ formation by antiinflammatory drugs in carrageenin-in-duced granuloma. Biochem. Pharmacol. 27, 109–111.

32. Cho, M. J., and Allen, M. A. (1976) Chemical stability of prostacyclin (PGI_2) in aqueous solutions. Prostaglandins 15(6), 943.

33. Dales, G. R., Piras, M. M., and Piras, R. (1974) The presence of phospholipids and diglyceride kinase activity in microtubules from different tissues. Biochem. Biophys. Res. Commun. 61(3), 1043–1050.

34. Dawson, W., Boot, J. R., Cockerill, A., Mallen, D. N. B., and Osborne, D. J. (1976) Release of novel prostaglandins and thromboxanes after immunological challenge of guinea pig lung. Nature (London) 262, 699–702.

35. Dazard, A., Morera, A. M., Bertrand, J., and Saez, J. M. (1974) Prostaglandin receptors in human and ovine adrenal glands; Binding and stimulation of adenylate cyclase in subcellular preparations. Endocrinology 95, 352–359.

36. de Deckre, E. A. M., Nugteren, D. H., and Tenhoor, F. (1977) Prostacyclin is the major prostaglandin released from the isolated perfused rabbit and rat heart. Nature (London) 268, 160–163.

37. Diczfalusy, U., Falardeau, P., and Hammarström, S. (1977) Conversion of prosta-glandin endoperoxides to C_{17}-hydroxy acids catalysed by human platelet thromboxane synthetase. FEBS. Lett. 84, 271–274.

38. Dorflinger, L. J. (1978) Evidence for the role of Ca^{2+} in the acute effect of $PGF_{2\alpha}$ on LH-stimulated adenylate-cyclase activity. Biol. Reprod. 18:62 A.

39. Eakins, K. E., and Kulkarni, P. S. (1976) N-0164 inhibits generation of thromboxane A_2-like activity from prostaglandin-endoperoxides by human platelet microsomes. Prostaglandins 12, 465–470.

40. Egan, R. W., Paxton, J., and Kuehl, F. A. (1976) Mechanism for irreversible self-deactivation of prostaglandin synthetase. J. Biol. Chem. 251, 7329–7335.

41. Elattar, R. M. A. (1978) Prostaglandins; Physiology, biochemistry, pharmacology and clinical applications. J. Oral Pathol. 7, 239–252.

42. Eliasson, R. (1959) Studies on prostaglandin occurrence, formation and biological actions. Acta Physiol. Scand. 46 (Suppl.) 158, 1–73.

43. Edmonds, J. W., and Duax, W. (1974) Molecular conformation of prostaglandin E_2. Prostaglandins 5, 275–281.

44. Falardeau, P., Hamberg, M., and Samuelsson, B. (1976) Metabolism of 8,11,14-eicos-atrienoic acid in human platelets. Biochim. Biophys. Acta 441, 193–200.

45. Fassina, G., and Contessa, A. R. (1967) Digitoxin and prostaglandin E_1 as inhibitors of catecholamine-stimulated lipolysis and their interaction with calcium in the process. Biochem. Pharmacol. 16, 1447–1453.

46. Fenwick, L., Jones, R. L., and Naylor, B. (1977) Production of prostaglandins by the pseudopregnant rat uterus in vitro and the effect of tamoxifen with the identification of 6-keto-prostaglandin $F_{1\alpha}$ as a major product. Br. J. Pharmacol. 59, 191–199.

47. Ferreira, S. H., and Vane, J. R. (1967) Prostaglandins; Their disappearance from and release into the circulation. Nature (London) 216, 868–869.

48. Fitzpatrick, F. A., and Gorman, R. R. (1977) Platelet rich plasma transforms exogenous plastaglandin endoperoxide H_2 into thromboxane A_2. Prostaglandins 14(5), 881–889.

49. Flores, A. G. A., and Sharp, G. W. G. (1972) Endogenous prostaglandins and osmotic water flow in toad bladder. Am. J. Physiol. 233(6), 1392–1397.

50. Flower, R. J., and Blackwell, G. J. (1979) Anti-inflammatory steroids induce biosynthesis of a phospholipase A_2 inhibitor which prevents prostaglandin generation. Nature (London) 278, 456–459.

51. Flower, R. J. (1974) Drugs which inhibit prostaglandin biosynthesis. Pharmacol. Rev. 26, 33–64.

52. Folco, G., Granström, E., and Kindahl, H. (1977) Albumin stabilizes thromboxane A_2. FEBS Lett. 82(2), 321–324.

53. Gandolfi, C. A., and Gryglewski, R. J. I. (1978) 20 Methyl-prostacyclin and analogs; A two-stage screening procedure for biological properties. Pharm. Res. Commun. 10(10), 885–896.

54. Gerrard, J. M., Butler, A. M., and White, J. G. (1977) Calcium release from a platelet calcium-sequestering membrane fraction by arachidonic acid and its prevention by aspirin. Prostaglandins 15, 703 (Abstr.).

55. Glatt, S., and Barenholz, Y. (1973) Enzymes of complex lipid metabolism. Annu. Rev. Biochem. 42, 61–90.

56. Glenn, E. M., Bowvrian, B. J., and Rohloff, N. A. (1977) Anti-inflammatory and prostaglandin inhibitory effects of phenacetin and acetaminophen. Agents. Actions 7, 513–516.

57. Goff, A. K., Zamecnik, J., Ali, M., and Armstrong, D. T. (1978) Prostacyclin stimulation of granulosa cell cyclic AMP production. Prostaglandins 15(5), 875–879.

58. Goldberg, V. J., and Ramwell, P. W. (1975) Role of prostaglandins in reproduction. Physiol. Rev. 55(3), 325–351.

59. Gordan, J. L., and Pearson, J. D. (1978) Effects of sulphinpyrazone and aspirin on prostaglandin I_2 (prostacyclin) synthesis by endothelial cells. Br. J. Pharmacol. 64, 481–483.

60. Gordan, J. L., Pearson, J. D., and MacIntyre, D. E. (1979) Effects of prostaglandin E_2 on prostacyclin production by endothelial cells. Nature (London) 278, 480.

61. Gorman, R. R., Hamberg, M., and Samuelsson, B. (1976) Biochim. Biophys. Acta 444, 596–603.

62. Gorman, R. R., and Miller, O. V. (1973) Specific prostaglandin E_1 and A_1 binding sites in rat adipocyte plasma membranes. Biochim. Biophys. Acta 323, 560–572.

63. Gorman, R. R., Wierenga, W., and Miller, O. V. (1979) Independence of the cyclic-AMP lowering activity of thromboxane A_2 from the platelet release reaction. Biochim. Biophys. Acta 572, 95–104.

64. Granström, E., Inger, U., and Samuelsson, B. (1965) The structure of a urinary metabolite of prostaglandin $F_{1\alpha}$ in the rat. J. Biol. Chem. 240, 457–461.

65. Granström, E., Kindahl, H., and Samuelsson, B. (1976) A method for measuring the unstable thromboxane A_2; Radioimmunoassay of the derived mono-o-methylthromboxane B_2. Prostaglandin 12(6), 929–941.

66. Granström, E., and Samuelsson, B. (1971) On the metabolism of prostaglandin $F_{2\alpha}$ in female subjects. J. Biol. Chem. 246(24), 7470–7485.

67. Greaves, M. W., Sondergaard, J., and McDonald-Gibson, W. (1971) Recovery of prostaglandins in human cutaneous inflammation. Br. Med. J. 2, 258–260.

68. Gréen, K. (1971) Metabolism of PGE_2 in the rat. Biochemistry 10(6), 1072–1086.

69. Grinwich, D. L., Hichens, M., and Behrman, H. R. (1976) Binding of human chorionic gonadotropin and response of cyclic nucleotides to LH in luteal tissue from rats treated with $PGF_{2\alpha}$. Endocrinology 98, 146–150.

70. Grotjan, H. E., Jr., Heindal, J. J., and Steinberger, E. (1978) Prostaglandin inhibition of testosterone production induced by luteinizing hormone, dibutyryl cyclic AMP or

3-isobutyl-methyl-xanthine in dispersed rat testicular interstitial cells. Steroids 32(3), 307–322.

71. Grunnet, I. (1976) PGE$_1$ high affinity binding sites of rat thymocytes. In: B. Samuelsson and R. Paoletti (eds.), Advances in Prostaglandin and Thromboxane Research, Vol. 1, Raven Press, New York, pp. 265–270.

72. Gryglewski, R. J., Bunting, S., Moncada, S., Flower, R. J., and Vane, J. R. (1976) Arterial walls are protected against deposition of thrombi by substance (prostaglandin X) which they make from prostaglandin endoperoxides. Prostaglandins 12, 685–708.

73. Gryglewski, R. J., and Korbut, R. (1975) Prostaglandin feedback mechanism limits vasoconstrictor action of norepinephrine in perfused rabbit ear. Experientia 31, 89–91.

74. Gryglewski, R. J., Korbut, R., and Ocetkiewicz, A. (1978) Generation of prostacyclin by lungs in vivo and its release into the arterial circulation. Nature (London), 273–265.

75. Gryglewski, R. J., Panczenko, B., Korbut, R., Grodzinska, L., and Ocetkiewicz, A. (1975) Corticosteroids inhibit prostaglandin release from perfused mesenteric blood vessels of rabbit and from perfused lungs of sensitised guinea pig. Prostaglandins 10, 343–355.

76. Guerignian, J. L. (1976) Prostaglandin-macromolecular interactions. Noncovalent binding of prostaglandins A$_1$, E$_2$, F$_{2\alpha}$, and E$_2$ by human and bovine serum albumin. J. Pharm. Exp. Ther. 197(2), 391.

77. Haas, de, G. H., Slotboom, A. J., Verheiji, H. M., Jansen, E. H. J. M., de Araujo, P. S., and Vidal, J. C. (1978) Interaction of phospholipase A$_2$ with lipid-water interfaces. In: C. Galli, G. Galli, and G. Porcellati (eds.), Advances in Prostaglandin and Thromboxane Research, Vol. 3, Raven Press, New York, pp. 11–21.

78. Hall, A. K., Merry, B. J., and Robinson, J. (1978) Luteolytic effects of prostaglandin F$_{2\alpha}$ and 16-aryloxy-prostaglandin F$_{2\alpha}$ in the hormonally induced pseudopregnant rat in vitro and in vivo. J. Endocrinol. 77, 19P–20P (Abstr.).

79. Haluska, P. V., Lurie, D., and Colwell, J. A. (1977) Increased synthesis of PGE-like material by patients with diabetes mellitus. New Engl. J. Med. 297, 1306–1310.

80. Ham, E. A., Oien, H. C., Ulm, E. H., and Kuehl, F. A., Jr., (1975) The reaction of PGA$_1$ with sulfydryl groups; A component in the binding of A-type prostaglandins to proteins. Prostaglandins 10, 217.

81. Hamberg, M. (1968) Metabolism of prostaglandins in rat liver mitochondria. Eur. J. Biochem. 6, 135–146.

82. Hamberg, M., and Samuelsson, B. (1969) The structure of a urinary metabolite of prostaglandin E$_2$ in guinea pig. Biochem. Biophys. Res. Commun. 34, 22–27.

83. Hamberg, M., and Samuelsson, B. (1973) Detection and isolation of an endoperoxide intermediate in prostaglandin biosynthesis. Proc. Natl. Acad. Sci. (U.S.) 70, 899–903.

84. Hamberg, M., and Samuelsson, B. (1974) Prostaglandin endoperoxides; Novel transformations of arachidonate in human platelets. Proc. Natl. Acad. Sci. (U.S.) 71, 3400–3404.

85. Hamberg, M., Svensson, J., and Samuelsson, B. (1974) Prostaglandin endoperoxides; A new concept concerning the mode of action and release of prostaglandins. Proc. Natl. Acad. Sci. (U.S.) 71, 3824–3828.

86. Hamberg, M., Svensson, J., and Samuelsson, B. (1975) Thromboxanes; A new group of biologically active compounds derived from prostaglandin endoperoxides. Proc. Natl. Acad. Sci. (U.S.) 72, 2994–2998.

87. Hammarström, S., and Falardeau, P. (1977) Resolution of prostaglandin endoperoxide synthetase and thromboxane synthetase of human platelets. Proc. Natl. Acad. Sci. (U.S.) 74, 3691–3698.

88. Hansen, H. S. (1974) Inhibition by indomethacin and aspirin of 15-hydroxyprostaglandin dehydrogenase in vitro. Prostaglandins 8(2), 95–105.

89. Hansen, H. S. (1976) 15-Hydroxyprostaglandin dehydrogenase: A review. Prostaglandins 12(4), 647–679.

90. Harris, R. H., Ramwell, P. W., and Gilmer, P. J. (1979) Cellular mechanisms of prostaglandin action. Annu. Rev. Physiol. 41, 653–668.

91. Hedqvist, P. (1976) Prostaglandin action transmitter release at adrenergic neuroeffector junctions. In: B. Samuelsson and R. Paoletti (eds.), Advances in Prostaglandin and Thromboxane Research, Vol. 1, Raven Press, New York, pp. 357–363.

92. Heggeness, M. H., Simon, M., and Singer, S. J. (1978) Association of mitochondria with microtubules in cultured cells. Proc. Natl. Acad. Sci. (U.S.) 75(8), 3863–3866.

93. Hensby, C. N. (1974) The reduction of prostaglandin E_2 to prostaglandin $F_{2\alpha}$ by various animal tissues. Br. J. Pharmacol. 52, 109 P (Abstr.).

94. Henderson, K. M., and McNatty, K. P. (1975) A biochemical hypothesis to explain the mechanism of luteal regression. Prostaglandins 9(5), 779–797.

95. Hirata, R., Strittmatter, W. J., and Axelrod, J. (1979) β-Adrenergic receptor agonists increase phospholipid methylation, membrane fluidity, and β-adrenergic receptor–adenylate cyclase coupling. Proc. Natl. Acad. Sci. (U.S.) 76, 368–372.

96. Ho, P. P. K., and Esterman, M. A. (1974) Fenoprofen: Inhibitor of prostaglandin synthesis. Prostaglandins 6, 107–113.

97. Ho, P. P. K., Walters, P., and Sullivan, H. R. (1976) Biosynthesis of thromboxane B_2: Assay isolation and properties of the enzyme system in human platelets. Prostaglandins 12(6), 951–969.

98. Hope, W. C., Dalton, C., Machlin, L. J., Filipski, R., and Vane, J. R. (1975) Influence of dietary vitamin E on prostaglandin biosynthesis in rat blood. Prostaglandins 10(4), 557–571.

99. Hoppen, H. O., and Findlay, J. K. (1976) The effect of luteolytic doses of prostaglandin $F_{2\alpha}$ on pregnenolone metabolism by the autotransplanted ovary of the ewe. In: B. Samuelsson and R. Paoletti (eds.), Advances in Prostaglandin and Thromboxane Research, Vol. 2, Raven Press, New York, p. 949.

100. Horrobin, D. F. (1979) Tricyclic antidepressants, anxiety, thromboxane A_2 and dipyridamole. Am. J. Psychiat. 136(1), p. 124 (letter).

101. Horrobin, D. F., Manku, M. S., Karmali, R. A., Oka, M., Ally, A. I., Morgan, R. O., Karmazyn, M., and Cunnane, S. C. (1978) Thromboxane A_2; A key regulator of prostaglandin biosynthesis and of interactions between prostaglandins, calcium and cyclic nucleotides. Med. Hypoth. 4, 178–186.

102. Horton, E. W., and Poyser, N. L. (1976) Uterine luteolytic hormone; A physiological role for prostaglandin $F_{2\alpha}$. Physiol. Rev. 56(4), 595–651.

103. Hynie, S., Čepelik, J., Černohorsky, M., Klenerové, V., Skřivanová, J., and Wenke, M. (1975) 7-Oxa-13-prostanoic acid and polyphloretin phosphate as nonspecific antagonists of the stimulatory effects of different agents on adenylate cyclase from various tissues. Prostaglandins 10(6), 971–981.

104. Isakson, P. C., Raz, A., Denny, S. E., Pure, E., and Needleman, P. (1977) A novel prostaglandin is the major product of arachidonic acid metabolism in rabbit heart. Proc. Natl. Acad. Sci. (U.S.) 74, 101–105.

105. Jackson-Roberts, L., II, Sweetman, B. J., and Oates, J. A. (1978) Metabolism of thromboxane B_2 in the monkey. J. Biol. Chem. 253, 5305–5318.

106. Jaffe, B. M. (1974) Prostaglandins and cancer: An update. Prostaglandins 6, 453–461.

107. Jaffe, R. A., and Castro-Apitz, R. (1979) Effect of colchicine on human blood platelets under conditions of short term incubation. Biochem. J. 178, 449–454.

108. Jaffe, E. A., and Weksler, B. B. (1979) Recovery of endothelial cell prostaglandin I_2 production after inhibition by low doses of aspirin. J. Clin. Invest. 53, 532–535.

109. Janssen, P. A. J. (1975) Suprofen (R25-061); A new potent inhibitor of prostaglandin biosynthesis. Arzneim.-Forsch., 25, 1495–1500.

110. Johnson, M., Jessup, R., Jessup, S., and Ramwell, P. W. (1974) Correlation of PGE_1 receptor binding with evoked uterine contraction; Modification by disulphide reduction. Prostaglandins 6(5), 433–449.

111. Johnson, R. A., Morton, D. R., Kinner, J. H., Gorman, R. R., McGuire, J. C., Sun, F. F., Whittaker, N., Bunting, S., Salmon, J., Moncada, S., and Vane, J. R. (1976) The chemical structure of prostaglandin X (prostacyclin). Prostaglandins 12, 915–928.

112. Johnson, R. A., Morton, D. R., and Nelson, N. A. (1978) Nomenclature for analogues of prostacyclin (PGI_2). Prostaglandins 15(5), 737–750.

113. Johnson, M., and Ramwell, P. W. (1973) Prostaglandin modification of membrane-bound enzyme activity; A possible mechanism of action? Prostaglandins 3, 703–719.

114. Kadowitz, P. J., Joiner, P. D., Greenberg, S., and Hyman, A. L. (1976) Comparison of the effects of prostaglandins A, E, F and B on the canine pulmonary vascular bed. In: B. Samuelsson and R. Paoletti (eds.), Advances in Prostaglandin and Thromboxane Research, Vol. 1, Raven Press, New York, pp. 403–415.

115. Karim, S. M., and Hillier, K. (1976) Physiological roles and pharmacological actions of prostaglandins in relation to human reproduction. In: S. M. M. Karim (ed.), Prostaglandins and Reproduction, MTP Press, Lancaster, pp. 23–75.

116. Khan, I., Rosberg, S., and Ahren, K. (1976) Suppressive action of $PGF_{2\alpha}$ in vitro on LH-induced rise of cyclic-AMP in rat corpora lutea of different ages. Acta Physiol. Scand. (Suppl.) 440–446.

117. Kimball, F. A., Kirton, K. T., Spilman, C. H., and Wyngarden, L. J. (1975) Prostaglandin E_1 specific binding in human myometrium. Biol. Reprod. 13, 482–489.

118. Kimball, F. A., and Wyngarden, L. J. (1975) Prostaglandin specific binding in hamster low speed supernatants. Prostaglandins 9, 413–429.

119. Kimball, F. A., and Wyngarden, L. J. (1977) Prostaglandin $F_{2\alpha}$ specific binding in equine corpus luteum. Prostaglandins 13, 553–564.

120. Kirtland, S. J., and Baum, H. (1972) PGE_1 may act as a calcium ionophore. Nature (London) 236, 926–934.

121. Klein, D. C., and Raisz, L. G. (1970) Prostaglandins; Stimulation of bone resorbtion in tissue culture. Endocrinology 84, 1436.

122. Kloeze, J. (1967) Influence of prostaglandins on platelet adhesiveness and aggregation. In: S. Bergström and B. Samuelsson (eds.), Prostaglandins (Proceedings of the Second Nobel Symposium), Interscience, London, p. 241.

123. Knapp, H. R., Oelz, O. L., Roberts, J., Sweetman, B. J., Oates, J. A., and Reed, P. W. (1977) Ionophores stimulate prostaglandin and thromboxane biosynthesis. Proc. Natl. Acad. Sci. (U.S.) 74, 4251–4255.

124. Kornberg, R. D., and McConnell, H. M. (1971) Inside-outside transitions of phospholipids in vesicle membranes. Biochemistry 10, 1111–1120.

125. Kuehl, F. A., Jr., and Humes, J. (1972) Direct evidence for a prostaglandin receptor and its application to prostaglandin measurements. Proc. Natl. Acad. Sci. (U.S.) 69, 480–484.

126. Kuehl, F. A., Jr. (1974) Prostaglandins, cyclic nucleotides and cell function. Prostaglandins 5(4), 325–340.

127. Kunze, H., and Vogt, W. (1971) Significance of phospholipase A_2 for prostaglandin formation. Ann. NY Acad. Sci. 180, 122–125.

128. Kury, P. G., Ramwell, P. W., and McConnell, H. M. (1974) The effect of prostaglandins E_1 and E_2 on the human erythrocyte as monitored by spin-labels. Biochem. Biophys. Res. Commun. 56, 478–483.

129. Kwon, T. W., and Olcott, H. S. (1966) Reduction and modification of ferritochrome C by malonaldehyde. Biochim. Biophys. Acta 130, 528–531.

130. Lacy, P. E. (1975) Endocrine secretory mechanisms. Am. J. Pathol. 79(1), 170–187.

131. Lahav, M., Freud, A., and Lindner, H. R. (1976) Abrogation by prostaglandin $F_{2\alpha}$ of LH-stimulated cyclic-AMP accumulation in isolated rat corpora lutea of pregnancy. Biochem. Biophys. Res. Commun. 68(4), 1294.

132. Lamprecht, S. A., Zor, U., Tsafriri, A., and Lindner, H. R. (1973) Action of prostaglandin E_2 and of luteinizing hormone on ovarian adenylate cyclase, protein kinase,

and ornithine decarboxylase activity during postnatal development and maturity in the rat. J. Endocrinol. 57, 217–233.

133. Lands, W., Lee, R., and Smith, W. (1971) Factors regulating the biosynthesis of various prostaglandins. Ann. NY Acad. Sci. 180, 107.

134. Lands, W. E. M. (1979) The biosynthesis and metabolism of prostaglandins. Annu. Rev. Physiol. 41, 633–652.

135. Lapetina, E. G., and Cuatrecasas, P. (1979) Rapid inactivation of cyclooxygenase activity after stimulation of intact platelets. Proc. Natl. Acad. Sci. (U.S.) 76(1), 121–125.

136. Lee, J. B. (1974) Cardiovascular-renal effects of prostaglandins. Arch. Intern. Med. 133, 56.

137. Lee, S. C., and Levine, L. (1975) Prostaglandin metabolism; identification of two types of 15-hydroxy-prostaglandin dehydrogenase. J. Biol. Chem. 250, 548.

138. Lee, S. C., and Levine, L. (1974) Purification and properties of chicken heart prostaglandin Δ^{13}-reductase. Biochem. Biophys. Res. Commun. 61, 14–21.

139. Lee, S. C., and Levine, L. (1975) Purification and regulatory properties of chicken heart prostaglandin E-9-ketoreductase. J. Biol. Chem. 250(12), 4549–4555.

140. Lerner, L. J., and Carminati, P. (1976) Effect of L-10503 (a novel antifertility compound) on the synthesis and metabolism of prostaglandins in vivo and in vitro in the pregnant rat placenta, ovary, kidney, and lung and rat deciduomata. In: B. Samuelsson and R. Paoletti (eds.), Advances in Prostaglandin and Thromboxane Research, Vol. 2, Raven Press, New York, p. 645.

141. Leslie, C. A., and Levine, L. (1973) Evidence for the presence of a prostaglandin E_2-9-ketoreductase in rat organs. Biochem. Biophys. Res. Commun. 52(3), 717–724.

142. Liedtke, M. P., and Seifert, B. (1978) Biosynthesis of prostaglandins in human ovarian tissue. Prostaglandins 16(5), 825–833.

143. Limas, C. J., and Cohn, J. N. (1973) Regulation of myocardial prostaglandin dehydrogenase activity; the role of cyclic-AMP and calcium ions. Proc. Soc. Exp. Biol. Med. 142, 1230–1234.

144. Lin, M. T., and Rao, C. V. (1977) [³H]Prostaglandins binding to dispersed bovine luteal cells; Evidence for discrete prostaglandin receptors. Biochem. Biophys. Res. Commun. 78(2), 510–516.

145. Lindgren, J. A., Claessan, H. E., Kindahl, H., and Hammarström, S. (1979) Effects of adenosine 3'5'-monophosphate and platelet aggregation upon thromboxane biosynthesis in human platelets. FEBS Lett. 98(2), 247–250.

146. Lord, J. T., Ziboh, V. A., and Warren, S. (1976) Prostaglandin binding to membrane fractions from rat skin. In: B. Samuelsson and R. Paoletti (eds.), Advances in Prostaglandin and Thromboxane Research, Vol. 1, Raven Press, New York, pp. 291–296.

147. MacIntyre, D. E., and Gordan, J. L. (1977) Discrimination between platelet prostaglandin receptors with a specific antagonist of bisenoic prostaglandins. Thromb. Res. 11, 705–713.

148. MacIntyre, D. E., and Willis, A. L. (1978) Trimethoquinol is a potent prostaglandin antagonist. Br. J. Pharmacol. 63, 316 (P).

149. Maddox, I. S. (1973) The role of copper in prostaglandin synthesis. Biochim. Biophys. Acta 306, 75–81.

150. Makheja, A. N., Vanderhoek, J. V., and Baily, J. M. (1979) Inhibition of platelet aggregation and thromboxane synthesis by onion and garlic. Lancet 8119(1), 781 (Abstr.).

151. Malstem, C., Granström, E., and Samuelsson, B. (1976) Cyclic-AMP inhibits the synthesis of prostaglandin endoperoxide (PGG_2) in human platelets. Biochem. Biophys. Res. Commun. 68(2), 569–576.

152. Marcum, J. M., Dedman, J. R., Brinkley, B. R., and Means, A. R. (1978) Control of microtubule assembly-disassembly by calcium-dependent regulator protein. Proc. Natl. Acad. Sci. (U.S.) 75(8), 3771–3775.

153. Markelonis, G., and Garbus, J. (1975) Alterations of intracellular oxidative metabolism evoking prostaglandin biosynthesis. Prostaglandins 10(6), 1087–1106.

154. Marnett, M., and Samuelsson, B. (1974) Light emission during the action of prostaglandin synthetase. Biochem. Biophys. Res. Commun. 60, 1286–1294.

155. Marrazzi, M. A., and Anderson, N. H. (1974) Prostaglandin dehydrogenase. In: P. W. Ramwell (ed.), The Prostaglandins, Vol. 2, Plenum Press, New York, p. 99.

156. Marsh, J. M., and LeMaire, W. J. (1974) Cyclic-AMP accumulation and steroidogenesis in the human corpus luteum: Effects of gonadotropins and prostaglandins. J. Clin. Endocrinol. Metab. 38, 99.

157. Marrazzi, M. A., and Matschinsky, F. M. (1972) Properties of 15-hydroxy-prostaglandin dehydrogenase. Structural requirements for substrate binding. Prostaglandins 1, 373–388.

158. Miller, O. V., and Gorman, R. R. (1976) Modulation of platelet cyclic nucleotide content by PGE_1 and the prostaglandin endoperoxide PGG_2. J. Cyclic Nucl. Res. 2, 79–87.

159. Miller, O. V., Johnson, R. A., and Gorman, R. (1977) Inhibition of PGE_1-stimulated cAMP accumulation in human platelets by thromboxane A_2. Prostaglandins 13, 599–609.

160. Milton, A. S., and Wendlandt, S. (1970) A possible role for prostaglandin E_1 as a modulator for temperature regulation in the central nervous system of the cat. J. Physiol. (London) 207, 76–77.

161. Minkes, M. Unpublished observations.

162. Minkes, M., Stanford, N., Chi, M. M. Y., Roth, G. J., Raz, A., Needleman, P., and Majerus, P. (1977) Cyclic adenosine 3'5'-monophosphate inhibits the availability of arachidonate to prostaglandin synthetase in human platelet suspensions. J. Clin. Invest. 59, 449–454.

163. Mitchell, M. D. Unpublished observations.

164. Mitchell, M. D., Flint, A. P. F., Hicks, B. R., Kingston, E. J., Thorburn, G. D., and Robinson, J. S. (1978) Uterine tissues from pregnant goats produce 6-oxo-prostaglandin $F_{1\alpha}$ in vitro. J. Endocrinol. 79, 401–402 (Abstr.).

165. Mitchell, M. D., Flint, A. P. F., Kingston, E. J., Thorburn, G. D., and Robinson, J. S. (1978) Production of thromboxane B_2 by intrauterine tissues from pregnant goats in vitro. J. Endocrinol. 78, 159–160.

166. Mitra, A. (1977) The Synthesis of Prostaglandins, Wiley, New York.

167. Miyamoto, T., Yamamoto, S., and Hayashi, O. (1974) Prostaglandin synthetase system; Resolution into oxygenase and isomerase. Proc. Natl. Acad. Sci. (U.S.) 71, 3645.

168. Miyamoto, T., Ogino, S., Yamamoto, S., and Nayaishi, O. J. (1976) Purification of prostaglandin endoperoxide synthetase in bovine vesicular gland microsomes. J. Biol. Chem. 251, 2629.

169. Moore, W. V., and Wolff, J. (1973) Binding of prostaglandins E_1 to beef thyroid membranes. J. Biol. Chem. 248, 5705–5711.

170. Moncada, S., Bunting, S., Mullane, K., Thorogood, P., Vane, J. R., Raz, A., and Needleman, P. (1977) Imidazole: A selective potent antagonist of thromboxane synthetase. Prostaglandins 13, 611.

171. Moncada, S., Higgs, E., and Vane, J. R. (1977) Human arterial and venous tissues generate prostacyclin (PGI_2) a potent inhibitor of platelet aggregation. Lancet 1, 18–21.

172. Moncada, S., Needleman, P., Bunting, S., and Vane, J. R. (1976) Prostaglandin endoperoxide and thromboxane generating systems and their selective inhibition. Prostaglandins 12(3), 323–335.

173. Moncada, S., and Korbut, R. (1978) Dipyridamole and other phosphodiesterase inhibitors act as antithrombotic agents by potentiating endogenous prostacyclin. Lancet 1, 1286–1289.

174. Moncada, S., Korbut, R., Bunting, S., and Vane, J. R. (1978) Prostacyclin is a circulating hormone. Nature (London) 273, 767–768.

175. Moncada, S., and Vane, J. R. (1978) Unstable metabolites of arachidonic acid and their role in hemostasis and thrombosis. Br. Med. Bull. 34, 129–135.

176. Mozzi, R., Orlacchio, A., Andreoli, V., Solinas, N., and Porcellati, G. (1978) The effect of prostaglandin $F_{2\alpha}$ on arachidonate and lipid-choline metabolism in rat brain slices in vitro. In: C. Galli, G. Galli, and G. Porcellati (eds.), Advances in Prostaglandin and Thromboxane Research, Vol. 3, Raven Press, New York, pp. 85–88.

177. Mullane, K. M., Dusting, G. J., Salmon, J. A., Moncada, S., and Vane, J. R. (1979) Biotransformation and cardiovascular effects of arachidonic acid in the dog. Eur. J. Pharmacol. 54, 217–228.

178. Nakano, J. (1973) Cardiovascular actions. In: P. W. Ramwell (ed.), The Prostaglandins, Vol. 2, Plenum Press, New York, pp. 239–316.

179. Needleman, P., Bronson, S. D., Wyche, A., and Sivakoff, M. (1977) Cardiac and renal prostaglandin I_2. J. Clin. Invest. 61, 839–849.

180. Needleman, P., Bryan, B., Wyche, A., Bronson, S., Eakins, K., Ferrendelli, J. A., and Minkes, M. (1977) Thromboxane synthetase inhibitors as pharmacological tools; Differential biochemical and biological effects on platelet suspensions. Prostaglandins 14(5), 897–907.

181. Needleman, P., Minkes, M., and Raz, A. (1976) Thromboxanes; Selective biosynthesis and distinct biological properties. Science 193, 163–165.

182. Needleman, P., Raz, A., Ferrendelli, J. A., and Minkes, M. (1977) Application of imidazole as a selective inhibitor of thromboxane synthetase in human platelets. Proc. Natl. Acad. Sci. (U.S.) 74, 1716.

183. Needleman, P., Raz, A., Kulkarni, P. S., Pure, E., Wyche, A., Denny, S. E., and Isakson, P. C. (1977) Biological and chemical characterisation of a unique endogenous vasodilator prostaglandin produced in isolated coronary artery and in intact perfused heart. In: Interscience Symposium on Prostaglandins, Academic Press, New York, pp. 199–215.

184. Needleman, P., Wyche, A., and Raz, A. (1979) Platelet and blood vessel arachidonate metabolism and interactions. J. Clin. Invest. 63, 345–349.

185. Nelson, N. A. (1974) Nomenclature and structure of prostaglandins. J. Med. Chem. 17, 911–919.

186. Nugteren, D. H. (1975) Arachidonate lipoxygenase in blood platelets. Biochim. Biophys. Acta 380, 299–307.

187. Nugteren, D. H., and Hazelhof, E. (1973) Isolation and properties of intermediates in prostaglandin and biosynthesis. Biochim. Biophys. Acta 326, 448–461.

188. Oelz, O., Knapp, H. R., Roberts, L. J., Oetz, R., Sweetman, B. J., Oates, J. A., and Reed, P. W. (1978) Calcium-dependent stimulation of thromboxane and prostaglandin biosynthesis by ionophores. In: C. Galli, G. Galli, and G. Porcellati (eds.), Advances in Prostaglandin and Thromboxane Research, Vol. 3, Raven Press, New York, pp. 147–158.

189. Oien, H. G., Mandel, L. R., Humes, J. L., Taub, D., Hoffsemmer, R. D., and Kuehl, F. A., Jr. (1975) Structural requirements for the binding of prostaglandins. Prostaglandins 9(6), 985–992.

190. Okamura, H., Yang, S., Wright, K., and Wallach, E. (1972) The effect of prostaglandin $F_{2\alpha}$ on the corpus luteum of the pregnant rat—An ultrastructural study. Fertil. Steril. 23, 475–483.

191. Oliw, E., Lundén, I., and ÄnggÅard, E. (1976) Affinity chromatography of 15-hydroxyprostaglandin dehydrogenases from swine kidney. In: B. Samuelsson and R. Paoletti (eds.), Advances in Prostaglandin and Thromboxane Research, Vol. 1, Raven Press, New York, pp. 147–151.

192. Ostlund, R., Jr., Pfleger, B., and Schonfeld, G. (1979) Role of microtubules in low density lipoprotein processing by cultured cells. J. Clin. Invest. 63, 75–84.

193. Pace-Asciak, C. (1976) A new prostaglandin metabolite of arachidonic acid. Formation of 6-keto-$PGF_{1\alpha}$ by the rat stomach. Experientia 32, 291–292.

194. Pace-Asciak, C. (1976) Biosynthesis and catabolism of prostaglandins during animal development. In: B. Samuelsson and R. Paoletti (eds.), Advances in Prostaglandin and Thromboxane Research, Vol. 1, Raven Press, New York, pp. 35–46.

195. Pace-Asciak, C., and Cole, S. (1975) Inhibition of prostaglandin catabolism; Differential sensitivity of 9-PGDH, 13-PGR and 15-PGDH to low concentrations of indomethacin. Experientia 31, 143–145.

196. Paulsrud, J. R., Miller, O. N., and Schlegel, W. (1974) Inhibition of 15-hydroxyprostaglandin dehydrogenase by several diuretic drugs. Fed. Proc. 33, 590 (Abstr.).

197. Pickett, W. C., Jesse, R. L., and Cohen, P. (1977) Initiation of phospholipase A_2 activity in human platelets by calcium ion ionophore A23187. Biochim. Biophys. Acta 486, 209–213.

198. Piper, O., and Vane, J. R. (1977) The release of prostaglandins from lung and other tissues. Ann. NY Acad. Sci. 180, 363.

199. Polis, D. B., Pakoskey, A. M., and Schmukler, H. W. (1969) Regeneration of oxidative phosphorylation in aged mitochondria by prostaglandin B_1. Proc. Natl. Acad. Sci. (U.S.) 63, 229 (Abstr.).

200. Powell, W. S., Hammarström, S., Kylden, U., and Samuelsson, B. B. (1976) In: R. A. Bradshaw, W. A. Frazier, R. C. Merrell, D. I. Gottlieb, and R. A. Hogue-Angelletti (eds.), Surface Membrane Receptors, Interface Between Cells and Their Environment, Plenum Press, New York, pp. 455–472.

201. Powles, I. J., Clark, S. A., Easty, D. M., Easty, G. C., and Neville, A. M. (1973) Inhibition by aspirin and indomethacin of osteolytic tumor deposits and hypercalcemia in rats with Walker tumor and its possible application to human breast cancer. Br. J. Cancer 38, 316.

202. Poyser, N. L., Horton, E. W., Thompson, C. J., and Los, M. (1971) Identification of $PGF_{2\alpha}$ released by distension of the guinea pig uterus in vitro. Nature (London) 230, 526–527.

203. Puglisi, L., Berti, F., Bosisio, E., Longiave, D., and Nicosia, S. (1976) Ascorbic acid and $PGF_{2\alpha}$ antagonism on tracheal smooth muscle. In: B. Samuelsson and R. Paoletti (eds.), Advances in Prostaglandin and Thromboxane Research, Vol. 1, Raven Press, New York, pp. 503–506.

204. Rabinowitz, I. N., Wolf, P. L., Berman, S., Shikuma, N., and Edwards, P. (1975) Prostaglandin E_2 effects on cation flux in sickle erythrocyte ghosts. Prostaglandins 9(4), 545–555.

205. Ramwell, P. W., Leovey, E. M. K., and Sintetos, A. O. (1977) Regulation of the arachidonic acid cascade. Biol. Reprod. 16, 70–87.

206. Rane, L. H., Lands, W. E. M., Roth, G. J., and Majerus, P. W. (1976) Aspirin as a quantitative acetylating reagent for fatty acid oxygenase that forms prostaglandins. Prostaglandins 11, 23–30.

207. Rasmussen, H. (1966) Mitochondrial ion transport; Mechanism and physiological significance. Fed. Proc. 25, 903–911.

208. Rasmussen, H., Lake, W., and Allen, J. (1975) The effects of catecholamines and prostaglandins upon human and rat erythrocytes. Biochim. Biophys. Acta 411, 63–73.

209. Reed, P. W., and Lardy, H. A. (1972) A23187; A divalent cation ionophore. J. Biol. Chem. 247(2), 6970–6977.

210. Rees, D. A., Lloyd, C. W., and Than, D. (1977) Control of grip and stick in cell adhesion through lateral relationships of membrane glycoproteins. Nature (London) 267, 124–128.

211. Roa, C. V. (1974) Differential properties of prostaglandin and gonadotropin receptors in the bovine corpus luteum cell membranes. Prostaglandins 6, 313–328.

212. Roa, C. V. (1976) Discrete prostaglandin receptors in the outer cell membranes of bovine corpora lutea. In: B. Samuelsson and R. Paoletti (eds.), Advances in Prostaglandin and Thromboxane Research, Vol. 1, Raven Press, New York, pp. 247–258.

213. Robert, A. (1976) Antisecretory, antiulcer, cytoprotective and diarrheogenic properties of prostaglandins. In: B. Samuelsson and R. Paoletti (eds.), Advances in Prostaglandin and Thromboxane Research, Vol. 2, Raven Press, New York, pp. 507–520.

214. Robinson, J., Merry, B. J., and A. K. Hall (1979) Prostaglandin-induced functional luteolysis in the pseudopregnant rat. J. Endocrinol. 80, 39–40P (Abstr.).

215. Robinson, J., and Vane, J. R. (1974) Prostaglandin Synthetase Inhibitors. Raven Press, New York.

216. Roseman, T. J., and Yaikausky, S. H. (1973) Physicochemical properties of $PGF_{2\alpha}$. J. Pharm. Sci. 62, 1680–1685.

217. Samuelsson, B. (1976) New trends in prostaglandin research. In: B. Samuelsson and R. Paoletti (eds.), Advances in Prostaglandin and Thromboxane Research, Vol. 1, Raven Press, New York, pp. 1–6.

218. Samuelsson, B. B., Granström, E., Green, K., Hamberg, M., and Hammarström, S. (1975) Prostaglandins. Annu. Rev. Biochem. 44, 669–695.

219. Samuelsson, B. B., Hamberg, M., Malmsten, C., and Svensson, J. (1976) The role of prostaglandin endoperoxides and thromboxanes in platelet aggregation. In: B. Samuelsson and R. Paoletti (eds.), Advances in Prostaglandin and Thromboxane Research, Vol. 2, Raven Press, New York, pp. 737–746.

220. Salzman, E. W. (1976) Prostaglandins and platelets function. In: B. Samuelsson and R. Paoletti (eds.), Advances in Prostaglandin and Thromboxane Research, Vol. 2, Raven Press, New York, pp. 767–780.

221. Schaumburg, B. (1973) Binding of prostaglandin E_1 to rat thymocytes. Biochim. Biophys. Acta 326, 127–133.

222. Schillinger, E., and Prior, C. (1976) Characteristics of prostaglandin receptor sites in human uterine tissue. In: B. Samuelsson and R. Paoletti (eds.), Advances in Prostaglandin and Thromboxane Research, Vol. 1, Raven Press, New York, pp. 259–263.

223. Schlegel, W., Demers, L. M., Hildebrandt-Stark, H. E., Behrman, H. R., and Greep, R. O. (1974) Partial purification of human placental 15-hydroxyprostaglandin dehydrogenase; Kinetic properties. Prostaglandins 5(5), 417–434.

224. Schneider, W. P., and Murray, H. C. (1973) Microbiological reduction and resolution of prostaglandins. Synthesis of natural $PGF_{2\alpha}$ and ent-$PGF_{2\beta}$ methyl esters. J. Org. Chem. 38, 397–398.

225. Siegl, A. M., Smith, B. J., Silver, M. J., Nicolaou, K. C., and Ahern, D. (1979) Selective binding site for [^{3}H]prostacyclin on platelets. J. Clin. Invest. 63, 215–220.

226. Siggins, G. R., Hoffer, B., and Bloom, F. (1971) Prostaglandin-norepinephrine interactions in brain; Microelectrophoretic and histochemical correlates. Ann. NY Acad. Sci. 180, 303–323.

227. Sih, C. J., Takeguchi, C., and Foss, P. J. (1970) Mechanisms of prostaglandin biosynthesis III. Catecholamine and serotonin as coenzymes. J. Am. Chem. Soc. 92, 6670.

228. Silver, M. J., and Smith, J. B. (1975) Minireview; Prostaglandins as intracellular messengers. Life Sci. 16, 1635–1648.

229. Smigel, M., and Fleischer, S. (1974) Characterisation and localization of prostaglandin E_1 receptor in rat liver plasma membranes. Biochim. Biophys. Acta 332, 358–373.

230. Smith, J. B., Ingerman, C. M., and Silver, M. J. (1976) Persistence of thromboxane A_2-like material and platelet release-inducing activity in plasma. J. Clin. Invest. 58(5), 1119–1122.

231. Smith, J. B., and MacFarlane, D. E. (1974) In: P. W. Ramwell (ed.), The Prostaglandins, Vol. 2, Plenum Press, New York, p. 293.

232. Spooner, P. M., Chernick, S. C., Garrison, M. M., and Scow, R. O. (1979) Development of lipoprotein lipase activity and accumulation of triacylglycerol in differentiating 3T3-L1 adipocytes. J. Biol. Chem. 254(4), 1305–1311.

233. Steiner, M., and Ikeda, Y. (1979) Quantitative assessment of polymerized and depolymerized platelet microtubules. J. Clin. Invest. 63, 443–448.

234. Stjarne, L. (1973) Inhibitory effects of prostaglandin E_2 on noradrenaline secretion from sympathetic nerves as a function of external calcium. Prostaglandins 3, 105–109.

235. Stone, K. J., Mather, S. J., and Gibson, P. P. (1975) Selective inhibition of prostaglandin biosynthesis by gold salts and phenylbutazone. Prostaglandins 10(2), 241–249.

236. Strauss, J. F., III., Seifter, E., Lien, E. L., Goodman, D. B. P., and Stambaugh, R. L. (1977) Lipid metabolism in regressing rat corpora lutea of pregnancy. J. Lipid Res. 18, 246.

237. Strickland, S., and Beers, W. (1976) Studies on the role of plasminogen activator in ovulation. J. Biol. Chem. 251, 5694–5702.

238. Sun, F. F., Armour, S. B., Bockstanz, V. R., and McGuire, J. C. (1976) Studies on 15-hydroxyprostaglandin dehydrogenase from monkey lung. In: B. Samuelsson and R. Paoletti (eds.), Advances in Prostaglandin and Thromboxane Research, Vol. 1, Raven Press, New York, pp. 163–169.

239. Sun, F. F., Chapman, J. P., and McGuire, J. C. (1977) Metabolism of prostaglandin endoperoxides in animal tissues. Prostaglandins 14, 1055–1074.

240. Sun, F. F., McGuire, J. C., and Taylor, B. M. (1978) Metabolism of prostacyclin (PGI$_2$). Prostaglandins 15, 724.

241. Tai, H. H. (1976) Mechanism of prostaglandin biosynthesis in rabbit kidney medulla. A rate-limiting step and different stimulatory actions of L-adrenaline and glutathione. J. Biol. Chem. 160, 577.

242. Tai, H. H., and Hollander, C. S. (1976) Regulation of prostaglandin metabolism: Activation of 15-hydroxyprostaglandin dehydrogenase by chlorpromazine and imipramine related drugs. Biochem. Biophys. Res. Commun. 68(3), 814–820.

243. Tai, H. H., and Hollander, C. S. (1976) Kinetic evidence for a distinct regulatory site on 15-hydroxyprostaglandin and thromboxane research. In: B. Samuelsson and R. Paoletti (eds.), Advances in Prostaglandin and Thromboxane Research, Vol. 1, Raven Press, New York, pp. 171–182.

244. Takequchi, C. E., Kohno, E., and Sih, C. J. (1971) Mechanism of prostaglandin biosynthesis. I. Characterisation and assay of bovine prostaglandin synthetase. Biochemistry 10, 2372.

245. Takequchi, C. E., and Sih, C. J. (1972) A rapid spectrophotometric assay for prostaglandin synthetase; application to the study of nonsteroidal antiinflammatory drugs. Prostaglandins 2, 169.

246. Thomas, J. P., Dorflinger, L. J., and Behrman, H. R. (1978) Mechanism of the rapid antigonadotropic action of prostaglandins in cultured luteal cells. Proc. Natl. Acad. Sci. (U.S.) 75, 1344–1348.

247. Tse, J., and Coceani, F. (1979) Does 15-hydroxyprostaglandin dehydrogenase contribute to prostaglandin inactivation in the brain? Prostaglandins 17(1), 76–77.

248. Turner, S. R., Tainer, J. A., and Lynn, W. S. (1975) Biogenesis of chemotactic molecules by the arachidonate lipoxygenase system of platelets. Nature (London) 257, 680.

249. Vane, J. R. (1976) Prostaglandins as mediators of inflammation. In: B. Samuelsson and R. Paoletti (eds.), Advances in Prostaglandin and Thromboxane Research, Vol. 2, Raven Press, New York, pp. 971–801.

250. Wakeling, A. E., Kirton, K. T., and Wyngarden, L. J. (1974) Prostaglandin receptors in the hamster uterus during the estrous cycle. Prostaglandins 4, 1–8.

251. Wakeling, A. E., and Spilman, C. H. (1973) Prostaglandin specific binding in rabbit the oviduct. Prostaglandins 4, 405–414.

252. Wakeling, A. E., and Wyngarden, L. J. (1974) Prostaglandin receptors in the human, monkey and hamster uterus. Endocrinology 95, 55–64.

253. Weeks, J. R. (1976) Introduction to cardiovascular research on prostaglandins. In: B. Samuelsson and R. Paoletti (eds.), Advances in Prostaglandin and Thromboxane Research, Vol. 1, Raven Press, New York, pp. 395–401.

254. Weissman, G., Goldstein, I., and Hoffstein, S. (1976) Prostaglandins and the modulation by cyclic nucleotides of lysosomal enzyme release. In: B. Samuelsson and R. Paoletti (eds.), Advances in Prostaglandin and Thromboxane Research, Vol. 2, Raven Press, New York, pp. 803–814.

255. Wennmalm, ÅA. (1978) Effects of nicotine on cardiac prostaglandin and platelet thromboxane synthesis. Br. J. Pharmacol. 64, 559–563.

256. White, J. G. (1969) Effects of colchicine and vinka-alkaloids on human platelets. III. Influence on primary internal contraction and secondary aggregation. Am. J. Pathol. 54, 467.

257. Whittle, B. J. R., Moncada, S., and Vane, J. R. (1978) Comparison of the effects of prostacyclin (PGI_2), PGE_1 and PGD_2 on platelet aggregation in different species. Prostaglandins 16(3), 373–388.

258. Wilson, D. E. (1974) Prostaglandins; Their actions on the gastrointestinal tract. Arch. Intern. Med. 133, 112–118.

259. Williams, K. I., Dembińska-Kieć, A., Amuda, A., and Gryglewski, R. J. (1978) Prostacyclin formation by myometrial and decidual fractions of the pregnant rat uterus. Prostaglandins 15(2), 343–350.

260. Wolf, L. S., Rostwonowski, K., and Marion, J. (1976) Endogenous formation of the prostaglandin endoperoxide metabolite, thromboxane B_2, by brain tissue. Biochem. Biophys. Res. Commun. 70, 907–913.

261. Woollard, P. M., Lagnado, P. J., and Lascelles, P. T. (1978) Microtubules. Lancet 1, 8069, 873 (letter).

262. Wong, P. Y. K., Sun, F. F., and McGiff, J. C. (1978) Metabolism of prostacyclin in blood vessels. J. Biol. Chem. 253, 5555–5557.

263. Wong, P. Y. K., Terragno, A., Terragno, N. A., and McGiff, J. C. (1977) Dual effects of bradykinin on prostaglandin metabolism; dissimilar vascular actions of kinins. Prostaglandins 13, 1113–1125.

264. Wright, K., Luborsky-Moore, J. L., and Behrman, H. R. (1979) Specific binding of prostaglandin $F_{2\alpha}$ to membranes of rat corpora lutea. Mol. Cell. Endocrinol. 13, 25–34.

265. Zor, U., Lamprecht, S. A., Kaneko, T., Schneider, H. P. G., McCann, S. M., Field, J., Tsafriri, A., and Lindner, H. R. (1972) Functional relationships between cyclic-AMP, prostaglandins and LH in rat pituitary and ovary. In: P. Greengard, and J. Robinson (eds.), Advances in Cyclic Nucleotide Research, Vol. 1, Raven Press, New York, p. 503.

266. Zor, U., and Lamprecht, S. A. (1977) Mechanism of prostaglandin action in endocrine glands. In: G. Litivich (ed.), Biochemical Actions of Hormones, Vol. 4, Academic Press, New York, London, pp. 86–133.

267. Zor, U., Strulovici, B., and Lindner, H. R. (1978) Implication of microtubules and microfilaments in the response of the ovarian adenylate cyclase–cyclic AMP system to gonadotropins and prostaglandin E_2. Biochem. Biophys. Res. Commun. 80(4), 983–992.

268. Phospholipases and prostaglandins. In: C. Galli, G. Galli, and G. Porcellati (eds.), Advances in Prostaglandin and Thromboxane Research, Vol. 3, Raven Press, New York, 1978.

WILLIAM F. STENSON, M.D.
CHARLES W. PARKER, M.D.

PROSTAGLANDINS AND THE IMMUNE RESPONSE

PROSTAGLANDINS AND THE IMMUNE RESPONSE

The Immune Response

COMPONENTS OF THE IMMUNE RESPONSE

One of the fundamental questions in immunology involves the means by which an immunologic stimulus (the binding of an antigen to a receptor on the lymphocyte surface) causes an immune response (blastogenesis, antibody production, lymphokine production). During an immune response small subpopulations of lymphocytes are stimulated selectively by antigen to divide and differentiate. The elucidation of the biochemical events that translate antigen binding into lymphocyte activation is important both for the understanding of the immune response and as a model for cell activation and differentiation [68].

The process of lymphocyte activation is complicated by the existence of two major lymphocyte subclasses, T- and B-cells, plus several further

From the Division of Gastroenterology, Jewish Hospital of St. Louis, Washington University School of Medicine, and the Howard Hughes Medical Institute and Department of Medicine, Division of Allergy and Immunology, Washington University School of Medicine, St. Louis, Missouri.

divisions of the major subclasses. T-cells make lymphokines (soluble mediators that regulate other cells in the immune system), divide to form antigen-specific cells that serve as effectors of the cell-mediated response, and regulate antibody production by B-cells. T-Cells that enhance antibody production by B-cells are called helper cells, while those that inhibit it are called suppressor cells. Cytotoxic T-cells are also produced and serve to ablate pathogenic microorganisms and neoplastic cells. B-Cells function by producing antibody in response to antigen. They can respond to some antigens (T-independent antigens) without the participation of T-cells, but for most antigens B-cell antibody production is enhanced by T-cell "help." The other major cell type of the immune system is the macrophage. The macrophage binds antigen on its surface and presents it to antigen-sensitive T- and B-lymphocytes. Macrophage function can be controlled to some extent by lymphokines produced by activated T-cells. Macrophages also act as phagocytic cells in the same way as polymorphonuclear leukocytes and are particularly important in the control of slowly replicating intracellular microorganisms.

The different cell types of the immune system interact with one another both by producing soluble mediators and by cell-cell interaction. The interrelationship of these cell types is not yet fully defined, but it appears that they may act on one another both as positive amplification systems to enhance cell differentiation or to recruit more cells into a response, or as negative feedback systems in which one cell type acts to turn off another, serving to limit the response. This system of positive and negative feedback controls is analogous to hormonal regulation of endocrine and peripheral tissues, although in contrast to endocrine systems much of the control appears to be exerted locally rather than through the bloodstream.

METABOLIC EVENTS DURING THE IMMUNE RESPONSE

During the past decade, a number of laboratories including our own have been interested in the metabolic changes that occur when T- and B-lymphocytes are treated with antigens or other stimuli [2,157]. A complex series of alterations in cellular transport and metabolism begins within a few minutes after exposure to the stimulus, continues for several days, and leads to changes in cell morphology, to increases in synthesis of protein, RNA, and DNA and, often, to mitosis and cell division [122,206]. As the response progresses, the cells synthesize new enzymes and secrete lymphokines. Lymphocyte activation is often studied by measurement of [3H]thymidine incorporation into DNA or release of lymphokine activity; however, many marked alterations in lymphocyte metabolism, morphology, or function suggest lymphocyte activation. Since lymphocytes are heterogeneous, subpopulations of cells may respond to stimulation differently, creating a very complex situation, and simultaneous assays in several systems are necessary to adequately describe the response.

Current dogma holds that both major lymphocyte subclasses contain a great number of immunologically distinguishable clones of cells, each programmed to respond to one or a limited number of antigens. Since only cells that recognize the antigen respond, the percentage of lymphocytes activated by a single antigen is very small, and the biochemistry of the response is difficult to study, particularly in its early phases. For this reason, many investigators have used polyclonal activators to increase the number of responding cells. The most popular polyclonal activators are the lectins, proteins, or glycoproteins of plant origin with binding affinity for cell surface carbohydrates; effective activators of lymphocyte metabolism include jack bean concanavalin A (Con A), *Phaseolus vulgaris* (kidney bean) phytohemagglutinin (PHA), and pokeweed mitogen (PWM). Since these agents induce mitosis in lymphocytes they are also termed mitogens.

A series of specific biochemical events occurs in lymphocytes at varying times after binding of antigen or lectin to the respective surface receptors:

1. Membrane changes. The rate of transport of amino acids, sugars, and nucleosides is increased. Changes in amino acid uptake, particularly of amino acids transported through the alanine (A) system, occur within 30 minutes and last for many hours. Increased Ca^{2+} uptake has been observed as early as 1 minute after exposure to the lectin PHA [211]. Beginning at about 10 minutes there is a very rapid turnover of phosphate and fatty acid molecules in phospholipid [157]. There is activation of an acyl transferase that favors the incorporation of unsaturated fatty acids into phospholipid [33]. Although further studies are needed, at least one report indicates that the distribution of fatty acid in membrane phospholipids changes markedly within a few hours after mitogen activation with increased incorporation of unsaturated fatty acids, including arachidonate [33]. Studies in a variety of cell types including mutant bacterial strains, which are particularly susceptible to manipulation, indicate that increased levels of unsaturated fatty acids lead to less constrained packing of phospholipids and increased membrane fluidity [6,76]. These changes in phospholipid fatty acid composition may be an important factor in the changes in membrane permeability to water, ions, sugars, and other substances that accompany lymphocyte activation, although it is doubtful that they are the sole cause. In addition to turnover of phospholipid fatty acids there is a rapid increase in turnover of phospholipid phosphate [35,100,158] similar to that in other tissues whose cells are subjected to external stimulation.

2. Cytoplasmic changes. Increased incorporation of labeled amino acids into protein is detectable by 2 hours and continues for 48 hours, a net increase in protein synthesis is detected at 12 hours [65]. The activities of a large number of cytoplasmic enzymes is increased with increased glucose utilization, pyruvate, and lactate production and fatty acid synthesis rising twofold within the first few hours [66].

3. Nuclear changes. There are early (15–30 minute) increases in incorporation of phosphate and acetate into histones. There are also early

(30 minute) increases in incorporation of uridine into nuclear RNA with much larger changes later at 24 to 72 hours. Beginning at 20 hours there is a marked increase in radiolabeled thymidine incorporation into DNA. This is the most commonly used measure of lymphocyte activation. However, the increase in thymidine uptake far exceeds the increase in the number of cells undergoing division (reviewed in Ref. 138).

INTRACELLULAR MEDIATORS IN LYMPHOCYTE ACTIVATION

The metabolic changes occurring during lymphocyte activation involve biochemical events leading to enzyme activation and DNA replication. It is generally assumed that lymphocyte function is controlled at the plasma membrane. Since lymphocytes contain surface receptors for antigens and lectins, this is a reasonable assumption, although rigorous proof is not yet available. Assuming the validity of the cell surface activation model, some mechanism must exist to transmit a stimulus into the interior of the cell and orchestrate the events that take place once activation is under way [130,133]. Several mechanisms have been proposed:

1. Changes in plasma membrane function due to alterations in lipid, protein, or glycoprotein composition, configuration, or organization, or their interactions with the cytoskeletal elements. For example, the binding of antigen with receptor causes changes in the lipid phase of the plasma membrane, resulting in changes in membrane fluidity, membrane permeability, and the activity of membrane proteins [157].
2. Altered uptake of essential nutrients and ions by the cell. For example, binding of the antigen to receptor appears to open up Ca^{2+} channels. Elevated intracellular Ca^{2+} levels may be sufficient to cause gene activation [159].
3. Activation of a membrane-bound enzyme resulting in the generation of a second messenger, which in turn is responsible for gene activation and various pleiotypic effects on cellular metabolism. Candidates for the role of second messenger in lymphocyte activation include cyclic AMP (cAMP), cyclic GMP (cGMP), arachidonic acid (AA) metabolites, subunits of membrane-bound enzymes with protein kinase and other activities, and as yet undefined modulatory molecules [60,138].

Obviously these mechanisms are not mutually exclusive, and it is likely that all play significant roles in lymphocyte activation. Since prostaglandins appear to produce their effects on cells primarily by stimulating or inhibiting adenylate cyclase with resultant changes in cAMP levels, we concentrate initially on the role of changes in cyclic nucleotide levels in the control of lymphocyte function. The discussion of membrane lipids is deferred; however it should be kept in mind that changes in turnover of fatty acids in membrane phospholipids in turn affect the availability of free arachidonate as a substrate for prostaglandin synthesis, indicating the marked interdependence of these systems.

ROLE OF CYCLIC AMP IN LYMPHOCYTE ACTIVATION

It is now abundantly clear that prostaglandins have the capability of exerting modulatory effects at virtually every level of the immune response (reviewed in Refs. 28, 102, and 147). As discussed below, lymphoid cells both produce and respond to prostaglandins, creating a situation where involvement of prostaglandins in local regulation of immune responses is clearly possible [56].

Before considering the role of prostaglandins in lymphocyte function in more detail, a brief discussion of cAMP metabolism in lymphocytes is desirable. The only well-established biochemical effect of the prostaglandins is their ability to alter cAMP (and in some tissues cGMP) levels. A 3- to 30-fold increase in the cAMP levels in intact lymphocytes can be obtained with a variety of prostaglandins. Members of the E, A, and F series are all stimulatory, with PGE_1 being most effective and PGF_2 the least effective on a molar basis [173]. Although other mechanisms are possible, it seems likely that most or all of the effects of prostaglandins in the immune response are mediated through adenylate cyclase. Adenylate cyclase generates cAMP from ATP by splitting off pyrophosphate and linking the 5'-phosphate group to the 3'-hydroxy group of the ribose ring to produce a phosphodiester. Under ordinary circumstances this reaction is irreversible. In most cells much or all of the adenylate cyclase is located in the plasma membrane, although there is now evidence that other subcellular fractions may also contain this enzyme [207].

All lymphocyte or thymocyte populations that have been studied to date contain cAMP. Human peripheral blood lymphocytes have been particularly carefully examined in regard to their cAMP metabolism [134,138]. Freshly isolated human lymphocytes obtained by dextran sedimentation and isopycnic centrifugation over a Ficoll-Hypaque gradient have resting cAMP levels of about 25 pmole per 10^7 cells. This is a high level relative to that found in other tissues. A diverse group of agents have been shown to increase cAMP either in human or animal lymphocytes (reviewed in Ref. 133): (1) β-adrenergic agonists such as isoproterenol and epinephrine, (2) prostaglandins, particularly the E and D prostaglandins and to a lesser extent the F prostaglandins, (3) histamine, apparently through an action on H-2 receptors, (4) lectins, including PHA, concanavalin A, and wheat germ agglutinin, (5) the divalent cation ionophore A23187, (6) phosphodiesterase inhibitors such as theophylline and isobutylmethylxanthine, (7) proteolytic enzymes, particularly trypsin, (8) arachidonic acid, but not other long chain fatty acids, (9) short chain aliphatic and aromatic alcohols, (10) certain nonmetabolizable particles such as latex beads, (11) a lymphokine termed "inhibitor of DNA synthesis" (IDS), which increases cAMP in lectin-stimulated cells shortly before the onset of the S phase, (12) certain of the polypeptide hormones, which induce thymocyte differentiation, (13) lipopolysaccharide, a B-cell mitogen [171], (14) adenosine [117], and (15) calcitonin [107].

The only substances that consistently lower lymphocyte cAMP levels are eicosatetraynoic acid (ETYA), a triple unsaturated analogue of arachidonic acid [159], and reagents that alkylate sulfhydryl groups such as N-ethylmaleimide and iodoacetate. The most marked effects of sulfhydryl reagents are at concentrations in the millimolar range. Part of the effect may be due to nonspecific cytotoxicity, but this does not appear to be the whole explanation.

The cAMP response to prostaglandins in mixed human peripheral blood lymphocytes develops rapidly. Marked (five- to tenfold) increases in cAMP are demonstrable within 30 to 60 seconds. The E and D prostaglandins are much more effective in raising cAMP than the F prostaglandins [173]. The most marked responses are obtained at micromolar prostaglandin concentrations, but, with the E prostaglandins at least, responses are detectable at concentrations as low as 10 nM [118]. The duration of the response depends in part on the culture medium used. When lymphocytes undergoing a near-maximal prostaglandin response are then suspended in Gey's balanced salt solution, the response peaks at 5 to 15 minutes and is already markedly decreased by 1 hour. This diminution with time is apparently due to some form of cellular desensitization, since adding fresh prostaglandin to the medium does not restore the response. Cells that have been desensitized to prostaglandin continue to respond to isoproterenol, indicating either that different pools of cAMP are involved (see below) or that the loss of prostaglandin sensitivity is at the receptor level [137]. The failure to sustain prostaglandin responses in lymphocytes at their original high level suggests that prostaglandin effects on lymphocyte responses such as mitogenesis are exerted relatively early in the activation process.

Information on the responses of lymphocyte subpopulations to these diverse agents is limited. Peripheral blood lymphocytes show higher basal cAMP levels than spleen, lymph node, or thymus lymphocytes. Thymocytes have a much more marked cAMP response to PGE_1 than do spleen, lymph node, or peripheral blood lymphocytes [3]. Obviously, the in vivo environment of the lymphocyte population under study could affect its behavior in vitro. Moreover, the effects of the purification procedures used to obtain these subpopulations, and the influence of contaminating cells, cannot be disregarded.

The existence of selective cAMP responses to prostaglandins suggests the presence of specific receptors. The most convincing evidence for prostaglandin receptors in tissue is in rat liver [58], where isolated plasma membrane preparations with apparently specific binding for the E prostaglandins with an estimated K_d of 1.0×10^{-9} to 2.5×10^{-8} M have been demonstrated. Receptor binding activity for prostaglandins has been reported in thymocytes and human lymphocytes [56,81]. Goodwin et al. have reported the existence of a high affinity receptor for PGE in human lymphocytes. This receptor has a K_d of approximately 2×10^{-9} [54].

A number of the agents that raise cAMP have been shown to inhibit mitogenesis. These include the E prostaglandins, catecholamines, histamine, theophylline [173], and the "inhibitor of DNA synthesis" described above. Inhibitory effects are seen on both T- and B-cell proliferation as well as on the production of lymphokines such as migration inhibitory factor (MIF). Several of these agents, including the prostaglandins, also inhibit lymphocyte-mediated cytolysis and T-lymphocyte rosette formation. In view of the inhibition by prostaglandins and histamine and the undoubted presence of these substances in lymphoid tissues undergoing stimulation with antigen, it has been suggested that these molecules may serve as natural regulators of lymphocyte responsiveness in vivo.

Even though pharmacologic agents that increase intracellular cAMP generally inhibit immune responses, it is now apparent that cAMP can also have a stimulatory effect. The earliest detectable metabolic change in lymphocytes stimulated by PHA or Con A is a rise in intracellular cAMP [173]. Increases in intracellular cAMP are demonstrable at 10 seconds, become maximal at 5 to 15 minutes, and persist for 45 to 120 minutes. In some cell systems agents that increase cAMP potentiate B-cell responses, particularly if the increase in cAMP is produced very early in the response and the cAMP agonist is then removed [138].

Since agents that raise cAMP may exert extraneous pharmacologic actions, investigators have studied the effect of adding exogenous cAMP or its lipophilic derivatives to the incubation medium. In interpreting these experiments it should be kept in mind that cAMP penetrates into viable cells poorly, and much of it is degraded in the medium. While lipophilic cAMP derivatives penetrate more readily, they do not fully mimic the action of cAMP intracellularly.

It is also apparent that the effects of exogenous cAMP on lymphocyte activation vary with the dose. High concentrations of cAMP inhibit DNA synthesis while low doses stimulate. The effects of exogenous cAMP depend not only on the concentration used but also on the stage of lymphocyte activation at which it is added. Kishimoto and Ishizaka found that moderate concentrations of cAMP enhanced antibody production by primed B-cells if added early in the course of lymphocyte activation but diminished antibody production if added more than 24 hours after the addition of antigen [86]. Whether the stimulatory phase of the biphasic response to cAMP involves an induction of differentiation in immature precursor cells or a distinctive stimulatory action of cAMP during a particular phase of the cell cycle remains to be established.

If cAMP does have a stimulatory action, the apparent paradox that pharmacologic agents that raise cAMP levels generally inhibit rather than stimulate mitogenesis must be explained. One explanation is that functionally distinct pools of cAMP are involved. The existence of discrete pools is suggested by cAMP immunofluorescence localization studies, which indicate that cAMP produced in response to PHA is localized to patchy areas in or near the plasma membrane, whereas the response to PGI_1 or isoproterenol occurs in different areas of the cell [9]. Other evidence suggesting distinct adenylate cyclases, hence distinct cAMP pools, comes from studies showing that the increases in cAMP induced by PHA, PGE_2, and isoproterenol are additive [138,173]. Moreover when the same three stimuli are evaluated in homogenized lymphocytes, they can be shown to activate adenylate cyclases in different subcellular fractions. Interestingly, the PGE_1-responsive cyclase is probably in the microsomal fraction, although since this fraction is contaminated with heavy plasma membrane fragments, the latter may be contributing importantly to the response.

Perhaps the most convincing evidence for a functionally distinct cAMP pool responsive to prostaglandins comes from the observation that the prostaglandins inhibit lectin-induced protein phosphorylation in lymphocytes, but isoproterenol does not [23]. The effects of cAMP in mammalian cells appear to be exerted through increases or decreases in protein phosphorylation. If cAMP is, indeed, involved in the initial action of lectin on lymphocytes, protein phosphorylation should change during the early stages of the response. Chaplin et al. have demonstrated in our laboratory that when intact human lymphocytes are preincubated with [^{32}P]orthophosphate (to prelabel intracellular ATP), stimulated with lectin, and then lysed, rapid increases in protein phosphorylation are demonstrable after separation of the proteins by polyacrylamide-gel electrophoresis [23]. In most systems, cAMP modulates phosphorylation of one or a few proteins, but in PHA-stimulated lymphocytes it appears to affect a larger number of proteins. In early studies it was shown that during the first few minutes of the response, increased phosphorylation occurs in proteins that fractionate in the 30,000-dalton to 100,000-dalton region of the gel. The increases in phosphorylation of most of these proteins is modest (of the order of 25%). In recent studies, however, one protein in particular (MW = 65,000) is much more heavily labeled in the presence than in the absence of lectin [22]. Three other lymphocyte mitogens—Con A, calcium ionophore A23187, and sodium metaperiodate—produce responses similar or identical to those produced by PHA. In contrast, isoproterenol, prostaglandin E_1, and theophylline, which are not mitogenic but do increase whole cell cAMP, either fail to enhance phosphorylation of proteins with high molecular weights or actually inhibit it. Of particular interest for this discussion, PGE_1 inhibits protein phosphorylation, although neither isoproterenol nor theophylline has this effect, and even though the increases in whole cell cAMP concentrations produced by these agents are comparable [23]. The fact that prostaglandins seem to act on selected adenylate cyclases adds complexity to the interpretation of experiments studying the effects of exogenous prostaglandins in mitogen-induced lymphocyte activation.

Arachidonate metabolites also affect the synthesis of cyclic GMP in the immune response. Graff et al. demonstrated that reactive intermediates of arachidonate metabolism, both from the cyclooxygenase and lipoxygenase pathways, stimulate splenic guanylate cyclase [57].

Arachidonic Acid and Lymphocytes

ARACHIDONIC ACID METABOLISM IN LYMPHOCYTES

Lymphocytes contain very little free arachidonic acid. The arachidonic acid (AA) that serves as substrate for the production of prostaglandins and other metabolites must first be released from membrane phospholipids. Mammalian cells contain a series of phospholipid cleaving enzymes including phospholipase A_2, which has been considered to be the means of releasing arachidonate from phospholipids. The liberation of arachidonate from phospholipid is thought to be the rate-limiting step in prostaglandin synthesis. Agents that cause increases in prostaglandin production probably act by stimulating arachidonic acid release from phospholipid. Work done in our laboratory has shown that when lymphocytes whose phospholipids contain radiolabeled arachidonate are incubated with PHA or Con A, they release the radiolabeled arachidonate. The release of arachidonate begins within 60 to 120 seconds; PGE_1 produces an almost immediate inhibition of this response [143], as do other cAMP raising agents, in accord with the known inhibitory effects of increases in intracellular cAMP in other systems.

After being released from phospholipid, arachidonate can be metabolized by two different pathways: lipoxygenase and cyclooxygenase. The lipoxygenase pathway leads to the formation of hydroxylated fatty acids. The cyclooxygenase pathway leads to formation of prostacyclin, thromboxanes, and prostaglandins. In the cyclooxygenase pathway there are two short-lived but biologically very active endoperoxide intermediates, PGG_2 and PGH_2. Different cell types produce different products through the cyclooxygenase pathway (Fig. 1). Most of the work on arachidonic acid metabolism in lymphocytes has been confined to prostaglandins, but it is possible, even likely, that other intermediates or end products are of greater physiologic importance.

Attempts to determine the AA metabolites produced by lymphocytes have been confounded by the relatively low AA metabolizing activity of these cells in comparison with potential cellular contaminants such as platelets, neutrophils, and monocytes. Although contaminating cells may be largely removed, small numbers usually remain. Moreover, since the purification procedures that have to be employed considerably diminish overall lymphocyte yields, subpopulations of lymphocytes may be semiselectively depleted and the cells themselves may be sufficiently damaged to impair their response. Moreover, it is important to keep in mind that the nonlymphocytic cells themselves frequently make nonspecific contributions to the mitogenic response. Given these limitations, it appears that purified human lymphocytes (predominantly T-cells) probably make small amounts of 5-hydroxy-6,8,11,14-eicosatetraenoic acid (5-HETE) [144], a lipoxygenase product originally reported in neutrophils [13], and 12-hydroxy-5,8,10,14-eicosatetraenoic acid (12-HETE), a prominent product of AA metabolism in platelets [63]. Since the identification of these products was based only on their behavior in a number of thin-layer chromatography systems, further substantiation is needed. 12-HETE formation with mass spectroscopic identification has been reported in spleen cells, but whether splenic lymphocytes or some other cell type was the source is unknown [62].

As already indicated, work on AA metabolism in lymphocytes is plagued by the difficulty of obtaining pure cell populations. It is clear from the work of Ferraris and De Rubertis [34] and Gordon et al. [55]

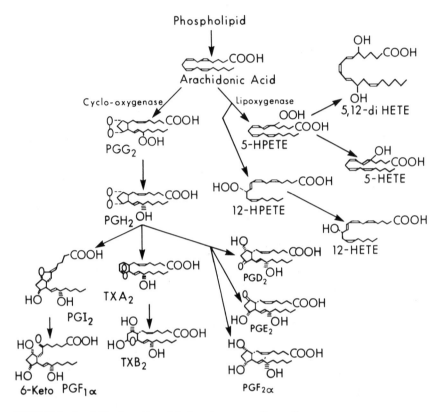

FIGURE 1. Arachidonic acid metabolism in mammalian cells.

that in cell populations containing both lymphocytes and macrophages, all or almost all of the prostaglandins produced are macrophage products (see "Prostaglandins and Macrophages," below). There is some evidence, however, that lymphocytes may also produce prostaglandins and other cyclooxygenase products. Lymphocytes have been reported to metabolize arachidonate both to PGE$_2$ and PGF$_{2\alpha}$ [126,148,154] through prostaglandin synthetase, and to thromboxane A$_2$ and its metabolite thromboxane B$_2$ through thromboxane synthetase [62,144]. Morley et al. reported that unstimulated human thoracic duct [109] lymphocytes make thromboxane B$_2$ and small amounts of PGE$_2$, but no detectable PGF$_2$. Bauminger reported prostaglandin E production in mouse thymocytes, a population considered to be free of macrophages and monocytes. In this study mature thymocytes (mature T-lymphocytes) were found to produce more PGE than immature thymocytes [7].

The effects of mitogen stimulation on the metabolism of both exogenous and endogenous radiolabeled arachidonate in human peripheral blood mononuclear cells were investigated in our laboratory [144]. Stimulation with PHA increases the metabolism of both exogenous and endogenous arachidonate to 5-HETE, 12-HETE, thromboxane B_2, and prostaglandins E_2 and $F_{2\alpha}$. When lymphocytes were purified by passing them over a nylon wool column (a procedure that removes monocytes and platelets in addition to B-cells), the stimulation of endogenous arachidonate metabolism by PHA was still observed, but exogenous AA metabolism was no longer increased by the lectin. Moreover, the overall level of AA metabolism was considerably below that in the original mononuclear cell population. This suggests that even with a known lymphocyte stimulant such as PHA, much of the response may be occurring in nonlymphocytic cells. It has been amply demonstrated that monocytes, neutrophils, and platelets bind and are metabolically stimulated by lectins (reviewed in Ref. 138). Alternatively, perhaps by complexing with lymphocytes in the presence of lectin, these cells may be potentiating the lymphocyte response. Since the purified lymphocytes metabolize exogenous AA at the same rate whether PHA is present or absent, whereas endogenous AA is metabolized faster, it appears that the major action of the lectin is to increase AA availability rather than to stimulate the enzymes that metabolize unesterified AA. In these studies thromboxane B_2 is a quantitatively more prominent product than the prostaglandins. This is in accord with the gas chromatographic–mass spectroscopic analysis of Morley et al. in human thoracic duct lymphocytes [109].

AA release and metabolism can be induced by specific antigen as well as by lectin. Webb and Osheroff have examined prostaglandin production in primed and unprimed mice [125,205]. Within 2 minutes following the intravenous injection of sheep red blood cells into mice there was a 20- to 80-fold increase in $PGF_{2\alpha}$ levels in the spleen, with smaller increases in PGE_2. This response is not made in nude mice (athymic) or in NZB mice (functionally deficient T-cells), suggesting that this is a T-cell-dependent process, but a number of other interpretations are possible. The elevation in $PGF_{2\alpha}$ concentrations does not occur in mice given indomethacin or Ro 20-5720, both of which markedly diminish prostaglandin synthesis at low concentrations. These agents can therefore be used to evaluate the role of the burst in prostaglandin synthesis in later immunologic events (for further discussion, see below). For example, these inhibitors of prostaglandin synthesis enhance the number of plaque-forming (antibody-producing) cells induced over several days in response to sheep red blood cells. This all suggests that prostaglandins may play a negative feedback role in proliferative responses of B-cells and ultimately in the control of antibody production.

Osherhoff and Webb have also studied the response of primed mice to hapten-substituted proteins [125]. Again they found large increases in splenic $PGF_{2\alpha}$ that were dependent on the number and chemical structure of the protein-bound hapten groups but independent of carrier protein. Unprimed mice that were passively immunized with dinitrophenyl–bovine γ-globulin (DNP-BGG) hyperimmune serum and then challenged with DNP-BGG also had a large rise in $PGE_{2\alpha}$, suggesting that it is the antigen-antibody interaction that induces the prostaglandin production. Recent work by Passwell et al. [146] showing prostaglandin production by macrophages incubated with aggregated immunoglobulin G may give some insight into this area. It is possible that the large rise in splenic prostaglandin production found by Webb and Osheroff is arising from splenic macrophages. Regardless of the cell source, some form of amplification mechanism appears to be needed to explain the magnitude of the response. One major source may be mast cells pre-sensitized with antibody. Rapid release of histamine and other mast cell products may affect prostaglandin synthesis when antigen is infused [150]. In accord with this possibility, appropriate antihistamines considerably inhibit the increase in prostaglandin formation. Histamine release also appears to be important in the burst of prostaglandin synthesis in lung fragments following anaphylactic stimulation [150].

Changes in prostaglandin formation in the later stages of lymphocyte responses have been less well studied. Ferraris and De Rubertis [34] reported severalfold increases in PGE synthesis 48 hours after initiation of lectin stimulation. However, as discussed in more detail below, the cell source of the prostaglandins was not identified, and after filtration of the cells through nylon wool to remove monocytes and neutrophils, little or no response was observed.

EFFECTS OF ARACHIDONIC ACID ON LYMPHOCYTE ACTIVATION

Effect of High Dose Exogenous Arachidonate. The possibility of modulatory effects of free fatty acids, especially arachidonate, on lymphocyte responses to lectins and antigen has been studied in a number of laboratories including our own. The addition of high dose (30–100 μM) arachidonate inhibits lectin-induced mitogenesis [104,105] and myoinositol incorporation [119]. The inhibition is nonselective and has been seen with a number of long chain fatty acids in addition to arachidonate. Meade and Mertin [101] found that mice treated with high doses of subcutaneous unsaturated fatty acids had an impaired immune response, as manifested by delayed rejection of skin allografts and reduced cell-mediated cytotoxicity. The physiologic significance of inhibition of mitogenesis by high doses of fatty acid is not clear. The doses used are many times the normal plasma concentrations of free arachidonate—the normal plasma concentration of arachidonate is 8–13 μM and almost all that amount is protein bound [61].

Effect of Low Dose Exogenous Arachidonate. Using much lower concentrations of AA (0.3–3 μM), we have seen substantial stimulation of mitogen-induced DNA synthesis [83]. The addition of low doses of AA to cells cultured in lipid-free or lipid-poor medium resulted in two- to fourfold increases in thymidine uptake in response to Con A or PHA. Linoleic and linolenic acids were less effective than arachidonate in stimulating thymidine uptake; oleic and arachidic acids were largely or completely inactive. Low dose exogenous AA also promoted blast transformation and the increased number of viable lymphocytes present after several days in culture, indicating that the effect is not on thymidine uptake or pool size alone. It is known that at least part of the stimulatory effects of low dose exogenous arachidonate occur early because if addition is delayed for 24 hours after the mitogen, there is considerable diminution in the response. Effects are observed in ordinary serum-containing media as well as media with lipid-poor proteins or no protein at all. These observations indicate that AA is needed for optimal lymphocyte responses to lectin but do not distinguish between effects on cell viability or a more direct role in the stimulatory process per se. Nor do they indicate whether the effect involves AA metabolites, free AA, or AA esterified in phospholipids or triglycerides. Low dose (8 μM) exogenous arachidonate has also been shown to stimulate chemokinesis in human T-lymphocytes [98]. This effect is apparently dependent on metabolism of the arachidonate, as demonstrated by inhibition of arachidonate-induced chemokinesis by indomethacin.

EFFECTS OF INHIBITORS OF ARACHIDONIC ACID METABOLISM ON LYMPHOCYTE ACTIVATION

One way to evaluate the role of AA and its metabolites in lymphocyte activation is to inhibit arachidonate metabolism at various points and observe the effects of lymphocyte activation. No studies to date have used inhibitors to block arachidonate release from lymphocyte phospholipid, even though this step is central to the control of prostaglandin production. On the other hand, a number of reports have evaluated the effects of aspirin and indomethacin, which are cyclooxygenase inhibitors. The results of these studies have been conflicting, ranging from marked inhibition [27,121,128,129], to no inhibition [174], to enhancement [53,127].

A number of groups, including our own, have reported inhibition of mitogenesis. In vitro studies by Panush and Anthony showed almost complete inhibition of thymidine incorporation by aspirin [129]. Human volunteers taking therapeutic doses of aspirin had a 60% diminution in lymphocyte reactivity. On the other hand, other groups found little inhibition by aspirin or indomethacin. Some of the differences in these studies may be explained by variations in the amount of protein in the incubation media. This affects not only the availability of the inhibitor but also the supply of arachidonate, which is the enzyme substrate. Despite the variation in results, the preponderance of the evidence suggests some inhibition of mitogenesis by the cyclooxygenase inhibitors aspirin and indomethacin. The concentrations of the inhibitors required for substantial effects on DNA synthesis are: aspirin, 330 μM [84] and indomethacin, 140 μM [128].

It is difficult to reconcile the inhibitory effects of indomethacin and aspirin on mitogenesis with the well-established inhibition of mitogenesis by prostaglandin unless it is assumed that aspirin and indomethacin also block the synthesis of stimulatory arachidonate products.

To investigate this possibility, we examined the effects of a variety of inhibitors of arachidonate metabolism on lectin-induced thymidine incorporation [84]. As mentioned earlier, problems with cell contamination create problems in interpretation, but human lymphocytes appear to convert arachidonate into PGE_2, $PGF_{2\alpha}$, and thromboxane A_2, all products of the cyclooxygenase pathway, plus 5-HETE and perhaps 12-HETE, products of the lipoxygenase pathway [144]. Whether these products are made by each of the lymphocyte subpopulations present remains to be established. Although it is well known that prostaglandins inhibit lymphocyte responses to mitogens, the role of the other arachidonate metabolites has not been investigated. Selective or partially selective inhibitors of thromboxane synthetase such as imidazole, benzylimidazole, N-0164, and L-8007 inhibited the mitogenic response.

To establish that these agents were indeed affecting thromboxane synthesis in our cell preparations, the cells were incubated with [^{14}C]AA in the presence and absence of inhibitors and lectin. Pretreatment of the cells with inhibitors of arachidonate metabolism yielded the expected results. Indomethacin, ETYA, and aspirin all inhibited the production of cyclooxygenase products at low concentrations, whereas the putative thromboxane inhibitors selectively inhibited thromboxane synthesis. As expected, since indomethacin and aspirin act by inhibiting cyclooxygenase, both prostaglandin and thromboxane production were diminished. However, indomethacin had approximately 30-fold greater inhibitory potency for prostaglandin synthesis as opposed to thromboxane synthesis, presumably because of a difference in K_m for the enzymes, which convert the endoperoxides to prostaglandins and thromboxanes through their respective pathways. At concentrations of indomethacin that inhibit prostaglandin but not thromboxane production, there was no effect on mitogen-induced thymidine incorporation. However, when enough indomethacin was given to inhibit thromboxane production, thymidine incorporation was markedly inhibited. It is axiomatic that no inhibitor can be assumed to be exerting its effects solely on the pathway of interest to the investigator. For example, indomethacin has been reported to affect cAMP metabolism, lysophospholipid acylation, and even phospholipase activity. Nonetheless the ability of several inhibitors of thromboxane biosynthesis to inhibit mitogenesis in a concentration range where thromboxane biosynthesis is inhibited suggests a role for thromboxanes in the response.

Because there are no truly selective inhibitors of the lipoxygenase pathway available, it is difficult to determine the effects of the products of this pathway on mitogenesis. However, eicosatetraynoic and nordihydroguaiaretic acids, both of which inhibit cyclooxygenase and lipoxygenase, inhibit mitogenesis at concentrations that exert little or no effect on thromboxane synthesis, suggesting that lipoxygenase products may also stimulate mitogenesis. Thus, in addition to the inhibitory effects of prostaglandins, other products of arachidonate metabolism, thromboxane A_2, and perhaps hydroperoxy- or hydroxyeicosatetraenoic acids may have a stimulatory action. However, to establish such a role conclusively, we need more selective antagonists, as well as reasonably stable agonists that can be added exogenously to cells and can be shown to stimulate a response. It is also necessary to study early activation events in lectin-stimulated cells to get a better idea of the mechanism. In this regard recent studies in our laboratory by Mark Udey indicate that thromboxane synthetase and cyclooxygenase inhibitors inhibit the lectin-stimulated transport of the nonmetabolizable amino acid aminoisobutyric acid within the first several hours of the response, indicating that the inhibition is exerted very early in the response. Unfortunately, apart from their effects on platelet aggregation and smooth muscle contraction, little is known about the action of thromboxanes on cell metabolism, and elucidation of the biochemical mechanism may be difficult.

Effects of Prostaglandins on the Immune Response

DIFFERENTIATION

Although most of the effects on the immune response of agents that elevate cAMP levels are inhibitory, these agents have a stimulatory effect on differentiation. During the process of differentiation lymphocytes (both B and T) pass through discrete phases that are recognized by the selective expression of cell surface markers. Murine T-cells acquire the surface marker Thy-1, while an early step in B-cell maturation is the appearance of complement receptors. Exogenous cAMP and agents that increase cAMP levels, including PGE_1, induce the development of early maturation antigens in both T- and B-cells [167,168]. The stimulatory effect of cAMP on antigen-induced antibody production when cAMP is added very early may be explained by cAMP-induced B-cell differentiation [86].

Exogenous PGE_2 (10^{-5} M) raises cAMP to comparable levels in mouse spleen and thymus cell populations [201]. Studies of separated splenic lymphocyte subpopulations show that both B- and T-cells respond to exogenous prostaglandins. Thymocytes from animals treated with cortisone to eliminate the less mature thymocytes have a markedly decreased response to prostaglandins. The cortisone-resistant cells have many properties of more mature cells, including ability to respond to PHA and to serve as helper cells in the development of the antibody response. They also have relatively high cAMP levels. Because substances that induce the appearance of maturation antigens on thymocytes (prostaglandin, histamine, and theophylline [167]) increase cAMP levels, it has been suggested that the mature, cortisone-resistant, thymocytes have an adenylate cyclase that is already maximally stimulated and cannot be stimulated further.

Having described some of the general features of prostaglandin action and metabolism in lymphocytes, we now consider their effects in individual lymphocyte subpopulations in more detail.

T-CELLS

Mitogenesis. It has been well established that exogenous prostaglandins block lymphocyte activation by T-cell mitogens such as PHA and Con A apparently by raising intracellular cAMP concentrations [50, 118,172,173]. Mediation by cAMP is likely because isoproterenol and theophylline, which also raise cAMP levels, also inhibit the lymphocyte response to mitogen. Prostaglandins have been shown to inhibit the growth of malignant cells [116] and to enhance the differentiation of tumor cells in culture [152], presumably by the same mechanism. A number of studies in PHA-stimulated human lymphocytes have shown inhibition of [^{3}H]thymidine uptake by PGE_1, but the lowest doses of PGE_1 capable of producing inhibition have varied considerably. The lowest concentration has varied from approximately 1×10^{-4} M [118,173] to as low as 3×10^{-8} M [50]. The lower limit of the inhibitory range of PGE_1 is of interest in attempting to define a role for prostaglandins as intracellular modulators of lymphocyte activation. If an argument is to be made for a role for PGE as an intracellular mediator, it is important to show that lymphocyte activity can be altered by physiologic PGE concentrations. It is probably the local concentration of prostaglandin in the lymphoid tissue that is relevant to the control of lymphoid function. Ferraris and De Rubertis found that lymphocytes stimulated with PHA produced 1×10^{-8} M PGE_2 [34]. Although it might be argued that this is a minimal value because of the nonphysiological nature of in vitro cell cultures, it is important to keep in mind that such cultures are a closed system and that prostaglandins synthesized in vivo are rapidly removed by diffusion and catabolism.

Detailed examination of the results of Goodwin and his colleagues [50,52], who see inhibition of mitogenesis at low concentrations (3×10^{-8} M) of exogenous PGE_1 or PGE_2, suggests an explanation for the differing sensitivities to prostaglandin observed in various laboratories. A high degree of sensitivity to inhibition by prostaglandin is seen only at suboptimal concentrations of lectin on cell preparations that have been partially enriched with respect to T-cells [52]. It may be that the increased sensitivity to inhibition by prostaglandin is due to monocyte depletion rather than to T-cell enrichment. One possible explanation is that since monocytes synthesize considerable amounts of prostaglandin, when they are present, small amounts of added exogenous prostaglandin exert little or no additional effect.

Novogrodsky and colleagues have largely confirmed the observation of Goodwin et al. that prostaglandin effects are more marked in partially purified T-cells [118] and have expanded it by looking at different lectins. They demonstrated that the blastogenic response of lymphocytes to lectins that bind to galactosyl residues (peanut agglutinin, soybean agglutinin) was markedly enhanced by depletion of cells that adhere to Sephadex G-10 (monocytes stick to Sephadex G-10), whereas the response to lectins that do not bind to galactosyl residues (PHA, Con A) was not changed. The cells that adhere to Sephadex G-10 accounted for almost all the endogenous prostaglandin production. The addition of very low concentrations of PGE_1 (3×10^{-9} M) to lymphocytes depleted of adherent cells markedly inhibited their response to galactosyl binding lectins, but much higher concentrations of PGE_1 (3×10^{-5} M) are required to inhibit the response of unfractionated cells to non-galactosyl binding lectins. Inhibition similar to that seen with PGE_1 was achieved with other agents that raise cAMP levels, including methyl isobutyl xanthine.

There is strong evidence that different mitogens stimulate different subpopulations of lymphocytes. In vitro responsiveness to PHA is a property of T-cells; lymphocytes from animals without T-cells do not respond to PHA. B-cells, however, respond to pokeweed mitogen (PWM), and both T- and B-cells respond to Con A. Stockman and Mumford [182] looked at the effects of PGE_2 on mitogenesis induced by these three lectins in human peripheral blood lymphocytes. They found that PGE_2 (1×10^{-5} to 1×10^{-7} M) inhibited mitogenesis stimulated by PHA and Con A but had no effect on PWM-induced mitogenesis. This supports that the prime effect of prostaglandins is on T-cells.

Lymphocyte activation can be measured by changes in assays other than thymidine incorporation. Offner and Clausen have studied activation by measuring the incorporation of tritiated inositol into phosphatidylinositol. They showed that PGE_1 and PGE_2 inhibit PHA and PPD-tuberculin induced inositol incorporation [119].

Prostaglandins and Suppressor Cells. There is considerable evidence that the mitogenic response of T-cells to lectins can be modulated by soluble mediators produced by other cells in the immune system. Cells producing soluble mediators that inhibit the mitogenic response are termed suppressor cells. A number of laboratories have identified populations of glass adherent cells that suppress lymphocyte response. Goodwin has shown that glass adherent mononuclear cells from human peripheral blood suppress T-cell mitogenic activity through production of prostaglandins of the E series. The prostaglandins were apparently produced by a subset of mononuclear cells that could be depleted by adherence to glass wool or by T-cell enrichment achieved by passage over beads coated with antihuman IgG-IgG. These glass wool adherent suppressor cells could be monocytes, B-cells, or glass adherent T-cells. The addition of indomethacin (3–30 µM) to unfractionated cells gave a 70% increase in the blastogenic response to PHA. When the cell preparation was depleted of glass wool adherent cells, there was no stimulation of blastogenesis by indomethacin. This was taken to indicate the existence of a population of glass wool adherent cells that suppress mitogenesis by producing prostaglandins. It is possible, however, that the suppressor substance is some other arachidonate metabolite whose synthesis is also blocked by indomethacin.

Patients with Hodgkin's disease are known to have depressed cellular immunity manifested by skin test anergy and impaired response in vitro to such T-cell mitogens as PHA. Goodwin and co-workers studied PHA-induced mitogenesis in normal individuals and in patients with Hodg-kin's disease [51]. When normal lymphocytes are treated with indo-methacin there is a 40% increase in the mitogenic response to PHA, whereas in Hodgkin's disease the increase is 100 to 280%. Goodwin et al. also demonstrated increased levels of prostaglandin production in Hodgkin's disease mononuclear cell cultures. The increase can be elim-inated by depleting the culture of glass adherent cells. All this suggests that the defect in cellular immunity in Hodgkin's disease is due to a population of glass adherent prostaglandin-producing suppressor cells.

In contrast to Goodwin, who suggested that prostaglandins might be directly responsible for suppressor effects, Webb has identified a sup-pressor cell that was activated by exogenous prostaglandin to make a protein suppressor substance. Webb's suppressor cells were a glass ad-herent fraction of mouse spleen cells that were phenotypically Thy-1 and Ly-1$^+$2$^+$3$^+$ [202,204]. This is characteristic of relatively undifferen-tiated T-cells. The protein suppressor was found to be heat stable with a molecular weight of 38,000. Suppressor activity was also present in a small polypeptide, which may be a fragment of the larger molecule. The suppressor has been termed PITS (prostaglandin-induced T-cell sup-pressor). The same investigators have shown that both glass wool ad-herent and nonadherent cells make prostaglandins in response to PHA. They have suggested a mechanism of feedback inhibition in which lym-phocyte-synthesized prostaglandin regulates the activity of a suppressor cell population, which responds to this prostaglandin stimulus by se-creting a soluble suppressor substance. Thus both direct and indirect effects of prostaglandins may result in suppression.

Lymphokine Production. Lymphokines, a diverse group of soluble mediators involved in the regulation of immune and inflammatory re-sponses, are released in response to antigens and other stimuli. They have a broad range of biological actions, one of which is the capacity to induce DNA synthesis in nonsensitized lymphocytes. This provides an amplification system or positive feedback in the delayed hypersensitivity reaction. The operation of such an amplification system demands the existence of a negative feedback system to limit the response. The work of Gordon, Bray, and Morley suggests that prostaglandins produced by macrophages may play an essential role in the negative regulation of macrophage migration inhibition factor (MIF) production by guinea pig lymphocytes [55]. Added PGE$_1$ (0.3–3.0 μM) inhibited lymphokine pro-duction by antigen stimulated sensitized guinea pig lymphocytes but did not affect the action of preformed MIF on macrophage migration. On the other hand, indomethacin, a cyclooxygenase inhibitor, enhanced antigen-induced lymphokine production without affecting the action of preformed lymphokine. Since MIF is thought to be an important me-diator of the delayed hypersensitivity reaction, these observations sug-gest an important role of prostaglandins in the control of this response. Lomnitzer et al. found very similar results regarding effects of PGE$_1$ and PGE$_2$ in the production of another lymphokine, leukocyte inhibitory factor (LIF) by PHA-stimulated human lymphocytes [96].

Lymphocyte-Mediated Cytotoxicity. The ability of sensitized cytotoxic T-lymphocytes to destroy target cells is subject to regulation by cAMP and possibly cGMP. Agents that raise intracellular cAMP, including prostaglandins and dibutyryl cAMP, inhibit the lysis of target cells by sensitized killer cells. In a mouse mastocytoma allogeneic system the E prostaglandins were the most efficient inhibitors of cytolysis as well as the most effective cAMP agonists [67,95].

Because of the ability of prostaglandins to inhibit lymphocyte-mediated cytolysis, their ability to affect allograft survival in vivo has been evaluated. Strom et al. used synthetically prepared prostaglandin derivatives with long biologic half-lives to study lymphocyte-mediated cytotoxicity in vitro and also the survival of renal allografts in vivo [184]. They found that the prostaglandin analogues inhibited cytolysis and prolonged graft survival in rat renal allograft recipients. Quagliata et al. studied the effect of E-type prostaglandins on mouse skin allograft survival [153]. Exogenous prostaglandins when used alone had no effect on graft survival, but prostaglandins did prolong graft survival in mice also treated with procarbazine, a powerful T-cell depressant. However, they found that the number of B-cells, but not T-cells, was decreased in the spleens of mice treated with PGE_1 and concluded that the primary inhibitory effect of PGE_1 was on B-cells. Although there is much to be learned about the role of endogenous prostaglandins in graft survival, there is evidence that prostaglandin metabolism may be markedly affected in animals undergoing chronic allograft reactions. Anderson et al. measured serum PGE levels in dogs after skin transplant and found that serum PGE rose tenfold over baseline by 2 months. However, no conclusions were drawn as to the relationship of the PGE level to transplant inflammation and survival [1]. Loose and DiLuzio have examined the effects of PGE_1 on the graft versus host reaction. Mice of one strain, C3H/fMai, were treated with intravenous PGE_1. Their spleen cells were isolated and injected into mice of another strain, C57BL/6fMai. After 8 days the spleens of the recipient mice were weighed. The spleens of the mice that had received cells from PGE_1-treated animals were heavier, suggesting enhancement of the graft-host response by prostaglandins [97].

B-CELLS

There is considerable evidence that exogenous prostaglandins inhibit B-cell function either directly or through actions on other cells. Several studies have demonstrated inhibition by prostaglandins of formation of plaque-producing cells by mouse spleen lymphocytes [103,203,214]. In the plaque-forming assay, sensitized lymphocytes are incubated in medium with complement and indicator red cells containing the antigen. Red cells in the immediate vicinity of antibody-producing cells are lysed, resulting in the formation of a plaque. This permits the number of antibody-producing cells to be determined directly. Melmon et al. found that agents that raise cAMP levels in lymphocytes (histamine, β-adrenergic agents, and PGE_2) inhibit the induction of plaque-forming cells.

The prostaglandin concentrations that were found to be effective were 1×10^{-6} to 1×10^{-4} M [103]. Webb and Nowowiejski [203] showed that exogenous PGE_2 reduces the number of plaque-forming cells in vitro if it is added at the beginning of the culture or just a few hours before the end of the culture. The late inhibition suggests a direct action on B-cells, whereas the early effect of prostaglandins is consistent with inhibition of the inductive phase either on helper T-cells or B-cell responsiveness to helper cells. To support these conclusions, they showed that the addition of prostaglandin synthetase inhibitors stimulated plaque formation whether added early or late in the culture.

The mechanism of the inhibition of the formation of plaque-forming cells by the early addition of prostaglandins can be evaluated by studying the response to T-independent antigens, which are less dependent on helper T-cells for induction. Again using plaque formation as an assay, Zimecki and Webb observed that early additions of exogenous PGE_1 (1×10^{-5} M) inhibited the response to the T-independent antigen, polyvinyl pyrolidone [214]. As expected, prostaglandin synthetase inhibitors increased the response to T-independent antigens. They concluded that prostaglandins act directly on antigen-stimulated B-cells.

Other authors, using different experimental systems, have also demonstrated a primary effect of exogenous prostaglandins on B-cells. In addition to the study of Quagliata et al. [153] on mouse skin allograft survival discussed above, Zurier and Quagliata showed a small decrease in antibody titer to sheep red blood cells in mice treated with PGE_1 [216].

Plescia et al. found that mice bearing syngeneic tumors became immunologically unresponsive as determined by measuring antibody response to sheep red blood cells [151] and concluded that prostaglandins were playing a major role in the suppression. They cultured tumor cells with normal spleen cells in vitro at a 1:1000 ratio in the presence of sheep red blood cells and assayed for the induction of plaque-forming cells. They found that even this small number of tumor cells could inhibit the response and that PGE_2 exerted a similar effect. Indomethacin and aspirin reversed the immunosuppression in vitro and retarded tumor growth in vivo, presumably because immune resistance was enhanced.

In contrast to the mass of evidence that exogenous prostaglandins inhibit B-cell function, there are two reports of enhancement of humoral immune responses by prostaglandins. Loose and DiLuzio [97] noted an increased secondary hemagglutination response to red blood cells in PGE_1-treated mice. This suggests that PGE either enhances B-cell or T-helper cell response or depresses suppressor cells. Bach and Bach [4] found that when thymectomized mice are treated with agents that elevate cAMP (PGE_1, PGE_2, dibutyryl cAMP, isoproterenol, and theophylline), their low spleen rosette-forming sensitivity to azathioprine and anti-θ serum is corrected.

An important consideration in interpreting all work on the effects of exogenous prostaglandins is suggested by the study of Berenbaum et al. [8]. Using a sensitive assay of cell viability, the ability to take up and hydrolyze fluorescein diacetate, they found that some agents, including isoprenaline, inhibit plaque formation in parallel with their cytotoxic effect on lymphocytes. Although these changes may be mediated by cAMP, alternative explanations must be considered. In addition, it is important to keep in mind that pulsing a cell preparation with a cAMP agonist may produce very different results from continuous exposure. As already discussed, brief exposures to cAMP agonists may enhance rather than inhibit B-cell proliferation. It is important to remember that prostaglandins secreted in vivo are quickly removed and metabolized. Thus, in vitro experiments in which secreted prostaglandins accumulate in the media over a period of hours do not reflect in vivo conditions. The inhibitory effects of prostaglandins seen in these circumstances need to be interpreted cautiously.

Prostaglandins and Macrophages

ROLE OF MACROPHAGES AND MONOCYTES

There is much evidence that macrophages are derived from peripheral blood monocytes that have undergone further differentiation in tissue. Monocytes cultured in vitro for 3 days acquire many of the characteristics of macrophages [146]. Macrophages have a dual function. They have an important role in what is termed "antigen processing." For many antigens, lymphocyte recognition of and response to antigen are not initiated unless the antigen is presented by the macrophage. This enhancing effect of macrophages on responses to antigen appears to require the participation of certain major histocompatibility antigens, indicating that a specific recognition process is involved. Lymphocytes in turn may regulate macrophage function by the production of soluble mediators, largely proteins, termed lymphokines. The best studied of the lymphokines is MIF, which inhibits macrophage motility. Release of MIF in response to antigen is presumed to be the major explanation for the large number of monocytes and macrophages that accumulate in cellular immune responses. Macrophages have a second function as phagocytic cells not unlike neutrophils. Macrophages are capable of ingesting particles including bacteria and zymosan granules; they are also capable of responding to soluble stimuli including immunoglobulins and C3b. Like neutrophils, they have specific receptors that recognize these reactants.

Arachidonic acid metabolism appears to play an important role both in macrophage-lymphocyte interactions and in the macrophage's role as a phagocytic cell [180]. A critical role for prostaglandin in the inflammatory process is suggested by the fact that the tissue concentration of prostaglandins correlates well with the intensity of the local inflammatory response. Moreover, inhibitors of prostaglandin synthesis markedly decrease inflammation [36,69,196]. As active producers of prostaglandin and prominent participants in cellular immune responses, macrophages are almost certainly a major source of these inflammatory mediators.

As with lymphocytes, there are two major problems associated with the study of AA metabolism in macrophages—cell contamination and subtype heterogeneity. Very few studies have been carried out with pure macrophage populations. Peritoneal exudates, a frequently utilized macrophage source, include neutrophils, lymphocytes, platelets, peritoneal epithelial cells, and mast cells, in addition to macrophages. Preparations of peripheral blood monocytes contain contaminating platelets and lymphocytes. Even seemingly trivial levels of contamination with other cell types, especially those that avidly take up and metabolize arachidonate, can lead to the production of substantial quantities of arachidonate metabolites by nonmacrophages. Contamination with platelets is a particular problem because platelets are difficult to count in a mixed-cell preparation and because they metabolize arachidonate effectively.

The biochemical and functional properties of macrophage populations are influenced by the method of harvesting and the treatment of the donor animal prior to harvesting. Normal ("resident") peritoneal macrophages obtained by simple lavage are different from "elicited" peritoneal macrophages induced by irritants (thioglycollate, caseinate, etc.) [26]. These in turn are different from "activated" macrophages obtained by peritoneal lavage of animals infected with BCG, Listeria monocytogenes, or other appropriate organisms [26]. The lessened prostaglandin production seen in elicited as compared to resident macrophages [75] may be caused by activation of macrophage arachidonate metabolism in vivo during the production of the "elicited" exudate. Thus, elicited macrophages may have passed through a cycle of phospholipase activation and prostaglandin production in vivo, being in a refractory state when harvested. Consistent with this notion is the observation that PGE_2 activates adenylate cyclase, resulting in increased cyclic AMP levels, which in turn may inhibit phospholipase activity [106]. Phospholipase inhibition could leave the cell refractory to further stimulation.

A macrophage population can also be heterogeneous with regard to degree of differentiation and to physical and functional variations among the cells of the macrophage population itself [74]. Goldyne and Stobo fractionated a population of human peripheral blood monocytes by discontinuous gradient centrifugation [49]. They found significant differences among these monocyte subpopulations in their synthesis of PGE_1 and PGE_2. There was no simple correlation between the synthesis of prostaglandin by a subpopulation and its degree of differentiation. Differences among macrophage subpopulations with respect to synthesis of other arachidonate products are likely but have not yet been established.

Macrophages have been reported to metabolize arachidonate to PGE_2 [19,146] and $PGF_{2\alpha}$ [208]. It has also been reported that mouse peritoneal and bone marrow macrophages make thromboxane B_2 [17]. Rigaud et al. reported the production of the lipoxygenase product, 12-HETE, by mouse peritoneal macrophages [160]. Using gas–liquid chromatography–mass spectroscopy techniques, Morley et al. determined PGE_2 and thromboxane B_2 (TXB_2) production by in human peripheral blood monocytes, human alveolar macrophages, and guinea pig peritoneal macrophages [109]. Although both PGE_2 and TXB_2 were present in all the macrophage preparations, TXB_2 was always the predominant product [109,112]. On a per cell basis the highest levels of these substances were produced by alveolar macrophages. No PGD_2, $PGF_{2\alpha}$, or 6-keto-$PGF_{1\alpha}$ was detected.

CONTROL OF PROSTAGLANDIN PRODUCTION IN MACROPHAGES

When cell cultures containing macrophages and lymphocytes are exposed to antigen or lectin, prostaglandins are released into the medium [29]. Ferraris and De Rubertis found increased prostaglandin production in antigen- and lectin-stimulated mouse spleen cell cultures and also in lectin-stimulated unpurified human peripheral leukocytes [34]. When the human peripheral leukocytes were depleted of glass adherent cells, stimulation of prostaglandin production by lectin was no longer seen, even though [^{3}H]thymidine incorporation was still stimulated. Thus a leukocyte population depleted of macrophages by glass bead adherence does not produce prostaglandins in response to lectin. The work of Gordon et al. has helped explain the mechanism of lectin- or antigen-induced prostaglandin synthesis [16,55]. These authors have shown that lymphokines produced by incubating sensitized lymph node lymphocytes with antigen are capable of inducing prostaglandin production in macrophages. The level of prostaglandin production induced in macrophages by lymphokine is similar to that in mixed leukocyte populations stimulated by antigen. In view of the known inhibitory effects of prostaglandins on the immune response, the investigators (Gordon, Bray, and Morley) have suggested that lymphokine-induced prostaglandin synthesis by macrophages may be an important mechanism for control of the immune response.

Macrophages produce prostaglandins in response to a number of phagocytic and soluble stimuli in addition to lymphokines. Prostaglandin formation can be stimulated by zymosan [38,40,208], *Corynebacterium parvum* [59], colchicine [41], antigen-antibody complexes [10], endotoxin [88], the calcium ionophore A23187 [39], and Con A [146]. In the cases in which it was studied, indomethacin inhibited PGE_2 production [18]. The induction of PGE_2 synthesis by Con A may be relevant to the induction of suppressor cells by Con A and the inhibitory effect of high concentrations of Con A on lymphocyte mitogenesis.

Macrophages and monocytes have receptors for the Fc portion of IgG permitting them to bind and internalize immune complexes. Since this processing of immune complexes is a function of macrophages, and since immune complexes have been reported to suppress T-cell activation, the effects of immunoglobulins on macrophage prostaglandin metabolism are of particular interest with regard to how macrophages affect lymphocyte function. This subject has been studied extensively by Passwell et al. [146]. Addition of Fc fragments of IgG to human monocyte monolayer cultures resulted in an increase in PGE_2 release. Heat-aggregated IgG also induced prostaglandin release, whereas Fab fragments, monomeric IgG, and human serum albumin had no effect. Although the response to Fc fragments might seem surprising, these preparations are known to undergo aggregation, providing a possible mechanism for the stimulation. The quantity of prostaglandin released with Fc fragments was 10 times that for zymosan, endotoxin, or Con A. Stimulation of PGE_2 release with Fc fragments of IgG and aggregated IgG suggests that binding of a ligand to the Fc receptor may play an important role in macrophage activation even in the absence of phagocytosis.

The mechanism by which stimuli induce prostaglandin production is best demonstrated by the work of Humes et al. [75]. They labeled macrophage phospholipids with [³H]AA and stimulated the cells with phagocytic stimuli. Zymosan caused a 23-fold increase in PGE_2 production as measured by incorporation of ³H counts into a thin-layer chromatography band corresponding to PGE_2. This technique shows that stimuli act by causing the release of AA from phospholipid, with subsequent metabolism to prostaglandin. This study confirmed other reports that zymosan stimulates prostaglandin production whereas another phagocytic particle, latex, does not. It seems likely that it is not the act of phagocytosis that stimulates PG production but the nature of the interaction between the particle and the cell membrane.

EFFECTS OF PROSTAGLANDINS ON MACROPHAGES

Gemsa et al. have done extensive studies on the interrelationships between phagocytosis, PGE_1, and the production of cAMP in rat peritoneal macrophages [38]. Macrophages phagocytosing zymosan have a more marked and more prolonged cAMP response to exogenous PGE_1 than do resting macrophages. As noted earlier, ingestion of zymosan also leads to release of endogenous prostaglandin. Thus enhanced prostaglandin sensitivity and increased prostaglandin release may be important components of a sensitive feedback control mechanism that regulates activated and potentially destructive macrophages in the inflammatory response. As further evidence for a regulatory effect of prostaglandin on macrophages, Weidemann et al. have demonstrated inhibition of zymosan-induced chemiluminescence by exogenous prostaglandin E_1 and E_2 (2.8×10^{-7} to 2.8×10^{-6} M) [208]. Exogenous prostaglandins also inhibit macrophage spreading, adherence, and migration [21]. On the other hand, low doses of PGE_2 (1×10^{-8} M) have been reported to increase phagocytosis of sheep red blood cells by mouse peritoneal macrophages [156]. Exogenous prostaglandin augments endotoxin-induced collagenase production, which may increase the destruction of connective tissue associated with inflammatory lesions [197]. The numbers of Fc and Con A receptors on macrophages are increased by prostaglandins [155]. Finally, exogenously added PGE_1 and PGE_2, but not $PGF_{2\alpha}$, have been shown to inhibit the tumoricidal actions of interferon-activated macrophages. Since prostaglandins of the E series increase intracellular concentrations of cAMP in macrophages and treatment of interferon-activated macrophages with dibutyryl cAMP inhibits expression of the tumoricidal function, prostaglandin-induced inhibition is presumably exerted through cAMP [170].

Macrophage-derived prostaglandin E_2 has also been shown to have an inhibitory effect on the clonal proliferation of the committed granu-locyte-macrophage stem cell [89–91]. Myelopoiesis is stimulated by col-ony-stimulating factor (CSF). Increases in CSF beyond a critical concen-tration within the local environment of the monocyte induce the elaboration of PGE_2, a self-regulated response that seems to limit the unopposed humoral stimulation of myelopoiesis. Thus macrophage-pro-duced prostaglandins may have an inhibitory effect on proliferation of the macrophage progenitor cell as well as on lymphocyte and monocyte function.

Overview of Prostaglandins and the Immune Response

Although the effects of pharmacologic doses of exogenous prostaglan-dins on the immune system are fairly clear, it is difficult to determine precisely the physiologic role of prostaglandins in immunity. When trying to draw conclusions from the data accumulated, it is important to keep certain potential problems in mind:

1. Because of the difficulty in studying the biochemistry of a response in a small number of stimulated cells against a background of a large population of unstimulated cells, most studies have not utilized specific antigen as the stimulus. Instead, lectins have been used to stimulate a large fraction of cells. Although lectin stimulation is a good model for lymphocyte activation, it is only a model.

2. When studies are done with mixed cell populations (unfractionated peripheral leukocytes or whole spleen preparations), it is difficult to determine which cells are producing prostaglandins and which cells are modulating prostaglandin production by other cells. Standard methods of fractionation (glass adherence, nylon wool adherence) yield cell prep-arations that are frequently little better defined than unfractionated cells. Until recently a scarcity of reliable surface markers has made precise definition of cellular composition difficult when analyzing human cell preparations. Careful attention must be paid to techniques of cell sep-aration and techniques for cell identification. One must be especially critical when interpreting experiments in which a substance (e.g., PGE_2) is produced in an unfractionated population and is no longer produced when certain cell types are depleted. This may mean that the producing cell has been depleted, but it could also mean that a cell controlling the function of the producing cell has been removed or that the producing cell has been altered by the purification process.

3. The inadequacies of our knowledge of the immune system are also evident in trying to compare experiments done with cells derived from different organs. Some differences between lymphocytes derived from spleen, thymus, bone marrow, lymph node, and peripheral blood are understood, but it is likely that there are others that are not. It is not clear which of these sources provides the most valid model for antigen-

specific lymphocyte activation. Lymphocyte preparations from different organs are subject to different degrees of contamination with nonlymphoid cells. Depending on both the organ chosen and the method of purification, lymphocytes may be contaminated with polymorphonuclear leukocytes, platelets, erythrocytes, monocytes, and macrophages. The accessory role of macrophages in lymphocyte activation is well established if not well understood. There is evidence however that platelets, monocytes, erythrocytes, and polymorphonuclear leukocytes may enhance lymphocyte response to lectin [138]. The magnitude of the effect of these accessory cells depends on the lectin, its affinity for the cells in question, its concentration, and the precise culture conditions.

4. Most studies measure the production of only one product, frequently PGE_2. Usually the product to be measured has been not chosen because of its physiologic importance but because it is the easiest to measure. It is likely that AA metabolites other than the prostaglandins will be found to be as important or more important than the prostaglandins in the regulation of the immune response. It is now clear that prostaglandins are products of highly active but short-lived endoperoxide intermediates. Pharmacologic investigations carried out with prostaglandins may be studies of the effects of relatively inactive analogs of the true physiologic mediators.

The following points summarize certain basic areas of our knowledge of the relationship between prostaglandins and immunity:

1. Prostaglandins appear to act by activating adenylate cyclase and raising cAMP levels. However, although cAMP is generally thought to act by activating protein kinase with resulting increases in protein phosphorylation, no convincing increase in protein phosphorylation has been demonstrated in prostaglandin-treated lymphocytes.

2. Exogenous prostaglandins in pharmacologic doses inhibit lymphocyte function—mitogenesis, cytolysis, lymphokine production. It has not been clearly shown that this is a physiologically important control mechanism, nor is it known whether these effects are specific to prostaglandins or are shared by other AA metabolites.

3. Exogenous AA in low concentrations stimulates mitogen-induced lymphocyte activation even though exogenous prostaglandin inhibits it. Aspirin and indomethacin inhibit lectin-induced mitogenesis even though their effects on prostaglandin production would be expected to result in stimulation. The combination of these observations suggests that there is a nonprostaglandin arachidonate metabolite that stimulates mitogenesis and that the synthesis of this metabolite can be blocked by inhibiting cyclooxygenase. The inhibition of lectin-induced mitogenesis by thromboxane synthetase inhibitors suggests that the stimulatory arachidonate metabolite may be thromboxane A_2. A stimulatory role for products of the lipoxygenase pathway is also suggested.

4. Macrophages appear to be the major site of prostaglandin synthesis in the immune response. Macrophages produce prostaglandins in response to some phagocytic stimuli, as well as to lymphokines and other soluble activators. It may be that macrophage-derived prostaglandins

have a physiologically important inhibitory role in the immune response. Morley, Bray, and Gordon have proposed a model in which antigen-stimulated lymphocytes produce lymphokines, which activate macrophages. The activated macrophages in turn produce prostaglandins, which act as inhibitors of lymphocyte function (Fig. 2A) [108]. Webb and Nowowiejski, on the other hand, propose a model in which activated lymphocytes produce prostaglandins that stimulate suppressor lymphocytes to make a suppressor peptide [204]. The suppressor peptide acts as an inhibitor of the lymphocyte response (Fig. 2B). These models are not incompatible and can be combined in a third model (Fig. 2C), which accommodates both interpretations.

FIGURE 2. Models for the physiologic role of prostaglandins in immune regulation; parts A–C described in text. [Modified from Fig. 1a in Morley, J. (1974) Prostaglandins and the lymphokines in arthritis. Prostaglandins 8, 315–326. Used by permission.]

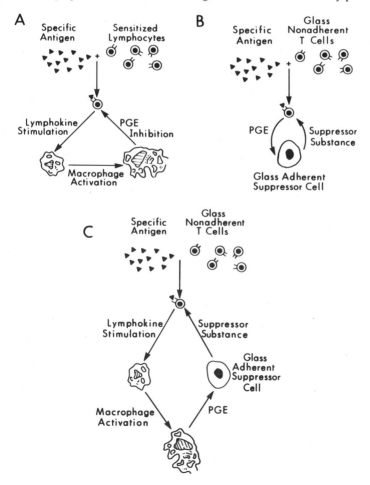

PROSTAGLANDINS AND NEUTROPHILS

Neutrophils and Prostaglandins

Prostaglandins have been implicated as mediators in inflammatory responses. They are found in increased levels in inflamed tissues [149], and their presence correlates with neutrophil infiltration [176]. There is, however, some confusion concerning the role of prostaglandins in inflammation. Prostaglandins have been shown to induce some of the properties of inflammation: vasodilation, hyperemia, pain, and leukocyte accumulation [108]. Conversely, prostaglandins have been shown to act by generating cAMP, which acts as an inhibitor of metabolic events in leukocyte activation [15,218]. A more complete review of the role of AA metabolites in inflammation can be found in the chapter by Zurier in this volume ("Prostaglandins and Inflammation"); here we review some of the work relating AA metabolism to neutrophil activation.

Neutrophils are capable of responding to particulate stimuli by phagocytosis. They can also respond to a number of soluble stimuli. Neutrophils have specific membrane receptors for certain of these soluble stimuli, including C5a and the Fc portion of IgG. Other soluble stimuli including sodium fluoride and the divalent cation ionophore A23187 [165] do not have specific receptors. The response of the neutrophil to these stimuli includes (reviewed in Refs. 24, 166, and 183):

1. Phagocytosis of particulate stimuli.
2. Degranulation with release of enzymes from specific and azurophilic granules.
3. Increased migration, including both increased random motion (chemokinesis) and motion in the direction of increased stimulus concentration (chemotaxis).
4. Activation of the respiratory burst with increased oxygen consumption, formation of superoxide, hydroxyl radicals, and other highly reactive molecules, and increased activity of the hexose monophosphate shunt.
5. Aggregation.

Most of these responses occur very rapidly in neutrophils. They also occur in macrophages; although the tempo of the response is considerably slower. Different stimuli show considerable selectivity for different portions of the neutrophil response. Most of the stimuli appear to activate by interacting with the neutrophil plasma membrane, some through a specific receptor and some not. It seems reasonable to assume that the neutrophil responses are directed by intracellular mediators that transduce stimulus-membrane interactions into cell function. Many of the stimuli that induce neutrophil activation also activate AA metabolism. AA metabolites may be intracellular mediators of neutrophil activation [12,47,99,178,181].

Arachidonic Acid Metabolism in Neutrophils

In neutrophils as in other cell types, there is essentially no intracellular pool of free AA. Arachidonate is stored esterified into phospholipids and triglycerides and can be released in response to stimuli by cleavage of the ester linkage [72]. The usual pathway for the release of arachidonate from phospholipids has been thought to be by activation of phospholipase A_2. Work in our laboratory has shown that at least in response to A23187, the AA released and metabolized comes from the phospholipid pool, not from triglycerides [178]. Arachidonate is also released from neutrophil phospholipids in response to phagocytosis of opsonized zymosan [198] and chemotactic peptides [72].

After AA is released it is metabolized by both the cyclooxygenase and lipoxygenase pathways. Both our laboratory and Borgeat and Samuelsson have prelabeled phospholipids and triglycerides in neutrophils with [14C]arachidonate and stimulated the cells with A23187 [12,178,181]. After stimulation the quantitatively most significant metabolite is 5-hydroxy-6,8,11,14-eicosatetraenoic acid (5-HETE), a hydroxylated fatty acid formed by the lipoxygenase pathway [12,13,178,181]. A second lipoxygenase product is 5,12-dihydroxy-6,8,10,14-eicosatetraenoic acid (5,12-di-HETE) [11,12,178]. Neutrophils also make several other lipoxygenase products in small quantities, including 8-HETE, 9-HETE, and 11-HETE [43]. The most prominent cyclooxygenase products are PGE_2 [178, 210,215] and thromboxane B_2 [20,48,71,154]. In the absence of a stimulus, only small quantities of these products are made. These observations hold using exogenous [14C]AA as a substrate unless very high AA concentrations are employed. Neutrophils also release PGE_2 in response to zymosan [215], a phagocytic stimulus. More recently zymosan has also been reported to cause the release of thromboxane B_2 [48] and 5-HETE [181] from neutrophils. Thus, products of both the lipoxygenase and the cyclooxygenase pathways are produced in response to external stimulation.

During the course of our studies in A23187-stimulated neutrophils we noted that the quantity of 5-HETE in the medium peaked at 1 to 2 minutes and then decreased. In investigating this phenomenon further, it was found that neutrophils and platelets could take up radiolabeled 5-HETE and 12-HETE into phospholipids and triglycerides [178] (Fig. 3). Although the significance of this observation is not yet clear, we believe that it is potentially of considerable interest. The incorporation of hydroxylated fatty acids into these lipids would be expected to change their overall polarity, thus their packing properties within the lipid bilayer. Although the net change in fatty acid composition of these normal membrane components is likely to be small, even limited changes at strategic locations in the plasma membrane might considerably affect membrane function. Selective effects on the catalytic activity of specific membrane enzymes must be considered. Despite the existence of numerous studies of the cyclooxygenase pathway in many organs, the

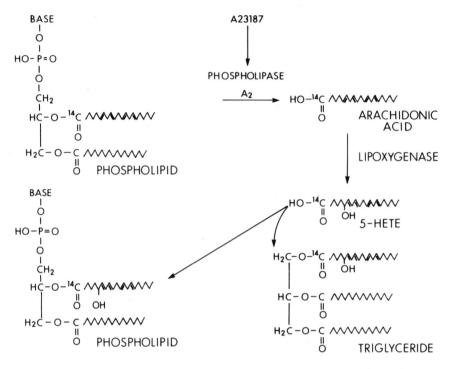

FIGURE 3. Scheme for release of arachidonate, conversion to 5-HETE, and esterification of 5-HETE.

lipoxygenase system has been largely ignored, and the function of the hydroxylated fatty acids has not been extensively studied.

Another conceivable role of the lipoxygenase pathway in activated neutrophils is to provide a portion of the energy that drives the hexose monophosphate shunt. The initial products formed in this pathway are hydroperoxy fatty acids, which are subsequently reduced to the corresponding hydroxy fatty acids. In the presence of NADPH, glutathione peroxidase is able to utilize long chain fatty acid hydroperoxides as a substrate, generating NADP and the hydroxylated fatty acid [24]. This enzyme is present in rat neutrophils and probably in human neutrophils as well. While the quantity of 5-HETE generated appears to be insufficient to account for more than a relatively small proportion of the increase in shunt activity, by virtue of its low polarity, 5-hydroperoxy-HETE might be able to penetrate intracellular membranes, providing substrate to drive the shunt in selected intracellular compartments.

Most of the AA stored in cells is bound at the 2 position of phospholipids. As already discussed, it is generally believed that the metabolism of AA is controlled by the rate of release of arachidonate from membrane phospholipids and as a consequence, the production of arachidonate metabolites is closely tied to events that result in alterations in membrane phospholipids. In the case of the calcium ionophore A23187, the likely sequence of events is understood: ionophore increases intracellular calcium levels, elevated calcium levels activate phospholipase A_2 [161] (which acts selectively at the 2 position), and activated phospholipase stimulates fatty acid turnover [193] with net release of arachidonate [178]. Ionophore also causes other alterations in neutrophil phospholipid metabolism with increased [^{32}P] incorporation into phosphatidic acid, phosphatidyl inositol, and phosphatidyl serine [192]. Elsbach has extensively reviewed the changes that occur in the neutrophil membrane during phagocytosis [30]. It is not clear exactly how the biochemical alterations in the membrane during phagocytosis relate to the functional responses of the neutrophil. Among the biochemical events that occur in the membrane during phagocytosis are activation of an esterase [114], and alterations in phospholipid fatty acid composition in the phagocytic vesicles with a fall in their AA content. The fall in AA content is presumably due to activation of phospholipase [175], although conversion of membrane phospholipids to diacylglycerol by phospholipase C followed by its deacylation to monoacylglycerol by diacylglycerol lipase is another plausible mechanism [85]. Some of the diacylglycerol would be recycled into phospholipid, explaining the increase in phospholipid labeling. Human neutrophils have not been studied for these enzymes, but phospholipase C is demonstrable in many different cell types, and purified rat mast cells contain high levels of diacylglycerol lipase activity [85]. It is attractive to postulate that this pathway is involved in AA release because it would provide a direct link between the increase in [^{32}P] incorporation into phospholipid and the formation of AA metabolites. On the other hand, the phospholipase A_2 in hog pancreas exists as a proenzyme that reaches its full activity only after removal of N-terminal oligopeptides by enzymatic digestion, and it is possible that a major role of the esterase in neutrophils is to modulate this reaction.

Recent work done showing esterification of 5-HETE in phospholipid suggests a mechanism for negative feedback inhibition of AA metabolism on the membrane [178]. 5-HETE is incorporated into the plasma membrane phospholipid as efficiently as AA on a molar basis. To the extent to which 5-HETE replaces AA in the plasma membrane or AA is otherwise exhausted, the further formation of AA metabolites will be inhibited. In addition, as already discussed, the incorporation of 5-HETE may alter the functional properties of the membrane. Thus, a diverse group of influences may operate to regulate AA metabolism once a response has been initiated.

Effects of Exogenous Arachidonate and Arachidonate Metabolites on Neutrophil Function

One of the most interesting effects of AA metabolites on neutrophils is chemotaxis. Two products of AA metabolism in platelets have been shown to be chemotactic for neutrophils: 12-HETE [44,194,195] and 12-hydroxy-5,8,10-heptadecatrienoic acid (HHT), a cyclooxygenase product

[42]. More recently, 5-HETE, the neutrophil lipoxygenase product, has also been shown to be chemotactic at concentrations lower than for the platelet products [45]. We have biosynthesized both 5-HETE and 12-HETE, incubated them with neutrophils, and demonstrated their esterification into phospholipids and triglycerides [177,178]. Significant incorporation occurs at concentrations at or below those that stimulate chemotaxis. However, it is not yet established that the esterification is related to chemotaxis. Goetzl et al. have shown that the methyl esters of 12-HETE and HHT are specific inhibitors of chemotaxis induced by 12-HETE and HHT [46]. This inhibition could be consistent with either a blockade of specific membrane receptor or an inhibition of esterification. The chemotactic properties of prostaglandins are disputed. One group has found a chemotactic action of PGE_1 but not PGE_2 or $PGF_{2\alpha}$ [70]. Another group reports inhibition of chemotaxis by PGE_2 [162]. A third group has found both chemotactic and chemokinetic effects of PGE_2 and a chemotactic effect of PGE_2, but only in the presence of albumin [191].

Arachidonate and arachidonate metabolites also have effects on neutrophil degranulation. Naccache et al. [115] demonstrated that exogenous AA in low concentrations induces degranulation of rabbit neutrophils. This degranulation could be blocked by inhibitors of arachidonate metabolism. More recently, we have shown that 5-HETE and 12-HETE can induce the release of specific but not azurophilic granules from human neutrophils while arachidonate is inactive [179]. Prostaglandins, on the other hand, block zymosan-induced degranulation [209,217]. Prostaglandins also inhibit neutrophil aggregation [120].

ARACHIDONIC ACID METABOLISM AND IMMEDIATE HYPERSENSITIVITY

Immediate Hypersensitivity

Immediate hypersensitivity reactions may affect the lungs, nasal passages, conjunctiva, skin, or multiple organs simultaneously. Important causes include airborne pollens, foods, and drugs. The clinical manifestations vary widely depending on antigen, dose, and route of exposure. Nasal congestion, asthma, and urticaria are particularly common. The process is mediated by IgE antibodies. Allergic individuals make particularly large quantities of these antibodies. Once IgE antibodies have been produced, the IgE molecule binds to a 45,000-dalton glycoprotein on the surface of mast cells (and basophils), sensitizing them to stimulation by antigen [87]. When the antigen is reintroduced, it binds to IgE antibody on the mast cell surface cross-linking receptors. The antigen-antibody interaction at the cell exterior leads to the noncytotoxic release of a number of biologically active molecules that function as mediators of the immediate hypersensitivity response. Some of these mediators, of which histamine is the most prominent, are contained in storage granules. During mast cell activation most of these granules are extruded from the cell [185]. Others remain inside the cell but develop channels communicating to the exterior. Channel formation and granule extrusion are preceded by lysis of perigranular membranes, which begins within a few seconds after the stimulus is applied to the cell surface. Stimulated mast cells also release newly synthesized mediators, including at least four arachidonate metabolites: PGE_2, $PGF_{2\alpha}$, PGD_2, and SRS-A (slow reacting substance of anaphylaxis) [92,163]. In addition to specific antigen, several other agents have been shown to induce histamine release from mast cells. Two of these stimuli, Con A [82], which binds to plasma membrane glycoproteins, and anti-IgE antibody, which cross-links surface-bound IgE molecules, initiate a response through receptors on the cell surface. Ionophore A23187 and 48/80 [73] induce histamine release without interacting with specific surface receptors.

The mechanism by which the surface interaction of antigen and antibody is translated into histamine release is not fully understood. There is considerable evidence that calcium and cyclic nucleotides are involved, but their roles are ill-defined. Antigen-induced release from human leukocytes [93], human lung [80], and rat mast cells [73] is dependent on the presence of calcium in the medium. Cells preincubated with chelators of Ca^{2+} such as EDTA are refractory to 48/80 but regain their responsiveness if calcium is added to the medium [25,29]. However, evidence of this kind cannot clearly distinguish a permissive from a causal role for calcium in mediator release. Cyclic nucleotides also modulate histamine release but, again, the exact nature of that relationship is not clear. In rat mast cells each of the histamine-releasing stimuli studied caused changes in cyclic nucleotide levels [185]. The two agents that clearly act at specific sites on the cell surface, Con A and anti-IgE, caused a transient rise in cAMP levels followed by a marked fall [189]. A23187 and 48/80, which do not bind to specific cell surface sites and presumably stimulate by a mechanism other than perturbation of cell surface macromolecules, caused the fall but not the early rise in cAMP [187,188]. One interpretation is that the binding of Con A or anti-IgE antibody activates a plasma membrane adenylate cyclase with a local rise in cAMP, resulting in changes in protein phosphorylation that help initiate the response. Once the response is under way, a fall in cAMP occurs inside the cell similar to that produced by A23187 and 48/80. A fall in cAMP in or near the granule membrane may be the final common stimulus leading to granule release [185]. As will be discussed later, a variety of pharmacologic agents that raise cAMP, including prostaglandins, inhibit histamine release.

Arachidonic Acid Metabolism in Mast Cells

As in the other cell types discussed here, there is no significant pool of free arachidonate in mast cells, and the first step in arachidonate metabolism is release of AA from phospholipids. The usual mechanism for cleavage of arachidonate from phospholipids is thought to be activation of phospholipase A_2. However, recent work in our laboratory suggests that mast cell stimulation results in activation of phospholipase C with production of diacylglycerol [85], which in turn is deacylated by a diacylglycerol lipase to yield AA and other free fatty acids. This pathway may be important in another respect in that diacylglycerol and its cleavage product monoacylglycerol are potent stimuli of granule fusion and may be directly responsible for the early changes in granule structure that precede and accompany mediator release.

After arachidonate is released, it is metabolized by both the cyclooxygenase and lipoxygenase pathways. Lewis and co-workers incubated purified rat peritoneal mast cells with the calcium ionophore A23187. Analysis of the products by gas chromatography–mass spectroscopy revealed five cyclooxygenase products: thromboxane B_2, PGD_2, PGE_2, and $PGF_{2\alpha}$, and the prostacyclin metabolite 6-keto-$PGF_{1\alpha}$ [92,163]. Ionophore-treated cells made more of these products than did untreated cells. Ionophore also stimulated the production of three lipoxygenase products, 12-HETE, 11-HETE, and 15-HETE.

In addition to the products already mentioned, there is now convincing evidence that SRS-A is an AA metabolite formed in mast cells and other cell types through the lipoxygenase pathway (reviewed in Refs. 132 and 136). SRS-A was first described by Feldberg and Kellaway in 1938 as a smooth muscle contracting agent released during the perfusion of rat and guinea pig lungs with cobra venom [132]. It was later demonstrated that a substance with similar properties was released during stimulation of perfused sensitized guinea pig lungs with antigen. SRS-A production has now been demonstrated in human, guinea pig, and bovine lung, mixed human peripheral blood leukocytes, mixed peritoneal leukocytes, a strain of rat basophilic leukemia cells (RBL-1 cells), cat paws, and several other tissues. In addition to antigen and cobra venom, other stimuli of SRS release include anti-IgE antibody, the histamine-releasing agent 48/80, and the calcium ionophore A23187.

The first report that AA is the precursor of SRS came from studies in our laboratory performed with RBL-1 cells [77,78]. Eicosatetraynoic acid (ETYA), an analogue of AA with triple bonds instead of double bonds at the 5, 8, 11, and 14 positions, was found to markedly diminish SRS formation. ETYA is an inhibitor of both the major pathways of arachidonate metabolism—the lipoxygenase and cyclooxygenase pathways. Since indomethacin, an inhibitor of the cyclooxygenase but not the lipoxygenase pathway, did not inhibit SRS production, it appeared that SRS was a lipoxygenase product. The relation of arachidonate to SRS was further shown by the ability of arachidonate to increase SRS synthesis in concentrations as low as 0.01 μg/ml [79]. Dihomo-γ-linolenic acid (a precursor of PGE_1 and PGD_1 that lacks the 5 double bonds of AA but is otherwise identical to AA) was much less stimulatory, and other long chain fatty acids, such as linoleic and linolenic ($C_{18:2}$ and $C_{18:3}$), were inhibitory. This specificity argued against a nonselective detergent action for AA and suggested instead that AA is an SRS precursor. This was convincingly demonstrated by radiolabel incorporation studies in which [14C] radioactivity from [14C]AA was found to comigrate with SRS bioreactivity after extensive purification, including preparative two-dimensional thin-layer chromatography (TLC) [5,77,78]. Correspondence of bioreactivity and radioactivity was demonstrated in nine one-dimensional TLC systems as well as by column chromatography on DEAE cellulose. Incubation of the cells with other radioactive long chain fatty acids was not associated with incorporation of radioactivity into biologically active products. Since stimulation of RBL-1 cells with A23187 produced a marked parallel increase in 5-HETE biosynthesis, and since neutrophils but not platelets also made SRS, we suggested that a lipoxygenase acting selectively at one of the carbons of the 5,6 double bond of AA was required for SRS synthesis [131].

We later showed that RBL-1 cells make little or no thromboxane A_2 and that the relatively selective lipoxygenase inhibitors, pyrogallol and nordihydroguaiaretic acid, markedly inhibited both SRS and 5-HETE synthesis [31]. Moreover, synthetic exogenous 5-hydroperoxyeicosatetraenoic acid (5-HPETE), the initial product of the 5-lipoxygenase pathway, markedly enhanced SRS synthesis even in the absence of A23187, and radiolabeled 5-HPETE was demonstrated to be incorporated into SRS [145]. We also showed that AA was incorporated into SRS in antigen-stimulated guinea pig lung fragments, human basophils, and rat peritoneal mast cells [200,212,213]. As discussed below, other laboratories soon confirmed that AA was an SRS precursor in several of these systems.

As far as other components of the SRS molecule are concerned, it had been suggested on the basis of preliminary microanalytic studies of partially purified SRS and inactivation of SRS by arylsulfatase that SRS might contain sulfur, presumably in the form of a sulfate ester [124]. Although later studies by our laboratory showed that the inactivation by arylsulfatase was due to contaminating proteases (Parker et al., submitted for publication), these observations led to further studies showing that the addition of exogenous thiols at the time of stimulation of SRS biosynthesis in mononuclear cells and antigen-stimulated lung fragments considerably increased SRS formation [123]. Although this effect was not observed in RBL-1 cells and attempts by others to demonstrate that sulfur was incorporated into the SRS molecule had been unsuccessful, in early 1979, at meetings of the Federated Biological Societies in Atlanta [140] and the American Society for Clinical Investigation in Washington, D.C. [139], we reported that when RBL-1 cells were incubated for 16 hours in tissue culture with [35S]-labeled cysteine (and to a lesser extent [35S]methionine or sulfate) or [3H]cysteine, radiolabel was incorporated into the SRS molecule. Using a series of chromatographic purification procedures including high pressure liquid chromatography (HPLC) on C_{18} reverse phase columns, the SRS could be subfractioned into three distinct species, arbitrarily termed types I, II, and III in decreasing order of their total spasmogenic activities. Each of these species could be radiolabeled with [1-14C]AA or [3H]- or [35S]cysteine and had a 280 nm ultraviolet absorption maximum as reported previously for SRS from anaphylactically stimulated guinea pig lungs by Morris, Piper, and their colleagues [110]. By conducting parallel studies with [^{14}C]- and [^{35}S]-labeled SRS, the two major SRS species (types I and II) were shown to be broken down by thioether cleaving reagents such as cyanogen bromide, sodium metal in liquid ammonia, and Raney nickel, indicating that the sulfur-containing side chain of the SRS molecule was attached to the lipid moiety through a thioether bond [139]. Since radioactivity was incorporated from [^{3}H]cysteine as well as [^{35}S]cysteine, it was apparent that one or more of the cysteine carbons was also being incorporated. However, since the efficiency of incorporation of cysteine label was much greater in cells preincubated with the labeled amino acid for many hours before addition of the SRS stimulus, it seemed likely that the side chain was not cysteine itself but one of its metabolites. This was quickly confirmed by TLC studies of the sodium metal cleavage product. These observations were reported in greater detail in the summer and fall of 1979 [112,141].

The evidence that each of the three SRS types had a sulfur-containing side chain, taken together with the already strongly suggestive evidence that SRS was a product of the lipoxygenase pathway, was of considerable interest because Gardner and his colleagues [37] had reported some time previously that low molecular weight thiols such as N-acetylcysteine react with lipid hydroperoxides under mild conditions to form thiolipids in which the sulfur-containing moiety is bound in thioether linkage. In our initial cleavage studies with sodium metal, the major fatty acid cleavage product from both [^{14}C]-labeled type I and type II SRS had been free AA. By the time of our presentation at the meeting of the American Society for Clinical Investigation in early May 1979, however, we were using less severe conditions for cleavage and, as we reported at that time, the major lipid cleavage product was a fatty acid with a 270–280 nm absorption maximum, migrating very closely or identically with 5-HETE in multiple TLC systems. Although we had not yet fully substantiated this structure by mass spectroscopy, we later showed that after further reduction with hydrazine and derivatization to promote volatilization, the saturated hydroxylated C_{20} fatty acid 5-hydroxyarachidic acid could be identified by combined gas chromatography–mass spectroscopy. Moreover, when SRS was synthesized in the presence of $^{18}O_2$, ^{18}O was found to be incorporated at the 5 position [141]. This confirmed that both type I and type II SRS have a C_{20} fatty acid core substituted with oxygen from molecular oxygen at the 5 position [141], as would be expected for a 5-lipoxygenase product.

About one month after the second of these presentations our results were confirmed and significantly extended by Samuelsson and his colleagues in an oral presentation at the International Prostaglandin Meeting in Washington, D.C. Incorporation of radiolabel from AA and cysteine into SRS was demonstrated in mouse mastocytoma cells stimulated with A23187. After reduction and cleavage with Raney nickel, 5-hydroxyarachidic acid was demonstrated by mass spectroscopy. Digestion with soybean lipoxygenase produced a shift in the absorption maximum from 280 to 308 nm, indicating that the double bonds were at the 7, 9, 11, and 14 positions. Although the side chain was not characterized, Samuelsson et al. proposed that SRS was a 6-cysteinyl-thioether of 5-OH-7,9,11,14-eicosatetraenoic acid. However, their later, more detailed report [113] considered the possibility that the side chain might not be cysteine.

The first indication of the true nature of the side chain in the two major forms of SRS was provided by our laboratory. As we indicated at the International Meeting on Clinical Applications of Prostaglandins in Paris in September 1979 [135], and in more detail in the November 1979 issue of Prostaglandins [141], amino acid analysis studies of SRS from RBL-1 cells indicated that the major side chain in SRS was not cysteine but glutathione (type II) or a mixture of cysteinyl-glycine with smaller amounts of glutathione (type I). Type II SRS contained 0.96 mole of glycine, 0.91 mole of glutamic acid, and 0.21 mole of cysteine (as half cystine) per mole of SRS, whereas type I SRS contained 0.85 mole of glycine, 0.30 mole of glutamic acid, and 0.14 mole of cysteine per mole of SRS. (Presumably the low yield of cysteine was due to its attachment to the fatty acid chain.) The presence of glutathione and cysteinyl-glycine was supported by chromatographic studies of the sodium metal cleavage products of [^{35}S]-labeled SRS. One early type I SRS preparation in particular contained substantial amounts of type II material, but later type I SRS preparations were largely or entirely cysteinyl-glycyl SRS. Subsequent studies by two other laboratories confirmed the existence of the cysteinyl-glycyl [111] and glutathionyl [64] forms of SRS. Morris, Piper, and their colleagues [111] were able to directly characterize the uncleaved SRS molecule by mass spectroscopy, which was the first time this had been accomplished.

Hammarström, Samuelsson, Corey, and their colleagues [64] compared naturally occurring glutathionyl SRS from mouse mastocytoma cells with different isomers of glutathionyl SRS prepared by organic synthesis. The results indicated that the side chain was substituted at the 6 position and that the double bonds were 7 (trans), 9 (trans), 11 (cis), and 14 (cis). Rokach et al. [164] independently drew similar conclusions with respect to double bond structure based on their own synthetic studies of the glutathionyl SRS molecule. These synthetic studies were important in that the double bond configuration would have been very difficult to establish by direct analysis of the naturally occurring SRS molecule. It thus appears that the structure of these two major forms of SRS has been definitely characterized. While we originally suggested that there may be a reducible function in the SRS molecule other than the double bond system such as a marked peroxy group this now appears unlikely.

The initial product formed when a lipoxygenase acts on an unsaturated fatty acid is a hydroperoxide. We had originally proposed that glutathione might be coupled to the 5-hydroperoxide of eicosatetraenoic acid through the action of glutathione S-transferase and that the cysteinyl-glycyl form of SRS might arise from glutathionyl SRS by the action of

γ-glutamyltranspeptidase, which cleaves the γ-glutamyl linkage in glutathione [141]. We later showed that glutathionyl SRS is produced first
during the initial phase of stimulation by A23187 and is subsequently
degraded to cysteinyl-glycyl SRS, which is the major SRS species, at 15
to 20 minutes. Studies in progress in collaboration with H. J. Wedner
in our laboratory confirm this sequence in that if intracellular glutathione
levels are markedly depleted by preincubating RBL-1 cells with cyclo-
hexene-1-one or diethyl maleate, SRS synthesis is almost completely
inhibited. Cysteinyl-glycyl SRS is also the predominant form of SRS in
anaphylactically stimulated guinea pig lung fragments [200] (Fig. 4). If
RBL-1 cells are incubated longer with A23187 most of the cysteinyl-glycyl
SRS is eventually degraded to cysteinyl SRS.

   In the guinea pig ileal smooth muscle bioassay system used in our
laboratory, the various SRS species have (usually) similar slopes al-

FIGURE 4. Proposed sequence for the formation of several major SRS species beginning
with glutathionyl SRS (type II), with subsequent conversion to cysteinyl-glycyl SRS (the
major component of type Ia) and cysteinyl SRS (type Ib). Based on the studies of Hammarström et al. (64), the double bond configurations are presumably 7-trans, 9-trans, 11-
cis, and 14-cis. The 5-O is shown as a hydroxyl group, although there is indirect evidence
to indicate that SRS may contain a reducible function, possibly in the form of a masked
peroxy group at the 5 position [141].

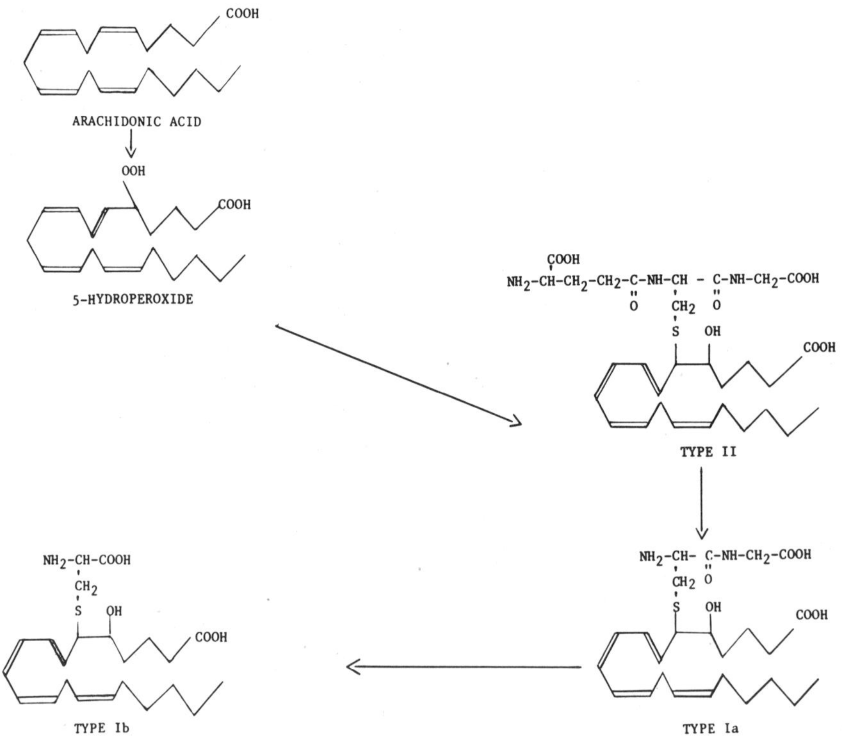

though the glutathionyl SRS has a longer latent period. In our hands their relative molar spasmogenic potencies in the guinea pig ileal muscle bioassay system are cysteinyl-glycyl SRS (1.0), glutathionyl SRS (0.3–0.75), and cysteinyl SRS (0.1). The cysteinyl-glycyl form of SRS is approximately 60 to 70 times more potent on a molar basis than histamine in this system. Depending on the particular ileal smooth muscle preparation, as little as 0.1 pmole of cysteinyl-glycyl SRS may produce an easily demonstrable contractile response. Even the partial inactivation product, cysteinyl SRS, is more effective than histamine in the ileal system.

A new nomenclature has been established for the various compounds in the SRS system. The glutathionyl form of SRS (Type II) is termed leukotriene C_4, the cysteinyl-glycyl form (Type Ia) is termed leukotriene D_4 and the cysteinyl form (Type Ib) is termed leukotriene E_4.

There is still much to be learned about the spectrum of physiologic and pharmacologic actions of SRS. It is already clear that SRS can affect the central and peripheral airways, intestinal and uterine smooth muscle, the cardiovascular system, and the skin, as well as potentiate the release of thromboxanes in perfused lung system. Preliminary evidence indicates that the various SRS species will differ quite significantly in their relative activities in some of these systems. It seems very possible that as-yet undefined but important physiologic and pharmacologic actions of SRS will be discovered. Of particular interest will be the determination of the importance of SRS in human bronchial asthma, where a major role in the bronchoconstrictor response has long been suspected.

Effects of Prostaglandins on Immediate Hypersensitivity

There is evidence, most of it somewhat indirect, that AA plays a role in control of mediator release in mast cells. Incubation of mast cells with ETYA has been shown to inhibit histamine release induced by anti-IgE, Con A, and A23187, with ID_{50} values of 65, 50, and 17 μM, respectively [186]. Aspirin (60 μM) and indomethacin (60 μM) do not inhibit. This suggests the possibility that a lipoxygenase product is involved in control of mediator release. However, substantiation by direct measurements of AA metabolites in ETYA-treated mast cells has not been carried out. Attempts to demonstrate that SRS influences release have thus far been unsuccessful, but SRS may not readily penetrate cells, and again further studies are needed.

The effects of exogenous arachidonate on mediator release are somewhat confusing and difficult to interpret. Exogenous arachidonate by itself does not cause mediator release, perhaps because both inhibitory and stimulatory products are produced. Preincubation of mast cells with AA (1–10 μM) inhibits subsequent release by anti-IgE or Con A [186]. This inhibition can be blocked by low concentrations of aspirin or indomethacin, suggesting that the inhibition is mediated by a cyclooxygenase product. If instead of preincubating the cells with AA, the AA is added after stimulation, either there is no inhibition or even enhancement of release may be observed. Interestingly, Lichtenstein et al. have reported that aspirin blocks the inhibition of release normally produced by cAMP agonists [95].

Pharmacological agents that elevate intracellular cAMP levels in human peripheral blood leukocytes inhibit the release from mast cells of preformed mediators such as histamine. In 1936 Schild reported that epinephrine inhibited the anaphylactic release of histamine from guinea pig lung [169]. Bourne and co-workers [14] and Lichtenstein and Margolis [94] have found that β-stimulants, prostaglandins, and theophylline inhibit antigen-induced histamine release from human peripheral blood leukocytes. Walker has shown inhibition of anaphylactic histamine release from human lung tissue by prostaglandin [199]. In a similar study by Tauber and co-workers involving a number of cAMP agonists, the concentrations of PGE_1, theophylline, isoproterenol, and norepinephrine required to cause inhibition of histamine release were sufficient to significantly increase cAMP levels [190]. It has also been shown that prostaglandins are released during antigen-stimulated responses in this tissue and that levels of cGMP also rise. This result raises the possibility that the alterations in cyclic nucleotides might be produced by prostaglandins. However Platshon and Kaliner have presented three lines of evidence suggesting that the rise in cyclic nucleotide levels is due to histamine rather than to the prostaglandins [150]: (1) histamine-receptor blockers prevented antigen-induced rises in cyclic nucleotide concentrations, (2) exogenous histamine raised both cAMP and cGMP levels, and (3) anaphylactically produced histamine caused similar changes in guinea pig and dog lung. By contrast, suppression of prostaglandin synthesis during anaphylaxis did not alter the rise in cyclic nucleotides. In the same study H_1 histamine receptor antagonists markedly inhibited the production of $PGF_{1\alpha}$ during anaphylaxis. Thus it appears that the production of prostaglandins in anaphylactically stimulated lung fragments is in large part a secondary event that follows histamine release and is dependent on it. It is not clear whether the prostaglandin synthesis is occurring in mast cells or in cells of another type.

In the interpretation of studies in heterogeneous tissues such as lung fragments or peripheral blood leukocytes, it is very important to consider the complexities in interpretation of the data. It is difficult to know whether stimuli are acting directly on mast cells or whether their effects are mediated through other cells. Similarly, one cannot identify the cells that synthesize the arachidonate products found in the medium. Studies in isolated mast cells avoid many of these difficulties.

REFERENCES

1. Anderson, C. B., Newton, W. T., and Jaffe, B. M. (1975) Circulating prostaglandin E and allograft rejection. Transplantation 19, 527–529.
2. Averdunk, R., and Lauf, P. K. (1975) Effects of mitogens on sodium-potassium transport, ^{3}H-ouabain binding, and adenosine triphosphatase activity in lymphocytes. Exp. Cell Res. 93, 331–342.

3. Bach, M.-A. (1975) Differences in cyclic AMP changes after stimulation by prosta-glandins and isoproterenol in lymphocyte subpopulations. J. Clin. Invest. 55, 1074–1081.

4. Bach, M.-A., and Bach, J. F. (1973) Studies of thymus products. VI. The effects of cyclic nucleotides and prostaglandins on rosette-forming cells. Interactions with thymic factor. Eur. J. Immunol. 3, 778–783.

5. Bach, M. K., Brashler, J. R., and Gorman, R. R. (1977) On the structure of slow reacting substance of anaphylaxis. Evidence for arachidonic acid. Prostaglandins 14, 21–38.

6. Barnett, R. E., Scott, R. E., Furcht, L. T., and Kersey, J. H. (1974) Evidence that mitogenic lectins induce changes in lymphocyte membrane fluidity. Nature (London) 249, 465–466.

7. Bauminger, S. (1978) Differences in prostaglandin formation between thymocyte sub-populations. Prostaglandins 16, 351–355.

8. Berenbaum, M. C., Purves, E. C., and Addison, I. E. (1976) Intercellular immunological controls and modulation of cyclic AMP levels. Immunology 30, 815–823.

9. Bloom, F. E., Wedner, H. J., and Parker, C. W. (1973) The use of antibodies to study cell structure and metabolism. Pharmacol. Rev. 25, 343–358.

10. Bonney, R. J., Naruns, P., Davies, P., and Humes, J. L. (1979) Antigen-antibody complexes stimulate the synthesis and release of prostaglandins by mouse peritoneal macrophages. Prostaglandins 18, 605–616.

11. Borgeat, P., and Samuelsson, B. (1979) Transformation of arachidonic acid by rabbit polymorphonuclear leukocytes. Formation of a novel dihydroxyeicosatetraenoic acid. J. Biol. Chem. 254, 2643–2646.

12. Borgeat, P., and Samuelsson, B. (1979) Arachidonic acid metabolism in polymor-phonuclear leukocytes: Effects of ionophore A23187. Proc. Natl. Acad. Sci. (US) 76, 2148–2152.

13. Borgeat, P., Hamberg, M., and Samuelsson, B. (1976) Transformation of arachidonic acid and homo-γ-linolenic acid by rabbit polymorphonuclear leukocytes. Monohy-droxy acids from novel lipoxygenases. J. Biol. Chem. 251, 7816–7820.

14. Bourne, H. R., Lichtenstein, L. M., and Melmon, K. L. (1971) Pharmacologic control of allergic histamine release in vitro: Evidence for an inhibitory role of 3',5'-adenosine monophosphate in human leukocytes. J. Immunol. 108, 695–705.

15. Bourne, H. R., Lichtenstein, L. M., Melmon, K. L., Henney, C. S., Weinstein, Y., and Shearer, G. M. (1974) Modulation of inflammation and immunity by cyclic AMP. Science 184, 19–28.

16. Bray, M. A., and Gordon, D. (1976) Effects of anti-inflammatory drugs on macrophage prostaglandin biosynthesis. Br. J. Pharmacol. 57, 466P–467P.

17. Bray, M. A., and Gordon, D. (1978) Prostaglandin production by macrophages and the effect of anti-inflammatory drugs. Br. J. Pharmacol. 63, 635–642.

18. Bray, M. A., Gordon, D., and Morley, J. (1978) Prostaglandins as regulators in cellular immunity. Prostaglandins Med. 1, 183–199.

19. Brune, K., Glatt, M., Kalin, H., and Peskar, B. A. (1978) Pharmacological control of prostaglandin and thromboxane release from macrophages. Nature (London) 274, 261–263.

20. Bunting, S., Higgs, G. A., Moncada, S., and Vane, J. R. (1976) Generation of throm-boxane A_2-like activity from prostaglandin endoperoxides by polymorphonuclear leu-kocyte homogenates. Br. J. Pharmacol. 58, 296P.

21. Cantarow, W. D., Cheung, H. T., and Sundharadas, G. (1978) Effects of prostaglandins on the spreading, adhesion and migration of mouse peritoneal macrophages. Pros-taglandins 16, 39–46.

22. Chaplin, D., Wedner, H. J., and Parker, C. W. (1980) Protein phosphorylation in human peripheral blood lymphocytes: Mitogen-induced increases in protein phos-phorylation in intact lymphocytes. J. Immunol. 124, 2390–2398.

23. Chaplin, D. D., Wedner, H. J., and Parker, C. W. (1980) Protein phosphorylation and lymphocyte activation. In: E. W. Gelfand and H. M. Dosch (eds.), Biological Basis of Immunodeficiency, Raven Press, New York, pp. 269–281.

24. Cheson, B. D., Curnutte, J. T., and Babior, B. M. (1977) The oxidative killing mechanisms of the neutrophil. Prog. Clin. Immunol. 3, 1–65.

25. Cochrane, D. E., and Douglas, W. W. (1974) Calcium induced extrusion of secretory granules (exocytosis) in mast cells exposed to 48/80 or the ionophores A23187 and X5374A. Proc. Natl. Acad. Sci. (US) 71, 408–412.

26. Cohn, Z. A. (1978) The activation of mononuclear phagocytes: Fact, fancy and future. J. Immunol. 121, 813–816.

27. Crout, J. E., Hepburn, B., and Ritts, R. E., Jr. (1975) Suppression of lymphocyte transformation after aspirin ingestion. New Engl. J. Med. 292, 221–223.

28. Davies, P., Bonney, R. J., Humes, J. L., and Kuehl, F. A., Jr. (1980) Secretion of arachidonic acid oxygenation products by mononuclear phagocytes: Their possible significance as modulators of lymphocyte function. In: E. R. Unanue and A. S. Rosenthal (eds.), Macrophage Regulation of Immunity, Academic Press, New York, pp. 347–360.

29. Douglass, W. W., and Ueda, Y. (1973) Mast cell secretion induced by 48/80: Calcium-dependent exocytosis inhibited strongly by cytochalasin only when glycolysis is rate-limiting. J. Physiol. 234, 97P–98P.

30. Elsbach, P. (1977) Cell surface changes in phagocytosis. In: G. Poste and G. L. Nicholson (eds.), The Synthesis, Assembly and Turnover of Cell Surface Components, Elsevier/North-Holland Biomedical Press, New York, pp. 363–402.

31. Falkenhein, S. F., MacDonald, H., Huber, M., Koch, D., and Parker, C. W. (1980) Effect of the 5-hydroperoxide of eicosatetraenoic acid and inhibitors of the lipoxygenase pathway on the formation of slow reacting substance by rat basophilic leukemia cells. Direct evidence that slow reacting substance is a product of the lipoxygenase pathway. J. Immunol. 125, 163–168.

32. Feldberg, W., Holden, H. F., and Kellaway, C. H. (1938) Liberation of histamine and formation of lysolecithin-like substances by cobra venom. J. Physiol. 94, 187.

33. Ferber, E., De Pasquale, G. G., and Resch, K. (1975) Phospholipid metabolism of stimulated lymphocytes. Composition of phospholipid fatty acids. Biochim. Biophys. Acta 398, 364–376.

34. Ferraris, V. A., and De Rubertis, F. R. (1974) Release of prostaglandin by mitogen- and antigen-stimulated leukocytes in culture. J. Clin. Invest. 54, 378–386.

35. Fisher, D. B., and Mueller, G. C. (1971) Studies on the mechanism by which phytohemagglutinin rapidly stimulated phospholipid metabolism of human lymphocytes. Biochim. Biophys. Acta 248, 434–448.

36. Flower, R. J. (1974) Drugs which inhibit prostaglandin synthesis. Pharmacol. Rev. 26, 33–67.

37. Gardner, H. W., Kleiman, R., Weisleder, D., and Inglett, G. E. (1977) Cysteine adds to lipid hydroperoxide. Lipids 12, 655–660.

38. Gemsa, D., Seitz, M., Kramer, W., Till, G., and Resch, K. (1978) The effects of phagocytosis, dextran sulfate, and cell damage of PGE_1 sensitivity and PGE_1 production of macrophages. J. Immunol. 120, 1187–1194.

39. Gemsa, D., Seitz, M., Kramer, W., Grimm, W., Till, G., and Resch, K. (1979) Ionophore A23187 raises cyclic AMP levels in macrophages by stimulating prostaglandin E formation. Exp. Cell Res. 118, 55–62.

40. Gemsa, D., Seitz, M., Menzel, J., Grimm, W., Kramer, W., and Till, G. (1979) Modulation of phagocytosis induced prostaglandin release from macrophages. Adv. Exp. Med. Biol. 114, 421–426.

41. Gemsa, D., Kramer, W., Brenner, M., Till, G., and Resch, K. (1980) Induction of prostaglandin E release from macrophages by colchicine. J. Immunol. 124, 376–380.

42. Goetzl, E. J., and Gorman, R. R. (1978) Chemotactic and chemokinetic stimulation of human eosinophil and neutrophil polymorphonuclear leukocytes by 12-L-hydroxy-5,8,10-heptadecatrienoic acid (HHT). J. Immunol. 120, 526–531.

43. Goetzl, E. J., and Sun, F. F. (1979) Generation of unique monohydroxy eicosatetraenoic acids from arachidonic acid by human neutrophils. J. Exp. Med. 150, 406–411.

44. Goetzl, E. J., Woods, J. M., and Gorman, R. R. (1977) Stimulation of human eosinophil and neutrophil polymorphonuclear leukocyte chemotaxis and random migration by 12-L-hydroxy-5,8,10,14-eicosatetraenoic acid. J. Clin. Invest. 59, 179–183.

45. Goetzl, E. J., Brash, A. R., Oates, J. A., and Hubbard, W. C. (1979) Functional determinants of the monohydroxy eicosatetraenoic acids (HETEs) which stimulate human neutrophil and eosinophil chemotaxis. Fed. Proc. 38, 1085.

46. Goetzl, E. J., Valone, F. H., Reinhold, V. N., and Gorman, R. R. (1979) Specific inhibition of the polymorphonuclear leukocyte chemotactic response to hydroxy–fatty acid metabolites of arachidonic acid by methyl ester derivatives. J. Clin. Invest. 63, 1181–1186.

47. Goldstein, I. M. (1978) Prostaglandins, thromboxanes and granulocytes. INFLO 11, 1–2.

48. Goldstein, I. M., Malmsten, C. L., Kindahl, H., Kaplan, H. B., Radmark, O., Samuelsson, B., and Weissmann, G. (1978) Thromboxane generation by human peripheral blood polymorphonuclear leukocytes. J. Exp. Med. 148, 787–792.

49. Goldyne, M. E. and Stobo, J. D. (1979) Synthesis of prostaglandins by subpopulations of human peripheral blood monocytes. Prostaglandins 18, 687–695.

50. Goodwin, J. S., Bankhurst, A. D., and Messner, R. P. (1977) Suppression of human T-cell mitogenesis by prostaglandin. J. Exp. Med. 146, 1719–1734.

51. Goodwin, J. S., Messner, R. P., Bankhurst, A. D., Peake, G. T., Saiki, J. H., and Williams, R. G., Jr. (1977) Prostaglandin producing suppressor cells in Hodgkin's disease. New Engl. J. Med. 297, 963–968.

52. Goodwin, J. S., Messner, R. P., and Peake, G. T. (1978) Prostaglandin suppression of mitogen-stimulated lymphocytes in vitro. Changes with mitogen dose and preincubation. J. Clin. Invest. 62, 753–760.

53. Goodwin, J. S., Selinger, D. S., Messner, R. P., and Reed, W. P. (1978) Effect of indomethacin in vivo on humoral and cellular immunity in humans. Infect. Immunol. 19, 430–433.

54. Goodwin, J. S., Wiik, A., Lewis, M., Bankhurst, A. D., and Williams, R. C., Jr. (1979) High-affinity binding sites for prostaglandin E on human lymphocytes. Cell. Immunol. 43, 150–159.

55. Gordon, D., Bray, M. A., and Morley, J. (1976) Control of lymphokine secretion by prostaglandins. Nature (London) 262, 401–402.

56. Gorman, R. R. (1978) Prostaglandins, thromboxanes, and prostacyclin. In: H. V. Richenberg (ed.), International Review of Biochemistry. Biochemistry and Mode of Action of Hormones, Part II, Vol. 20, University Park Press, Baltimore, pp. 81–107.

57. Graff, G., Stephenson, J. H., Glass, D. B., Haddox, M. I., and Goldberg, N. D. (1978) Activation of soluble splenic cell guanylate cyclase by prostaglandin endoperoxides and fatty acid hydroperoxides. J. Biol. Chem. 253, 7662–7676.

58. Greaves, M. W., Kingston, W. P., and Pretty, K. (1975) Actions of a series of nonsteroid and steroid anti-inflammatory drugs on prostaglandin synthesis by the microsomal fraction of rat skin. Br. J. Pharmacol. 53, 470P.

59. Grimm, W., Seitz, M., Kirchner, H., and Gemsa, D. (1978) Prostaglandin synthesis in spleen cell cultures of mice injected with Corynebacterium parvum. Cell. Immunol. 40, 419–426.

60. Hadden, J. W., Hadden, E. M., Haddox, M. K., and Goldberg, N. D. (1972) Guanosine 3'5'-cyclic monophosphate: A possible intracellular mediator of mitogenic influences in lymphocytes. Proc. Natl. Acad. Sci. (US) 69, 3024–3027.

61. Hagenfeldt, L., Hagenfeldt, K. H., and Weinnmalm, Å. (1975) Turnover of plasma free arachidonic and oleic acids in men and women. Hormone Metab. Res. 7, 467–480.

62. Hamberg, M. (1976) On the formation of thromboxane B_2 and 12-L-hydroxy-5,8,10,14-eicosatetraenoic acid (12 ho-20:4) in tissues from the guinea pig. Biochim. Biophys. Acta 431, 651–654.

63. Hamberg, M., and Samuelsson, B. (1974) Prostaglandin endoperoxides. Novel transformations of arachidonic acid in platelets. Proc. Natl. Acad. Sci. (US) 71, 3400–3404.

64. Hammarström, S., Murphy, R. C., Samuelsson, B., Clark, D. A., Mioskowski, D., and Corey, E. J. (1979) Structure of leukotriene C. Identification of the amino acid part. Biochem. Biophys. Res. Commun. 91, 1266–1272.

65. Hansen, P., Stein, H., and Peters, H. (1969) On the synthesis of RNA in lymphocytes stimulated by phytohemagglutinin; The activity of deoxyribonucleoprotein-bound and soluble DNA polymerase. Eur. J. Biochem. 9, 542–549.

66. Hedeskov, C. J. (1968) Early effects of phytohemagglutinin on glucose metabolism of normal human lymphocytes. Biochem. J. 110, 373–380.

67. Henney, C. S., Bourne, H. R., and Lichtenstein, L. M. (1972) The role of cyclic 3',5'-adenosine monophosphate in the specific cytolytic activity of lymphocytes. J. Immunol. 108, 1526–1534.

68. Hesketh, R. (1978) Early biochemical events in lymphocyte stimulation. In: J. C. Metcalfe (ed.), International Review of Biochemistry. Biochemistry of Cell Walls and Membranes, Part II. Vol. 19, University Park Press, Baltimore, pp. 63–91.

69. Higgs, G. A., and Salmon, J. A. (1979) Cyclo-oxygenase products in carrageenin-induced inflammation. Prostaglandins 17, 737–746.

70. Higgs, G. A., McCall, E., and Youlten, L. J. F. (1975) A chemotactic role for prostaglandins released from polymorphonuclear leucocytes during phagocytosis. Br. J. Pharmacol. 53, 539–549.

71. Higgs, G. A., Bunting, S., Moncada, S., and Vane, J. R. (1976) Polymorphonuclear leukocytes produce thromboxane A_2-like activity during phagocytosis. Prostaglandins 12, 749–757.

72. Hirata, F., Corcoran, B. A., Venkatasubramanian, K., Schiffman, E., and Axelrod, J. (1979) Chemoattractants stimulate degradation of methylated phospholipids and release of arachidonic acid in rabbit leukocytes. Proc. Natl. Acad. Sci. (US) 76, 2640–2643.

73. Hogberg, B., and Uvnas, B. (1960) Further observations on the disruption of rat mesentery mast cells caused by compound 48/80, antigen-antibody reaction, lectinase A and decylamine. Acta Physiol. Scand. 48, 133–145.

74. Hopper, K. E., Wood, P. R., and Nelson, D. S. (1979) Macrophage heterogeneity. Vox Sang. 36, 257–274.

75. Humes, J. L., Bonney, R. J., Pelus, L., Dahlgren, M. E., Sadowski, S. J., Kuehl, F. A., Jr., and Davies, P. (1977) Macrophages synthesize and release prostaglandins in response to inflammatory stimuli. Nature (London) 269, 149–151.

76. Inbar, M., and Shinitzky, M. (1975) Decrease in microviscosity of lymphocyte surface membrane associated with stimulation induced by concanavalin A. Eur. J. Immunol. 5, 166–170.

77. Jakschik, B., and Parker, C. W. (1976) Probable precursor role for arachidonic acid (AA) in slow reacting substance (SRS) biosynthesis. Clin. Res. 24, 575A (Abstr.).

78. Jakschik, B. A., Falkenhein, S., and Parker, C. W. (1977) Precursor role of arachidonic acid in slow reacting substance release from rat basophilic leukemia cells. Proc. Natl. Acad. Sci. (US) 74, 4577–4581.

79. Jakschik, B., Sullivan, T. J., Kulczycki, A., Jr., and Parker, C. W. (1977) Release of slow reacting substance (SRS) from rat mast cells. Fed. Proc. 36, 1328 (Abstr.).

80. Kaliner, M., and Austen, K. F. (1973) The immunological release of chemical mediators from nasal polyps. J. Allergy Clin. Immunol. 51, 105–106.

81. Kalisker, A., and Dyer, D. C. (1972) In vitro release of prostaglandins from the renal medulla. Eur. J. Pharmacol. 19, 305–309.

82. Keller, R. (1973) Concanavalin A, a model "antigen" for the in vitro detection of cell-bound reaginic antibody in the rat. Clin. Exp. Immunol. 13, 139–147.

83. Kelly, J. P., and Parker, C. W. (1979) Effects of arachidonic acid and other unsaturated fatty acids on mitogenesis in human lymphocytes. J. Immunol. 122, 1556–1562.

84. Kelly, J. P., Johnson, M. C., and Parker, C. W. (1979) Effect of inhibitors of arachidonic acid metabolism on mitogenesis in human lymphocytes: Possible role of thromboxanes and products of the lipoxygenase pathway. J. Immunol. 122, 1563–1571.

85. Kennerly, D. A., Sullivan, T. J., Sylwester, P., and Parker, C. W. (1979) Diacylglycerol metabolism in mast cells: A potential role in membrane fusion and arachidonic acid release. J. Exp. Med., 150, 1039–1044.

86. Kishimoto, T., and Ishizaka, K. (1976) Regulation of antibody response in vitro. X. Biphasic effect of cyclic AMP on the secondary anti-hapten antibody response to anti-immunoglobulin and enhancing soluble factor. J. Immunol. 116, 534–541.

87. Kulczycki, A., and Parker, C. W. (1979) The cell surface receptor for immunoglobulin E. I. The use of repetitive affinity chromatography for the preparation of a mammalian receptor. J. Biol. Chem. 254, 3187–3193.

88. Kurland, J. I., and Bockman, R. (1978) Prostaglandin E production by human blood monocytes and mouse peritoneal macrophages. J. Exp. Med. 147, 952–957.

89. Kurland, J. I., Bockman, R. S., Broxmeyer, H. E., and Moore, M. A. S. (1978) Limitation of excessive myelopoiesis by the intrinsic modulation of macrophage-derived prostaglandin E. Science 197, 552–555.

90. Kurland, J. I., Broxmeyer, H. E., Pelus, L. M., Bockman, R. S., and Moore, M. A. S. (1978) Role for monocyte-macrophage-derived colony-stimulating factor and prostaglandin E in the positive and negative feedback control of myeloid stem cell proliferation. Blood 52, 388–407.

91. Kurland, J. I., Pelus, L. M., Ralph, P., Bockman, R. S., and Moore, M. A. S. (1979) Induction of prostaglandin E synthesis in normal and neoplastic macrophages: Role for colony-stimulating factor(s) distinct from effects of myeloid progenitor cell proliferation. Proc. Natl. Acad. Sci. (US) 76, 2326–2330.

92. Lewis, R. A., Roberts, L. J., II, Lawson, J. A., Austen, K. F., and Oates, J. A. (1979) Generation of oxidative metabolites of arachidonic acid from rat serosal mast cells. J. Allergy Clin. Immunol. 63, 220 (Abstr.).

93. Lichtenstein, L. M. (1971) The immediate allergic response. In vitro separation of antigen activation, decay and histamine release. J. Immunol. 107, 1122–1130.

94. Lichtenstein, L. M., and Margolis, S. (1968) Histamine release in vitro: Inhibition by catecholamines and methyl xanthines. Science 161, 902–903.

95. Lichtenstein, L. M., Gillespie, E., Bourne, H. R., and Henney, C. S. (1972) The effects of a series of prostaglandins on in vitro models of the allergic response and cellular immunity. Prostaglandins 2, 519–528.

96. Lomnitzer, R., Rabson, A. R., and Koornhof, H. J. (1976) The effects of cyclic AMP on leucocyte inhibitory factor (LIF) production and on the inhibition of leucocyte migration. Clin. Exp. Immunol. 24, 42–48.

97. Loose, I. D., and Di Luzio, N. R. (1973) Effect of prostaglandin E_1 on cellular and humoral immune responses. J. Reticuloendothel. Soc. 13, 70–77.

98. McCarty, J., and Goetzl, E. J. (1979) Stimulation of human T-lymphocyte chemokinesis by arachidonic acid. Cell. Immunol. 43, 103–112.

99. Mapes, C. A., George, D. T., and Sobocinski, P. Z. (1977) Possible relations of prostaglandins to PMN-derived mediators of host metabolic responses to inflammation. Prostaglandins 13, 73–85.

100. Masuzawa, Y., Osawa, T., Inoue, K., and Nojima, S. (1973) Effects of various mitogens on the phospholipid metabolism of human peripheral lymphocytes. Biochim. Biophy. Acta 326, 339–344.

101. Meade, C. J., and Mertin, J. (1976) The mechanism of immunoinhibition by arachidonic and linoleic acid: Effects on the lymphoid and reticuloendothelial systems. Int. Arch. Allergy Appl. Immunol. 51, 2–24.

102. Meade, C. J., and Mertin, J. (1978) Fatty acids and immunity. Adv. Lipid Res. 16, 127–166.

103. Melmon, K. L., Bourne, H. R., Weinstein, Y., Shearer, G. M., Kram, J., and Bauminger, S. (1974) Hemolytic plaque formation by leukocytes in vitro. J. Clin. Invest. 53, 13–21.

104. Mertin, J., and Hughes, D. (1975) Specific inhibitory action of polyunsaturated fatty acids on lymphocyte transformation induced by PHA and PPD. Int. Arch. Allergy Appl. Immunol. 48, 203–210.

105. Mihas, A. A., Gibson, R. G., and Hirschowitz, B. I. (1975) Suppression of lymphocyte transformation by 16,(16)-dimethyl prostaglandin E_2 and unsaturated fatty acids. Proc. Soc. Exp. Biol. Med. 149, 1026–1028.

106. Minkes, M., Stanford, N., Chi, M. M-Y., Roth, G. J., Raz, A., Needleman, P., and Majerus, P. W. (1977) Cyclic adenosine 3',5'-monophosphate inhibits the availability of arachidonate to prostaglandin synthetase in human platelet suspensions. J. Clin. Invest. 59, 449–454.

107. Moran, J., Hunziker, W., and Fischer, J. A. (1978) Calcitonin and calcium ionophores: Cyclic AMP responses in cells of a human lymphoid line. Proc. Natl. Acad. Sci. (US) 75, 1984–1988.

108. Morley, J. (1974) Prostaglandins and lymphokines in arthritis. Prostaglandins 8, 315–326.

109. Morley, J., Bray, M. A., Jones, R. W., Nugteren, D. H., and van Dorp, D. A. (1979) Prostaglandin and thromboxane production by human and guinea-pig macrophages and leucocytes. Prostaglandins 17, 730–736.

110. Morris, H. R., Taylor, G. W., Piper, P. J., Sirois, P., and Tippins, J. R. (1978) Slow reacting substance of anaphylaxis. Purification and characterisation. FEBS Lett. 87, 203–206.

111. Morris, H. R., Taylor, G. W., Piper, P. J., Samhoun, M. N., and Tippins, J. R. (1980) Slow reacting substances (SRSs): The structure identification of SRSs from rat basophil leukaemia (RBL-1) cells. Prostaglandins 19, 185–201.

112. Murota, S.-I., Kawamura, M., and Morita, I. (1978) Transformation of arachidonic acid into thromboxane B_2 by the homogenates of activated macrophages. Biochim. Biophys. Acta 528, 507–511.

113. Murphy, R. C., Hammarström, S., and Samuelsson, B. (1979) Leukotriene C: A slow-reacting substance from murine mastocytoma cells. Proc. Natl. Acad. Sci. (US) 76, 4275–4279.

114. Musson, R. A., and Becker, E. L. (1977) The role of an activatable esterase in immune-dependent phagocytosis by human neutrophils. J. Immunol. 118, 1354–1364.

115. Naccache, P. H., Showell, H. J., Becker, E. L., and Sha'afi, R. I. (1979) Arachidonic acid induced degranulation of rabbit peritoneal neutrophils. Biochem. Biophys. Res. Commun. 87, 292–299.

116. Nasseen, S. M., and Hollander, V. P. (1973) Insulin reversal of growth inhibition of plasma cell tumor by prostaglandin or adenosine 3',5'-monophosphate. Cancer Res. 33, 2909.

117. Nordeen, S. K., and Young, D. A. (1978) Refractoriness of the cyclic AMP response to adenosine and prostaglandin E_1 in thymic lymphocytes. J. Biol. Chem. 253, 1234–1239.

118. Novogrodsky, A., Rubin, A. L., and Stenzel, K. H. (1979) Selective suppression by adherent cells, prostaglandin, and cyclic AMP analogues of blastogenesis induced by different mitogens. J. Immunol. 122, 1–7.

119. Offner, H., and Clausen, J. (1974) Inhibition of lymphocyte response to stimulants induced by unsaturated fatty acids and prostaglandins. Lancet 2, 400–401.

120. O'Flaherty, J. T., Kreutzer, D. L., and Ward, P. A. (1979) Effect of prostaglandins E_1, E_2, and $F_{2\alpha}$ on neutrophil aggregation. Prostaglandins 17, 201–210.

121. Opelz, G., Terasaki, P. I., and Hirata, A. A. (1973) Suppression of lymphocyte transformation by aspirin. Lancet 2, 478–480.

122. Oppenheim, J. J., and Rosenstreich, D. L. (1976) Signals regulating in vitro activation of lymphocytes. Prog. Allergy 20, 65–194.

123. Orange, R. P., and Chang, P. L. (1975) The effect of thiols on immunologic release of slow reacting substance of anaphylaxis. J. Immunol. 115, 1072–1077.

124. Orange, R. P., Murphy, R. C., and Austen, K. F. (1974) Inactivation of slow reacting substance of anaphylaxis (SRS-A) by arylsulfatase. J. Immunol. 113, 316–322.

125. Osheroff, P. L., and Webb, D. R. (1978) Stimulation of splenic prostaglandin levels by DNP-protein antigens. Cell. Immunol. 38, 319–327.

126. Osheroff, P. L., Webb, D. R., and Paulsrud, J. (1975) Induction of T-cell dependent splenic prostaglandin $F_{2\alpha}$ by T-cell dependent antigen. Biochem. Biophys. Res. Commun. 66, 425–429.

127. Pachman, L. M., Esterly, N. B., and Peterson, R. D. A. (1971) The effect of salicylate on the metabolism of normal and stimulated human lymphocytes in vitro. J. Clin. Invest. 50, 226–230.

128. Panayi, G. S., and Rix, A. (1974) The effect of phenylbutazone, indomethacin and ibuprofen on lymphocyte stimulation by phytohaemagglutinin in vitro. Rheumatol. Rehabil. 13, 179–183.

129. Panush, R. S., and Anthony, C. R. (1976) Effects of acetylsalicylic acid on normal human peripheral blood lymphocytes. Inhibition of mitogen- and antigen-stimulated incorporation of tritiated thymidine. Clin. Exp. Immunol. 12, 114–125.

130. Parker, C. W. (1976) Control of lymphocyte function. New Engl. J. Med. 295, 1180–1186.

131. Parker, C. W. (1977) Aspirin sensitive asthma. In: L. M. Lichtenstein, K. F. Austen, and A. S. Simon (eds.), Asthma: Physiology, Immunopharmacology, and Treatment. Second International Symposium, Academic Press, New York, pp. 301–313.

132. Parker, C. W. (1979) Prostaglandins and slow-reacting substance. J. Allergy Clin. Immunol. 63, 1–14.

133. Parker, C. W. (1979) The role of intracellular mediators in the immune response. In: E. Pick, J. Oppenheim, and S. Cohen (eds.), Biology of the Lymphokines, Academic Press, New York, pp. 541–583.

134. Parker, C. W. (1979) Role of cyclic nucleotides in regulating lymphocytes. Ann. NY Acad. Sci. 332, 255–261.

135. Parker, C. W. (1980) Pulmonary effects of inhibitors. In: Prostaglandin Synthetase Inhibitors in Clinical Medicine. Proceedings of the International Meeting on Prostaglandins, Paris, September 1979, Alan R. Liss, New York, Vol. 6, pp. 30–43.

136. Parker, C. W. (1981) SRS-A of rat basophil leukemia and rat mast cells. In: Proceedings of the Fourth International Kroc Foundation Symposium on the Biochemistry of the Acute Allergic Reaction, Alan R. Liss, New York, in press.

137. Parker, C. W., Baumann, M. L., and Huber, M. G. (1973) Alterations in cyclic AMP metabolism in human bronchial asthma. J. Clin. Invest. 52, 1336–1341.

138. Parker, C. W., Sullivan, T. J., and Wedner, H. J. (1974) Cyclic AMP and the immune response. In: P. Greengard and G. A. Robison (eds.), Advances in Cyclic Nucleotide Research. Vol. 4, Raven Press, New York, pp. 1–79.

139. Parker, C. W., Huber, M. G., and Falkenhein, S. (1979) Evidence that slow reacting substance (SRS) is a fatty acid thioether formed through a previously undefined pathway of arachidonate metabolism. Clin. Res. 27, 473A (abstr.).

140. Parker, C. W., Huber, M., and Falkenhein, S. (1979) Incorporation of ^{35}S into slow reacting substance (SRS). Fed. Proc. 38, 1167 (abstr.).

141. Parker, C. W., Huber, M. M., Hoffman, M. K., and Falkenhein, S. F. (1979) Characterization of the two major species of slow reacting substance from rat basophilic

leukemia cells as glutathionyl thioethers of eicosatetraenoic acids oxygenated at the 5 position. Evidence that peroxy groups are present and important for spasmogenic activity. Prostaglandins 18, 673–686.

142. Parker, C. W., Jakschik, B. A., Huber, M. G., and Falkenhein, S. F. (1979) Characterization of slow reacting substance as a family of thiolipids derived from arachidonic acid. Biochem. Biophys. Res. Commun. 89, 1186–1192.

143. Parker, C. W., Kelly, J. P., Falkenhein, S. F., and Huber, M. G. (1979) Release of arachidonic acid from human lymphocytes in response to mitogenic lectins. J. Exp. Med. 149, 1487–1503.

144. Parker, C. W., Stenson, W. F., Huber, M. G., and Kelly, J. P. (1979) Formation of thromboxane B_2 and hydroxyarachidonic acids in purified human lymphocytes in the presence and absence of PHA. J. Immunol. 122, 1572–1577.

145. Parker, C. W., Koch, D., Huber, M. M., and Falkenhein, S. F. (1980) Incorporation of radiolabel from [1-^{14}C]5-hydroxy-eicosatetraenoic acid into slow reacting substance. Biochem. Biophys. Res. Commun. 94, 1037–1043.

146. Passwell, J. H., Dayer, J.-M., and Merler, E. (1979) Increased prostaglandin production by human monocytes after membrane receptor activation. J. Immunol. 123, 115–120.

147. Pelus, L. M., and Strausser, H. R. (1977) Prostaglandins and the immune response. Life Sci. 20, 903–914.

148. Phillips, C. A., Girit, E. Z., and Kay, J. E. (1978) Changes in intracellular prostaglandin content during activation of lymphocytes by phytohaemagglutinin. FEBS Lett. 94, 115–119.

149. Piper, P., and Vane, J. (1971) Release of prostaglandins from lung and other tissues. Ann. NY Acad. Sci. 180, 363–385.

150. Platshon, L. F., and Kaliner, M. (1978) The effects of the immunologic release of histamine upon human lung cyclic nucleotide levels and prostaglandin generation. J. Clin. Invest. 62, 1113–1121.

151. Plescia, O. J., Smith, A. H., and Grinwich, K. (1975) Subversion of immune system by tumor cells and role of prostaglandins. Proc. Natl. Acad. Sci. (US) 72, 1848–1851.

152. Prasad, K. N. (1972) Morphological differentiation induced by prostaglandin in mouse neuroblastoma cells in culture. Nature (London) (New Biol.) 236, 49–52.

153. Quagliata, F., Lawrence, V. J. W., and Phillips-Quagliata, J. M. (1973) Prostaglandin D_1 as a regulator of lymphocyte function. Selective action of B lymphocytes and synergy with procarbazine in depression of immune responses. Cell. Immunol. 6, 457–465.

154. Rapoport, B., Pillarisetty, R. J., Herman, E. A., and Congco, E. G. (1977) Evidence for prostaglandin production by human lymphocytes during culture with human thyroid cells in monolayer: A possible role for prostaglandins in the pathogenesis of Graves' disease. Biochem. Biophys. Res. Commun. 77, 1245–1250.

155. Razin, E., and Globerson, A. (1979) The effect of various prostaglandins on plasma membrane receptors and function of mouse macrophages. Adv. Exp. Med. Biol. 114, 415–419.

156. Razin, E., Bauminger, S., and Globerson, A. (1978) Effect of prostaglandins on phagocytosis of sheep erythrocytes by mouse peritoneal macrophages. J. Reticuloendothel. Soc. 23, 237–242.

157. Resch, K. (1976) Membrane associated events in lymphocyte activation. In: P. Cuatrecasas and M. F. Greaves (eds.), Receptors and Recognition, Vol. 1, Chapman and Hall, London, pp. 59–117.

158. Resch, K., Ferber, E., Odenthal, J., and Fischer, H. (1971) Early changes in the phospholipid metabolism of lymphocytes following stimulation with phytohemagglutinin and with lysolecithin. Eur. J. Immunol. 1, 162–165.

159. Resch, K., Bouillon, D., and Gemsa, D. (1978) The activation of lymphocytes by the ionophore A23187. J. Immunol. 120, 1514–1520.

160. Rigaud, M., Durand, J., and Breton, J. C. (1979) Transformation of arachidonic acid into 12-hydroxy-5,8,10,14-eicosatetraenoic acid by mouse peritoneal macrophages. Biochim. Biophys. Acta 573, 408–412.

161. Rittenhouse-Simmons, S., and Deykin, D. (1977) The mobilization of arachidonic acid in platelets exposed to thrombin or ionophore A23187. J. Clin. Invest. 60, 495–498.

162. Rivkin, I., Rosenblatt, J., and Becker, E. L. (1975) Role of cyclic AMP in the chemotactic responsiveness and spontaneous motility of rabbit peritoneal macrophages. J. Immunol. 115, 1126–1134.

163. Roberts, L. J., II, Lewis, R. A., Lawson, J. A., Sweetman, B. J., Austen, K. F., and Oates, J. A. (1978) Arachidonic acid metabolism by rat mast cells. Prostaglandins 15, 717.

164. Rokach, J., Girard, Y., Guindon, Y., Atkinson, J. G., Larue, M., Young, R. N., Masson, P., and Holme, G. (1980) The synthesis of a leukotriene with SRS-like activity. Tetrahedron Lett. 21, 1485–1488.

165. Romeo, D., Zabucchi, G., Miani, N., and Rossi, F. (1975) Ion movement across leukocyte plasma membrane and excitation of their metabolism. Nature (London) 253, 542–544.

166. Rossi, F., Patriarca, P., Romeo, D., and Zabucchi, G. (1976) The mechanism of control of phagocytic metabolism. In: S. H. Reichard, M. R. Escobar, and H. Friedman (eds.), The Reticuloendothelial System in Health and Disease, Plenum Press, New York, pp. 205–223.

167. Scheid, M. P., Goldstein, G., Hammerling, U., and Boyse, E. A. (1975) Lymphocyte differentiation from precursor cells in vitro. Ann. NY Acad. Sci. 249, 531–540.

168. Scheid, M. P., Goldstein, G., and Boyse, E. A. (1978) The generation and regulation of lymphocyte populations. Evidence from differentiative induction systems in vitro. J. Exp. Med. 147, 1727–1743.

169. Schild, H. (1936) Histamine release and anaphylactic shock in isolated lungs of guinea pigs. Q. J. Exp. Physiol. 26, 165.

170. Schultz, R. M., Pavlidis, N. A., Stylos, W. A., and Chirigos, M. A. (1978) Regulation of macrophage tumoricidal function: A role for prostaglandins of the E series. Science 202, 320–321.

171. Shenker, B. J., and Gray, I. (1979) Cyclic nucleotide metabolism during lymphocyte transformation. I. Enzymatic mechanisms in changes in cAMP and cGMP concentration in Balb/c mice. Cell. Immunol. 43, 11–22.

172. Sims, T., Clagett, J. A., and Page, R. C. (1979) Effects of cell concentration and exogenous prostaglandin on the interaction and responsiveness of human peripheral blood leukocytes. Clin. Immunol. Immunopathol. 23, 150–161.

173. Smith, J. W., Steiner, A. L., Newberry, W. M., Jr., and Parker, C. W. (1971) Cyclic adenosine 3',5'-monophosphate in human lymphocytes. Alterations after phytohemagglutinin stimulation. J. Clin. Invest. 50, 432–441.

174. Smith, M. J., Hoth, M., and Davis, K. (1975) Aspirin and lymphocyte transformation. Ann. Intern. Med. 83, 509–511.

175. Smolen, J. E., and Shohet, S. B. (1974) Remodeling of granulocyte membrane fatty acids during phagocytosis. J. Clin. Invest. 53, 726–734.

176. Sondergaard, J., and Wolf-Jurgensen, P. (1972) The cellular exudate of human cutaneous inflammation induced by prostaglandins E_1 and $F_{1\alpha}$. Acta Dermatovenerol. 52, 361–364.

177. Stenson, W. F., and Parker, C. W. (1979) 12-L-Hydroxy-5,8,10,14-eicosatetraenoic acid, a chemotactic fatty acid, is incorporated into neutrophil phospholipids and triglyceride. Prostaglandins 18, 285–292.

178. Stenson, W. F., and Parker, C. W. (1979) Metabolism of arachidonic acid in ionophore stimulated neutrophils. Esterification of an hydroxylated metabolite into phospholipids. J. Clin. Invest. 64, 1457–1465.

179. Stenson, W. F., and Parker, C. W. (1980) Monohydroxyeicosatetraenoic acids (HETEs) induce degranulation of human neutrophils. J. Immunol. 124, 2100–2104.

180. Stenson, W. F., and Parker, C. W. (1980) Opinion: Prostaglandins, macrophages and immunity. J. Immunol. 125, 1–5.

181. Stenson, W. F., Atkinson, J. P., Kulczycki, A., Jr., and Parker, C. W. (1978) Stimulation of hydroxylated fatty acid and thromboxane synthesis in human neutrophils by phagocytic and other stimuli. Fed. Proc. 37, 1318.

182. Stockman, G. D., and Mumford, D. M. (1974) The effect of prostaglandins on the in vitro blastogenic response of human peripheral blood lymphocytes. Exp. Hematol. 2, 65–72.

183. Stossel, T. (1974) Phagocytosis. New Engl. J. Med. 290, 717–723, 774–782, 833–839.

184. Strom, T. B., Carpenter, C. B., Cragoe, D. J., Jr., Norris, S., Devlin, R., and Perper, R. J. (1977) Suppression of in vivo and in vitro alloimmunity by prostaglandins. Trans. Proc. 9, 1075–1079.

185. Sullivan, T. J., and Parker, C. W. (1976) Pharmacologic modulation of inflammatory mediator release by rat mast cells. Am. J. Pathol. 85, 437–463.

186. Sullivan, T. J., and Parker, C. W. (1979) Possible role of arachidonic acid and its metabolites in mediator release from rat mast cells. J. Immunol. 122, 431–436.

187. Sullivan, T. J., Parker, K. L., Eisen, S. A., and Parker, C. W. (1975) Modulation of cyclic AMP in purified rat mast cells. II. Studies on the relationship between intracellular cyclic AMP concentrations and histamine release. J. Immunol. 114, 1480–1485.

188. Sullivan, T. J., Parker, K. L., Stenson, W., and Parker, C. W. (1975) Modulation of cyclic AMP in purified rat mast cells. I. Responses to pharmacologic, metabolic, and physical stimuli. J. Immunol. 114, 1473–1479.

189. Sullivan, T. J., Parker, K. L., Kulczycki, A., and Parker, C. W. (1976) Modulation of cyclic AMP in purified rat mast cells. III. Studies on the effects of anti-IgE and concanavalin A on cyclic AMP concentrations during histamine release. J. Immunol. 117, 713–716.

190. Tauber, A. I., Kaliner, M., Stechschulte, D. J., and Austen, K. F. (1973) Immunologic release of histamine and slow reacting substance of anaphylaxis from human lung. V. Effects of prostaglandins on the release of histamine. J. Immunol. 111, 27–32.

191. Till, G., Kownatzki, E., Seitz, M., and Gemsa, D. (1979) Chemokinetic and chemotactic activity of various prostaglandins for neutrophil granulocytes. Clin. Immunol. Immunopathol. 12, 111–118.

192. Tou, J.-S. (1978) Modulation of $^{32}P_i$ incorporation into phospholipids of polymorphonuclear leukocytes by ionophore A23187. Biochim. Biophys. Acta 531, 167–178.

193. Tou, J.-S. (1979) Fatty acid and glycerol labeling of glycerolipids of leukocytes in response to ionophore A23187. Biochim. Biophys. Acta 572, 307–313.

194. Turner, S. R., Campbell, J. A., and Lynn, W. S. (1975) Polymorphonuclear leukocyte chemotaxis toward oxidized lipid components of cell membranes. J. Exp. Med. 141, 1437–1441.

195. Turner, S. R., Tainer, J. A., and Lynn, W. S. (1975) Biogenesis of chemotactic molecules by the arachidonate lipoxygenase system of platelets. Nature (London) 257, 680–681.

196. Vane, J. R. (1976) Prostaglandins as mediators of inflammation. In: B. Samuelsson and R. Paoletti (eds.), Advances in Prostaglandin and Thromboxane Research, Vol. 2, Raven Press, New York, pp. 791–801.

197. Wahl, L. M., Olsen, C. E., Sandberg, A. L., and Mergenhagen, S. E. (1978) Prostaglandin regulation of macrophage collagenase production. Proc. Natl. Acad. Sci. (US) 74, 4955–4958.

198. Waite, M., De Chatelet, L. R., King, L., and Shirley, P. S. (1979) Phagocytosis-induced release of arachidonic acid from human neutrophils. Biochem. Biophys. Res. Commun. 90, 984–992.

199. Walker, J. L. (1973) The regulatory role of prostaglandins in the release of histamine and SRS-A from passively sensitized human lung tissue. Adv. Biosci. 9, 235–240.

200. Watanabe, S., and Parker, C. W. (1980) Role of arachidonic acid in the biosynthesis of slow reacting substance of anaphylaxis (SRS-A) from sensitized guinea pig lung fragments. Evidence that SRS-A is very similar or identical structurally to nonimmunologically induced forms of SRS. J. Immunol. 125, 946–955.

201. Webb, D. R. (1978) The effects of prostaglandins of cAMP levels in subpopulations of mouse lymphocytes. Prostaglandins Med. 1, 441–453.

202. Webb, D.R., and Jamieson, A. T. (1976) Control of mitogen-induced transformation: Characterization of a splenic suppressor cell and its mode of action. Cell. Immunol. 24,45–57.

203. Webb, D. R., and Nowowiejski, I. (1977) The role of prostaglandins in the control of primary 19S immune response to sRBC. Cell. Immunol. 33, 1–10.

204. Webb, D. R., and Nowowiejski, I. (1978) Mitogen-induced changes in lymphocyte prostaglandin levels: A signal for the induction of suppressor cell activity. Cell. Immunol. 41, 72–85.

205. Webb, D. R., and Osheroff, P. L. (1976) Antigen stimulation of prostaglandin synthesis and control of immune responses. Proc. Natl. Acad. Sci. (US) 73, 1300–1304.

206. Wedner, H. J., and Parker, C. W. (1976) Lymphocyte activation. Prog. Allergy 20, 195–300.

207. Wedner, H. J., and Parker, C. W. (1977) Adenylate cyclase activity in lymphocyte subcellular fractions. Biochem. J. 162, 483–491.

208. Weidemann, M. J., Peskar, B. A., Wrogemann, K., Rietschel, E. T., Staudinger, H., and Fischer, H. (1978) Prostaglandin and thromboxane synthesis in a pure macrophage population and the inhibition, by E-type prostaglandins, of chemiluminescence. FEBS Lett. 89, 136–140.

209. Weissmann, G., Goldstein, I., and Hoffstein, S. (1976) Prostaglandins and the modulation by cyclic nucleotides of lysosomal enzyme release. In: B. Samuelsson and R. Paoletti (eds.), Advances in Prostaglandin and Thromboxane Research, Vol. 2, Raven Press, New York, pp. 803–814.

210. Wentzell, B., and Epand, R. M. (1978) Stimulation of the release of prostaglandins from polymorphonuclear leukocytes by the calcium ionophore A23187. FEBS Lett. 86, 255–258.

211. Whitney, R. B., and Sutherland, R. M. (1973) Kinetics of calcium transport in lymphocytes before and after stimulation by phytohemagglutinin. In: Proceedings of the Seventh Leukocyte Culture Conference, Academic Press, New York, pp. 63–74.

212. Yecies, L. D., Wedner, H. J., Johnson, S. M., Jakschik, B. A., and Parker, C. W. (1979) Slow reacting substance (SRS) from ionophore A23187-stimulated peritoneal mast cells of the normal rat. J. Immunol. 122, 2083–2089.

213. Yecies, L. D., Wedner, H. J., and Parker, C. W. (1979) Slow reacting substance (SRS) from ionophore A-23187 stimulated human leukemic basophils. I. Evidence for a precursor role of arachidonic acid and initial purification. J. Immunol. 123, 2814–2916.

214. Zimecki, M., and Webb, D. R. (1976) The regulation of the immune response to T-independent antigens by prostaglandins and B cells. J. Immunol. 117, 2158–2164.

215. Zurier, R. B. (1976) Prostaglandin release from human polymorphonuclear leukocytes. In: B. Samuelsson and R. Paoletti (eds.), Advances in Prostaglandin and Thromboxane Research, Vol. 2, Raven Press, New York, pp. 815–818.

216. Zurier, R. B., and Quagliata, F. (1971) Effect of prostaglandin E_1 on adjuvant arthritis. Nature (London) 234, 304–305.

217. Zurier, R. B., Weissmann, G., Hoffstein, S., Kammerman, S., and Tai, H. H. (1974) Mechanisms of lysosomal enzyme release from human leukocytes. II. Effects of cAMP and cGMP, autonomic agonists, and agents which affect microtubule function. J. Clin. Invest. 53, 297–309.

218. Zurier, R. B., Doty, J., and Goldenberg, A. (1977) Cyclic AMP response to prostaglandin E_1 in mononuclear cells from peripheral blood and synovial fluid of patients with rheumatoid arthritis. Prostaglandins 13, 25–31.

ROBERT B. ZURIER, M.D.

PROSTAGLANDINS AND INFLAMMATION

INTRODUCTION

Although the precise role of the prostaglandins in inflammation is not clear, abundant experimental evidence supports the view that prostaglandins participate in development of the inflammatory response [121]. All the criteria presented by Dale a half-century ago [23], which must be met before a compound may be classified as a mediator of inflammation, have been satisfied by the prostaglandins. These include (1) induction of the signs of inflammation, (2) release of the substance during an inflammatory reaction in a concentration capable of inducing inflammation, and (3) reduction of release by known antiinflammatory drugs. This chapter examines the prostaglandins accordingly.

The term "prostaglandins" is very widely employed but should be used to describe only the products of metabolism of the C_{20} polyenoic fatty acids (homo-γ-linolenic acid, arachidonic acid, eicosapentanoic acid) that contain the five-membered carbon ring. The other products of their metabolism are also pharmacologically active, and their role in inflammation—and that of the fatty acid precursors—must also be con-

From the Department of Medicine, Rheumatology Section, University of Pennsylvania School of Medicine, Philadelphia, Pennsylvania

sidered. Since arachidonate is the most abundant of the three precursors, it and its metabolites have been studied most thoroughly, and this chapter focuses on the "arachidonic acid cascade." However, the other precursors and their products may also prove to be important to the inflammatory response.

INDUCTION AND RELEASE OF PROSTAGLANDINS DURING INFLAMMATION

Induction of Inflammation

The four classical cardinal signs of inflammation outlined by Celsus in the first century A.D.—redness and swelling with heat and pain—are all induced by prostaglandins. This is due in large part to the ability of these substances to dilate vessels [74] and increase vascular permeability. Prostaglandin E_1 (PGE_1) increases vascular permeability (an invariable concomitant of acute inflammation, which leads to swelling) in the skin of experimental animals [22,56,61]. Intradermal injections of PGE_1 into normal human skin in concentrations of less than 10 ng/ml cause pronounced and sustained erythema, which is painful when touched. Although prostaglandins induce wheal and flare responses in human skin [22], it is not yet clear whether the permeability effects in man are due to a direct action on the microvasculature [130] or to release of vasoactive substances [68]. It appears not unlikely that a combination of these effects is responsible. Experimental evidence now also indicates that prostaglandins are probably better at potentiating the effects of other mediators of inflammation than they are at inducing inflammation directly. Prostaglandins (unlike histamine and bradykinin) are poor at eliciting plasma exudation when injected into guinea pig [56,128,129] or rabbit [129] skin, but they do potentiate plasma exudation produced by other mediators [82,128,129]. In addition, the stable prostaglandins E and F appear late in development of carrageenan edema [29,86], indicating that this inflammatory response is due to earlier release of other mediators, the effects of which are subsequently potentiated by the prostaglandins.

Kuehl and his colleagues [68] suggest that since E and F prostaglandins do not always fully mimic inflammatory reactions, other products of arachidonic acid should be considered to be mediators. Their work indicates that edema provoked by phorbol myristate acetate is induced by the free radical formed by conversion of the endoperoxide PGG_2 to PGH_2 [68,69], and that PGG_2 has a pivotal role in inflammation.

Williams and Peck [130], on the other hand, have suggested that the capacity of products derived from arachidonic acid to provoke modest edema and to potentiate edema induced by bradykinin and histamine reflects enhanced vasodilation. Results of their studies indicate that the rank order of prostaglandins for "exudation-potentiation potency" is the same as for "blood flow increasing potency": PGE > PGF > PGD. They also found that other compounds (isoprenaline, adenosine, adenosine diphosphate) that increase skin blood flow when injected locally also had exudation-potentiating activity. In contrast, substances that reduce skin blood flow (noradrenalin, angiotensin II) also reduce exudation. These authors concluded that prostaglandins potentiate histamine- and bradykinin-induced exudation by virtue of vasodilation rather than by increasing vascular permeability. Thus, the quantity of inflammatory exudate appears to be governed in large part by the level of vasodilator substance produced when generated concomitantly with substances that increase vessel wall permeability [131].

Arachidonic acid can cause vasodilation [30] and does potentiate carrageenan-induced edema [86]. The prostaglandin endoperoxides PGG_2 and PGH_2 are weak potentiators of edema provoked by carrageenan, by bradykinin, and by histamine [85,130]. Their effect on vascular smooth muscle, like that of thromboxane A_2 [30], is vasoconstrictive. If their transformation to PGI_2 (prostacyclin) is not prevented, however, vasodilatation follows the vasoconstriction [74,83].

Prostacyclin induces local vasodilation and increased plasma exudation when injected into rabbit skin [96] and is 5 to 10 times less potent than PGE_2 in potentiating (local injection) carrageenan-induced edema in the rat paw [55]. Prostacyclin also potentiates bradykinin edema; in this respect it resembles PGE and PGF, which in low doses potentiate edema induced by croton oil, carrageenan, histamine, and bradykinin [54,86,128,130].

The prostaglandin precursors (arachidonate, homo-γ-linolenate, and eicosapentanoate) also yield hydroperoxides by a lipoxygenase reaction that is not blocked by aspirin. Some of these compounds, such as hydroxyeicosatrienoic acid (HETE) are leukotactic and may therefore help mediate inflammation [120]. In addition, products of the lipoxygenase pathway enhance IgE-induced histamine release from human neutrophils [112].

Whereas pain is transitory when produced in man by intradermal injections of the hydroperoxide of arachidonic acid, by acetylcholine, bradykinin, and histamine, pain produced by PGE_1 lasts more than 2 hours. In addition, PGE compounds and intermediate hydroperoxides of arachidonic acid increase pain sensitivity to other chemical mediators such as bradykinin and histamine [37]. The effects of PGE are cumulative depending on concentration, time, or both. Therefore, even very small amounts of prostaglandins, if allowed to persist at the site of injury, may in time cause pain.

Although prostacyclin does not by itself provoke pain, it does induce pain upon addition of bradykinin or histamine [39]. The prostacyclin-induced pain lasts approximately 30 minutes. Cyclic AMP and theophylline also provoke long-lasting pain similar to that induced by PGE_2 [38], whereas morphine (which increases cellular cGMP) diminishes hyperalgesia induced by PGE_2, but not by cAMP. These studies suggest that agents that increase cellular cGMP antagonize agents that raise cAMP concentrations in cells. At any rate, as is the case for induction of swelling (edema), most of the oxidation products of arachidonic acid appear more readily able to potentiate pain induced by other mediators than to induce severe pain directly.

The overwhelming influence Rudolph Virchow exerted over the world of pathology led to acceptance of his concept that disturbance of function resulting from tissue injury must be included as a cardinal sign of inflammation. Thus the fifth cardinal sign, "functio laesa," was introduced by Virchow in his treatise on cellular pathology. Prostaglandins also cause disturbance of function. Repeated injections of PGE_1 into rat paws elicit—in a dose-dependent manner—inflammatory edema, which interferes with ambulation [133]. Moreover, injection of PGE_1 or PGE_2 into knee joints of dogs results in severe disabling arthritis.

Prostaglandins are able to resorb bone as measured by their effects on the release of previously incorporated ^{45}Ca from cultured fetal rat long bones. The endoperoxides PGG_2 and PGH_2 cause a rapid transient increase in ^{45}Ca release, but do not stimulate prolonged resorption [102]. PGE_2 is the most potent stimulator of bone resorption among the prostaglandins tested in vitro, but its 13,14-dihydro derivative is nearly as potent [102]. Addition of serum to the culture medium stimulates bone resorption [113], a process that is complement dependent and may be prostaglandin mediated [101]. This mechanism may help explain bone resorption in the rheumatoid joint, for example, where complement is activated and PGE_2 concentrations are high.

Osteoclast activating factor (OAF) is also a potent local mediator of bone resorption produced by cells involved in immune responses. The production of OAF by human lymphocytes stimulated by phytohemagglutinin (PHA) is inhibited by indomethacin and flufenamic acid, and OAF production is restored by addition to the lymphocytes of PGE [134,135]. The studies indicate that prostaglandin synthesis is necessary for OAF production.

Release During Inflammation

Among the earliest studies to implicate prostaglandins in the inflammatory response were those that showed that mechanical irritation of rabbit eyes evoked release of "irin" into the anterior chamber. In subsequent studies irin was identified as PGE_2 and $PGF_{2\alpha}$. Willis [132] was the first to discover prostaglandins in inflammatory exudate. There is evidence that prostaglandins are not stored within any subcellular compartment but are formed upon physiological demand, probably to act close to the site of synthesis. Most processes that disturb membrane function—such as inflammation—activate the hydrolysis of fatty acids from membrane phospholipids and thereby favor synthesis of prostaglandins. There is experimental evidence that $PGF_{2\alpha}$ can be transported across a biological membrane against a concentration gradient. The movement of prostaglandins into and out of cells is therefore not passive, but requires energy-dependent carrier systems. Alterations in these active transport processes could conceivably influence cell function profoundly and adversely.

The prostaglandinlike substances associated with several experimental models of inflammation have been regarded as terminal mediators of the acute response. Carrageenan, a sulfated mucopolysaccharide derived from Irish sea moss (Chondrus), induces an acute inflammatory reaction when injected into the paw of a rat. Carrageenan-induced edema of the rat foot is used widely as a model of inflammation in the search for new antiinflammatory agents. In fact, the model has been credited with forming the basis for the discovery of indomethacin. A number of substances, including histamine, 5-hydroxytryptamine (5-HT), kinins, and prostaglandins, are involved in the development of carrageenan edema. There appear to be three distinct phases of mediator release: an initial simultaneous release of histamine and 5-HT, a second phase mediated by kinins, and a third phase, the mediator of which is suspected to be prostaglandins. In experiments using histamine and 5-HT antagonists, or polymonine, which depletes tissue stores of both vasoactive amines, there is a marked reduction in paw edema during the first 90 minutes of the inflammatory response [29], indicating that simultaneous release of histamine and 5-HT mediates the initial phase of inflammation. Treatment of rats with cellulose sulfate (CS) lowers the plasma kininogen level about 50% and reduces the edema during 1½ to 2½ hours after carrageenan injection. Thus kinin appears to mediate the second phase of this particular inflammatory response. Treatment of rats with polymonine (to deplete stores of histamine and 5-HT) combined with injection of CS (to reduce kininogen) leads to total suppression of carrageenan-induced edema up to 2½ hours. Willis has demonstrated the presence of prostaglandins in inflamed paws 2½ to 6 hours after carrageenan injection, suggesting that prostaglandins mediate the later phase of this inflammatory reaction. Activation of this third phase of inflammation requires the presence of the complement system. Depletion or blockade of the complement system prevents formation of the prostaglandinlike substance.

In the foregoing experiments, however, edema fluid was squeezed from the paws, and it was not certain how much of the prostaglandinlike activity was due to trauma. The carrageenan air bleb was therefore developed as a convenient atraumatic method for obtaining inflammatory exudate free from contamination with blood: a suspension of carrageenan in saline is injected into a subcutaneous air bleb that has been raised on the back of a rat. An inflammatory reaction ensues, and samples of bleb fluid are withdrawn at various time intervals. In bleb fluid, as in exudate from the inflamed paw, histamine and kinin are found shortly after carrageenan injection, whereas prostaglandins (mainly PGE_2) appear after 3 hours and reach maximum concentrations at 12 to 24 hours. Moreover, carrageenan induces prostaglandin accumulation in a dose-response manner. The concentrations of PGE_2 recovered are far in excess of those necessary to produce cutaneous inflammation. Concentrations in the bleb fluid of lysosomal β-glucuronidase and PGE_2 increase in parallel during the 24 hours after carrageenan injection, and it was suggested that inflammatory cells phagocytose carrageenan, consequently releasing lysosomal phospholipases that hydrolyze phospholipids of cell membranes to yield arachidonic acid, which in turn is converted to PGE_2.

Human skin possesses substrates and enzymes for the formation and metabolism of prostaglandins and prostaglandins have in fact been recovered from skin inflamed by a variety of stimuli. Prostaglandins have been identified in the inflamed skin of patients with allergic contact eczema and have been recovered from areas of delayed inflammation in skin exposed to ultraviolet radiation. PGD_2 is just beginning to be studied, but this compound is also a major skin prostaglandin and has the ability to produce inflammation. The carrageenan-induced granuloma pouch is a model for chronic inflammation. That thromboxane B_2 and $6\text{-keto-}PGF_{1\alpha}$ (the stable breakdown product of prostacyclin) are major products formed in the pouch after addition of arachidonic acid, suggests that these compounds are produced during chronic inflammation.

Synovium obtained at surgery from patients with rheumatoid arthritis (RA) and maintained in culture produces larger amounts of prostaglandin than synovium from patients with osteoarthritis [106]. RA synovial cell culture media promote bone resorption, whereas supernates from indomethacin-treated cultures do not [107]. Thus in addition to mediating rheumatoid inflammation, prostaglandins may be responsible for the periarticular bone demineralization characteristic of RA.

In addition to tissue cells, cells that invade sites of inflammation are also a potential source of prostaglandins. First, of course, these cells must get from the circulation to the area of inflammation. The possible role of prostaglandins in vasodilation and vasopermeability has been mentioned. Egress of inflammatory cells from blood vessels is undoubtedly aided by increased permeability of vessel walls, but the mysterious and mystical phenomenon whereby cells arrive at appropriate sites remains unexplained. Directed migration of cells toward an attractant (chemotaxis) and their increased random locomotion due to a chemical agent (chemokinesis) appear to be influenced by prostaglandins. Unfortunately, no precise pattern of prostaglandin effects on chemotaxis has been defined, and prostaglandins have been observed to increase [29,40,61] and suppress or have no effect [50,104] on neutrophil chemotaxis. In one study PGE_1, but not PGE_2 or $PGF_{2\alpha}$, was chemotactic for rabbit peritoneal polymorphonuclear leukocytes (PMNs). In another study the effects on chemotaxis-kinesis of PGE and PGF compounds depended on the presence or absence in the in vitro system of bovine serum albumin (BSA). In the absence of BSA, which is itself chemokinetically active, PGF induced a chemokinetic and chemotactic response in rabbit peritoneal PMN. Under the same conditions PGE and PGA had no effect. However, in the presence of BSA, PGE and PGA induced chemotactic responses [118]. The mechanism whereby albumin allows PGE and PGA to be chemotactic is unknown. In the absence of BSA, PGE_1 increased cellular cyclic AMP, which was not observed when BSA was present. Cyclic AMP has been shown to be weakly chemotactic for rabbit neutrophils [103]. Dibutyryl cyclic AMP effects were biphasic: weakly chemotactic at low concentrations and inhibitory at high concentrations. The weak effect of cyclic AMP on chemotaxis may help explain why results vary among laboratories.

Arachidonic acid is chemotactic [91,120], but the chemotactic activity of the endoperoxides PGG_2 and PGH_2 has not been determined. Prostacyclin has been shown to inhibit chemotaxis [127] and thromboxane A_2 has weak chemotactic properties [64]. Products of the lipoxygenase pathway are potent chemotactic agents for leucocytes of several species [43,120].

A new mechanism for generation of chemotactic activity has been presented [99]: when arachidonate is acted on by a superoxide-generating system (xanthine oxidase plus acetaldehyde), a lipid product is formed that has potent chemotactic activity for human neutrophils. Generation of superoxide within and at the surface of neutrophils follows exposure of these cells to chemotactic stimuli and to immune complexes. Thus neutrophils are able to generate products from arachidonate that will call forth more PMN to the site of inflammation.

Evidence has been presented [81] that PGE_2 enhances the chemotactic responsiveness of human monocytes to complement activated human serum by almost 200%. Interestingly, PGE_1 had no effect, and none of the E, F, A, or B prostaglandins was directly chemotactic for monocytes.

Platelets are often overlooked in discussions of cellular elements that help initiate inflammation. The extraordinary rapidity with which platelets adhere to damaged tissue and aggregate and release potent biologically active materials suggests that the platelet—like the mast cell—is well suited to be a cellular trigger for the inflammatory process. The role of platelets in inflammation has been well reviewed [132]. A wide variety of arachidonic acid metabolites are produced by platelets.

In man, intestinal mucosa, lungs, and skin have a relatively high histamine content, and mast cells are most abundant in these tissues. Mast cells release a wide variety of mediators of inflammation [5], and products of arachidonate metabolism may now be added to the list. Activation of mast cells by antigen-IgE interactions leads to release of preformed histamine from the granule matrix, and secretion of newly synthesized inflammatory mediators such as slow reacting substances (SRS). A number of arachidonic acid metabolites are formed by mast cells, including PGD_2, hydroxyheptadecatrienoic acid, $PGF_{2\alpha}$, thromboxane B_2, and PGE_2 [105], and arachidonate appears to be the principal precursor of mast cell or basophil SRS [4,60]. Evidence has been presented that enzymatic conversion of arachidonic acid to some active metabolites may be an integral reaction in the processes leading to release of inflammatory mediators from mast cells. When free arachidonic acid was added to resting mast cells, they became less responsive (histamine release) to anti-IgE, and the effect was blocked by aspirin or indomethacin. Thus arachidonate metabolites appear to be able to mediate histamine release.

The neutrophil is of course the cell type most characteristic of acute inflammation. PMNs do release prostaglandins and thromboxanes during phagocytosis and when there is plasma membrane stimulation [45,143]. The small amounts of stable prostaglandins released (PGE > PGF in ratio of approximately 3 : 1) are not due to platelet contamination. Platelets also were eliminated as a source of thromboxanes.

The lipoxygenase pathway is also very active in rabbit and human PMNs [12,13]. Products of this pathway synthesized in the PMNs include monohydroperoxy acids, and a novel dihydroxy fatty acid [(5S,12R)-dihydroxy-6,8,10,14-icosatetranenoic acid], which has been designated leukotriene B.

The essential role of mononuclear phagocytes in chronic inflammation is well established [24]. In response to inflammatory stimuli, mononuclear phagocytes release products of diverse nature, including oxygenation products of arachidonic acid. Although most studies indicate that the major products of arachidonate metabolism produced by macrophages are PGE_2 and 6-keto-$PGF_{1\alpha}$, the stable metabolite of PGI_2 [15, 25,46,58,87], others have shown increased transformation of PGE_2 into $PGF_{2\alpha}$ in mouse peritoneal exudate macrophages stimulated with *Corynebacterium parvum* [35]. Increases in $PGF_{2\alpha}$ seen in exudates of resolving inflammatory reactions [123] may therefore be due to the late arrival of macrophages.

EFFECTS OF ANTIINFLAMMATORY DRUGS

The original and now classical observations of Vane [122] and of Smith and Willis [109] documenting the dose-related inhibition of prostaglandin synthesis in both cell-free and single-cell systems have been confirmed in many experimental models. Moreover, prostaglandin production is abolished in platelets one hour after ingestion of 10 grains of aspirin, an effect that persists for as long as 3 days [65]. Ingestion of 20 grains of aspirin also prevents phagocytosis-induced release of prostaglandins from PMNs within 12 hours [143] and inhibits prostaglandin synthesis by mononuclear cells in culture (Dore-Duffy and Zurier, unpublished observations). Nearly all the nonsteroidal antiinflammatory substances now available inhibit prostaglandin synthesis. Furthermore, gold salts, which are antiinflammatory and "antirheumatic," also inhibit prostaglandin synthesis [97,114]. One new nonsteroidal antiinflammatory compound (2-aminomethyl-4-t-butyl-6-iodophenol; MK 447) is inactive as an inhibitor in the routine prostaglandin synthetase assay. Rather, MK 447 stimulates overall prostaglandin synthesis, apparently by facilitating conversion of PGG_2 to primary prostaglandins. In the process, MK 447 reduces PGG_2 levels. It has therefore been suggested [68] that the primary prostaglandins PGE_2 and $PGF_{2\alpha}$ are not the important inflammation-inducing agents obtained from arachidonic acid. Instead, the endoperoxide PGG_2 itself or a nonprostaglandin product derived from it during enzymatic oxidation of arachidonic acid, or the free radical formed in its metabolism, would fill that role. Hydroxy radicals such as those formed during conversion of PGG_2 to PGH_2 have been linked to inflammatory processes [41,92]. The superoxide free radical (O_2^-) can also induce inflammation [90].

In addition to MK 447, other readily oxidizable materials such as lipoic acid and sodium iodide have been demonstrated to increase both the extent and rate of the in vitro prostaglandin cyclooxygenase reaction. Both these compounds also exhibit antiinflammatory effects in PMA-induced mouse ear edema [34]. As a result of catalyzing the oxygenation of these compounds, the cyclooxygenase is deactivated [110]. The oxidative radicals released during the conversion of PGG_2 to PGH_2 are oxidizing equivalents of these compounds, and it was therefore proposed [31] that cyclooxygenase deactivation results from an irreversible reaction between the enzyme and the radical released. If these radicals are "scavenged" and their activity inhibited by the new breed of antiinflammatory compounds, then deactivation of cyclooxygenase is inhibited and the conversion of PGG_2 to PGH_2 is increased. Reducing agents (those that are readily oxidizable) thus enhance reduction of PGG_2 to PGH_2 and undergo oxidative metabolism [32,77,78]. Sodium iodide, lipoic acid, phenol, and MK 447 are all antiinflammatory agents. Despite gross structural differences, they all decrease PGG_2 levels and all appear to be scavengers of radicals. A direct interaction of these compounds with cyclooxygenase is also possible [33].

Glucocorticosteroids are the drugs most commonly used to suppress undesirable immune or inflammatory processes. Although there exists a vast body of descriptive detail dealing with these steroids, relatively little is known about the exact mechanisms whereby their antiinflammatory benefits are achieved. It is therefore of interest that corticosteroids inhibit release from cells of prostaglandins [62,72]. Corticosteroids appear to reduce prostaglandin production by limiting the availability to the prostaglandin synthetase system of the substrates (fatty acids) for prostaglandin biosynthesis [47,88,116]. Goldstein and his colleagues have shown [45] that preincubation with hydrocortisone sodium succinate of both normal human peripheral blood neutrophils and those treated with cytochalasin B significantly reduced thromboxane generation when these cells were exposed to serum-treated zymosan. They also found that arachidonic acid was capable of restoring thromboxane generation by neutrophils treated with hydrocortisone and then with serum-treated zymosan. Thus it is likely that corticosteroids, by stabilizing neutrophil membranes, interfere with the release of membrane phospholipids from which fatty acid substrates for the cyclooxygenase system are derived. On the other hand, it has been demonstrated [19] that dexamethasone pretreatment of cultured cells enhances cyclooxygenase activity, which leads to increased conversion of arachidonate to prostaglandins. It is conceivable that the steroid, like MK 447, also facilitates conversion of PGG_2 to prostaglandins. These events need further investigation.

Robinson and his colleagues have shown [107] that despite their alleged action in other tissues, glucocorticoids have no demonstrable effect on the release of arachidonic acid from membranes of synovial cells.

Treatment of rheumatoid synovial organ cultures with 10^{-7} M dexamethasone caused 80–90% inhibition of PGE_2 synthesis, but no significant difference in free arachidonic acid compared with untreated tissue. Their studies indicate that dexamethasone does not inhibit PG synthesis at the level of the phospholipase reaction, but does reduce cyclooxygenase activity, although not directly interacting with this enzyme.

The sensitivity of cyclooxygenase to inactivation of drugs varies from tissue to tissue. There is evidence [76] that platelet cyclooxygenase is less resistant to aspirin than is the enzyme in other tissues. The dose of aspirin that is necessary to inhibit prostaglandin synthesis in different tissues can vary from 325 mg/day to 7 g/day [49,57,95]. Also, the effect of antiinflammatory agents on prostaglandin synthesis in a particular tissue is not predictable from in vitro studies. For example, whereas prostaglandin synthetase activity in the microsomal fraction of synovial tissue from rheumatoid arthritis patients is abolished even by low doses (600 mg/day) of aspirin, considerable synthetase activity persists in synovial tissue from RA patients treated with indomethacin, ibuprofen, or naproxen. Addition to tissue in vitro, however, of these nonsteroidal antiinflammatory agents resulted in more potent inhibition of enzyme activity than addition of aspirin [21].

PROSTAGLANDINS AS MODULATORS
OF INFLAMMATION

That prostaglandins suppress diverse effector systems of inflammation suggests that they may have *antiphlogistic* actions. Thus PGE compounds, which increase levels of cyclic AMP in human leukocytes, reduce extrusion of lysosomal enzymes from human PMNs [141], prevent release of histamine from basophiles and lung fragments [75,91], and inhibit lymphocyte-mediated cytotoxicity [52]. Pharmacological doses of prostaglandins E_1 and E_2 suppress adjuvant-induced arthritis and cartilage degradation in rats [3,10,42], and cyclic AMP treatment suppresses acute and chronic inflammation in several experimental models [138,140]. The data suggest that PGE compounds, perhaps acting via cyclic AMP, may suppress as well as mediate acute and chronic inflammation. It is possible that as concentrations of prostaglandins in inflammatory exudates increase to approach "pharmacological" levels, they may help retard inflammation.

A regulatory effect of prostaglandins is not without precedent in other systems. For example, PGE inhibits the release of noradrenaline from the spleen in response to sympathetic nerve stimulation [51]. PGE is released from spleen when it contracts in response to sympathetic nerve stimulation. Thus by a feedback mechanism the contracting smooth muscle can reduce the stimulus that is leading to the contraction. Prostaglandin release may therefore be a defense mechanism [20] aimed at minimizing potential injury. Pertinent to a view of prostaglandins as local regulators of the inflammatory response is the observation [59] that whereas large amounts of cyclic AMP (500 mg/kg body weight daily for

5 days) reduce the size of preformed granulomata in rats, similar treatment with smaller amounts of cyclic AMP (1 or 10 mg/kg) increases granulomata size.

Local control of inflammation might also result from preferential biosynthesis of one or another of the prostaglandins or PG intermediates. For example, $PGF_{2\alpha}$ inhibits PGE-induced increases in vascular permeability in skin [22]. Moreover, as inflammatory exudate develops in rats with carrageenan-induced pleuritis and peritonitis, PGE rises relative to PGF (increased PGE : PGF ratio). As inflammation wanes, the PGE : PGF ratio drops toward preexudate values [123], suggesting that an appropriate balance of prostaglandins is important to regulation and restraint of the inflammatory response. A regulatory action might also be exerted through a mechanism whereby the 9-keto group of PGE_2 is reduced by PGE keto-reductase, resulting in formation of $PGF_{2\alpha}$. Indeed, constriction of bovine mesenteric veins evoked by bradykinin appears to depend on increased prostaglandin synthesis and conversion of PGE (vasodilator) to PGF (vasoconstrictor), both steps being affected by the kinin. Thus the ratio of PGE to PGF within a tissue has functional consequences.

The term "inflammation," of course, includes the acute and the chronic conditions. The emphasis in prostaglandin research to date has been on the role of prostaglandins in the acute inflammatory response. Prostaglandins, however, may also help modulate the chronic phase of inflammation. Whereas acute inflammation is characterized by neutrophil infiltrate and exudate, tissue proliferation is the hallmark of chronic inflammation. Appropriate control of cell proliferation is crucial to improved management of a disease such as rheumatoid arthritis, for example, in which synovium develops into granulation tissue (pannus), which invades and erodes articular cartilage. Proliferation of human fibroblasts and synovial cells (assessed by [3H]thymidine incorporation and direct cell counts) is suppressed by supernatants from human peripheral blood mononuclear cells [26,66]. The growth suppression seen is due in part to stimulation of fibroblast prostaglandin synthesis, suggesting that fibroblasts can modulate their own growth in vitro through a prostaglandin-mediated mechanism.

Prostaglandins also appear to play a role in many inflammatory conditions of skin [148]. Skin of patients with psoriasis is characterized by excessive proliferation of epidermal cells. Although the mechanisms whereby epidermal cell function is regulated have not been defined precisely, it is clear that prostaglandins are important to maintenance of epithelial homeostasis. The accumulation of cyclic AMP in psoriatic epidermis after PGE_1 stimulation is substantially less than in normal skin [124]. A similar lack of sensitivity to PGE_1 has been found in mononuclear cells from synovial fluid of patients with rheumatoid arthritis [144]. Thus an altered prostaglandin–cyclic nucleotide relation in rheumatoid joint might lead to abnormal synovial cell proliferation. PGE_1 causes a dose-dependent rise of cyclic AMP levels in cultured fibroblasts, which is followed by a dose-dependent increase in glycosaminoglycan (GAG) secretion, and reduced proliferation [100,108]. $PGF_{2\alpha}$ also increases synthesis of GAG in cultured fibroblasts, hyaluronic acid being the most stimulated of the hexosamine-containing substances. It appears that $PGF_{2\alpha}$ is able to induce activity of hyaluronic acid synthetase [84]. Prostaglandins may therefore help limit chronic inflammation by restraining fibroblast proliferation.

INFLUENCE OF PROSTAGLANDINS IN EXPERIMENTAL ANIMAL MODELS OF INFLAMMATION AND DISORDERED IMMUNITY

Essential Fatty Acid Deficient (EFAD) Animals

The EFAD rat has been a useful model for studying the role of prostaglandins in inflammation. When animals are kept on essential fatty acid deficient (EFAD) food, tissue arachidonic acid and bishomo-γ-linolenic acid (the prostaglandin precursors) are replaced by 5,8,11-eicosatrienoic acid [136], which is not a substrate for cyclooxygenase activity [137]. Collagen-induced aggregation of platelets from EFAD rats results in negligible release of thromboxane A_2, prostaglandin endoperoxides, and prostaglandins [18]. Thus arachidonate metabolites do not participate in a major way in inflammatory and other cellular responses in EFAD rats.

When injected into the rat paw, EFAs potentiate carrageenan-induced edema, but 5,8,11-eicosatrienoic acid does not. Carrageenan-induced edema (rat paw) is partly suppressed in EFAD rats and is restored by local administration of arachidonic acid [9] probably because of inadequate substrate for cyclooxygenase [6]. In EFAD rats, the poorly developed delayed phase of carrageenan-induced paw edema is not further suppressed by indomethacin, whereas aspirin and dexamethasone exhibit their characteristic antiinflammatory actions [9]. The results of the studies suggest that the antiinflammatory effects of aspirin and dexamethasone in this model are independent of inhibition of prostaglandin biosynthesis. It is not unlikely that the antiinflammatory activity of aspirin does not rest solely in its ability to inhibit cyclooxygenase activity [17].

Sponge-Induced Granuloma Formation

Inhibition of granuloma formation was observed when carrageenan-injected sponges were impregnated with large amounts of PGE_2 [28]. In EFAD rats, which produce only very small amounts of prostaglandins because they lack precursors, granuloma formation is enhanced [7]. The increased chronic inflammatory response is associated with increased collagen synthesis [93]. Thus, endogenous prostaglandins might act to suppress chronic inflammation in this model. PGE_1 injection (1 μg/sponge) upon implantation enhanced the acute inflammation and the subsequent production of granuloma, whereas PGE_1 administration on days 4 to 7 inhibited subsequent growth of granuloma [11]. In EFAD rats as little as 0.05 μg of PGE_1 per sponge reduced granuloma formation.

During kaolin-induced granuloma pouch inflammation in the rat the concentration of malondialdehyde (MDA) in the exudate increased steadily, whereas the concentration of PGE reached a maximum at day 1 and returned to control levels by day 4 [14]. MDA is a product of both cyclooxygenase-dependent and -independent metabolism of arachidonic acid. Thus, products of the lipoxygenase pathway appear to play a role in this animal model of acute and chronic inflammation.

Adjuvant Arthritis

Release of lysosomal enzymes from synovial cells and invading poly-morphonuclear leukocytes engaged in phagocytosis of immune complexes help initiate and perpetuate inflammation and joint tissue injury in patients with RA [126]. Reduction by PGE of endocytosis-induced enzyme release in vitro [141] suggested that PGE might suppress inflammation in vivo. It was then shown that PGE_1 and PGE_2, which increase cellular levels of cyclic AMP, do in fact prevent progression of adjuvant-induced arthritis and cartilage destruction in rats [138–140]. Cyclic AMP treatment also suppresses acute and chronic inflammation in several experimental animal models [8,59]. $PGF_{2\alpha}$, which does not increase cellular cyclic AMP in vitro, does not influence adjuvant arthritis [138]. Furthermore, when doses of theophylline (a compound that serves to maintain cellular cyclic AMP) and PGE_1, which alone do not affect adjuvant arthritis, were used together, inflammation and cartilage damage were prevented [10].

Although these studies suggest that PGE suppresses adjuvant disease by virtue of its ability to increase cyclic AMP, the precise mechanisms whereby PGE protects these animals remain unexplained. That PGE prevents pannus formation suggests an effect on the immune response itself. Since adjuvant disease is exacerbated by depletion of suppressor T-cells [63], PGE may enhance or substitute for T-suppressor activity. PGE treatment increases a cell-mediated response–skin reaction to injected PPD$^-$ and reduces a humoral response–antibody formation to sheep red blood cells [138].

NZB/W F_1 Mice

Although PGE_1 reduces lymphocyte-mediated cytotoxicity in vitro [52], it enhances monocyte-mediated cytotoxicity [142]. Thus PGE_1 appears to be capable of exerting different actions on different cells that help initiate the immune response. It is also likely that PGE_1 affects immunodeficient cells and normal cells differently. Because of the evidence that PGE can enhance cell-mediated responses and suppress humoral responses, we treated NZB/W F_1 mice with PGE_1. The NZB/W mouse is considered a good model for human systemic lupus erythematosus (SLE), and the animals, like the patients, exhibit impaired cell-mediated and exuberant humoral immune responses [115]. Unlike human SLE patients, all NZB/W mice succumb to immune complex nephritis. PGE_1 treatment prevents progression of nephritis in these mice and increases their survival dramatically [144–146]. The reasons for these benefits are not known. T-cell proportions decrease with age in NZB/W mice. There appears to be a specific loss of suppressor T-cells in these animals, and there is loss of spleen cell responsiveness to T-cell mitogens [115]. PGE_1 treatment maintains an appropriate balance among T- and B-cells, and preserves spleen cell responses to PHA [67]. Reflecting their impaired cell-mediated responses, NZB/W mice do not respond to intradermal injections of native DNA with classic delayed hypersensitivity (DH) reactions, and their splenic lymphocytes do not produce migration-inhibitory factor (MIF) following in vitro stimulation with DNA [1]. In contrast, NZB/W mice treated with PGE_1 (200 μg twice daily) are capable of mounting DH skin reactions to DNA, and a majority of spleen cell cultures derived from PGE_1-treated mice release MIF after DNA stimulation [1]. Thus PGE_1 treatment of NZB/W mice significantly alters the immunological reactivity of these animals toward DNA, one of the antigens implicated in the pathogenesis of systemic lupus erythematosus.

Immune Complex Vasculitis (Reversed Passive Arthus Reaction)

The reversed passive arthus (RPA) reaction is induced in rat skin by intravenous administration of antigen and intradermal injection of antibody. Formation of immune complexes in vessel walls leads to activation of complement and local generation of C_5-derived chemotactic peptides. Neutrophils respond to the chemotactic products, infiltrate the skin site, ingest the immune complexes, and release lysosomal enzymes and other mediators of inflammation and tissue injury. Injury to vessels can be measured by the great increase in vascular permeability (leakage into tissue of [^{125}I] albumin) and by development of hemorrhage. Treatment of rats with PGE_1 or with its more stable analogue 15(S)-15-methyl-PGE_1 inhibits increased vascular permeability and tissue injury, even though intra- and perivascular depositions of antigen and complement are not prevented [70]. Immunofluorescence microscopy studies suggest that immune complexes form in PGE-treated animals, and the complement sequence is activated. However, egress of leukocytes from blood vessels appears to be impaired in these animals. Electron microscopy studies indicate that neutrophils that do leave the circulation and find their way to the reaction site do not ingest immune complexes. Biochemical studies indicate that peripheral blood PMNs from PGE-treated animals have a reduced response to a chemotactic peptide and do not release lysosomal enzymes when treated in vitro with cytochalasin B and exposed to the peptide (PMNs from untreated control rats release 54% of total enzyme under similar in vitro conditions). Thus the cytoprotective effects of PGE demonstrated in this model appear to be due in part to interference with directed motion of neutrophils and with degranulation of these cells. Of great interest in these studies is the finding that 15(S)-15-methyl-PGE$_1$ exhibits potent antiinflammatory activity even after oral administration.

SUMMARY

Despite the complexity of the role of prostaglandins in immunological responses and inflammatory reactions, these ubiquitous compounds appear to be important to the regulation of cell function and host defenses. The challenge to be met in an effort to better treat diseases characterized by acute and chronic inflammation will be to determine whether and when to inhibit or stimulate the production of prostaglandin (and which prostaglandins or endoperoxides or thromboxanes to select). It is likely that observations of prostaglandin concentrations in experimental systems (in vitro and in vivo) over time will prove more useful to understanding biological events than manipulation of prostaglandin levels in tissue. Temporal changes in prostaglandin levels may be more important than absolute levels at any one time. The therapeutic potential of the prostaglandins appears to be great, and their use for a wide variety of diseases is just beginning. Whether they will prove to be helpful clinically as modulators of the immune response is not yet clear.

ACKNOWLEDGMENT

Supported in part by NIH grant AM 17309.

REFERENCES

1. Adelman, N., Ksiazek, J., Cohen, S., Yoshida, T., and Zurier, R. B. (1980) Prostaglandin E$_1$ treatment of NZB/W F$_1$ hybrid mice. Induction of in vitro and in vivo cell mediated immune responses to DNA. Clin. Immunol. Immunopathol. 17, 353–362.

2. Adkinson, N. F., Barron, T., Powell, S., and Cohen, S. (1977) Prostaglandin production by human peripheral blood cells in vitro. J. Lab. Clin. Med. 90, 1043–1053.

3. Aspinall, R. L., and Cammarata, P. S. (1969) Effect of prostaglandin E$_2$ on adjuvant arthritis. Nature (London) 224, 304–305.

4. Bach, M. K., Brashler, J. R., and Gorman, R. R. (1977) Slow reacting substance of anaphylaxis (SRS-A) is a metabolite of arachidonic acid. Fed. Proc. 36, 376.

5. Becker, E. L., and Henson P. M. (1973) In vitro studies of immunologically induced secretion of mediators from cells and related phenomena. Adv. Immunol. 17, 93–118.

6. Bonta, I. L., Bult, H., van der Ven, L. L. M., and Noordhoek, J. (1976) Essential fatty acid deficiency: A condition to discriminate prostaglandin and non-prostaglandin mediated components of inflammation. Agents Actions 6, 154–158.

7. Bonta, I. L., Parnham, M. J., and Adolfs, M. J. P. (1977) Reduced exudation and increased tissue proliferation during chronic inflammation in rats deprived of endogenous prostaglandin precursors. Prostaglandins 14, 295–307.

8. Bonta, I. L., Parnham, M. J., Adolfs, M. J. P., and Van Vliet, L. (1977) Dual function of E type prostaglandins in models of chronic inflammation. In: D. A. Willoughby, J. P. Giroud, and G. P. Velo (eds.), Perspectives in Inflammation; Future Trends and Developments, MTP Press, Lancaster.

9. Bonta, I. L., and Bult, H. (1977) Effects of antiinflammatory drugs on the carrageenin-induced hind paw inflammation of rats deprived of endogenous precursors of prostaglandins. In: I. L. Bonta (ed.), Recent Developments in the Pharmacology of Inflammatory Mediators, Birkhäuser Verlag, Basel, pp. 77–83.

10. Bonta, I. L., Parnham, M. J., and Van Vliet, L. (1978) Combination of theophylline and prostaglandin E₁ as inhibitors of the adjuvant induced arthritis syndrome of rats. Ann. Rheum. Dis. 37, 212–217.

11. Bonta, I. L., and Parnham, M. J. (1979) Time dependent stimulatory and inhibitory effects of prostaglandin E₁ on exudative and tissue components of granulomatous inflammation in rats. Br. J. Pharmacol. 65, 465–472.

12. Borgeat, P., Hamberg, M., and Samuelsson, B. (1976) Transformation of arachidonic acid and homo-gamma-linolenic acid by polymorphonuclear leukocytes. J. Biol. Chem. 251, 2816–2828.

13. Borgeat, P., and Samuelsson, B. (1979) Arachidonic acid metabolism in polymorphonuclear leukocytes: Effects of ionophore A23187. Proc. Natl. Acad. Sci. (US) 76, 2148–2152.

14. Bragt, P. C., Schenkelaars, E. P. M., and Bonta, I. L. (1979) Dissociation between prostaglandin and malondialdehyde formation in exudate and increased levels of malondialdehyde in plasma and liver during granulomatous inflammation in the rat. Prostaglandins Med. 2, 51–61.

15. Bray, M. A., and Gordon, D. (1978) Prostaglandin production by macrophages and the effect of antiinflammatory drugs. Br. J. Pharmacol. 63, 635–642.

16. Bray, M. A., and Franco, M. (1978) Prostaglandins and inflammatory cell movement in vitro. Int. Arch. Allergy Appl. Immunol. 56, 500–506.

17. Brune, K. (1974) How aspirin might work: A pharmacokinetic approach. Agents Actions 4, 230–232.

18. Bult, H., and Bonta, I. L. (1976) Rat platelets aggregate in the absence of endogenous precursors of prostaglandin endoperoxides. Nature (London) 264, 449–451.

19. Chandrabose, K. A., Lapetina, E. G., Schmitges, C. J., Siegel, M. J., and Cuatrecasas, P. (1978) Action of corticosteroids in regulation of prostaglandin biosynthesis in cultured fibroblasts. Proc. Natl. Acad. Sci. (US) 75, 214–217.

20. Collier, H. O. J. (1971) Prostaglandins and aspirin. Nature (London) 232, 17–19.

21. Cook, D., Collins, A. J., Bacon, P. A., and Chan, R. (1976) Prostaglandin synthetase activity from human rheumatoid synovial microsomes. Effect of "aspirinlike" drug therapy. Ann. Rheum. Dis. 35, 327–332.

22. Crunkhorn, P., and Willis, A. L. (1971) Interaction between prostaglandins E and F given intradermally in the rat. Br. J. Pharmacol. 41, 507–512.

23. Dale, H. H. (1929) Some chemical factors in the control of the circulation. Lancet 1, 1285–1290.

24. Davies, P., and Allison, A. C. (1976) Secretion of macrophage enzymes in relation to the pathogenesis of chronic inflammation. In: D. S. Nelson (ed.), Immunobiology of the Macrophage, Academic Press, New York, pp. 427–461.

25. Davies, P., Bonney, R. J., Humes, J. L., and Kuehl, F. A. (1977) Synthesis and release of oxygenation products of arachidonic acid by mononuclear phagocytes in response to inflammatory stimuli. Inflammation 2, 335–344.

26. Dayer, J. M., Robinson, D. R., and Krane, S. M. (1977) Prostaglandin production by rheumatoid synovial cells. Stimulation by a factor from human mononuclear cells. J. Exp. Med. 145, 1399–1404.

27. Diaz-Perez, J. L., Goldyne, M. E., and Winkelmann, R. K. (1976) Prostaglandins and chemotaxis: Enhancement of polymorphonuclear leukocyte chemotaxis by prostaglandin F₂α. J. Invest. Dermatol. 66, 149–152.

28. Di Pasquale, G., Rassaert, C., Righter, R., Welaj, P., and Tripp, L. (1973) Influence of PGE₂ and PGF₂α on the inflammatory process. Prostaglandins 3, 741–757.

29. Di Rosa, M., Giroud, J. P., and Willoughby, D. A. (1971) Studies of the mediators of acute inflammatory response induced in rats in different sites by carrageenan and turpentine. J. Pathol. 104, 15–29.

30. Dusting, G. J., Moncada, S., and Vane, J. R. (1978) Vascular actions of arachidonic acid and its metabolites in perfused mesenteric and femoral beds of the dog. Eur. J. Pharmacol. 49, 65–72.

31. Egan, R. W., Paxton, J., and Kuehl, F. A. (1976) Mechanism for irreversible self-deactivation of prostaglandin synthetase. J. Biol. Chem. 251, 7329–7335.

32. Egan, R. W., Gale, P. H., and Kuehl, F. A. (1977) The influence of oxidizing radicals and radical scavengers on prostaglandin biosynthesis. Prostaglandins 14, 183–184.

33. Egan, R. W., Humes, J. L., and Kuehl, F. A. (1978) Differential effects of prostaglandin synthetase stimulators on inhibition of cyclooxygenase. Biochemistry 17, 2230–2234.

34. Egan, R. W., Gale, P. H., Beveridge, G. C., Phillips, G. B., and Marnett, L. J. (1978) Radical scavenging as the mechanism for stimulation of prostaglandin cyclooxygenase and depression of inflammation by lipoic acid and sodium iodide. Prostaglandins 16, 861–869.

35. Farzad, A., Penneys, N. S., Ghaffar, A., Zibooh, V. A., and Schlossberg, J. (1977) PGE_2 and $PGF_{2\alpha}$ biosynthesis in stimulated and non-stimulated peritoneal preparations containing macrophages. Prostaglandins 14, 829–837.

36. Ferraris, V. A., De Rubertis, F. R., Hudson, T. H., and Wolfe, L. S. (1974) Release of prostaglandin by mitogen and antigen-stimulated leukocytes in culture. J. Clin. Invest. 54, 539–546.

37. Ferreira, S. H. (1972) Prostaglandins, aspirin-like drugs and analgesia. Nature (London) New Biol. 240, 200–203.

38. Ferreira, S. H., and Nakamura, M. (1979) Humoral mediators of pain. In: G. Weissman, R. Paoletti, and B. Samuelsson (eds.), Advances in Inflammation Research, Raven Press, New York.

39. Ferreira, S. H., Nakamura, M., and Castro, M. S. A. (1978) The hyperalgesic effects of prostacyclin and prostaglandin E_2. Prostaglandins 16, 31–37.

40. Ford-Hutchinson, A. W., Smith, M. J. H., and Walker, J. R. (1976) Effects of indomethacin on prostaglandin levels and leucocyte migration in an inflammatory exudate in vivo. J. Pharmacol. 57, 467.

41. Fridovich, I. (1975) Superoxide dismutases. Annu. Rev. Biochem. 44, 147–159.

42. Glenn, E. M., and Rohloff, N. (1972) Antiarthritic and anti-inflammatory effects of certain prostaglandins. Proc. Soc. Exp. Biol. Med. 139, 290–294.

43. Goetzl, E. J., and Gorman, R. R. (1978) Chemotactic and chemokinetic stimulation of human eosinophil and neutrophil polymorphonuclear leukocytes by 12-L-hydroxy-5,8,10-heptadecatrienoic acid (HHT). J. Immunol. 120, 526–531.

44. Goetzl, E. J., and Sun, F. F. (1979) Generation of unique monohydroxyeicosatetraenoic acids from arachidonic acid by human neutrophils. J. Exp. Med. 150, 406–412.

45. Goldstein, I. M., Malmsten, C. L., Samuelsson, B., and Weissmann, G. (1977) Prostaglandins, thromboxanes and polymorphonuclear leukocytes. Mediation and modulation of inflammation. Inflammation 2, 309–317.

46. Gordon, D., Bray, M. A., and Morley, J. (1976) Control of lymphokine production by prostaglandins. Nature (London) 262, 401–402.

47. Gryglewski, R. J., Panczenko, B., Korbut, R., Grodzinska, L., and Ocetkiewicz, A. (1975) Corticosteroids inhibit prostaglandin release from perfused mesenteric blood vessels of rabbit and from perfused lungs of sensitized guinea pig. Prostaglandins 10, 343–355.

48. Hahn, B. H. (1975) Cell mediated immunity in systemic lupus erythematosus. Clin. Rheum. Dis. 1, 497.

49. Halushka, P. V., Daniell, H. B., Miller, W. L., and Thibodeaux, H. (1977) Increased coronary sinus prostaglandin E-like material (iPGE) during myocardial infarction: Beneficial effects of aspirin. Clin. Res. 25, 225A.

50. Hatch, G. E., Nichols, W. K., and Hill, H. R. (1977) Cyclic nucleotide changes in human neutrophils induced by chemoattractants and chemotactic modulators. J. Immunol. 119(2), 450–456.

51. Hedqvist, P. (1970) Studies on the effect of prostaglandins E_1 and E_2 on the sympathetic neuromuscular transmission in some animal tissues. Acta Physiol. Scand. 345 (Suppl. 79), 1–40.

52. Henney, C. S., Bourne, H. R., and Lichtenstein, L. M. (1972) The role of cyclic AMP in the specific cytolytic activity of lymphocytes. J. Immunol. 108, 1526–1534.

53. Higgs, G. A., Vane, J. R., Hart, F. D., and Wojtulewski, J. A. (1974) Effects of antiinflammatory drugs on prostaglandins in rheumatoid arthritis. In: H. J. Robinson and J. R. Vane (eds.), Prostaglandin Synthetase Inhibitors—Their effects on Physiological Functions and Pathological States, Raven Press, New York, p. 165.

54. Higgs, G. A., Moncada, S., and Vane, J. R. (1978) Prostacyclin as a potent dilator of arterioles in the hamster cheek pouch. J. Physiol. 275, 30P.

55. Higgs, G. A., Moncada, S., and Vane, J. R. (1978) Inflammatory effects of prostacyclin (PGI_2) and 6-oxo-$PGF_{1\alpha}$ in the rat paw. Prostaglandins 16, 153–162.

56. Horton, E. W. (1963) Action of prostaglandin E_1 on tissues which respond to bradykinin. Nature (London) 200, 892–893.

57. Horton, E. W., Jones, R. L., and Marr, C. G. (1973) Effects of aspirin on prostaglandin and fructose levels in human semen. J. Reprod. Fertil. 33, 385–392.

58. Humes, J. L., Bonney, R. J., Pelus, L., Dahlgren, M. E., Kuehl, F. A., and Davies, P. (1977) Macrophages synthesize and release prostaglandins in response to inflammatory stimuli. Nature (London) 269, 149–151.

59. Ichikawa, A., Nagasaki, M., Umezu, K., Hayashi, H., and Tomita, K. (1972) Effect of cyclic AMP on edema and granuloma induced by carrageenan. Biochem. Pharmacol. 21, 2615–2626.

60. Jakschik, B. A., Falkenhein, S., and Parker, C. W. (1977) Precursor role of arachidonic acid in slow reacting substance release from rat basophilic leukemia cells. Proc. Natl. Acad. Sci. (US) 74, 4577–4581.

61. Kaley, G., and Weiner, R. (1971) Effect of prostaglandin E_1 on leukocyte migration. Nature (London) New Biol. 234, 114.

62. Kantrowitz, F., Robinson, D. R., McGuire, M. B., and Levine, L. (1975) Corticosteroids inhibit prostaglandin production by rheumatoid synovia. Nature (London) 258, 737–739.

63. Kayashima, K., Koga, T., and Onoue, K. (1976) Role of T lymphocytes in adjuvant arthritis. I. Evidence for the regulatory function of thymus-derived cells in induction of the disease. J. Immunol. 117, 1878–1882.

64. Kitchen, E. A., Boot, J. R., and Dawson, W. (1978) Chemotactic activity of thromboxane A_2 for polymorphonuclear leukocytes. Prostaglandins 16, 239–244.

65. Kocsis, J. J., Hernandovich, J., Silver, M. J., Smith, J. B., and Ingerman, C. (1973) Duration of inhibition of platelet prostaglandin formation and aggregation by ingested aspirin or indomethacin. Prostaglandins 3, 141–144.

66. Korn, J. H., Halushka, P. V., and LeRoy, E. C. (1978) Suppression of growth and the phenotype expression of fibroblasts by peripheral blood mononuclear cell supernatants: A role for prostaglandins. Arthritis Rheum. 21, 571.

67. Krakauer, K. A., Torrey, S. B., and Zurier, R. B. (1978) Prostaglandin E_1 treatment of NZB/W mice. III. Preservation of spleen cell concentrations and mitogen-induced proliferative responses. Clin. Immunol. Immunopathol. 11, 256–266.

68. Kuehl, F. A., Humes, J. L., Egan, R. W., Ham, E. A., Beveridge, G. C., and Van Arman, C. G. (1977) Role of prostaglandin endoperoxide in inflammatory processes. Nature (London) 265, 170–173.

69. Kuehl, F. A., Humes, J. L., Torchiana, M. L., Ham, E. A., and Egan, R. W. (1979) Oxygen centered radicals in inflammatory processes. In: G. Weissmann, R. Paoletti, and B. Samuelsson (eds.), Advances in Inflammation Research, Raven Press, New York, pp. 419–430.

70. Kunkel, S. L., Thrall, R. S., McCormick, J. R., Ward, P. A., and Zurier, R. B. (1979) Suppression of immune complex vasculitis in rats by prostaglandins. J. Clin. Invest. 64, 1525–1529.

71. Kurland, J. I., and Bockman, R. (1978) Prostaglandin E production by human blood monocytes and mouse peritoneal macrophages. J. Exp. Med. 147, 952–957.

72. Lewis, G. P., and Piper, P. J. (1975) Inhibition of release of prostaglandins as an explanation of some of the actions of anti-inflammatory corticosteroids. Nature (London) 254, 308–310.

73. Lewis, A. J., Nelson, D. J., and Sugrue, M. F. (1975) On the ability of prostaglandin E_1 and arachidonic acid to modulate experimentally-induced oedema in the rat paw. Br. J. Pharmacol. 55, 51–56.

74. Lewis, G. P., Westwick, J., and Williams, T. J. (1977) Microvascular responses produced by the prostaglandin endoperoxide PGG_2 in vivo. Br. J. Pharmacol. 59, 442P.

75. Lichtenstein, L. M., and Di Bernardo, R. (1971) The immediate allergic response: In vitro action of cyclic AMP active and other drugs on the two stages of histamine release. J. Immunol. 107, 1131–1136.

76. Majerus, P. W., and Stanford, N. (1977) Comparative effects of aspirin and diflusional on prostaglandin synthetase from human platelets and sheep seminal vesicles. Br. J. Clin. Pharmacol. 4, 155–185.

77. Marnett, L. J., Wlodawer, P., and Samuelsson, B. (1975) Co-oxygenation of organic substrates by the prostaglandin synthetase of sheep vesicular gland. J. Biol. Chem. 250, 8510–8517.

78. Marnett, L. J., and Wilcox, C. L. (1977) Stimulation of prostaglandin biosynthesis by lipoic acid. Biochim. Biophys. Acta 487, 222–230.

79. McCall, E., and Youlten, L. J. F. (1973) Prostaglandin E_1 synthesis by phagocytosing rabbit polymorphonuclear leucocytes: Its inhibition by indomethacin and its role in chemotaxis. J. Physiol. 98P–99P.

80. McCall, E., and Youlten, L. J. F. (1974) The effects of indomethacin and depletion of complement on cell migration and prostaglandin levels in carageenan-induced air bleb inflammation. Br. J. Pharmacol. 52, 452P.

81. McClatchney, W., and Snyderman, R. (1976) Prostaglandins and inflammation: Enhancement of monocyte chemotactic responsiveness by prostaglandin E_2. Prostaglandins 12, 415–426.

82. Moncada, S., Ferreira, S. H., and Vane, J. R. (1973) Prostaglandins, aspirin-like drugs and the oedema of inflammation. Nature (London) 246, 217–219.

83. Moncada, S., and Vane, J. R. (1979) The role of prostacyclin in vascular tissue. Fed. Proc. 38, 66.

84. Murota, S. I., Abe, M., and Otsuka, K. (1977) Stimulatory effect of prostaglandins on the production of hexosamine-containing substances by cultured fibroblasts. III. Induction of hyaluronic acid synthetase by prostaglandin $F_{2\alpha}$. Prostaglandins 14, 983–991.

85. Murota, S., Morita, I., Tsurufuji, S., Sato, H., and Sugio, K. (1978) Effect of prostaglandin I_2 and related compounds on vascular permeability response in granuloma tissues. Prostaglandins 15, 297–301.

86. Murota, S., Chang, W. C., Tsurufuji, S., and Morita, I. (1979) The possible roles of prostacyclin (PGI_2) and thromboxanes in chronic inflammation. In: G. Weissman, R. Paoletti, and B. Samuelsson (eds.), Advances in Inflammation Research, Raven Press, New York, pp. 439–456.

87. Myatt, L., Bray, M. A., Gordon, D. A., and Morley, J. (1975) Macrophages on intra-uterine contraceptive devices produce prostaglandins. Nature (London) 257, 227–228.

88. Newcombe, D. S., and Ishikawa, Y. (1976) The effect of anti-inflammatory agents on human synovial fibroblast prostaglandin synthetase. Prostaglandins 12, 849–869.

89. Oelz, O., Oelz, R., Knapp, H. R., Sweetman, B. J., and Oates, J. A. (1977) Biosynthesis of prostaglandin D_2. Formation of prostaglandin D_2 by human platelets. Prostaglandins 13, 225–234.

90. Ohmori, H., Komoriya, K., Azuma, A., Hashimoto, Y., and Kurozumi, S. (1978) Xanthine oxidase-induced foot edema in rats: Involvement of oxygen radicals. Biochem. Pharmacol. 27, 1397–1400.

91. Orange, R. P., Austen, W. G., and Austen, K. F. (1971) Immunological release of histamine and slow reacting substance of anaphylaxis from human lung. I. Modulation by agents influencing cellular levels of cyclic AMP. J. Exp. Med. 134, 136S–148S.

92. Oyanagui, Y. (1976) Participation of superoxide anions at the prostaglandin phase of carrageenan foot oedema. Biochem. Pharmacol. 25, 1465–1472.

93. Parnham, M. J., Shoshan, S., Bonta, I. L., and Neiman-Wollner, S. (1977) Increased collagen metabolism in granulomata induced in rats deficient in endogenous prostaglandin precursors. Prostaglandins 14, 709–714.

94. Parnham, M. J., Bonta, I. L., and Adolfs, J. P. (1978) Cyclic AMP and prostaglandin E_1 in perfusates of rat hind paws during the development of adjuvant arthritis. Ann. Rheum. Dis. 37, 218–224.

95. Patrono, C., Ciabuttoni, G., Greco, F., and Grossi-Belloni, D. (1976) Comparative evaluation of the inhibitory effects of aspirin-like drugs on prostaglandin production by human platelets and synovial tissue. In: B. Samuelsson and R. Paoletti (eds.), Advances in Prostaglandin and Thromboxane Research, Vol. 1, Raven Press, New York, pp. 125–131.

96. Peck, M. J., and Williams, T. J. (1978) Prostacyclin (PGI_2) potentiates histamine-induced plasma exudation in rabbit skin. Br. J. Pharmacol. 62, 464P–465P.

97. Penneys, N. S., Ziboh, V., Gottlieb, N., and Katz, S. (1974) Inhibition of prostaglandin synthesis and human epidermal enzymes by aurothiomalate in vitro: Possible actions of gold in pemphigus. J. Invest. Dermatol. 63, 356–361.

98. Penneys, N. S., Simon, P., Ziboh, V. A., and Schlossberg, J. (1977) In vivo chemotaxis induced by polyunsaturated fatty acids. J. Invest. Dermatol. 69, 435–438.

99. Perez, H. D., Weksler, B. B., and Goldstein, I. M. (1979) A new mechanism for the generation of biologically active products from arachidonic acid. Clin. Res. 27, 464A.

100. Peters, H. D., Peskar, B. A., and Schönhöfer, P. S. (1977) Influence of prostaglandins on connective tissue cell growth and function. Naunyn-Schmiedebergs Arch. Pharmacol. 297, 589–593.

101. Raisz, L. G., Sandberg, A. L., Goodson, J. M., Simmons, H. A., and Mergenhagen, S. E. (1974) Complement dependent stimulation of prostaglandin synthesis and bone resorption. Science 185, 789–791.

102. Raisz, L. G., Dietrich, J. W., Simmons, H. A., Seyberth, H. W., Hubbard, W., and Oates, J. A. (1977) Effect of prostaglandin endoperoxides and metabolites on bone resorption in vitro. Nature (London) 267, 532–534.

103. Rivkin, I., and Becker, E. L. (1975) Effect of exogenous cyclic AMP and other adenine nucleotides on neutrophil chemotaxis and motility. Int. Arch. Allergy Appl. Immunol. 50, 95–102.

104. Rivkin, I., Rosenblatt, J., and Becker, E. L. (1975) The role of cyclic AMP in the chemotactic responsiveness and spontaneous motility of rabbit peritoneal neutrophils. The inhibition of neutrophil movement and the elevation of cyclic AMP levels by catecholamines, prostaglandins, theophylline and cholera toxin. J. Immunol. 115, 1126–1134.

105. Roberts, L. J., Lewis, R. A., Lawson, J. A., Sweetman, B. J., Austen, K. F., and Oates, J. A. (1978) Arachidonic acid metabolism by rat mast cells. Prostaglandins 15, 717.

106. Robinson, D. R., McGuire, M. B., and Levine, L. (1975) Prostaglandins in the rheumatic diseases. Ann. NY Acad. Sci. 256, 318–329.

107. Robinson, D. R., Bustian, D., and Servello, L. (1979) Mechanism of corticosteroid inhibition of prostaglandin synthesis by rheumatoid synovial tissue. Arthritis Rheum. 22:650 (abst).

108. Schönhöfer, P. S., Peters, H. D., Wasmus, A., Peskar, B. A., Von Figura, K., Klappstein, I., (1978) Prostaglandins, cyclic nucleotides, and glycosaminoglycan biosynthesis in cultured fibroblasts. Pol. J. Pharmacol. Pharm. 30, 183–193.

109. Smith, J. B., and Willis, A. L. (1971) Aspirin selectively inhibits prostaglandin production in human platelets. Nature (London) New Biol. 231, 235–237.

110. Smith, W. L., and Lands, W. E. M. (1972) Oxygenation of polyunsaturated fatty acids during prostaglandin biosynthesis by sheep vesicular gland. Biochemistry 11, 3276–3285.

111. Smith, M. J. H. (1975) Prostaglandins and aspirin: An alternative view. Agents Actions 5, 315–317.

112. Sobotka, R., Marone, G., and Lichtenstein, L. (1978) Arachidonic acid metabolism and basophil histamine release. Paper presented at National Institutes of Health Meeting on Asthma and Allergic Disease Program.

113. Stern, P. H., and Raisz, L. G. (1967) An analysis of the role of serum in parathyroid hormone-induced bone resorption in tissue culture. Exp. Cell Res. 46, 106–120.

114. Stone, K. J., Mather, S. J., and Gibson, P. P. (1975) Selective inhibition of prostaglandin biosynthesis by gold salts and phenylbutazane. Prostaglandins 10, 244–251.

115. Talal, N. (1975) Animal models for systemic lupus erythematosus. Clin. Rheum. Dis. 1, 485–492.

116. Tashjian, A. J., Voelkel, E. F., McDonough, J., and Levine, L. (1975) Hydrocortisone inhibits prostaglandin production by mouse fibrosarcoma cells. Nature (London) 258, 739–741.

117. Thomas, G., and West, G. B. (1973) Prostaglandins as regulators of bradykinin responses. J. Pharm. Pharmacol. 25, 747–748.

118. Till, G., Kownatzki, E., Seitz, M., Gemsa, D. (1979) Chemokinetic and chemotactic activity of various prostaglandins for neutrophil granulocytes. Clin. Immunol. Immunopathol. 12, 111–118.

119. Trang, L. E. (1977) Joint fluid levels of prostaglandins ($PGF_{2\alpha}$, PGE_2), thromboxanes (TxB_2), and cyclic nucleotides (cAMP, cGMP) in rheumatoid arthritis. Abstracts, Fourteenth International Congress on Rheumatology, San Francisco, p. 234.

120. Turner, S. R., Campbell, J. A., and Lynn, W. S. (1975) Polymorphonuclear chemotaxis toward oxidized lipid components of cell membranes. J. Exp. Med. 141, 1437–1441.

121. Vane, J. (1976) Prostaglandins as mediators of inflammation. In: B. Samuelsson and R. Paoletti (eds.), Advances in Prostaglandin and Thromboxane Research, Vol. 2, Raven Press, New York, p. 791.

122. Vane, J. R. (1971) Inhibition of prostaglandin synthesis as a mechanism of action for aspirinlike drugs. Nature (London) New Biol. 231, 232–235.

123. Velo, G. P., Dunn, C. J., Giroud, J. P., Timsit, J., and Willoughby, D. A. (1973) Distribution of prostaglandins in inflammatory exudate. J. Pathol. 111, 149–157.

124. Voorhees, J. J. (1977) Pathophysiology of psoriasis. Annu. Rev. Med. 28, 467–473.

125. Walker, J. R., Smith, M. J. H., and Ford-Hutchinson, A. W. (1976) Antiinflammatory drugs. Prostaglandins and leucocyte migration. Agents Actions 6, 602–606.

126. Weissmann, G. (1972) Lysosomal mechanisms of tissue injury in arthritis. New Engl. J. Med. 286, 141–144.

127. Weksler, B. B., Knapp, J. M., and Jaffe, E. A. (1977) Prostacyclin (PGI_2) synthesized by cultured endothelial cells modulates polymorphonuclear leukocyte functions. Blood 50 (Suppl. 1), 287–294.

128. Williams, T. J., and Morley, J. (1973) Prostaglandins as potentiators of increased vascular permeability in inflammation. Nature (London) 246, 215–217.

129. Williams, T. J. (1976) The pro-inflammatory activity of E-, A-, D- and F-type prostaglandins and analogues 16,16-dimethyl-PGE_2 and (15S)-15-methyl-PGE_2 in rabbit skin; The relationship between potentiation of plasma exudation and local blood flow changes. Br. J. Pharmacol. 56, 341P–342P.

130. Williams, T. J., and Peck, M. J. (1977) Role of prostaglandin mediated vasodilation in inflammation. Nature (London) 270, 530–532.

131. Williams, T. J. (1979) Prostaglandin E_2, prostaglandin I_2 and the vascular changes of inflammation. Br. J. Pharmacol. 65, 517–524.

132. Willis, A. L. (1978) Platelet aggregation mechanisms and their implications in haemostasis and inflammatory disease. In: S. H. Ferreira and J. R. Vane (eds.), Inflammation, Handbook of Experimental Pharmacology, Springer-Verlag, Berlin, pp. 138–205.

133. Willis, A. L., and Cornelsen, M. (1973) Repeated injections of prostaglandin E_2 in rat paw induces chronic swelling and marked decrease in pain threshold. Prostaglandins 3, 353–357.

134. Yoneda, T., and Mundy, G. R. (1979) Prostaglandins are necessary for osteoclast activating factor production by activated peripheral blood leukocytes. J. Exp. Med. 149, 279–283.

135. Yoneda, T., and Mundy, G. R. (1979) Monocytes regulate osteoclast-activating factor production by releasing prostaglandins. J. Exp. Med. 150, 338–350.

136. Ziboh, V. A., and Hsia, S. L. (1972) Effects of prostaglandin E_2 on rat skin: Inhibition of sterol ester biosynthesis and clearing of scaly lesions in essential fatty acid deficiency. J. Lipid Res. 13, 458–467.

137. Ziboh, V. A., Vanderhoek, J. T., and Lands, W. M. (1974) Inhibition of sheep vesicular gland oxygenase by unsaturated fatty acids from skin of essential fatty acid deficient rats. Prostaglandins 5, 233–240.

138. Zurier, R. B., and Quagliata, F. (1971) Effect of prostaglandin E_1 on adjuvant arthritis. Nature (London) 234, 304–305.

139. Zurier, R. B., and Ballas, M. (1973) Prostaglandin E_1 suppression of adjuvant arthritis: Histopathology. Arthritis Rheum. 16, 251–258.

140. Zurier, R. B., Hoffstein, S., and Weissmann, G. (1973) Suppression of acute and chronic inflammation in adrenalectomized rats by pharmacologic amounts of prostaglandins. Arthritis Rheum. 16, 606–615.

141. Zurier, R. B., Weissman, G., Hoffstein, S., Kammerman, S., and Tai, H. H. (1974) Mechanisms of lysosomal enzyme release from human leukocytes. II. Effects of cAMP and cGMP, autonomic agonists and agents which affect microtubule function. J. Clin. Invest. 53, 297–309.

142. Zurier, R. B., Cosgrove, J. M., and Hinz, C. F. (1975) Enhancement by cyclic AMP and prostaglandin E_1 of cytotoxicity mediated by human monocytes. Fed. Proc. 34:1029 (abst)

143. Zurier, R. B. (1976) Prostaglandin release from human polymorphonuclear leukocytes. In: B. Samuelsson and R. Paoletti (eds.), Advances in Prostaglandin and Thromboxane Research, Vol. 2, Raven Press, New York, pp. 815–818.

144. Zurier, R. B., Doty, J., and Goldenberg, A. (1977) Cyclic AMP response to prostaglandin E_1 in mononuclear cells from peripheral blood and synovial fluid of patients with rheumatoid arthritis. Prostaglandins 13, 25–31.

145. Zurier, R. B., Damjanov, I., Sayadoff, D. M., and Rothfield, N. F. (1977) Prostaglandin E_1 treatment of NZB/NZW F_1 hybrid mice. II. Prevention of glomerulonephritis. Arthritis Rheum. 20, 1449–1456.

146. Zurier, R. B., Damjanov, I., Miller, P. L., and Biewer, B. F. (1979) Prostaglandin E_1 treatment prevents progression of nephritis in murine lupus erythematosus. J. Clin. Lab. Immunol. 2, 95–98.

147. Zurier, R. B., and Ramwell, P. W. (1981) Prostaglandins in cutaneous pathophysiology. In: B. Safai and R. Good (eds.), Immunodermatology, Plenum Medical Book Company, New York, pp. 161–176.

ANDRE ROBERT, M.D., Ph.D.

MARY J. RUWART, Ph.D.

EFFECTS OF PROSTAGLANDINS ON THE DIGESTIVE SYSTEM

INTRODUCTION

Several prostaglandins that have been isolated from the gastrointestinal tract in rather large amounts in comparison to amounts extracted from other tissues have been found to influence gastrointestinal functions. Certain properties suggest a role for prostaglandins as therapeutic agents. This chapter reviews the effects of these substances on the morphology and functions of the gastrointestinal tract, and on bile and pancreatic secretion, and discusses the clinical implications of these findings.

PRESENCE OF PROSTAGLANDINS IN THE GASTROINTESTINAL TRACT

Several prostaglandins (PGs) have been identified in the gastrointestinal tract of several species. Table 1 lists the various PGs extracted from the major segments of the gastrointestinal tract. Enzymes responsible for generation as well as degradation of PGs have been identified in the

From the Department of Experimental Biology, The Upjohn Company, Kalamazoo, Michigan.

TABLE 1. Prostaglandins Identified in the Gastrointestinal Tract

	PGD_2	PGE	PGE_1	PGE_2	PGE_3	$PGF_{1\alpha}$	$PGF_{2\alpha}$	$PGF_{3\alpha}$	6-Keto-1 $PGF_{1\alpha}$	TXB_2
Stomach	26,232, 480	29	24,29	26,29, 79,232, 327, 334, 480			26,79, 232,327, 334,480		301, 328, 329	480
Jejunum	232	14,148								
Ileum		14,24, 29		254, 475			14,475			
Colon	232	29,297	29	29,232	29	29	29,232	29		
Gastric juice		10,11, 69,176, 435	24	79			79			
Small intestinal secretion		33								

Note: Numbers indicate literature cited in References.

stomach [17,419]. The PG cyclooxygenase was found exclusively in the lamina propria, not in the epithelial cells. In rabbits, the 15-hydroxy dehydrogenase, which transforms the 15-hydroxy into 15-keto derivatives, and the D^{13}-reductase, which reduces the 13,14 double bond, were nine times and seven times, respectively, more abundant in the antrum than in the fundus [419,420].

EFFECT OF PROSTAGLANDINS ON SECRETION

Salivation

Intravenous injection of $PGF_{2\alpha}$ (1–16 µg/kg) in the anesthetized dog produced dose-dependent increases in salivation that were augmented by physostigmine, abolished by atropine, and unaffected by phentolamine [166]. Injection of $PGF_{2\alpha}$ into the facial artery of anesthetized dogs caused salivation that could be blocked by tetrodotoxin [167,428] or 1-hyoscyamine [427]. $PGF_{2\beta}$ (10–500 µg/dog) was less potent in producing salivation than $PGF_{2\alpha}$, and 15-epi-$PGF_{2\alpha}$ (1–500 µg/dog) was ineffective [167]. $PGF_{1\alpha}$ (0.3–100 nmole/dog) was one one-hundredth as potent as $PGF_{2\alpha}$ in increasing salivation when administered via the glandular artery of dog mandibular gland. This response was also inhibited by 1-hyoscyamine and tetrodotoxin [426]. PGE_2 administered via the artery supplying the mandibular gland was about one three-hundredth as potent as $PGF_{2\alpha}$ in producing salivation that was blocked by tetrodotoxin pretreatment [426,429]. The salivary response to PGE_1 and PGE_2 could not

bated rat gastric mucosa secretes acid in response to histamine, pentagastrin, or methacholine added to the serosal bathing solution. Addition of PGE_1 or PGE_2 reduced the effect of these three secretogogues [275]. The uptake of aminopyrine by isolated canine parietal cells is a measure of acid secretion by these cells [413]. The increased aminopyrine uptake was inhibited by PGE_2, as well as the increase in cyclic AMP induced by histamine [414,415].

HUMAN STUDIES

PGE_1, PGE_2, and PGA_1, administered intravenously, inhibited both basal gastric acid secretion [76,449] and secretion stimulated by pentagastrin [75,313], tetragastrin [449], or histamine [467,468]. As in animals, the effect lasted as long as the PG was infused, and secretion returned to normal within 1 hour postinfusion. After oral administration, none of these natural prostaglandins (PGE_1, PGE_2, PGA_1) inhibited gastric acid secretion [34,185,217]; PGA_2 produced a transient inhibition of basal secretion [34]. $PGF_{2\alpha}$, given intravenously, had no effect on basal and maximal secretion (pentagastrin), although it produced a transient inhibition of submaximal acid secretion [313]. Oral administration of certain methyl analogues of PGE_2 inhibited both basal and stimulated (pentagastrin, histamine, food) secretion, and the effect lasted 3–5 hours, depending on the dose. Such inhibition was demonstrated for 15(R)-15-methyl PGE_2 [58,217,218,221,234,239,335], 15(S)-15-methyl PGE_2 [217, 239,320,323,366], and 16,16-dimethyl PGE_2 [219,220,233,239,320,366] against pentagastrin, for 16,16-dimethyl PGE_2 against histamine [469, 470] and food [194,239], and for 11,16,16-trimethyl PGE_2 against histamine [471]. These analogues also inhibited basal acid secretion [4,217]. Given orally, 15(R)-15-methyl PGE_2 inhibited acid secretion (basal and pentagastrin stimulated) in duodenal ulcer patients [68].

ROLE OF CYCLIC AMP IN THE ANTISECRETORY EFFECT
OF PROSTAGLANDINS

The initial observation [332] that PGE_1 stimulates adenylyl cyclase activity in the guinea pig gastric mucosa was confirmed with other PGs and in other species [473]. It has led to the hypothesis that the antisecretory effect of PGs may be mediated by an increase in gastric cyclic AMP. Prostaglandins known to inhibit gastric acid secretion increased adenyl cyclase activity in the dog corpus, whereas $PGF_{2\alpha}$, which is not antisecretory, produced very slight stimulation; arachidonic acid did not stimulate enzyme activity [108]. Human biopsy samples were examined for adenylyl cyclase activity. When either histamine or PGE_2 was added in vitro, enzyme activity was increased. Addition of cimetidine blocked the effect of histamine, but not that of PGE_2 [407].

More recently, PGE_1 and PGE_2, administered at gastric antisecretory doses either intravenously or directly into the gastric mucosal circulation, did not significantly alter antral or fundic mucosal cyclic nucleotide concentration (cyclic AMP and cyclic GMP) [266]. Using in vitro frog gastric mucosal preparations, no correlation was found between gastric acid secretion and cyclic AMP [68]. Moreover, neither dibutyryl cyclic AMP nor inhibitors of phosphodiesterase (theophylline and papaverine) initiated acid secretion in dogs [284]. These findings, plus the fact that the mucosal level of cyclic AMP can be raised by either inhibitors or stimulators of acid secretion [433], challenged the validity of the hypothesis invoking a mediating role for cyclic AMP in the antisecretory effect of PGs.

Improved techniques for obtaining isolated parietal cells have helped to clarify the role of PGE_2 on cyclic AMP and acid secretion. Acid secreted by viable isolated parietal cells was measured by the amount of aminopyrine picked up and trapped by these cells [413]. Histamine stimulated aminopyrine uptake and increased the cellular content of cyclic AMP, and these two effects were blocked by adding PGE_2 [414,415]. On the other hand, PGE_2 by itself stimulated cyclic AMP only in preparations that were poor in parietal cells, not in enriched preparations [415]. The increase in aminopyrine uptake by gastrin, carbachol, or dibutryl cyclic AMP was not inhibited by PGE_2. It was concluded that PGE_2 inhibits the response of isolated parietal cells to histamine by blocking histamine-stimulated cyclic AMP production.

Intestinal Secretion: Enteropooling and Diarrhea Produced by Prostaglandins

Most biologically active prostaglandins, when administered at high doses, can produce diarrhea in animals. This event occurs whether the PG is given orally or parenterally, usually 1–2 hours after treatment. Studies in dogs showed that the initial effect is a sudden and marked increase in accumulation of fluid in the small intestine. PGE_1 and $PGF_{2\alpha}$ given to dogs either intravenously or into the superior mesenteric artery supplying an isolated intestinal loop stimulated formation of intestinal fluid [159,339]. The concentrations of sodium, potassium, and chloride of this fluid were similar to those of plasma. These changes were later confirmed in humans with intrajejunal perfusion [90,286,287]. In these studies, PGE_1 and PGE_2 promoted active intestinal secretion and inhibited intestinal absorption of water and electrolytes. Absorption of glucose was also reduced by about 25% [287].

This phenomenon of fluid accumulation into the small intestine was called "enteropooling," and an assay was developed in rats to quantitate the enteropooling potency of PG [363]. The assay consists of administering a PG either orally or subcutaneously to rats previously fasted for 24 hours. The animals are killed 30 minutes later, at which time the entire small intestine, from the pylorus to the terminal ileum, is dissected out. Its contents, consisting of a thick fluid in controls and a very watery fluid in animals that received a high dose of PG, are collected into a graduated test tube by milking the whole length of the intestine with the fingers. The volume of fluid thus obtained is a direct measure of the enteropooling activity of the PG. The degree of enteropooling is related to the diarrheogenic property of a given PG. Although minimal diarrhea occurred during the 30 minutes required for the assay, diarrhea was observed when the animals were maintained for 1–2 hours after treatment with the PG, provided the dose was high enough. The incidence of diarrhea correlated well with the degree of enteropooling.

However, a contribution from increased propulsion must also be present, since in normal rats, transit from the stomach to the cecum is 2 hours (Ruwart, unpublished results) and movement from the cecum to excretion is in excess of 3 hours [382]. Thus, it is clear that in normal rats diarrhea one hour after PG treatment is indicative of accelerated small and large bowel transit in addition to an enteropooling effect. This stimulation of propulsion is probably attributable to a direct PG effect rather than to a distension phenomenon due to enteropooling, since tying the ileocecal junction did not alter the accelerated colonic transit seen after treatment with 16,16-dimethyl PGE_2 [381]. Antagonism of PG-induced stimulation of propulsion is discussed in the latter sections of this chapter dealing with the motility of the small and large bowel.

It appears, therefore, that after PG administration sudden enteropooling and increased gut transit occur; since the intestinal fluid keeps forming for 1–2 hours and is quickly propelled through the intestinal tract, reabsorption is limited and most of the fluid is expelled as diarrhea.

The mechanism of enteropooling by PG is similar to that of cholera toxin. Both agents stimulate function of cyclic AMP by the intestinal mucosa, and this latter compound is believed to be the mediator for enteropooling [230]. However, prostacyclin (PGI_2) and PGD_2, two other PGs that are potent stimulators of cyclic AMP in some other cells (e.g., blood platelets [151] and foreskin fibroblasts [151a]), are not enteropooling. In fact, PGI_2 and PGD_2 actually block the enteropooling caused by other PGs and even by cholera toxin [353,353a]. Whether PGI_2 and PGD_2 stimulate intestinal adenylyl cyclase is not known. If it is found they do, the postulate that PG-induced enteropooling is mediated by cyclic AMP must be reexamined.

Biliary Secretion

Various PGs affect biliary secretion differently depending on their chemical structure. Infusions of PGA_1 (2.5 µg/kg-min), for example, caused a ductal choleresis in dogs as evidenced by increased bicarbonate concentration accompanied by augmented sodium and chloride output [216]. The same dose of PGA_1 did not stimulate bile flow in isolated perfused canine liver [380], however, suggesting that the PG activity was mediated by extrahepatic factors such as release of other hormones, neural interaction, or modifications in mesenteric blood flow. PGA_1 probably does not act through secretin release, since it diminished choleresis produced by that hormone, but did not affect cholecystokinin-octapeptide-stimulated bile flow except to increase sodium output. PGA_1 (10 µg/kg-min) has been reported to increase bile flow in the anesthetized rat without modification of bile salt output [258]. Since bicarbonate was not measured in the latter study, the character of the choleretic increment (ductal or bile salt independent canalicular) is not known.

Both PGE_1 and PGE_2 (0.1 μg/kg-min) are ductal choleretics [252] in anesthetized cats. In anesthetized dogs, no choleresis or inhibition of secretin-stimulated bile flow was seen when PGE_2 was infused at 4.4 μg/kg-min [412], whereas a modest bicarbonate-enriched volume increase was observed in conscious dogs with PGE_1 (2.5 μg/kg-min) [216]. In isolated rat liver, however, PGE_1 (100–200 μg/hr) did not stimulate bile flow [265]. Intraperitoneal injection of PGE_1 or PGE_2 (0.1 μg) on alternate days for 2 weeks in guinea pigs resulted in lower volumes of bile flow than in vehicle-treated controls. Total biliary lipids were significantly lower in animals treated with PGE_1 than in the other two groups, although cholesterol concentration in bile was unaltered [376]. Intraarterial or intravenous infusions of $PGF_{2\alpha}$ (1, 2, 4, or 8 μg/kg-min) induced a canalicular choleresis in conscious dogs as evidenced by increased bile volume, chloride concentration and output, and lack of bicarbonate concentration increases [212]. Cyclic AMP concentration and output was also increased by $PGF_{2\alpha}$ [213,214]. Similar infusions of $PGF_{2\alpha}$ produced spasm in hepatic venous sphincters in perfused canine livers, which resulted in engorgement of the liver with blood, and had no choleretic effect on perfused porcine liver [380], again suggesting that the increases in bile flow due to in vivo administration of PG were mediated by an extrahepatic factor or changes in vascular blood flow, which was kept constant in perfusion experiments.

In unanesthetized dogs, 16,16-dimethyl PGE_2 (0.01, 0.1, or 1.0 μg/kg-min) did not produce any effect on bile flow or composition [215], while 16,16-dimethyl $PGF_{2\alpha}$ (0.01, 0.1, or 1.0 μg/kg-min) increased bile volume, bicarbonate concentration, and chloride concentration, while lowering bile salt and sodium concentrations. Erythritol clearance, however, was increased by 16,16-dimethyl $PGF_{2\alpha}$ [215]. These data suggest that 16,16-dimethyl $PGF_{2\alpha}$ stimulates a mixed choleresis, having both ductal- and bile salt–independent components.

Thus, acute PG administration appears to cause choleresis in most whole animal models, probably by a mechanism other than direct action on the hepatic biliary secretory apparatus. The changes in biliary composition appear to differ depending on the PG type.

Pancreatic Secretion

EFFECT OF PROSTAGLANDINS ON EXOCRINE SECRETION (PANCREATIC JUICE)

E-type Prostaglandins. PG infusion decreases basal, acid-stimulated, or secretin-stimulated pancreatic volume and bicarbonate output while elaborating enzyme secretion in vivo. Infusion of PGE_1 (2 μg/kg-min), for example, depressed acid-stimulated pancreatic volume and bicarbonate output in unanesthetized dogs with pancreatic fistulas. At least part of this antagonism could have been due to the observed depression of plasma secretin during the PG infusion [451]. When secretin was used as the pancreatic stimulus, PGE_1 infusions still inhibited the increased volume and bicarbonate output. Protein output during secretin infusion was enhanced by a bolus of PGE_1 (10 μg/kg), but the effect was not as dramatic as that seen with cholecystokinin (1 U/kg). The ED_{50} for these effects was 1.8 μg/kg-min for infusion; for a single injection it was 23 μg/kg [379]. 16,16-Dimethyl PGE_2, administered in graded intravenous doses (0.1, 0.3, 0.5, and 1.0 μg/kg), or intraduodenally (15, 30, 50, and 100 μg/kg), also inhibited volume and bicarbonate output in resting and secretin-stimulated canine pancreas, while elaborating enzyme output [377]. In rat, basal and ethanol-stimulated volume, bicarbonate output, and protein concentration were inhibited by intraduodenal, intravenous, or intraperitoneal injections of 16,16-dimethyl PGE_2 (0.5–20 μg/rat) [41]. Another synthetic PG, 15(S)-15-methyl-PGE_2 methyl ester (1 μg/kg-hr), did not affect pancreatic response to exogenous secretin or duodenal acidification in conscious cats [241]. However, the dose used was probably much smaller per unit time than that used in the aforementioned studies with bolus injection of 16,16-dimethyl PGE_2, a fact that might account for its lack of effect. In anesthetized cats, intraarterial injections of PGE_1 and PGE_2 (0.5–10 μg) diminished secretin-stimulated pancreatic secretion [59].

In humans, intragastric administration of 140 μg of 16,16-dimethyl PGE_2 decreased the amount of lipase recovered from the jejunum, suggesting a decrease in basal pancreatic output [115]. Konturek et al. [238], however, found no decrease in duodenal volume or bicarbonate during secretin infusion of patients treated with intragastric administration of 15(R)-15-methyl PGE_2 methyl ester or 16,16-dimethyl PGE_2 (1.5 μg/kg), although the enzyme output was increased.

The mechanism of PG effects on the pancreas is ill defined because other activities of these compounds, such as reduction of pancreatic blood flow, are known to occur [59,261,396]. Furthermore, PGE_1 and PGE_2 infused into the isolated perfused cat pancreas at a concentration of 3×10^{-7} M increased rather than decreased pancreatic volume and electrolytes. These effects were enhanced by the addition of theophylline, suggesting cyclic nucleotides as possible mediators of PG activity [59]. PGE_1 and PGE_2 (10^{-8} to 10^{-5} M) did not alter basal pancreatic protein secretion in isolated rat pancreas [174], in contrast to their in vivo effects [141]. Incubation of guinea pig pancreatic slices with PGE_1 (100 ng/ml), with or without cholecystokinin, did not produce a significant elevation of enzyme secretion [141]. The distinction between the in vitro and in vivo results suggests that the effects of PGE_1 and PGE_2 in vivo are not solely a function of direct PG action on the pancreas.

F-type Prostaglandins. Intraarterial $PGF_{2\alpha}$ (100 μg) antagonized secretin-induced pancreatic flow, but not dopamine-induced increases in anesthetized dogs [199]. In cats, intravenous or intraarterial injections of

$PGF_{1\alpha}$ and $PGF_{2\alpha}$ (0.5–10 µg) did not diminish secretin-induced pancreatic secretion or blood flow [59,400]. $PGF_{2\alpha}$ (10^{-8} to 10^{-5} M) did not alter protein release from exocrine rat pancreas [174]. PGF appears to be less potent than PGE in depressing pancreatic secretion in vivo.

Prostacyclin (PGI_2). In vivo studies with intravenous PGI_2 (1.25–20 µg/kg-hr) showed that this compound is capable of stimulating bicarbonate and enzyme secretion in the resting canine pancreas. The mild stimulation of bicarbonate contrasts with the inhibitory effects of the PGE compounds in the basal state. However, PGI_2 competitively inhibited secretin- and acid-induced bicarbonate secretion (ED_{50} was 9 µg/kg-hr for secretin and 4.5 µg/kg-hr for duodenal acid) [242].

EFFECT OF PROSTAGLANDINS ON ENDOCRINE SECRETION (PANCREATIC HORMONES)

Insulin. The effect of prostaglandins on insulin secretion is complex, but some generalizations can be made from existing data. The inhibition or release of insulin as a result of PG treatment is highly dependent on the preexisting glucose levels in vivo and in vitro. In humans, for example, intravenous PGE_2 (10 µg/min) [373] and PGE_1 (0.2 µg/kg-min) [146]) antagonized insulin release due to a glucose challenge, whereas $PGF_{2\alpha}$ (0.2 and 0.5 µg/kg-min) had no effect [146]. In fasted subjects, however, PGE_1 (0.2 µg/kg-min) exhibited no influence on insulin release [147], although plasma glucose increased [147] in one study and remained unchanged in another [53]. Glucose and insulin levels in fasted pregnant women were not affected by one-hour infusion of increasing doses of PGE_2 (0.3, 0.6, 1.2, and 2.4 µg/min) or $PGF_{2\alpha}$ (2.5, 5.0, 10.0, and 20.0 µg/min) [418]. Thus, at doses likely to be used clinically in fasted subjects, prostaglandins appear to have little effect on pancreatic insulin release. In dogs, intravenous PGA_1 (0.25 µg/kg-min) [388] and PGE_1 (10 µg/min) [374,375] decreased circulating insulin response to a glucose load. In fasted animals, however, increased insulin output was observed after cessation of a PGE_1 infusion (0.5 and 1 µg/kg-min), even though the output was unchanged during the infusion period [262].

In fasted rats, intravenous PGE_1 and PGE_2 (0.5 or 7 µg/kg-min) lowered plasma insulin and caused hyperglycemia [107,387]. Reserpine treatment did not block these effects [387]. PGA_1 infused at approximately 7 µg/kg-min but not at 0.5 µg/kg-min also depressed insulin release in fasted animals, but produced a hypoglycemic effect [107]. PGE_1 (0.5 µg/kg-min) did not modify insulin release following a glucose load in rats but did depress peripheral glucose uptake [107]. Insulin release during a glucose load was not altered by PGA_1 (0.5 µg/kg-min), but peripheral glucose uptake was enhanced [107]. In fasted rats, PGE_1 antagonized insulin responses to tolbutamide, glucagon, and aminophylline [387]. On the other hand, fasted mice treated with intraperitoneal PGE_1 (2.5 or 5 µg) exhibited hyperglycemia and increased plasma insulin. The latter effects were antagonized by β-adrenergic blockade [43]. Thus insulin responses to PG vary with species.

Changes in blood flow induced by PGs are unlikely to account for all these effects, since no correlation was found between the degree of hypotension produced by the PGs and their effects on insulin release [387,388]. Furthermore, insulin secretion was not influenced by hydralazine administered at a dose that induced a hypotension comparable to that of the PG [372]. Involvement of α-adrenergic activity is unlikely, since phentolamine did not affect insulin responses to PG [372,375,387]. The evidence for β-adrenergic involvement in insulin secretion [43] warrants further investigation.

In perfused rat pancreas, PGE_2 has been reported either to have no effect [257] or to cause release of [331] insulin. $PGF_{2\alpha}$ stimulated basal insulin release at low doses (1 μM) and inhibited it at high doses (10 μM) [257]. Glucose-stimulated insulin release was unaffected by $PGF_{2\alpha}$ but was inhibited by high doses (50 μg/ml) of indomethacin [257] and was stimulated by arachidonic acid [338]. The latter finding suggests the possibility of PG mediation of glucose-stimulated insulin release by perfused pancreas. Perhaps the hyperglycemia associated with PG administration in vivo is required for the depression of insulin release, since this hormone (1) was secreted by rat islets exposed to PGE_1 (10 μM) in the presence of a low glucose concentration (50 mg/100 ml) [51], (2) was unaffected by PGE_1 (10^{-8} to 10^{-5} M) at a moderate glucose concentration (150 mg/100 ml) [442], and (3) was depressed by PGE_1 (10^{-6} M) in the presence of 300 mg/100 ml of glucose [51]. Higher concentrations of PGE_1 and PGA_1 (10 μM) were reported to have no effect on insulin secretion by rat islets [378], but other investigators have suggested that such high doses may be less effective than lower doses in promoting insulin secretion in this model [206]. Interpretation of these results is further complicated by the observation that the addition of theophylline to the incubation media (containing glucose at 300 mg/ml) promotes rather than depresses release of insulin secretion when PGE_1, PGE_2, and $PGF_{2\alpha}$ (10^{-5} to 10^{-8} M) were added. In the presence of theophylline and 30 mg/100 ml glucose, no stimulation of insulin release was observed. PGA_1 did not affect insulin release at either glucose concentration [206]. Thus, cyclic nucleotides probably modulate PG effects. Adenylyl cyclase activity in isolated rat islets was stimulated by addition of PGE_1, PGE_2, and PGA_2, but not $PGF_{2\alpha}$, lending further support to this hypothesis [207].

There is some evidence that PGs may play a role in the glucose intolerance characteristic of adult-onset diabetes, since sodium salicylate, a PG synthesis inhibitor, restored the insulin response to a glucose pulse in such patients [289,373]. Indomethacin, however, lowered the insulin response to glucose in normal subjects but had no effect on those with maturity-onset diabetes [45]. The blood levels of PGE_2 and $PGF_{2\alpha}$, but not of PGE_1, were elevated in juvenile diabetes [64]. PG impairment of pancreatic insulin secretion or utilization may be a factor in disturbances of carbohydrate metabolism. There is also some evidence that PGE_2 may directly impair hepatic glucose utilization independent of its effects on pancreatic secretion [263,465]. More work needs to be done to determine the complex relationships between insulin secretion, prostaglandins, and glucose.

Glucagon. The effect of PGs on pancreatic glucagon secretion has not been well defined. In the fasted rat, PGE_1 infusion (2 $\mu g/min$) increased glucagon and glucose levels, whereas PGA_1 had no effect. The results were not altered by β-adrenergic blockade or sympathectomy [386]. In rat pancreas perfused with 100 mg/100 ml glucose, PGE_2 (10^{-6} M) resulted in increased glucagon levels, followed by a rise in insulin [331]. Arachidonic acid increased glucagon release by perfused rat pancreas [338]. In isolated rat islets bathed in 150 mg/100 ml glucose, PGE_1 (3 $\times$ 10^{-6} M) did not alter glucagon or insulin release [442]. In fasted humans, PGE_1 (0.2 $\mu g/kg$-min) increased glucagon and glucose levels without affecting plasma insulin [147]. PGE_1 at the same dose elevated glucagon responses to a glucose tolerance test while depressing insulin levels [375]. $PGF_{2\alpha}$ (0.2 and 0.5 $\mu g/kg$-min) had no effect on any of these parameters [375].

Thus, in all reports to date, PGE_1 appears to increase glucagon levels in perfused or in vivo pancreas. Elevations in plasma glucose accompany these increases in the fasted state. Insulin changes do not appear to be related to glucagon increases. In view of the stimulation of glucagon release from perfused pancreas treated with PG, direct action of these hormones on the pancreas is likely.

EFFECT OF PROSTAGLANDINS ON ULCER FORMATION

Since several prostaglandins inhibit gastric acid secretion, these substances were tested in experimental ulcer models and also in patients with peptic ulcer.

Animal Studies

Gastric ulcers were produced in rats and cats by various methods, and the prostaglandins were given orally, subcutaneously, or intravenously. Table 2, which lists the various studies performed and the PGs used, shows that PGs known to inhibit gastric acid secretion also inhibited ulcer formation. The same PGs were then tested against duodenal ulcers produced experimentally in animals. Table 3 lists the various studies performed, and the PGs used. As for gastric ulcers, PGs known to inhibit gastric acid secretion also prevented development of duodenal ulcers.

Human Studies

Several studies were performed in patients with either gastric or duodenal ulcers. Patients with gastric ulcers were given a single oral administration of 15(R)-15-methyl PGE_2 at a dose of 150 μg per patient. This

TABLE 2. Antiulcer Effects of Prostaglandins: Gastric Ulcers in Animals

Species	Ulcer model	Prostaglandin	Reference
Rat	Shay	15(R)-15-Methyl PGE$_2$	57
		PGE$_2$	260,368
		PGE$_1$	346,365
		16,16-Dimethyl PGE$_2$	355,368
		15(S)-15-Methyl PGE$_2$	368
			259
	Stress		
	Restraint	PGE$_1$	226
	Exertion	SC-24665	259
	Drugs		
	Bile salts	PGE$_2$	283
		15(R)-15-Methyl PGE$_2$	56
		15(S)-15-Methyl PGE$_2$	458
		16,16-Dimethyl PGE$_2$	66
	NOSAC*		
	Aspirin	PGE$_2$	84
		16,16-Dimethyl PGE$_2$	84,150,163,164,354
		15(R)-15-Methyl PGE$_2$	55a,84
		15(S)-15-Methyl PGE$_2$	55a
	Flurbiprofen	Various PGs	350
	Indomethacin	Various PGs	350
		PGE$_2$	12,101
		15(S)-15-Methyl PGE$_2$	457
		16,16-Dimethyl PGE$_2$	457
		PGI$_2$	459
	Reserpine	PGE$_2$	260
	Serotonin	PGE$_1$	124
	Steroids	PGE$_1$	365
		PGE$_2$	368
		16,16-Dimethyl PGE$_2$	368
Cat	Aspirin	16,16-Dimethyl PGE$_2$	224

*NOSAC: nonsteroidal antiinflammatory compounds.

resulted in prompt relief of the ulcer pain [139]. Since, however, no placebo control was used, it is not clear whether the effect was specific to the PG. In other studies, 15(R)-15-methyl PGE$_2$ or its methyl ester was administered to gastric ulcer patients three to four times a day for 14 days at a dose of 150 μg per patient. As judged by endoscopic measurement of the ulcer size, the treatment accelerated ulcer healing by comparison to a placebo group [137,138,140]. In a double blind study, three different methyl PGs were used in gastric and duodenal ulcer patients. These were 15(R)-15-methyl PGE$_2$ methyl ester, 15(S)-15-methyl PGE$_2$ methyl ester, and 16,16-dimethyl PGE$_2$, administered orally, three

TABLE 3. Antiulcer Effects of Prostaglandins: Duodenal Ulcers in Animals

Species	Ulcer model	Prostaglandin	Reference
Rat	Cysteamine	16,16-Dimethyl PGE$_2$	360
	Indomethacin plus bile duct ligation	16,16-Dimethyl PGE$_2$	357
	Propionitrile	16,16-Dimethyl PGE$_2$	358
	Secretogogues		
	Histamine	PGE$_2$	369
	Histamine + carbachol	PGE$_2$	347,370
		16,16-Dimethyl PGE$_2$	368
	Histamine + pentagastrin	PGE$_2$	347,370
	Pentagastrin + carbachol	PGE$_2$	347,370
Cat	Pentagastrin	PGE$_2$	241
		15(S)-15-Methyl PGE$_2$	241
Guinea pig	Histamine	PGE$_2$	260
	Pentagastrin	PGE$_2$	260

times a day, at doses ranging from 1.5 to 3 μg/kg for 14 days. A total of 117 patients were included. The healing rate of duodenal ulcers was accelerated, but not that of gastric ulcers [144,385]. In yet another study, PGE$_2$ was given orally at a dose of 1 mg four times a day to gastric ulcer patients. At the end of 2 weeks, the crater size had diminished more in the treated group than in the placebo group [138,222].

CYTOPROTECTION BY PROSTAGLANDINS

Gastric Cytoprotection

It was assumed that the antiulcer effect of prostaglandins was due to their antisecretory property. Such a conclusion was supported by the antiulcer effects of other inhibitors of gastric acid secretion (anticholinergics, histamine H$_2$ antagonists), as well as of antacids. However, recent studies, summarized below, led to a reexamination of this interpretation.

Oral administration of necrotizing agents such as absolute ethanol, 0.6 N HCl, 0.2 N NaOH, hypertonic solutions (25% NaCl), bile acids, and even boiling water, produce in rats extensive necrosis of the gastric mucosa [361,362]. These agents kill mucosal cells by direct contact with the mucosa. Such gastric necrosis was prevented by PGs, even by those that do not inhibit gastric acid secretion. In the case of PGs that are antisecretory, protection against necrotizing agents was obtained at doses less than one one-hundredth their antisecretory dose. Other inhibitors of gastric acid secretion, such as anticholinergics and histamine H$_2$ antagonists, did not protect against this type of gastric damage. This property of PGs was called "cytoprotection" [352,361,362]. It is defined as the property of many PGs to protect the gastric mucosa of the stomach from becoming inflamed and necrotic, when this mucosa is exposed to noxious agents. A large number of PGs were found to be cytoprotective; their effect was dose dependent, and the doses used were extremely small. Reviews have appeared recently on gastric and intestinal cytoprotection by PG [291,351].

Prostaglandins were cytoprotective after either oral or subcutaneous administration, the effect being three to five times more marked after oral treatment [362]. Although a large number of PGs are cytoprotective, their potency varies widely. For instance, the ED_{50} (dose reducing by 50% the number of ethanol-induced lesions per stomach) for 16,16-dimethyl PGE_2 was 50 ng/kg, whereas the ED_{50} for PGE_2 was 25 µg/kg, a ratio of 1 : 500 [362].

The mechanism of cytoprotection is unknown. Since PGE_2 stimulates gastric mucus formation in rats [35,36], dogs [34a], and humans [140a,379a], the sudden release of mucus may play a role in cytoprotection. Several PGs also stimulate the formation of cyclic AMP by gastric mucosal cells [108,202,332]; cyclic AMP could be a mediator by cytoprotection. Even if this were the case, however, one would still have to explain the mechanism by which cyclic AMP is cytoprotective. Several PGs influence the gastric mucosal circulation, and this effect may also play a role in cytoprotection. Finally, studies in dogs have shown that inhibitors of PG cyclooxygenase, such as indomethacin, block the active transport of sodium from the mucosal to the serosal side and also alter some of the electrophysiological parameters, such as mucosal electrical resistance and potential difference [65,202]. These effects were reversed by administration of theophylline, dibutyryl cyclic AMP, or 16,16-dimethyl PGE_2 [42,65,202]. It was suggested that this effect of PGs on the gastric sodium pump may be related to cytoprotection.

One of the initial effects of noxious agents (e.g. ethanol, salicylates, indomethacin, bile salts) placed directly on the gastric mucosa is to break the mucosal barrier. This is demonstrated by a decrease in hydrogen ion content and an increase in water, sodium, and potassium in gastric fluid [102]. Breaking of the gastric mucosal barrier was prevented by PGE_2 [82], 16,16-dimethyl PGE_2 [432], and PGI_2 [236]. This effect on the mucosal barrier may explain in large part the cytoprotective property of PG.

Nonsteroidal antiinflammatory compounds (NOSAC) can cause gastric mucosal damage in both animals and humans. This is expressed as pain and sometimes gastric bleeding and ulcerations. A variety of PGs, even those devoid of antisecretory activity, prevented NOSAC-induced gastric lesions in animals [12,54,101,164,350,354,457]. It was suggested that this gastric damage might result from a local (gastric) depletion of PG, since NOSAC inhibit the activity of PG cyclooxygenase [443]. Exogenous administration of PG prevents the tissue depletion of PG by NOSAC and therefore is believed to maintain gastric mucosal integrity through cytoprotection. The development of gastric damage following treatment with NOSAC is, however, a complex phenomenon. Not only is it related to inhibition of PG biosynthesis, but such lesions develop only if acid is present in the stomach [44]. This is why drugs other than PG, such as anticholinergic agents, histamine H_2 blockers, and antacids, can prevent development of NOSAC-induced lesions [12,44]. The unique feature of prostaglandins in this regard is that they prevent formation of NOSAC-induced gastric lesions even when the NOSACs are given together with acid. Thus, severe gastric lesions produced in rats by acidified aspirin or acidified bile salts are completely prevented by cytoprotective PGs, whereas they are not inhibited by antisecretory agents [55,56,66,354].

Antisecretory agents such as cimetidine and probanthine were reported to inhibit lesions produced by acidified aspirin given orally to pylorus-ligated rats [150,163,164,165]. It was concluded that these two drugs were cytoprotective. However, this conclusion was questioned [354] for the following reason: probanthine and cimetidine inhibit the lesions only if the concentration of acid, given with aspirin, is near physiological (0.15 N), but not when acidity exceeds 0.15 N, whereas 16,16-dimethyl PGE_2 is cytoprotective regardless of the concentration of acid given with aspirin [354]. Therefore, cytoprotection by PG is independent of any antisecretory activity, whereas the antiulcer effect of probanthine and cimetidine is linked to their antisecretory activity.

Cytoprotective PGs may eventually be of therapeutic value in various forms of gastritis, whether caused by drugs, microorganisms, or viruses, or of unknown etiology. Such PGs may also accelerate the healing of gastric ulcers and particularly prevent their recurrence, by maintaining gastric mucosal integrity and thus protecting against injurious agents present in the lumen.

Oral administration of PGE_2 was shown to prevent occult bleeding produced by aspirin (600 mg four times a day) [83] or indomethacin (50 mg three times a day) [205]. Since occult blood produced by these antiinflammatory drugs originates from the stomach, and since PGE_2 does not reduce gastric acid secretion when given orally [185], this effect of PGE_2 is due to gastric cytoprotection and constitutes the first demonstration of cytoprotection in humans.

Intestinal Cytoprotection

Another form of cytoprotection involves the intestine. Administration of most NOSACs commonly used in the treatment of arthritis (e.g. indomethacin, naproxen, flufenamic acid, phenylbutazone) can cause in animals a severe intestinal syndrome characterized by multiple necrotic patches of the small intestine followed by ulcerations, perforations, and fatal peritonitis [227,452]. Within 4 days, for instance, a single oral administration of a high dose (15 mg/kg) of indomethacin causes rats to die of peritonitis. Administration of a variety of PGs together with indomethacin completely prevented the development of this intestinal syndrome [348–350]. The intestinal lesions were ascribed to a PG deficiency induced by the NOSACs, since these chemicals block the activity of PG cyclooxygenase necessary for the synthesis of prostaglandins [130,443]. It is therefore the PG deficiency, not the NOSACs themselves, that causes the intestinal mucosal necrosis. Substitution therapy with a PG given either orally or parenterally prevents the PG depletion in intestinal tissue, and thus renders the NOSACs innocuous for the gut. This hypothesis is supported by the observation that a single treatment with a PG, if given at the time of indomethacin treatment, is sufficient to prevent the intestinal lesions [349]. Substitution therapy with a PG, during the few hours following indomethacin administration, precisely when the body contents of PGs are depleted [130], sufficed to block the damaging effect of indomethacin.

Intestinal lesions characterized by necrotic areas of the ileum were produced in rats by administering prednisolone for 5 to 8 days. These lesions were prevented by treatment with 16,16-dimethyl PGE_2 given orally twice a day [256]. Since corticosteroids also deplete the body stores of prostaglandins by preventing the release of the substrate arachidonic acid from the phospholipid pool [162], the pathogenesis of prednisolone-induced intestinal lesions is similar to that of NOSAC-induced lesions, although steroid-induced lesions develop later than NOSAC-induced intestinal lesions.

Clinical application of intestinal cytoprotection may include treatment of a variety of inflammatory bowel diseases such as Crohn's disease and ulcerative colitis.

EFFECT OF PROSTAGLANDINS ON BLOOD FLOW

Gastric Blood Flow

Most agents influencing gastric acid secretion also affect gastric blood flow. In general, gastric secretogogues (histamine, gastrin, acetylcholine) increase mucosal blood flow, whereas inhibitors decrease it. Since most PGs are vasoactive, their effects on gastric blood flow was measured. Prostaglandins of the E type decreased gastric mucosal blood flow in dogs [70,71,201,237,243,292,431,464], cats [134], and rats [12,276–279]. In contrast, PGI_2 (prostacyclin) increased mucosal blood flow in the resting stomach of rats [459] and dogs [237a]. When infused intravenously to Heidenhain pouch dogs stimulated with either a meal or intravenous pentagastrin, both PGI_2 and PGE_2 decreased acid secretion and mucosal blood flow [237a]. When infused intraarterially into the gastric artery (lucite chamber preparation) of dogs stimulated with histamine, PGI_2 and PGE_2 decreased acid secretion; however, PGI_2 increased mucosal blood flow and the R value (ratio of blood flow to gastric secretion), whereas PGE_2 decreased both end points [243]. In rats stimulated with intravenous pentagastrin, PGI_2 also decreased both acid secretion and gastric mucosal blood flow [459]. 6-Keto-$PGF_{1\alpha}$, the major metabolite of PGI_2, was inactive on gastric secretion and gastric mucosal blood flow [225,243,459]. 6-β-PGI_2 and an analogue of the endoperoxide PGH_2 (U-46619) also inhibited gastric acid secretion stimulated by his-

tamine and decreased gastric mucosal blood flow [225,431]. Two publications reported an increase in total gastric blood flow after either PGI_2
or PGE_2, using an anesthetized dog preparation stimulated with pentagastrin [142,143]. Different experimental conditions, including the
measurement of total rather than mucosal blood flow, may explain the
discrepancy from other published results.

In almost all studies, the ratio of gastric mucosal blood flow to gastric
secretion was unchanged or even increased, demonstrating that the
gastric antisecretory effect of PGs is not due to a diminution in the
amount of blood circulating through the mucosa; on the contrary, the
reduction in gastric mucosal blood flow is the result, not the cause, of
the antisecretory effect.

Mesenteric Blood Flow

PGE_2, PGI_2, and PGH_2 increased mesenteric blood flow in dogs and pigs
[61,62,187], whereas PGD_2, $PGF_{2\alpha}$, and U-46619 (an analogue of PGH_2)
decreased blood flow in dogs, cats, and pigs [61,62,187,330]. Arachidonic
acid also increased mesenteric blood flow, whereas 6-keto-$PGF_{1\alpha}$ was
inactive [62].

EFFECT OF PROSTAGLANDINS ON
GASTROINTESTINAL MOTILITY

Esophagus

ANIMAL STUDIES

Prostaglandin release from frog esophageal strips in the resting and
electrically stimulated states was demonstrated in 1971 [342]. Since that
time, the effects of PGs on esophageal motility and lower esophageal
sphincter (LES) pressure have been investigated primarily in lightly anesthetized opossums which, like humans, have smooth muscle in the
lower third of the esophagus [74]. Infusion of PGE_1 (1 µg/kg-min) in the
opossum lowered the velocity, but not the amplitude, of the peristaltic
wave in the upper and lower esophagus [304]. In this model, intravenous
PGE_1 [157,344], PGA_2 [157,344], or $PGF_{2\alpha}$ [344,345] (0.15–8 µg/kg) depressed, slightly depressed, or increased LES pressure, respectively
(mean rise = 36.2 mm Hg). PGE_2 was as potent as PGE_1 with a threshold
dose of 0.15 µg/kg and a maximal effect at 1 µg/kg [157]. The threshold
doses of PGA_2 [157] and $PGF_{2\alpha}$ [345] were much higher (1 µg/kg). Although the primary effect of $PGF_{2\alpha}$ was to increase LES pressure, decreases or biphasic responses were occasionally observed [345]. The effects were not attributable to the transient hypotension caused by certain
of these PGs, since the effect on the sphincter was more prolonged and
could not be produced by hemorrhage or intravenous sodium pentobarbital [157]. The action of PGE_1 on LES pressure was not altered by
adrenergic or cholinergic blockade, but was enhanced by compounds

favoring cyclic AMP accumulation [156]. Consistent with the hypothesis that PGE_1 activity and normal LES pressure fluctuations might be mediated through cyclic nucleotides, the adenylyl cyclase inhibitor nicotinic acid and the phosphodiesterase stimulator imidazole inhibited the fall in LES pressure occasioned by the PG or by esophageal distention [156].

The role of endogenous PGs in normal LES tone may be minimal, since indomethacin treatment did not modify basal LES tone or relaxation stimulated by vagal stimulation in the anesthetized opossum [100]. PGE_1 (0.125 µg/kg-min) also failed to affect vagally induced LES relaxation, suggesting that PGs do not modulate vagal inhibitory neurotransmission in this model [343].

Although gastrin administration increases LES pressure in dogs [269], serum gastrin following administration of intravenous 15-methyl PGE_2 (0.05–1.0 µg/kg) did not change [273] and is thought to be an unlikely mechanism of prostanoid activity. In cats, PGE_1 (0.15 µg/kg-min) given intraarterially caused a more significant and prolonged fall in LES pressure than did PGE_1 given intravenously. PGE_2 at the same dose had no effect on LES pressure. PGI_2 (0.15 µg/kg-min) given intraarterially, lowered LES pressure during infusion, but increased it postinfusion [409]. PGE_1 blocked the rise in LES pressure normally produced in cats by edrophonium, a cholinergic agent, suggesting that excess PGs may inhibit cholinergic regulation of LES pressure in cases of esophageal dysfunction [408].

Isolated circular LES strips from opossums contracted when exposed to $PGF_{2\alpha}$ or thromboxane B_2 (0.5–5 µg/ml), whereas similar doses of PGE_1 and PGE_2 either caused relaxation or contraction, or had no effect [97]. Stable endoperoxide analogues [15(S)-hydroxy-11α,9α-(epoxymethano)-prosta-5Z,13E-dienoic acid] and [15(S)-hydroxy-9α,11α-(epoxymethano)-prosta-5Z,13E-dienoic acid] caused stronger contractions at lower doses than $PGF_{2\alpha}$. PGI_2 relaxed (1–10 µg/ml) or contracted (100 µg/ml) LES strips, depending on the dose used [97]. Indomethacin and 5,8,11,14-eicosatetraenoic acid inhibited muscle tone, suggesting that PG synthesis was necessary for its maintenance. These agents also antagonized the relaxation of the sphincter caused by 0.5- and 5-msec field stimulation, suggesting that PG synthesis was necessary for this nonadrenergic, inhibitory effect [97,98]. Further evidence suggests that PGI_2, PGE_2, and an unknown prostanoid are responsible for in vitro LES tone [99].

HUMAN STUDIES

In human volunteers, 10-minute infusions of PGE_1 (0.02 µg/kg-min) lowered basal sphincter pressure from 14 to 6 mm Hg [416,417]. PGE_2 infusion (0.05–0.4 µg/kg-min) reduced LES pressure also, but did not affect the upper esophageal sphincter. The amplitude of peristaltic contractions was reduced in the lower, but not in the upper part of the esophagus [305]. In patients with achalasia treated with PGE_2 (0.01–0.8 µg/kg-min), LES pressure was reduced to control values [155]. In another study, low doses of PGE_2 (0.01–0.08 μg/kg-min) did not affect resting sphincter pressure, but pentagastrin-induced contractions of the sphincter were diminished [106]. Dose-related increases in LES pressure were produced by infusion (2.5–4.0 ng/kg-min) but not by bolus injection (2.5–4.0 μg/kg) of $PGF_{2\alpha}$ [106]. This PG augmented the amplitude of esophageal contractions without affecting plasma gastrin levels [106]. Oral 16,16-dimethyl PGE_2 (1.5–2.5 μg/kg), like infusion of PGE_2, did not affect basal LES pressure, but reduced the LES response to pentagastrin [288]. Indomethacin given intraarterially [106] or orally [253] to normal volunteers increased LES pressure, suggesting that PGs may play a role in the in vivo regulation of esophageal pressure in humans, in contrast to the opossum [343].

Since prostaglandins can increase or decrease LES pressure depending on their chemical structures, these compounds may play a role in the etiology and treatment of esophageal dysfunction (achalasia, dysphagia, reflux, etc.).

Stomach

CONTRACTILITY STUDIES

Endogenous Prostaglandin Effects. In vitro studies suggest that gastric contractility can be influenced by both endogenous and exogenous prostaglandins. The tone of isolated rat stomach strips was depressed by indomethacin and restored by PGE_2, suggesting that release of endogenous PG may be responsible, at least in part, for the smooth muscle tone of that organ [111,175,393]. Furthermore, indomethacin antagonized contractions produced by arachidonic acid [421], and aspirin antagonized those elicited by 4,5-epoxy-hexane-hydroperoxide and 3-methyl-3-hydroxymethyl-1,2-dioxolane [5], suggesting that PG production by the isolated tissue was responsible for the contractility elicited by addition of these precursors.

Rat stomach minces released PGE_2, PGD_2, and $PGF_{2\alpha}$ into their suspending media. This release was increased by hypertonic sucrose and by histamine [231]. The tone of rat stomach strips from animals fed a normal diet increased with time, presumably because of PG release. Rats fed a diet deficient in essential fatty acids, however, had stomach strips that exhibited decreased tone with time, presumably because of a lack of continued PG synthesis [135]. Prostaglandins were also released from isolated rat stomachs [24,472]. Cholinergic, but not adrenergic stimulation, increased release of the E and F types of PG. Anoxia inhibited PG release, whereas ascorbic acid increased it [79].

Exogenous Prostaglandin Effects. Exogenous PGs can either contract or relax isolated stomach strips, depending on the type of PG and the animal used. In the rat stomach strip, all PGs tested elicited contraction. The E-type PGs appeared to be more potent than the F type, which in turn were more potent than the A type. Furthermore, the "2" series was more potent than the "1" series [178]. PGE_2 methyl ester was less potent than PGE_2 itself [423]. Other prostanoids reported to contract the rat stomach strip were PGG_2 [169], PGH_2 [169], PGI_2 [299], thromboxane A_2 [299], alkyl hydroperoxides [5], PGD_2 [182], 19-hydroxy-PGA_1 [181], 19-hydroxy-PGB_1 [181], and ent-11,15-epi-PGE_2 [440]. In the isolated rat stomach, prostaglandins A_1, B_1, E_1, E_2, $F_{1\alpha}$, and $F_{2\alpha}$ caused stronger contractions when applied serosally than when applied mucosally [188].

Hamster stomach strips contracted when exposed to PGE_1, PGE_2, PGA_1, or $PGF_{2\alpha}$ [439]. PGE_1 produced relaxation, however, of the frog stomach [16]. In the rabbit transverse stomach strip, contraction with PGI_2, $PGF_{2\alpha}$, PGH_2, and thromboxane A_2, and relaxation with PGA_2, PGD_2, and PGE_2 have been reported [299,460]. Thus, species differences undoubtedly exist in the stomach strip model.

The type of muscle taken from the stomach also influences the result of PG application (contraction or relaxation). Unfortunately, details of the preparation are frequently not stated. For example, with guinea pig stomach strips, PGE_2 and, to a lesser extent PGE_1, produced tonic contractions of longitudinal muscle and phasic contractions of the circular muscle [198,450]. Similarly, in the human stomach, PGE_1 and PGE_2 relaxed circular muscle and contracted longitudinal muscle [26,298]. $PGF_{2\alpha}$ contracted both types of human stomach muscle [27].

Measurement of motility in whole stomach, in vivo and in vitro, has been performed in a variety of species with PGE_1 with diverging results. Rat gastric motility measured by telemetry in the unanesthetized animal was increased by daily intraperitoneal injections of PGE_1 (4.5 µg/kg) [405]. In situ rabbit stomach motor activity was stimulated by intravenous PGE_1 (500 µg/kg) [411]. In the isolated guinea pig stomach, PGE_1 increased internal pressure when applied serosally [450]. In other species, however, the E-type PGs tended to inhibit gastric motility. In healthy volunteers, for example, PGE_1 given intravenously (300 µg) depressed antral motility [77]. The frequency of antral contractions in human subjects measured with pressure transducers was increased by $PGF_{2\alpha}$ (0.08 µg/kg-min) but unaffected by PGE_2 (0.04 or 0.08 µg/kg-min) [313]. 16,16-Dimethyl PGE_2 (140 µg orally) depressed antral motility [321], while the motility index in dogs with antral pouches was also depressed by PGE_1 given intravenously (1 µg/kg-min) [67]. In the ex vivo perfused canine stomach, a bolus of PGE_2 (25 µg) into the gastric artery caused an increase, followed by a decrease, in antral contractions. Prolonged infusion (500 µg/kg) completely suppressed antral contractions [250]. Table 4 summarizes studies performed with exogenous prostaglandins.

Mechanism of Prostaglandin Activity. The mechanism by which exogenous PGs modulate the tone of stomach strips has not been adequately determined. A direct action on smooth muscle seems likely, since PGs can contract tissue in vitro even in the presence of cholinergic, adrenergic, serotonergic, and histaminergic blockers [178]. However, papaverine, which depresses smooth muscle activity, reduced rat stomach strip contraction elicited by acetylcholine but not by PGE_1 [472].

TABLE 4. Effect of Exogenous Prostaglandins on Stomach

Model	Species	PGF$_{2\alpha}$	PGF$_{1\alpha}$	PGE$_2$	PGE$_1$	PGD$_2$	PGA$_2$	PGA$_1$	Other	Reference
Perfused stomach strip (Longitudinal)	Man	27 298		26 27 298	26 298					
	Guinea pig	188	188	188 197 450	3 188 198 450			188	PGB$_1$	188
	Rat	27 40 78 135 182 188 299 421 454	188	25 27 111 175 182 188 299 421 448	2 78 80 81 135 181 188 405 454 472	182 299	181 299	181 188	15(S)-Hydroxy-9α,11α-(epoxymethano) prosta-5Z,13E-dienoic acid 15(S)-Hydroxy-11α,9α-(epoxymethano) prosta-5Z,13E-dienoic acid ent-11,15-Diepi-PGE$_2$ 19-Hydroxy PGA$_1$; 19-hydroxy PGB$_1$ PGB$_1$ PGH$_2$, PGG$_2$, TXA$_2$ PGF$_{1\beta}$ PGG$_2$, PGH$_2$ PGI$_2$	25 25 440 15 188 299 78 169 299,300
	Mouse	188	188	188	188			188	PGB$_1$	188
	Hamster		439	439	439			439		
	Frog				16					
(Transverse)	Rabbit	299 460		299 460		299 460	299 460		PGI$_2$, PGH$_2$, TXA$_2$	299 460
(Circular)	Man	27 298		26 27 298	26 298					

Preparation	Species	References	Compound	Ref
Superfused fundic strip	Guinea pig	178		
	Rat	178; 198, 450, 111, 170, 178, 454; 197, 450, 178; 178	PGE_2 Methyl ester	454
			15(S)-15-Methyl PGE_2	454
			1-Hydroperoxy-4,5-epoxyhexane	5
			3-Methyl-3-hydroxymethyl-1,2-dioxolane	5
			9-Hydroperoxy-cis,trans,cis-6,10,12-octadecatrienoic acid	5
	Gerbil	169; 169; 169	PGG_2, PGH_2	169
Isolated stomach	Guinea pig	450; 450		
	Dog	250		
In vivo (motility)	Man	313; 313; 77	16,16-Dimethyl PGE_2	321
			15(S)-15-Methyl PGE_2	321
	Dog	67	13-Hydroperoxy-cis,cis,trans-6,9,11-octadecatrienoic acid	5
	Rat	405		
	Rabbit	411		
Gastric emptying	Man	185	16,16-Dimethyl PGE_2	322
	Monkey		15(S)-15-Methyl $PGF_{2\alpha}$	317, 404
			15(S)-15-Methyl PGE_2	315
			PGI_2	404
			16,16-Dimethyl PGE_2	359
Pyloric pressure	Rat	314; 32		
Perfused pyloric ring	Dog	149; 149; 149		

Note: Numbers indicate literature cited in References.

There is no direct evidence that PGs affect gastric release of neurotransmitters (e.g. acetylcholine, norepinephrine), as has been demonstrated in the small intestine and the colon (see subsections entitled "Small Intestine" and "Colon," under "Effects of Prostaglandins on Motility."). PG activity can, however, be modulated by sympathetic nerve input. For example, drugs that inhibit sympathetic fibers or receptors potentiated PG action on rat stomach strips, whereas drugs stimulating adrenergic receptors inhibited PG-induced contractions [80,81]. Addition of epinephrine or norepinephrine to the bathing fluid also inhibited PG-induced contractions [472]. Atropine did not antagonize the response of rat stomach strips to PGE_1 [472], suggesting that PG effects are not cholinergically mediated. Oxygen is required for PG-induced effects, since anoxia inhibits contractions of rat stomach strips exposed to PGE_1 although anoxia does not block the effect of acetylcholine. Reducing agents such as ascorbic acid and glutathione potentiated PGE_1 effects on the stomach strips, presumably by delaying degradation [472].

PGE_1-induced contractions of rat fundic muscle were accompanied by a decrease in cyclic AMP and an increase in cyclic GMP tissue levels [405], indicating that cyclic nucleotides may be involved in PG effects.

In guinea pig stomach muscle, ATP-stimulated contractions were inhibited by indomethacin, suggesting possible mediation of ATP-induced contractility by the release of endogenous PG [211].

GASTRIC EMPTYING

The studies of prostaglandins on stomach muscle contractility described above are difficult to interpret in terms of physiological function (e.g. gastric emptying). This is partly because data on the effect of PGs on the pylorus are lacking. Since E-type PGs antagonize basal [149] and caerulein-induced [32] pyloric contraction, such contribution may be of great importance with respect to gastric emptying. Indomethacin did not alter basal or fluid-stimulated gastric emptying in monkeys [318] or rats [384], suggesting that endogenous PGs are not primary regulators of gastric emptying.

Exogenous PGs, however, do influence gastric emptying. In rats, 16,16-dimethyl PGE_2 [359] or $PGF_{2\alpha}$ [314] administered subcutaneously, delayed gastric emptying, but oral administration of the first compound was without effect [359]. In monkeys, intravenous or subcutaneous administration of 15(S)-15-methyl PGE_2 and 15(S)-15-methyl $PGF_{2\alpha}$ increased gastric emptying [315,317,319], whereas intravenous PGI_2 inhibited it [404]. In humans, 16,16-dimethyl PGE_2 given orally enhanced the rate of evacuation of a barium meal [204,322], whereas PGE_1 (20–40 μg/kg), also given orally, produced biliary reflux into the stomach [185].

CLINICAL IMPLICATIONS

Prostaglandins can retard or stimulate gastric emptying, depending on the experimental conditions. Nausea, a possible consequence of delayed emptying, has been reported after administration of PGs in humans

[53,136]. However, for patients with abnormally rapid emptying rates such as in duodenal ulcer [123] or postgastrectomy dumping syndrome [122], who might benefit from the cytoprotective or antiulcer effects of PGs, delayed gastric emptying could be a desirable effect.

In conditions of retarded gastric emptying (e.g. ileus [60]) certain PGs may be of use in stimulating normal function. For example, 16,16-dimethyl PGE_2 given intravenously to postoperative rats restored the ability of the stomach to evacuate a radioactive chromium solution. Subcutaneous or oral administration was ineffective. The ability of 16,16-dimethyl PGE_2 to enhance gastric emptying in ileus rats appears to be due to smooth muscle stimulation, not to enhancement of cholinergic effects or suppression of sympathetic ones [383].

Small Intestine

CONTRACTILITY STUDIES

Endogenous Prostaglandin Effects. Incubated intestinal strips, like those of the stomach, release prostaglandins into the bathing fluid. Isolated frog intestine, for example, released a muscle-contracting material known as *darmstoff*, which was identified as a mixture of PGE_2 and $PGF_{2\alpha}$ [446]. Strips of guinea pig ileum also released PGE_2 into the bathing fluid [39]. Removing the PG by changing the bathing fluid or blocking PG synthesis or action with indomethacin [39], polyphloretin phosphate [337], or 5,8,11,14-eicosatetraynoic acid [103,461] resulted in a decrease in the basal tone of the isolated muscle. Isolated rabbit jejunum also released PGE_2 and $PGF_{2\alpha}$ into the bathing fluid; this outflow was increased by mechanical trauma and inhibited by indomethacin and aspirin [111,125,126]. Therefore, the tone of isolated intestine appears to be related to PG synthesis and release.

Field stimulation of ileal strips [39] and distention of isolated guinea pig small intestine [474] increased the rate of PG release. The release of PG caused by field stimulation of guinea pig ileum, however, could be blocked by phentolamine, propranolol, a combination of the two drugs, or guanethidine, suggesting that norepinephrine release with subsequent stimulation of α- and β-adrenergic receptors may be responsible for the outflow of endogenous PGs [38]. This observation differs from those on the isolated rat stomach, where cholinergic, but not adrenergic stimulation, increased PG release [79]; confirmation is needed before this difference can be firmly established, however. Challenge of sensitized, superfused guinea pig ileum with ovalbumin, acetylcholine, or histamine resulted in liberation of PG-like materials. This release was blocked by the antihistamine mepyramine [254].

Coincidental with inhibiting PG release, indomethacin and aspirin decreased peristalsis in a perfused ileal segment isolated from guinea pig [22,133]. One group reported that the indomethacin inhibition could be overcome by the addition of PGE_1 or PGE_2 [133], whereas another showed that $PGF_{2\alpha}$, histamine, or acetylcholine prevented the inhibition induced by indomethacin [22]. Aspirin inhibition could be overcome by

PGE_2 [22]. These data imply that peristaltic activity in vitro is at least partially mediated by endogenous PG release, and that exogenous PGs can substitute effectively. The ability of acetylcholine and histamine to overcome indomethacin inhibition suggests that their effects may be mediated by PGs, or that the dose of indomethacin used was high enough to have caused nonspecific inhibition of peristalsis.

In rings of ileum from cat, the PG content of the muscle layer was increased by addition of acetylcholine to the bathing medium [391]. However, PG was not a necessary component for acetylcholine-induced contractions, since these were enhanced even when the tissue was pre-treated with indomethacin or 5,8,11,14-eicosatetraynoic acid [391]. In anesthetized cats, similar results were found. Intramesenteric arterial infusion of acetylcholine caused an increase in PGE content of the ileum. Indomethacin abolished this increase but enhanced the intraluminal pressure caused by acetylcholine [392]. The feline data differ from reports on other species cited above, where indomethacin depressed rather than enhanced tone and contractility. More work is needed to resolve these discrepancies.

Exogenous Prostaglandin Effects. PGE_1, PGE_2, and PGE_3 contract in vitro longitudinal strips from humans, rats, guinea pigs, rabbits, and chicks, whereas they relax the circular muscle [18,19,21,31,39,171,183, 184,395]. Longitudinal rat duodenum, but not jejunum, was exceptional in this regard, since it relaxed upon application of PGE_1 [229,411]. PGA_1, PGA_2, and PGD_2 also contracted longitudinal muscle from rats, mice, rabbits, and guinea pigs [181,182,188,248,341,455], but their effect on circular muscle is not known. $PGF_{1\alpha}$ and $PGF_{2\alpha}$ contracted longitudinal muscle strips from guinea pig ileum but had little effect on circular muscle rings [21,171,183]. These results contrast with the contractile effect of $PGF_{2\alpha}$ on both the longitudinal and circular muscle of human small intestine [30].

PGE compounds tended to contract guinea pig ileum more than PGF compounds [31,183]. PGE_1 and PGE_2 may have a common receptor site in this model [191]. Serosal application of PG to isolated ileum of rats, mice, and guinea pigs was more effective than mucosal administration in producing contractions [188]. Thus species differences, site of application, and muscle type need to be taken into account when evaluating the effects of PGs on intestinal tissue strips.

Certain synthetic analogues and racemic mixtures of the natural PGs [ent-PGE_1; ent-11,15-epi-PGE_2; ent-11-epi-PGE_2; ent-11,15-epi-$PGF_{2\beta}$; ent-11,15-epi-$PGF_{2\alpha}$; 15(S)-hydroxy-9α,11α-dienoic acid; and 15(S)-hydroxy-11α,9α-(epoxymethano)-prosta-5Z,13E-dienoic acid; racemic mixtures of PGE_1, 11-epi-PGE_1, 11,15-epi-PGE_1, $PGF_{1\alpha}$, and PGA_1] were less active on guinea pig ileum and rabbit jejunum than the parent PGs [25,341,440]. 15-Methyl and 16,16-dimethyl PGE_2 were as active as PGE_2 [280], whereas ent-11,15-epi-PGE_1 and racemic mixtures of 15-epi-PGE_1 or 15-epi-PGA_1 were more potent than the parent PGs in these systems [341].

The concentration of a PG in the bathing fluid of an isolated organ can determine whether the compound will be inhibitory or stimulatory. For example, peristalsis of isolated guinea pig ileum was stimulated by low concentrations (0.63–50 μg/l) of PGE_1 or PGE_2 [133,340,395] but inhibited by higher concentrations (250–1000 μg/l) [19,340]. The inhibition appears to be due to a rebound release of norepinephrine, since reserpine pretreatment was able to block it [340]. $PGF_{1\alpha}$ and $PGF_{2\alpha}$ increased propulsion of intraluminal fluid in isolated guinea pig ileum [116].

When injected intravenously, rather than applied serosally, PGE_1 and PGE_2 increased intraluminal pressure in anesthetized rats, but produced inconsistent results in guinea pigs [19]. 15-Methyl and 16,16-dimethyl PGE_2, given subcutaneously, were 20 times as potent as PGE_2 in raising intraluminal pressures in anesthetized rat duodenum, jejunum, and ileum [280]. In contrast, intraluminal pressure was generally depressed in canine small intestine by parenteral PGE_1 [324,406] (dose dependent) and in the cat small intestine (dose independent) [438]. $PGF_{2\alpha}$ increased intraluminal pressure in dogs [406]. Circular and longitudinal muscle contractions were markedly stimulated in the canine ileum by $PGF_{2\alpha}$, whereas circular tone was increased and longitudinal tone depressed [92].

Myoelectric activity was increased in conscious fasted dogs receiving PGE_2, whereas fed dogs did not respond to this PG [306]. Interdigestive myoelectric complexes, moreover, were blocked by PGE_2 and 15(S)-15-methyl PGE_2 in fasted dogs [235]. Both PGs induced the fasted-type pattern of spike activity in the fed animals [235]. Thus, PGs affect motility in vivo, but the direction of their effects depends on the animal, the intestinal region monitored, and the PG used. The literature dealing with these effects is summarized in Table 5.

Mechanism of Prostaglandin Activity. The interactions of PGs and other smooth muscle effectors on isolated intestine are complex. However, there are more data on small intestinal muscle than on gastric muscle. The current evidence on the mechanisms of PG stimulation of intestinal contractions points to direct smooth muscle stimulation [18,20,30,208], inhibition of sympathetic neurotransmitter release [1,78,172,192,208,209,285,333,394], and potentiation of cholinergic transmission [18,20,158,208–210,255,430,461]; it is likely that all these mechanisms contribute to PG activity. Postsynaptic sympathetic inhibition has also been observed [15] and may be due to accelerated autoxidation of norepinephrine by PGE compounds [114].

The stimulatory effect of morphine in isolated vascularly perfused canine intestine was antagonized by PGE_1, PGE_2, PGA_2, PGB_2, and $PGF_{2\alpha}$ [49,161]. Similar experiments demonstrated that PGE_1 methyl ester blocked the stimulatory effects of diphenoxylate and morphine [95]. PGE_1-induced contractions in guinea pig ileum were inhibited by the addition of methionine and leucine enkephalins [203]. Conversely, PGE_1, PGE_2, and $PGF_{2\alpha}$ reversed the inhibition of electrically induced contractions in guinea pig ileum by morphine; PGB_1 was less potent, and $PGF_{1\alpha}$

TABLE 5. Effects of Exogenous Prostaglandins on Small Intestine

Model	Species	PGF$_{2\alpha}$	PGF$_{1\alpha}$	PGE$_2$	PGE$_1$	PGD$_2$	PGA$_2$	PGA$_1$	Other	Reference
Perfused ileum (Longitudinal)	Man	27, 30, 171	30	18, 27, 30, 171	18, 30					
	Guinea pig	21, 184, 22, 188, 40, 210, 113, 255, 116, 336, 118, 337, 120, 448, 158, 454	21, 113, 116, 183, 188, 341	15, 183, 18, 188, 19, 191, 20, 208, 22, 209, 25, 210, 39, 280, 72, 285, 103, 333, 113, 398, 114, 448, 118, 454, 133, 455, 145, 461, 158	2, 183, 15, 184, 18, 188, 19, 191, 20, 203, 113, 333, 114, 336, 118, 337, 120, 340, 121, 394, 132, 395, 133, 398, 145, 455, 180, 461, 181, 482	455		188, 341	15(S)-15-Methyl PGE$_2$	280
									16,16-Dimethyl PGE$_2$	280
									rac-PGE$_1$; rac-PGF$_{1\alpha}$	341
									15-epi-PGE$_1$; rac-15-epi-PGE$_1$	341
									rac-11,15-diepi-PGE$_1$	341
									15(S)-Hydroxy-11α,9α-(epoxymethano)prosta-5Z, 13E-dienoic acid	25
									15(S)-Hydroxy-9α11α-(epoxymethano)prosta-5Z, 13E-dienoic acid	25
									ent-11,15-diepi-PGE$_2$; ent-11-epi-PGE$_2$; ent-11,15-diepi-1 PGF$_{2\beta}$; ent-11,15-diepi-PGF$_{2\alpha}$	440
									PGE$_3$	183
									PGF	31
									PGB$_1$	113,188
									PGE	31,255
									PGE, methyl ester	95
									PGB$_1$	188
	Rat	89, 112, 188	112, 188	18, 112, 188	18, 121, 188					
	Rabbit	188	1, 188	1, 188						
	Mouse	188	188	188	188				PGB$_1$	188

Preparation	Species							Other compounds	Ref.
(Circular)	Man	30	30	30	30	28			
	Guinea pig	28, 116	116	19, 21, 28, 398	19, 21, 398				
Perfused jejunum (longitudinal)	Rat	182				182		PGE, PGF	31
	Rabbit	183, 184, 246, 247, 341	125, 182, 183, 247	172, 183, 184, 192, 246, 333, 341	182	181, 248	181, 247, 248, 341	rac-PGE$_i$; ent-PGE$_i$; rac-PGF$_{2\alpha}$; rac-11-epi-PGE$_i$; rac-11, 15-diepi- PGE$_i$; rac-PGA$_i$; rac-15-epi-PGA$_1$	341
	Chick							PGE, PGF	31
Perfused duodenum (longitudinal)	Rat			180, 229, 411, 437				PGE, PGF	31
	Rabbit	454	455	73, 177, 454, 455	455	455		PGE	297
In vivo-in situ (Intraluminal pressure)	Man	294							
	Guinea pig	19, 398	19, 398						
	Dog	49, 161, 406	49, 161	49, 79, 161, 324, 406, 439	49, 161	49	161	PGB$_2$	49, 161
	Cat	445	445	445					

(continued)

TABLE 5. Effects of Exogenous Prostaglandins on Small Intestine (continued)

Model	Species	$PGF_{2\alpha}$	$PGF_{1\alpha}$	PGE_2	PGE_1	PGD_2	PGA_2	PGA_1	Other	Reference
	Rat			19	19				15(S)-15-Methyl PGE_2 methyl ester	280
				280					16,16-Dimethyl PGE_2	280
	Rabbit	128		128						
		129		129						
(Myoelectrical	Man	90							15(S)-15-Methyl PGE_2	321
motor activity)		136							16,16-Dimethyl PGE_2	115,321
	Dog	92		161	160				PGE_1, Methyl ester	95
		160		235	161		161		PG-S, PGA, PGF	235
		161		306	324				PGB_2	161
		405			405					
	Rabbit	128		128						
		129		129						
		310		310						
Peristalsis	Guinea pig	22	116	22						
		116								
Transit	Man	90			295				16,16-Dimethyl PGE_2	322
		294								
	Guinea pig								16,16-Dimethyl PGE_2	383
	Rat	314		52					16,16-Dimethyl PGE_2	381
		383		383					16,16-Dimethyl PGE_2	383
	Mouse	200								
Intestinal villae	Dog				190					

and PGA_1 were virtually inactive [113]. These results point to an antagonism between the effects of PGs and of morphinelike compounds on small bowel contractions.

Contractions in rabbit jejunal strips induced by PGA_1 [248], PGA_2 [248], PGE_1 [246], and $PGF_{1\alpha}$ [246] were antagonized by AMP and ATP. Similarly, contractions induced by PGE_2 [247], PGA_1 [247], and $PGF_{1\alpha}$ [247] were inhibited by NADP and β-NAD. It has been proposed that these nucleotides exert physiological control on the PGs. In guinea pig duodenum, jejunum, and ileum strips, ATP-induced contractions were inhibited by indomethacin, suggesting a mediation of ATP activity by PG. However, the dose of indomethacin may have been high enough to give nonspecific effects, since submaximal contractions due to acetylcholine and histamine were also inhibited [211].

In rat ileal strips, PGs have been implicated as mediators of bradykinin contractions. Indomethacin, aspirin, and the PG antagonist polyphloretin phosphate all inhibited bradykinin activity but did not affect contractions produced by acetylcholine [88,89].

The interaction of prostaglandins and serotonin are not clearly defined. Indomethacin antagonized contractions of isolated guinea pig ileum produced by serotonin, and PGE_1 reversed the inhibition [121]. The doses of indomethacin employed, however, have also been reported to antagonize contractions to nicotine [20,120], PGE_1 and $PGF_{2\alpha}$ [119], and electrical stimulation [118,182], suggesting that nonspecific inhibition of motility rather than inhibition of PG synthesis may have been responsible for the antagonism of serotonin effects. However, contractions of isolated guinea pig ileum induced by both serotonin and PGE_1 were antagonized by agents that blocked either serotonin or PG receptors. Contractions induced by acetylcholine were not affected by either type of blocking agent [337]. These results suggest either that the blocking agents are nonspecific or that there is a real relationship between serotonin and the effect of PGs on intestinal motility. In the dog, PGA_2, PGB_2, PGE_1, PGE_2, and $PGF_{2\alpha}$ inhibited the stimulated intestinal motility induced by serotonin [161], suggesting that such interaction, if present, is antagonistic.

Indomethacin inhibited contractions of guinea pig ileum elicited by angiotensin II. Addition of PGE_2 in doses too low to cause contractions restored activity of the tissue to subsequent doses of angiotensin II [72]. These data imply that PG may be involved in the angiotensin response. Indomethacin was reported to inhibit cholecystokinin contractions in isolated guinea pig ileum, but whether this is a specific effect of the drug is unclear [482].

TRANSIT STUDIES

As with gastric motility, studies measuring contractility or pressure changes are difficult to relate to the physiological role of small intestinal motile function (i.e. transit). Furthermore, in vivo and in situ studies suffer from the high probability that motile function is altered by laparotomy and handling; that is, excised or manipulated organs are in a state of "ileus" in which some, but not all, function is retained [60]. A few well-controlled investigations have been performed in vivo, however. $PGF_{2\alpha}$, given subcutaneously to anesthetized rats, retarded the transit through the small bowel of a charcoal meal given orally [314]. However, since the PG was given subcutaneously, gastric emptying was also inhibited [314], and this could have been entirely responsible for the delay in small intestinal transit. Mice receiving $PGF_{2\alpha}$ orally exhibited increased propulsion of an intragastric charcoal meal and a delayed transit with PGE_1 [200]. No measurements of gastric emptying were made, however; thus these results are difficult to interpret. PGE_2 given orally has been reported to increase transit in rats given a charcoal meal [52]. In our hands, rats receiving black ink through a preimplanted duodenal cannula showed increased small intestinal transit when given PGE_2 subcutaneously (Table 6). By delivering the transit marker directly to the duodenum, gastric emptying effects were excluded. Such a precaution is required to resolve the question of the effect of PG on small intestinal transit.

In humans, $PGF_{2\alpha}$ (0.28–0.86 µg/kg-min) inhibited motility and increased intestinal fluid secretion without affecting transit [90,294]. PGE_1 given orally (2 mg), however, accelerated transit through the small intestine of radiotelemetered capsules [295]. Duodenal administration of 15(S)-15-methyl PGE_2 methyl ester (80 µg) to normal volunteers caused an inhibition of duodenal motor activity; similar results were observed after oral administration of 16,16-dimethyl PGE_2 (140 µg) [321]. Nevertheless, an intragastric barium meal reached the colon faster than in vehicle-treated controls with the latter PG [322]. Since gastric emptying was also increased, however, it was not certain whether the observed increase in small intestinal transit was due entirely to direct effects on the small bowel [322]. Other investigators, in fact, found that transit along a 70-cm jejunal segment was delayed in subjects receiving 16,16-dimethyl PGE_2 (140 µg) orally, whereas gastric emptying was enhanced [115,204]. Again careful methodology will be necessary to assess the effect of PGs on intestinal transit in humans.

Evidence to date indicates that endogenous PGs probably do not contribute to small intestinal transit in the normal animal. In two studies,

TABLE 6. Effect of PGE_2 on Small Intestinal Transit (SIT) in Rats

Dose (mg/kg)	N	SIT*
0	7	62 ± 3
1	8	100 ± 0

*Expressed as percent of intestinal length traveled by the ink.

Note: Rats were fasted for 48 hours, then either PGE_2 or vehicle was administered subcutaneously. After 45 minutes, the rats were sacrificed by asphyxiation and the small intestine was excised.

one in monkeys [316] and one in rats [384], indomethacin did not affect small intestinal transit. Another study in rats reported increased small bowel propulsion after indomethacin [424], but measurements were taken after ulcerations had developed (see section entitled "Effect of Prostaglandins on Ulcer Formation"), complicating the interpretation of results.

CLINICAL IMPLICATIONS

In patients with depressed motility or transit, prostaglandins may be of benefit in restoring normal function. For example, $PGF_{2\alpha}$ but not PGE_1 reversed the inhibition of peristaltic contractions caused by the intraperitoneal injection of potassium iodide in conscious dogs with subcutaneous jejunal segments [160]. $PGF_{2\alpha}$, but not PGE_2, increased intraluminal pressure and peristaltic amplitude in mechanical ileus in rabbits [128,129]. $PGF_{2\alpha}$ infusions (0.3–0.5 μg/kg-min) given for 2 hours after surgery, served to stimulate electrical activity in the duodenum, jejunum, and ileum of the postoperative patients [136]. In the postoperative ileus rat, PGE_2 and 16,16-dimethyl PGE_2, but not $PGF_{2\alpha}$, were found to increase but not normalize delayed small intestinal transit [381]. 16,16-Dimethyl PGE_2 normalized small bowel propulsion in the laparotomized guinea pig [383]. Thus, PGs may be able to restore motile function to the traumatized small intestine.

Some evidence suggests that PGs may be involved in the etiology of delayed transit. Small bowel pseudoobstruction is sometimes accompanied by raised PG levels in peripheral blood and gastric juice [37, 73,270]. Resolution of this condition spontaneously or with administration of PG synthetase inhibitors resulted in a return to normal prostaglandin levels. The data suggest that different prostanoids may be able to decrease or increase small bowel transit.

Colon

CONTRACTILITY STUDIES

Endogenous Prostaglandin Effects. Much less is known about PG activity on the colon than on the upper gastrointestinal tract. Aspirin and indomethacin reduced tone and peristalsis in isolated guinea pig colon [22,111,211,389,476], chick rectum [111], and human longitudinal colonic strips [47], suggesting that PG play a significant role in these functions. The same concentration of indomethacin that inhibited spontaneous mechanical activity also depressed efflux of PGE from the isolated guinea pig *Taenia coli* and increased norepinephrine release [195]. Aspirin and 5,8,11,14-eicosatetraynoic acid behaved similarly [476]. PG synthetase inhibitors were more effective in blocking peristaltic activity when applied serosally than mucosally [22]. Calcium ions stimulate prostaglandin release [105]. Thus, tone and peristalsis of isolated gut appears to be dependent on PG release. Whether this phenomenon also occurs in vivo or is a response to the trauma of excision is uncertain.

Exogenous Prostaglandin Effects. $PGE_{1\alpha}$ and $PGF_{2\alpha}$ contracted superfused rat colonic tissue (presumably longitudinal) [170,178]. PGE_2 and PGE_1 did not contract the same preparation in one laboratory [170], but these two PGs, as well as PGA_1 and PGA_2, contracted isolated rat colon in another [198]. In this latter study, PG of the E type were more potent than PG of the F type, and the latter were more potent than PG of the A type. PGs from the "2" series were more active than PGs from the "1" series [198]. 15(S)-15-Methyl PGE_2 was as potent as PGE_2, but more potent than PGE_2 methyl ester, in contracting rat colon [423]. PGE_1, PGE_2, PGE_3, $PGF_{1\alpha}$, and $PGF_{2\alpha}$ also stimulated contractions of the isolated hamster colon [183,184]. The gerbil colon was contracted by PG and endoperoxides with the following potencies: $PGE_2 > PGG_2 = PGH_2$ $= PGF_{2\alpha} > PGD_2$ [169]. 16E-Fluoro-$PGF_{2\alpha}$ was 78% as active as $PGF_{2\alpha}$, whereas 16,16-difluoro-$PGF_{2\alpha}$ methyl ester was less potent [272]. 17-Phenyl trinor-PGE_2 was not as potent as PGE_2, but 16-phenyl trinor-$PGF_{2\alpha}$ was 1.7 times as active as $PGF_{2\alpha}$ [293]. Chick rectum was contracted by PGF compounds and was less affected by PGs of the E type [31,178]. Prostaglandins E_1, E_2, $F_{2\alpha}$, and A_1 contracted strips of human appendix [448]. Large intestinal segments from human fetus contracted upon application of PGE_2 [171]. Thus, PGs contract longitudinal colonic muscle from several species.

Serosally applied $PGF_{1\alpha}$ or $PGF_{2\alpha}$ increased circular muscle peristaltic activity and propulsion stimulated by artificially increased intraluminal pressure in isolated guinea pig colon [116]. PGA_1, PGD_2, $PGF_{1\alpha}$, and $PGF_{2\alpha}$ also contracted circular colonic muscle from rat, dog, guinea pig, and humans, whereas PGE_1 and PGE_2 caused a relaxation [28,131, 324,399,441]. PGE_1 and PGE_2 initially contracted the guinea pig longitudinal muscle and increased peristaltic activity of the circular and longitudinal muscle without significantly affecting propulsion. Mucosally applied PGs had little effect [116]. Thus, PGs of the E type relax circular colonic muscle, whereas other PGs contract it.

In longitudinal muscle strips from dogs and humans, PGE_1, PGE_2, $PGF_{1\alpha}$, $PGF_{2\alpha}$, and PGA increase the frequency and amplitude of electrical slow waves that were associated with augmented tone. Spike potentials associated with strong phasic contractions were also increased [441]. In vivo, however, $PGF_{2\alpha}$ (1 µg/kg-min) did not affect colonic motor activity in anesthetized dogs, although small intestinal muscle contraction was stimulated [92]. In human subjects, intravenous PGE_2 (0.08 µg/kg-min) but not $PGF_{2\alpha}$ (0.8 µg/kg-min) significantly inhibited sigmoid motility [189]. Thus, PGs have different effects on colonic muscle depending on chemical structure and tissue type. These data are summarized in Table 7.

Mechanism of Prostaglandin Activity. Three major mechanisms by which PGs cause in vitro contractility have been proposed: cholinergic

TABLE 7. Effect of Exogenous Prostaglandins on the Colon

Model	Species	PGF₂α	PGF₁α	PGE₂	PGE₁	PGD₂	PGA₂	PGA₁	Other	Reference
Perfused colon (Longitudinal)	Man	27 46 397 399 441	399 441	27 46 110 171 397 399 441	46 110 324 397 399 442				PGA	399,441
	Guinea pig	21 27 40 116 196 197	21 116	21 22 27 111 116 175	3 21 22 23 116 389 441					
	Rat	40 78 198	198		78 425		198	198	9-Hydroperoxy-cis,trans,cis-6,10,12-octadecatrienoic acid — 5 PGF₁β — 78 13-Hydroperoxy-cis,cis,trans-6,9,11-octadecatrienoic acid — 5 PGI₂ — 300	
	Gerbil	169 272 293 454		169 293	454	169			PGH₂, PGG₂ — 169 16-E-Fluoro PGF₂α — 272 16,16-Difluoro PGF₂α methyl ester — 272	
	Dog	399	399	399	399				PGA	399
	Hamster	184	183	183	184				PGE₃	183

(continued)

TABLE 7. Effect of Exogenous Prostaglandins on the Colon (continued)

Model	Species	PGF$_{2\alpha}$	PGF$_{1\alpha}$	PGE$_2$	PGE$_1$	PGD$_2$	PGA$_2$	PGA$_1$	Other	Reference
(Circular)	Man	27 131 399 440	131 399 441	131 399	131 324 399				PGA	399, 441
	Guinea pig	27 28 116 131	116 131	22 28 116 131	22 116 131	28 428			17 Phenyl trinor-PGE$_2$ 17 Phenyl trinor-PGF$_{2\alpha}$	293 293
	Rat	131	131	131	131					
	Dog	399	399	399	399				PGA	399
Superfused colon (longitudinal)	Rat	170 178	170 178	170 178	170 178		178	178	15(S)-15-Methyl PGE$_2$ PGE$_2$ Methyl ester	423 423
	Chick	170 178	170 178	111 170 178 423	170		170 178	170 178	PGE, PGF 15(S)-15-Methyl PGE$_2$ PGE$_2$ Methyl ester	31 423 423
	Gerbil	169		169					PGG$_2$, PGH$_2$	169
Perfused Taenia coli, appendix	Man	46 298 448		46 298 448	46 298 448			411		169

Preparation	Species				
	Guinea pig		105	198 389	
Taenia coli (sucrose gap)	Guinea pig	325 326	131	131 436	
Isolated colon (peristalsis)	Guinea pig	116	116	22 116	22 116
In situ–In vivo (motor activity)	Man	145 189	145 189		
	Dog	92			
	Rabbit	310		310	
(Transit)	Man			295	
	Rat	381	381; this chapter		
(Defecation; diarrhea)	Man	90 127 136		185 295	
	Mouse	2	2 95	2	
16,16-Dimethyl PGE_2				381, 383	
PGE_2 Methyl ester				95	

potentiation, antagonism of adrenergic transmission, and direct smooth muscle stimulation. In colonic muscle strips from humans and guinea pigs, atropine did not inhibit the activity of PGE_1 [3,397,436], PGE_2 [397], or $PGF_{2\alpha}$ [325,326,397]. Hyoscine either had no effect [131,441] or reduced contractions elicited by $PGF_{2\alpha}$ [21]. This suggests that PG activity on colonic muscle strips is not modulated by cholinergic nerves, but rather by direct smooth muscle stimulation, suppression of inhibitory stimuli, or possibly a noncholinergic excitatory pathway [21,441]. However, atropine did antagonize PGE_1- and $PGF_{2\alpha}$-induced propulsive activity in the isolated guinea pig colon [196,197]. Furthermore, atropine partially inhibited the increase in colonic transit stimulation by 16,16-dimethyl PGE_2 in postoperative ileus rats [383]. Such data suggest that the relationship between muscle strip contractility and the more organized propulsive movements of an organ segment or an in vivo organ may be too complex for extrapolation. In vivo evidence supports a role for a cholinergic component of PG stimulatory activity.

Adrenergic blockade did not affect guinea pig *Taenia coli* contractions to $PGF_{2\alpha}$ [325]. In fact, stimulation of adrenergic receptors antagonized the contractions induced by PGE_1 in the rat colon [425] and human *Taenia coli* strips [46]. When, however, epinephrine or norepinephrine was added to human *Taenia coli* strips that were stimulated by PGE_1 and β-blocked, tension was increased. This increase was presumably due to α-adrenergic stimulation by the added norepinephrine, since α-blockade with phentolamine reduced the tone to the levels seen with the PG and β-blockade alone [46]. Thus, α-adrenergic stimulation appears to augment the tone produced by PGs, whereas β-adrenergic stimulation decreases it. Whether these effects indicate a direct action of PGs on adrenergic receptors in this organ has not been determined. Evidence does suggest, however, that PGE_1 may inhibit norepinephrine release and desensitize its postjunctional site of action in guinea pig *Taenia coli* [195,389]. Indirect evidence for PG interaction with sympathetic effectors comes also from studies on postoperative ileus rats. Colonic transit was increased by 16,16-dimethyl PGE_2 or chemical sympathectomy, but combining these treatments did not produce further enhancement of transit. Thus the action of both agents might be similar, that is, countering the antipropulsive effects of sympathetic stimulation caused by laparotomy [383]. Direct action on smooth muscle cannot be ruled out.

Pentagastrin and cholecystokinin stimulation of peristaltic activity was suppressed by indomethacin [48]. Furthermore, indomethacin and polyphloretin phosphate have been shown to enhance the ATP-induced relaxation of the guinea pig colon, suggesting that PG activity may be linked with that of other mediators [211]. Indomethacin has also been reported to block the "rebound contraction" due to nonadrenergic, noncholinergic (presumably purinergic) nerve stimulation or exogenous ATP in the guinea pig *Taenia coli* [50]. This study suggests that PGs may mediate inhibitory purinergic responses. Thus, the mechanism(s) of PG activity on the colon is still unclear.

TRANSIT STUDIES

Very few direct measurements of colonic transit have been performed because of the inaccessibility of the proximal colon. Only one study in humans has been reported where colonic transit, measured by telemetry, was accelerated after oral ingestion of PGE_1 (2 mg) [295]. Watery stools were also reported after oral ingestion of PGE_1 (10–40 µg/kg) [185] or intravenous $PGF_{2\alpha}$ (0.28–0.86 µg/kg-min) [90]. These results, coupled with premature defecation in subjects treated with PGs [90,185], could be interpreted as a sign of accelerated colonic transit. However, PG activity in this organ may be an indirect effect of enteropooling and accelerated small bowel transit with subsequent entry of abnormally large amounts of fluid into the colon, which could stimulate peristalsis.

CLINICAL IMPLICATIONS

16,16-Dimethyl PGE_2 and PGE_2 increased colonic transit when administered to postoperative ileus rats immediately after surgery [381]. This is probably a direct action of prostaglandins on colonic transit, since tying the ileocecal junction in PG-treated animals did not interfere with the accelerated transit of a gelatinous bolus injected into the proximal colon [381]. These results suggest that PGs might be of benefit in states of slowed colonic transit (e.g., constipation, paralytic ileus). Two uncontrolled clinical studies with $PGF_{2\alpha}$ infusion indicate that resolution of postoperative adynamic ileus with this PG is possible [127,136].

Prostaglandins may play a role in ulcerative colitis, since patients with this disease show elevated levels of PG in stools, blood, urine, and rectal mucosa [152–154,401,410]. Sulfasalazine, the most common drug used in the treatment for ulcerative colitis, has been shown to inhibit PGE_2 synthesis in rat colon and in cultured mucosa from such patients [186]. The drug metabolite, 5-aminosalicylic acid, was even more effective in inhibiting PG synthesis [401]. These studies suggest that control of colonic PG production may be beneficial in reducing the inflammatory aspects of ulcerative colitis.

Gallbladder

PGE_2 and $PGF_{2\alpha}$ (0.1–1.0 µg/ml) contracted guinea pig gallbladder strips, while PGE_1 at the same doses caused relaxation [6–8]. Arachidonic acid also produced contractions, but these contractions were inhibited by indomethacin, whereas those caused by PGE_2 were not [8]. PGA_1 (50–400 µg/ml), PGE_1 (50–400 µg/ml), PGE_2 (500–4000 µg/ml), and $PGF_{2\alpha}$ (500–4000 µg/ml) contracted or increased pressure of the intact isolated gallbladder of guinea pig [173,303,447]. β-adrenergic agonists diminished contractions due to PGE_1, whereas β-blockers or α-agonists augmented it [422]. In anesthetized dogs gallbladder pressure increased after $PGF_{2\alpha}$ (4 µg/kg) given intravenously and, to a lesser extent, by similar doses of PGE_1 and PGE_2 when the cystic duct was clamped, thereby excluding pressure contributions from the sphincter of Oddi [311]. The cholecystokinetic action of pentagastrin was abolished by indomethacin treatment in this preparation, suggesting that PGs may mediate the gallbladder contractions caused by this hormone [311].

$PGF_{2\alpha}$ constricted the sphincter of Oddi in this model, whereas PGE_1 and PGE_2 relaxed it [311]. Similar results were obtained in rabbits [390]. PGE_1, PGE_2, and $PGF_{2\alpha}$ (10^{-5} to 10^{-8} M) caused a triphasic response in the isolated guinea pig of rabbit gallbladder: fluid loss followed by a dose-dependent inhibition of fluid transport, and finally net secretion [173,267,303]. Thus, PGs can affect fluid transport, gallbladder contractility, and relaxation of the sphincter of Oddi.

PGE_2 given intravenously (20, 50, or 75 µg per subject) in normal volunteers caused no change in gallbladder shape or size during oral cholecystography [245]. However, 16,16-dimethyl PGE_2 given intragastrically (140 µg per patient) in normal subjects greatly reduced the bile recovered from the jejunum, suggesting impairment of gallbladder emptying, hepatic biliary output, or relaxation of the sphincter of Oddi [115]. The effects of clinical doses of PG on the gallbladder are as yet poorly defined. However, indomethacin has been used successfully to treat attacks of biliary pain in patients with gallbladder disease, suggesting that endogenous PGs may play a significant role in this condition [434].

REFERENCES

1. Abdel-Aziz, A. (1974) Blockage by prostaglandins E_2 and $F_{1\alpha}$ of the response of the rabbit ileum to stimulation of sympathetic nerve and its reversal by some antihistamines, dexamphetamine and methylphenidate. Eur. J. Pharmacol. 25, 226–230.

2. Acharya, S. B., Debnath, P. K., Dey, C., and Sanyal, A. K. (1977) Effect of prostaglandins on gastrointestinal smooth muscle. Indian J. Med. Res. 66, 1004–1010.

3. Akanuma, M. (1970) Relationship between stimulating action of prostaglandin E_2 and calcium on the gastrointestinal smooth muscle from the guinea pig. Sapporo Med. J. 38, 53–59.

4. Amy, J. J., Jackson, D. M., Ganesan, P. A., and Karim, S. M. M. (1973) Prostaglandin 15(R)-15-methyl-E_2 methyl ester for suppression of gastric acidity in gravida at term. Br. Med. J. 4, 208–211.

5. Anderson, W. G., Porter, N. A., and Menzel, D. B. (1976) Activity of endoperoxides and hydroperoxides on smooth muscle. Fed. Proc. 35, 457.

6. Andersson, K. E., Andersson, R., Hedner, P., and Persson, C. G. A. (1972) Dual effects on gallbladder and sphincter of Oddi induced by cholecystokinin and prostaglandins. Acta Pharmacol. Toxicol. 31 (Suppl. 1), 44.

7. Andersson, K. E., Andersson, R., Hedner, P., and Persson, C. G. A. (1973) Analogous effects of cholecystokinin and prostaglandin E_2 on mechanical activity and tissue levels of cAMP in biliary smooth muscle. Acta Physiol. Scand. 87, 41A–42A.

8. Andersson, K. E., Hedner, P., and Persson, C. G. A. (1974) Differentiation of the contractile effects of prostaglandin E_2 and the C-terminal octapeptide of cholecystokinin in isolated guinea pig gallbladder. Acta Physiol. Scand. 90, 657–663.

9. Baker, R., Jaffe, B. M., Reed, J. D., Shaw, B., and Venables, C. W. (1978) Exogenous prostaglandins and gastric secretion in the cat. J. Physiol. 278, 441–450.

10. Baker, R., Jaffe, B. M., Reed, J. D., Shaw, B., and Venables, C. W. (1978) Endogenous prostaglandins and gastric secretion in the cat. J. Physiol. 278, 451–460.

11. Baker, R., Jaffe, B. M., Reed, J. D., Shaw, B., and Venables, C. W. (1978) Relationships between gastric acid, pepsin, and prostaglandin secretion. Gastroenterology 74, 1005.

12. Banerjee, A. K., Christmas, A. J., and Hall, C. E. (1975) Effects of H_2-receptor antagonists, prostaglandins E_2 and 16,16-dimethyl-E_2-methyl ester on gastric acid secretion, mucosal blood flow and ulceration. 6th Int. Congr. Pharmacol. 120 (Abstr.).

13. Banerjee, A. K., Phillips, J., and Winning, W. W. (1972) E-Type prostaglandins and gastric acid secretion in the rat. Nature (London) New Biol. 238, 177–179.

14. Bartels, J., Kunze, H., Vogt, W., and Willie, G. (1970) Prostaglandin: Liberation from and formation in perfused frog intestine. Naunyn-Schmiedebergs Arch. Pharmacol. 266, 199.

15. Barthó, L. (1978) Adrenergic responses of the guinea-pig ileum: Inhibition by prostaglandins and potentiation by non-steroid anti-inflammatory drugs (NSAIDs). Arch. Int. Pharmacodyn. Ther. 235, 238–247.

16. Baysal, F., and Gemalmaz, A. (1972) Effects of prostaglandin E_1 on the stomach muscles of a frog and related studies. Turk. Hij. Tecr. Biyol. Derg. 32, 116–121.

17. Bebiak, D. M., Miller, E. R., Huslig, R. L., and Smith, W. L. (1979) Distribution of prostaglandin-forming cyclooxygenase in the porcine stomach. Fed. Proc. 38, 884.

18. Bennett, A., Eley, K. G., and Scholes, G. B. (1968) Effects of prostaglandins E_1 and E_2 on human, guinea pig and rat isolated small intestine. Br. J. Pharmacol. 34, 630–638.

19. Bennett, A., Eley, K. G., and Scholes, G. B. (1968) Effect of prostaglandins E_1 and E_2 on intestinal motility in the guinea pig and rat. Br. J. Pharmacol. 34, 639–647.

20. Bennett, A., Eley, K. G., and Stockley, H. L. (1975) Modulation by prostaglandins of contractions in guinea pig ileum. Prostaglandins 9, 377–384.

21. Bennett, A., Eley, K. G., and Stockley, H. L. (1975) The effects of prostaglandins on guinea pig isolated intestine and their possible contribution to muscle activity and tone. Br. J. Pharmacol. 54, 197–204.

22. Bennett A., Eley, K. G., and Stockley, H. L. (1976) Inhibition of peristalsis in guinea pig isolated ileum and colon by drugs that block prostaglandin synthesis. Br. J. Pharmacol. 57, 335–340.

23. Bennett, A., and Fleshler, B. (1969) Action of prostaglandin E_1 on the longitudinal muscle of the guinea pig isolated colon. Br. J. Pharmacol. 35, 351P–352P.

24. Bennett, A., Friedmann, C. A., and Vane, J. R. (1967) Release of prostaglandin E_1 from the rat stomach. Nature (London) 216, 873–876.

25. Bennett, A., Jarosik, C., and Wilson, D. E. (1978) A study of receptors activated by analogs of prostaglandin H_2. Br. J. Pharmacol. 63, 358P.

26. Bennett, A., Murray, J. G., and Wyllie, J. H. (1968) Occurrence of prostaglandin E_2 in the human stomach, and a study of its effects on human isolated gastric muscle. Br. J. Pharmacol. Chemother. 32, 339–349.

27. Bennett, A., and Posner, J. (1971) Studies on prostaglandin antagonists. Br. J. Pharmacol. 42, 584–594.

28. Bennett, A., and Sanger, G. J. (1978) The effects of prostaglandin D_2 on the circular muscle of guinea pig isolated ileum and colon. Br. J. Pharmacol. 63, 357P–358P.

29. Bennett A., Stamford, I. F., and Stockley, H. L. (1977) Estimation and characterization of prostaglandins in the human gastrointestinal tract. Br. J. Pharmacol. 61, 579–586.

30. Bennett, A., and Stockley, H. L. (1977) The contribution of prostaglandins in the muscle of human isolated small intestine to neurogenic responses. Br. J. Pharmacol. 61, 573–578.

31. Bergström, S., Eliasson, R., von Euler, U. S., and Sjövall, J. (1959) Some biological effects of two crystalline prostaglandin factors. Acta Physiol. Scand. 45, 133–144.

32. Bertaccini, G., Impicciatore, M., and DeCaro, G. (1973) Action of caerulein and related substances on the pyloric sphincter of the anaesthetized rat. Eur. J. Pharmacol. 22, 320–324.

33. Beubler, E., and Juan, H. (1978) PGE release, blood flow and transmucosal water movement after mechanical stimulation of the rat jejunal mucosa. Arch. Pharmacol. 305, 91–95.

34. Bhana, D., Karim, S. M. M., Carter, D. C., and Ganesan, P. A. (1973) The effect of orally administered prostaglandins A_1, A_2, and 15-epi-A_2 on human gastric secretion. Prostaglandins 3, 307–316.

34a. Bolton, J. P., and Cohen, M. M. (1978) Stimulation of non-parietal cell secretion in canine Heidenhain pouches by 16,16-dimethyl prostaglandin E_2. Digestion 17, 291–299.

35. Bolton, J. P., Palmer, D., and Cohen, M. M. (1976) Effect of the E_2 prostaglandins on gastric mucus production in rats. Surg. Forum 27, 402–403.

36. Bolton, J. P., Palmer, D., and Cohen, M. M. (1978) Stimulation of mucus and non-parietal cell secretion by the E_2 prostaglandins. Am. J. Dig. Dis. 23, 359–364.

37. Book, L. S., Johnson, D. G., Jubiz, W., and Roberts, C. (1979) Elevated prostaglandin E in children with chronic idiopathic intestinal pseudo-obstruction syndrome (CIIPS): Effects of prostaglandin synthetase inhibitors on gastrointestinal motility. Clin. Res. 27, 100A.

38. Botting, J. H. (1977) The mechanism of the release of prostaglandin-like activity from the guinea pig isolated ileum. J. Pharm. Pharmacol. 29, 708–709.

39. Botting, J. H., and Salzmann, R. (1974) The effect of indomethacin on the release of prostaglandin E_2 and acetylcholine from guinea-pig isolated ileum at rest and during field stimulation. Br. J. Pharmacol. 50, 119–124.

40. Boullin, D. J., Hunt, T. M., and Rogers, A. T. (1978) Models for investigating the aetiology of cerebral arterial spasm: Comparative responses of the human basilar artery with rat colon, anococcygeus, stomach fundus, and aorta and guinea pig ileum and colon. Br. J. Pharmacol. 63, 251–257.

41. Bourry, J., Demol, P., and Sarles, H. (1979) Interaction of dimethyl prostaglandin E_2 and ethanol in rat pancreatic secretion. Can. J. Physiol. Pharmacol. 57, 152–156.

42. Bowen, J. C., Kuo Y.-Y., Pawlik, W., Williams, D., Shanbour, L. L., and Jacobson, E. D. (1975) Electrophysiological effects of burimamide and 16,16-dimethyl prostaglandin E_2 on the canine gastric mucosa. Gastroenterology 68, 1480–1484.

43. Bressler, R., Vargas-Cordon, M., Lebovitz, H. E., and Durham, N. C. (1968) Tranylcypromine: A potent insulin secretagogue and hypoglycemic agent. Diabetes 17, 617–624.

44. Brodie, D. A., and Chase, B. J. (1967) Role of gastric acid in aspirin-induced gastric irritation in the rat. Gastroenterology 53, 604–610.

45. Brodows, R. G. (1978) Endogenous prostaglandins as insulin secretagogues: Effect of indomethacin (INDO) on basal, glucose-, and arginine-stimulated insulin release in man. Clin. Res. 26, 677A.

46. Bruch, H.-P., Schmidt, E., and Laven, R. (1976) The modulation of the prostaglandin-induced (E_1, E_2, $F_{1\alpha}$) motility of the large intestine by the adrenergic system. Acta Hepatogastroenterol. 23, 430–434.

47. Bruch, H.-P., Schmidt, E., and Laven, R. (1978) Prostaglandins and peristalsis of the human colon. Eur. J. Physiol. 373 (Suppl.), R52.

48. Bruch, H.-P., Schmidt, E., and Laven, R. (1978) The role of prostaglandins and peristalsis of the human colon. Acta Hepatogastroenterol. 25, 303–307.

49. Burks, T. F., Heindel, J. J., and Grubb, M. N. (1976) Morphine interactions with intestinal prostaglandins. Pharmacologist 18, 175.

50. Burnstock, G., Cocks, T., Paddle, B., and Staszewska-Barczak, J. (1975) Evidence that prostaglandin is responsible for the "rebound contraction" following stimulation of non-adrenergic, non-cholinergic ("purinergic") inhibitory nerves. Eur. J. Pharmacol. 31, 360–362.

51. Burr, I. M., and Sharp, R. (1974) Effects of prostaglandin E_1 and of epinephrine on the dynamics of insulin release in vitro. Endocrinology 94, 835–839.

52. Calaprice, A., Lampa, E., Rosatti, F., Giordano, L., Maglicilo, S., Di Mezza, F., Spaziante, G., Ariello, B., and Marino, E. (1979) Analisi sperimentale comparativa degli effetti della PGE$_2$ sulla muscolatura uterina di bovine e di bufale (vuote e gravide) intestinale e cardiaca, e su quella striata di animali di laboratorio in funzione del suo impiego nella pratica ostetrico-ginecologica. XI Congresso Nazionale della Societa Italiana di Buiatria e Giornata Internazionale della Bufala.

53. Carlson, L. A., Ekelund, L.-G., and Oro, L. (1968) Clinical and metabolic effects of different doses of prostaglandin E$_2$ in man. Acta Med. Scand. 183, 423–430.

54. Carmichael, H. A., Nelson, L. M., and Russell, R. I. (1977) Cimetidine and prostaglandins: Evidence for different modes of action on the gastric mucosa. Gut 18, A404.

55. Carmichael, H. A., Nelson, L. M., and Russell, R. I. (1978) Cimetidine and prostaglandin: Evidence for different modes of action on the rat gastric mucosa. Gastroenterology 74, 1229–1232.

56. Carmichael, H. A., Nelson, L., Russell, R. I., Lyon, A., and Chandra, V. (1977) The effect of the synthetic prostaglandin analog 15(R)-15-methyl-PGE$_2$ methyl ester on gastric mucosal hemorrhage induced in rats by taurocholic acid and hydrochloric acid. Am. J. Dig. Dis. 22, 411–414.

57. Carter, D. C., Ganesan, P. A., Bhana, D., and Karim, S. M. M. (1974) The effect of locally administered prostaglandin 15(R)-15-methyl PGE$_2$ methyl ester on gastric ulcer formation in the Shay rat preparation. Prostaglandins 5, 455–463.

58. Carter, D. C., Karim, S. M. M., Bhana, D., and Ganesan, P. A. (1973) Inhibition of human gastric secretion by prostaglandins. Br. J. Surg. 60, 828–831.

59. Case, R. M., and Scratcherd, T. (1972) Prostaglandin action on pancreatic blood flow and on electrolyte and enzyme secretion by exocrine pancreas in vivo and in vitro. J. Physiol. 226, 393–405.

60. Catchpole, B. N. (1969) Ileus: Use of sympathetic blocking agents in its treatment. Surgery 66, 811–820.

61. Chapnick, B. M., Feigen, L. P., Flemming, J. M., Hyman, A. L., and Kadowitz, P. J. (1977) Comparison of the effects of prostaglandin H$_2$ and an analog of prostaglandin H$_2$ on the intestinal vascular bed of the dog. Pharmacologist 19, 148.

62. Chapnick, B. M., Feigen, L. P., Hyman, A. L., and Kadowitz, P. J. (1978) Differential effects of prostaglandins in the mesenteric vascular. Am. J. Physiol. 235, H326–H332.

63. Charters, A. C., Brown, B. N., and Orloff, M. J. (1975) Metiamide and prostaglandin E$_1$ inhibition of pentagastrin stimulated acid secretion. Gastroenterology 68, 872.

64. Chase, H. P., Williams, R. L., and Dupont, J. (1979) Increased prostaglandin synthesis in childhood diabetes mellitus. J. Pediatr. 94, 185–189.

65. Chaudhury, T. K., and Jacobson, E. D. (1978) Prostaglandin cytoprotection of gastric mucosa. Gastroenterology 74, 58–63.

66. Chaudhury, T. K., and Robert, A. (1980) Prevention by mild irritants of gastric necrosis produced in rats by sodium taurocholate. Dig. Dis. Sci. 25, 830–836.

67. Chawala, R. C., and Eisenberg, M. M. (1969) Prostaglandin inhibition of innervated antral motility in dogs. Proc. Soc. Exp. Biol. Med. 132, 1081–1086.

68. Chen, F. W. K., Teck, H. S., and Karim, S. M. M. (1977) The effect of 15(R)-15-methyl prostaglandin E$_2$ on gastric acid secretion in duodenal ulcer patients. Prostaglandins 13, 115–124.

69. Cheung, L. Y., Jubiz, W., Moore, J. G., and Frailey, J. (1975) Gastric prostaglandin E (PGE) output during basal and stimulated acid secretion in normal subjects and patients with peptic ulcer. Gastroenterology 68, 873.

70. Cheung, L. Y., and Lowry, S. F. (1976) Effect of prostaglandin E$_2$ (PGE$_2$) and 16,6-dimethyl PGE$_2$ (DMPGE$_2$) on gastric acid secretion and blood flow. Gastroenterology 70, 870.

71. Cheung, L. Y., Moody, F. G., Larson, K., and Lowry, S. F. (1978) Oxygen consumption during cimetidine and prostaglandin E$_2$ inhibition of acid secretion. Am. J. Physiol. 234, E445–E450.

72. Chong, E. K. S., and Downing, O. A. (1974) Reversal by prostaglandin E_2 of the inhibitory effect of indomethacin on contractions of guinea pig ileum induced by angiotension. J. Pharm. Pharmacol. 26, 729–730.

73. Chousterman, M., Petite, J. P., Housset, E., and Hornych, A. (1977) Prostaglandins and acute intestinal pseudo-obstruction. Lancet 2, 138–139.

74. Christensen, J., and Daniel, E. E. (1968) Effects of some autonomic drugs on circular esophageal smooth muscle. J. Pharmacol. Exp. Ther. 159, 243–249.

75. Classen, M., Koch, H., Bickhardt, J., Topf, G., and Demling L. (1971) The effect of prostaglandin E_1 on the pentagastrin-stimulated gastric secretion in man. Digestion 4, 333–344.

76. Classen, M., Koch, H., Deyhle, P., Weidenhiller, S., and Demling, L. (1970) Wirkung von prostaglandin E_1 auf die basale Magensekretion des Menschen. Klin. Wochenschr. 48, 876–878.

77. Classen, M., Sturzanhofecker, P., Koch, H., and Demling, L. (1973) The effect of prostaglandin E_1 on the secretion and the motility of the human stomach. Acta Hepatogastroenterol. 20, 159–162.

78. Clegg, P. C. (1966) Antagonism by prostaglandins of the responses of various smooth muscle preparations to sympathomimetics. Nature (London) 209, 1137–1139.

79. Coceani, F., Pace-Asciak, C., Volta, F., and Wolfe, L. S. (1967) Effect of nerve stimulation on prostaglandin formation and release from the rat stomach. Am. J. Physiol. 213, 1056–1064.

80. Coceani, F., and Wolfe, L. S. (1966) On the action of prostaglandin E_1 and prostaglandins from the brain on the isolated rat stomach. Can. J. Physiol. Pharmacol. 44, 933–950.

81. Coceani, F., and Wolfe, L. S. (1967) Pharmacological properties of prostaglandin E_1 and prostaglandins extracted from the brain. Prog. Biochem. Pharmacol. 3, 129–135.

82. Cohen, M. M. (1975) Prostaglandin E_2 prevents gastric mucosal barrier damage. Gastroenterology 68, 876.

83. Cohen, M. M. (1978) Mucosal cytoprotection by prostaglandin E_2. Lancet 2, 1253–1254.

84. Cohen, M. M., and Pollett, J. M. (1977) Treatment of gastric erosions with E_2 prostaglandins and metiamide. Gastroenterology 72, 1039.

85. Conolly, M. E., Bieck, P. R., Payne, N. A., Adkins, B., and Oates, J. A. (1977) Effect of the prostaglandin precursor, arachidonic acid, on histamine stimulated gastric secretion in the conscious dog, and observations on the effect of inhibiting endogenous prostaglandin synthesis. Gut 18, 429–437.

86. Corrado, A. P., and Grellet, M. (1976) Mechanism of the sialogogic effect induced by bradykinin in dogs: Possible mediation by endogenous prostaglandin. Adv. Exp. Med. Biol. 70, 81–95.

87. Corrado, A. P., Grellet, M., and Ribeiro, R. T. N. (1976) Possible mediation by endogenous prostaglandin of the sialogogic effect induced by bradykinin in dogs. Agents Actions 6, 419.

88. Crocker, A. D., Walker, R., and Wilson, N. A. (1978) Prostaglandins and the contractile action of bradykinin on the longitudinal muscle of rat isolated ileum. Br. J. Pharmacol. 64, 441P.

89. Crocker, A. D., and Willavoys, S. P. (1976) Possible involvement of prostaglandins in the contractile action of bradykinin on rat terminal ileum. J. Pharm. Pharmacol. 28, 78–79.

90. Cummings, J. H., Newman, A., Misiewicz, J. J., Milton-Thompson, G. J., and Billings, J. A. (1973) Effect of intravenous prostaglandin $F_{2\alpha}$ on small intestinal function in man. Nature (London) 243, 169.

91. Dajani, E. Z., Callison, D. A., and Bianchi, R. G. (1976) Gastric antisecretory effects of E-prostaglandins in conscious monkeys. Fed. Proc. 35, 539.

92. Dajani, E. Z., Bertermann, R. E., Rose, E. A. W., Schweingruber, F. L., and Woods, E. M. (1979) Canine gastrointestinal motility effects of prostaglandin $F_{2\alpha}$ in vivo. Arch. Int. Pharmacodyn. 237, 16–24.

93. Dajani, E. Z., Callison, D. A., Bianchi, R. G., and Driskill, D. R. (1976) Gastric antisecretory effects of E prostaglandins in rhesus monkeys. Am. J. Dig. Dis. 21, 1020–1028.

94. Dajani, E. Z., Driskill, D. R., Bianchi, R. G., Collins, P. W., and Pappo, R. (1976) SC-29333: A potent inhibitor of canine gastric secretion. Am. J. Dig. Dis. 21, 1049–1057.

95. Dajani, E. Z., Rose, E. A. W., and Bertermann, R. E. (1975) Effects of E prostaglandins, diphenoxylate and morphine on intestinal motility in vivo. Eur. J. Pharmacol. 34, 105–113.

96. Dalton, T. (1977) The effect of prostaglandin E_1 on cyclic AMP production in the salivary glands of *Calliphora erythrocephala*. Experientia 33, 1329–1330.

97. Daniel, E. E., Crankshaw, J., and Sarna, S. (1979) Prostaglandins and myogenic control of tension in the lower esophageal sphincter in vitro. Prostaglandins 17, 629–639.

98. Daniel, E. E., Crankshaw, J., and Sarna, S. (1979) Prostaglandins and tetrodotoxin-insensitive relaxation of opossum lower esophageal sphincter. Am. J. Physiol. 236, E153–E172.

99. Daniel, E. E., Crankshaw, J., Sarna, S., Jessup, R., Johnson, M., and Fitzgerald, D. A. (1980) Prostaglandins and lower esophageal sphincter tone in opossum. In: J. Christensen (ed.), Gastrointestinal Motility: Proceedings of the Seventh International Symposium, Raven Press, New York, pp. 21–28.

100. Daniel, E. E., Sarna, S., Waterfall, W., and Crankshaw, J. (1979) Role of prostaglandins in regulating the tone of opossum lower esophageal sphincter in vivo. Prostaglandins 17, 641–649.

101. Daturi, S., Franceschini, J., Mandelli, V., Mizzotti, B., and Usardi, M. M. (1974) A proposed role for PGE_2 in the genesis of stress-induced gastric ulcers. Br. J. Pharmacol. 52, 464P.

102. Davenport, H. W. (1969) Gastric mucosal hemorrhage in dogs. Effects of acid, aspirin, and alcohol. Gastroenterology 56, 439–449.

103. Davison, P., Ramwell, P. W., and Willis, A. L. (1972) Inhibition of intestinal tone and prostaglandin synthesis by 5,8,11,14-eicosatetraynoic acid. Br. J. Pharmacol. 46, 547P–548P.

104. Dickinson, R. G., O'Hagan, J. E., Schotz, M., Binnington, K. C., and Hegarty, M. P. (1976) Prostaglandin in the saliva of the cattle tick *Boophilus microplus*. Aust. J. Exp. Biol. Med. Sci. 54, 475–486.

105. Diegel, J., and Coburn, R. F. (1979) Site of the Ca^{++} effect on PGE_2 synthesis in guinea pig *Taenia coli*. Fed. Proc. 38, 180.

106. Dilawari, J. B., Newman, A., Poleo, J., and Misiewicz, J. J. (1975) Response of the human cardiac sphincter to circulating prostaglandins $F_{2\alpha}$ and E_2 and to anti-inflammatory drugs. Gut 16, 137–143.

107. D'Onofrio, F., Torella, R., Giugliano, D., Improta, L., and Grazioli, A. (1977) Effects of vaso-inactive doses of PGA_1 and PGE_1 on insulin secretion in the rat. Pharmacol. Res. Commun. 9, 427–436.

108. Dozois, R. R., Kim, J. K., and Dousa, T. P. (1978) Interaction of prostaglandins with canine gastric mucosal adenylate cyclase–cyclic AMP system. Am. J. Physiol. 235, E546–E551.

109. Dozois, R. R., and Wollin, A. (1975) Prostaglandine E_2, adénylate cyclase et sécrétion gastrique chez le chien. Biol. Gastroenterol. 8, 122.

110. Dupont, C., Laburthe, M., and Rosselin, G. (1978) Isolation of epithelial cells of human colon and demonstration of the action of V.I.P. Scand. J. Gastroenterol. 13, 51.

111. Eckenfels, A., and Vane, J. R. (1972) Prostaglandins, oxygen tension and smooth muscle tone. Br. J. Pharmacol. 45, 451–462.

112. Edery, H., and Shemesh, M. (1978) Release of prostaglandins mediating the potentiation of bradykinin by BPF and chymotrypsin in rat isolated ileum. Agents Actions 8, 159–160.

113. Ehrenpreis, S., Greenberg, J., and Belman, S. (1973) Prostaglandins reverse inhibition of electrically induced contractions of guinea pig ileum by morphine, indomethacin and acetylsalicylic acid. Nature (London) New Biol. 245, 280–282.

114. Ehrenpreis, S., Greenberg, J., and Comaty, J. E. (1978) Prostaglandin-norepinephrine interaction in guinea pig longitudinal muscle. Life Sci. 23, 11–16.

115. Ekelund, K., Johansson, C., and Nylander, B. (1977) Effects of 16,16-dimethyl prostaglandin E_2 on food stimulated pancreatic secretion and output of bile in man. Scand. J. Gastroenterol. 12, 457–460.

116. Eley, K. G., Bennett, A., and Stockley, H. L. (1977) The effects of prostaglandins E_1, E_2, $F_{1\alpha}$ and $F_{2\alpha}$ on guinea pig ileal and colonic peristalsis. J. Pharm. Pharmacol. 29, 276–280.

117. Evans, J., and Siegel, I. A. (1976) Effect of prostaglandins on dog submandibular gland function. J. Dent. Res. 55, B230.

118. Famaey, J. P., Fontaine, J., and Reuse, J. (1975) Inhibiting effects of morphine, chloroquine, non-steroidal and steroidal anti-inflammatory drugs on electrically induced contractions of guinea pig ileum and the reversing effect of prostaglandins. Agents Actions 5, 354–358.

119. Famaey, J. P., Fontaine, J., and Reuse, J. (1977) Effect of high concentrations of nonsteroidal and steroidal anti-inflammatory drugs on prostaglandin-induced contractions of the guinea pig isolated ileum. Prostaglandins 13, 107–114.

120. Famaey, J. P., Fontaine, J., and Reuse J. (1977) The effects of non-steroidal anti-inflammatory drugs on cholinergic and histamine-induced contractions of guinea pig isolated ileum. Br. J. Pharmacol. 60, 165–171.

121. Famaey, J. P., Fontaine, J., Seaman, I., and Reuse, J. 1977) A possible role of prostaglandins in guinea pig isolated ileum contractions to serotonin. Prostaglandins 14, 119–124.

122. Faxén, A., Berger, T., Kewenter, J., and Kock, N. G. (1977) Gastric emptying after different surgical procedures for duodenal ulcer. Scand. J. Gastroenterol. 12, 983–987.

123. Faxén A., Kewenter, J., and Kock, N. G. (1978) Gastric emptying of a liquid meal in health and duodenal ulcer disease. Scand. J. Gastroenterol. 13, 735–740.

124. Ferguson, W. W., Edmonds, A. W., Starling, J. R., and Wangensteen, S. L. (1973) Protective effect of prostaglandin E_1 (PGE_1) on lysosomal enzyme release in serotonin-induced gastric ulceration. Ann. Surg. 177, 648–654.

125. Ferreira, S. H., Herman, A. G., and Vane, J. R. (1972) Prostaglandin generation maintains the smooth muscle tone of the rabbit isolated jejunum. Br. J. Pharmacol. 44, 328P–330P.

126. Ferreira, S. H., Herman, A. G., and Vane, J. R. (1976) Prostaglandin production by rabbit isolated jejunum and its relationship to the inherent tone of the preparation. Br. J. Pharmacol. 56, 469–477.

127. Fiedler, L. (1980) $PGF_{2\alpha}$—A new therapy for paralytic ileus? In: B. Samuelsson, P. Ramwell, R. Paoletti (eds.), Advances in Prostaglandin and Thromboxane Research, Vol. 8, Raven Press, New York, pp. 1609–1610.

128. Fiedler, L., Lindenmaier, H., Hartung, H., Kohnlein, H. E., and Wiegend, G. (1975) Behavior of intestinal motility and serum gastrin level during prostaglandin administration in acute mechanical ileus of the rabbit. Langenbecks Arch. Chir. (Suppl.), 309–314.

129. Fiedler, L., Lindenmaier, H. L., Hartung, H., Trendelenburg, C., and Assfalg, W. (1976) Verhalten von Darmmotilitat und Serum-gastrinsprigel unter gabe von Prostaglandin A_1, E_1 und $F_{2\alpha}$ beim frischen mechanischen Ileus des Kaninchens. Langenbecks Arch. Chir. (Suppl.), 37–42.

130. Fitzpatrick, F. A., and Wynalda, M. A. (1976) In vivo suppression of prostaglandin biosynthesis by non-steroidal anti-inflammatory agents. Prostaglandins 12, 1037–1051.

131. Fleshler, B., and Bennett, A. (1969) Responses of human, guinea pig and rat colonic circular muscle to prostaglandin. J. Lab. Clin. Med. 74, 872–873.

132. Fontaine, J., Seaman, I., Famaey, J. P., and Reuse, J. (1978) The inhibitory effects of two mineralocorticoids (aldosterone and desoxycorticosterone) on the responses of the guinea pig isolated ileum to various agonists. Arch. Int. Pharmacodyn. 232, 336–338.

133. Fontaine, J., Van Neuten, J. M., and Reuse, J. J. (1977) Effects of prostaglandins on the peristaltic reflex of the guinea pig ileum. Arch. Int. Pharmacodyn. Ther. 266, 341–343.

134. Francis, H. P., Smy, J. R., and Sunderland, U. K. (1978) Comparison of intravenous and close arterial infusions of prostaglandins E_1 and E_2 on gastric acid secretion and mucosal blood flow in anaesthetized cats. J. Physiol. 285, 38P.

135. Frankhuijzer, A. L., and Bonta, I. L. (1975) Role of prostaglandins in tone and effector reactivity of the isolated rat stomach preparation. Eur. J. Pharmacol. 31, 44–52.

136. Fukunishi, S., Amano, S., Saijo, H., Matsumoto, K., Iriyama, K., and Fujino, T. (1977) The effects of prostaglandin $F_{2\alpha}$ on gastrointestinal tract motility following surgery, from the standpoint of electrophysiology. Jpn. J. Smooth Muscle Res. 13, 141–152.

137. Fung, W. P., and Karim, S. M. M. (1976) Effect of 15(R)-15-methyl prostaglandin E_2 on the healing of gastric ulcers—Double blind endoscopic study. Med. J. Aust. 2, 127–128.

138. Fung, W. P., and Karim, S. M. M. (1976) Effect of prostaglandin E_2 on the healing of gastric ulcers: A double-blind endoscopic trial. Aust. NZ J. Med. 6, 121–122.

139. Fung, W. P., Karim, S. M. M., and Tye, C. Y. (1974) Double-blind trial of 15(R)-15-methyl prostaglandin E_2 methyl ester in the relief of peptic ulcer pain. Ann. Acad. Med. 3, 375.

140. Fung, W. P., Karim, S. M. M., and Tye, C. Y. (1974) Effect of 15(R)-15-methyl prostaglandin E_2 methyl ester on healing of gastric ulcers. Controlled endoscopic study. Lancet 2, 10–12.

140a. Fung, W. P., Lee, S. K., and Karim, S. M. M. (1974) Effect of prostaglandin 15(R)-15-methyl-E_2-methyl ester on the gastric mucosa in patients with peptic ulceration. An endoscopic and histological study. Prostaglandins 5, 465–472.

141. Gabryelewicz, A., Szalaj, W., Kinalska, I., Stasiewicz, J., and Langiewicz, J. (1974) The effect of prostaglandin E_1 on exocrine pancreatic secretion (in vivo and in vitro). Pol. J. Pharmacol. Pharm. 26, 263–267.

142. Gerkens, J. F., Flexner, C., Oates, J. A., and Shand, D. G. (1977) Prostaglandin and histamine involvement in the gastric vasodilator action of pentagastrin. J. Pharmacol. Exp. Ther. 201, 421–426.

143. Gerkens, J. F., Gerber, J. G., Shand, D. G., and Branch, R. A. (1978) Effect of PGI_2, PGE_2 and 6-keto-$PGF_{1\alpha}$ on canine gastric blood flow and acid secretion. Prostaglandins 16, 815–823.

144. Gibinski, K., Rybicka, J., Mikos, E., and Nowak, A. (1977) Double-blind clinical trial on gastroduodenal ulcer healing with prostaglandin E_2 analogues. Gut 18, 636–639.

145. Gintzler, A. R., and Musacchio, J. M. (1974) Failure of prostaglandins to participate in the inhibitory response of the guinea pig ileum to morphine. Fed. Proc. 33, 502.

146. Giugliano, D., Torella, R. Improta, L., and D'Onofrio, F. (1978) Effects of prostaglandin E_1 and prostaglandin $F_{2\alpha}$ on insulin and glucagon plasma levels during the intravenous glucose tolerance test in man. Diabetes Metab. 4, 187–191.

147. Giugliano, D., Torella, R., Sgambato, S., and D'Onofrio, F. (1978) Prostaglandin E_1 induces basal glucagon in man. Pharmacol. Res. Commun. 10, 813–821.

148. Gold, M. H., Jr., Mathias, J. R., Carlson, G. M., Martin, J. L., and Jaffe, B. M. (1978) The relationship of tissue and portal vein blood prostaglandin levels to the migrating action potential complex of cholera. Gastroenterology 74, 1125.

149. Golenhofen, K., and Lüdtke, F. E. (1980) Excitatory and inhibitory effects on canine pyloric musculature. In: J. Christensen (ed.), Gastrointestinal Motility. Proceedings of the Seventh International Symposium, Raven Press, New York, pp. 203–212.

150. Gommelaer, G., and Guth, P. H. (1978) Protection by histamine antagonists and prostaglandin against gastric mucosal barrier disruption. Pharmacologist 20, 208.

151. Gorman, R. R., Bunting, S., and Miller, O. V. (1977) Modulation of human platelet adenylate cyclase by prostaglandin (PGX). Prostaglandins 13, 373–388.

151a. Gorman, R. R., Hamilton, R. D., and Hopkins, N. K. (1979) Stimulation of human foreskin fibroblast adenosine 3' : 5'-cyclic monophosphate levels by prostacyclin (prostaglandin I_2). J. Biol. Chem. 254, 1671–1676.

152. Gould, S. R. (1975) Prostaglandins, ulcerative colitis, and sulfasalazine. Lancet 2, 988.

153. Gould, S. R. (1976) Assay of prostaglandin-like substances in faeces and their measurement in ulcerative colitis. Prostaglandins 11, 489–497.

154. Gould, S. R., and Lennard-Jones, J. E. (1976) Production of prostaglandins in ulcerative colitis and their inhibition by sulfasalazine. Gut 17, 828.

155. Goyal, R. K., Mukhopadhyay, A., and Rattan, S. (1974) Effect of prostaglandin E_2 on the lower esophageal sphincter in normal subjects and patients with achalasia. Clin. Res. 22, 358A.

156. Goyal, R. K., and Rattan, S. (1973) Mechanism of the lower esophageal sphincter relaxation. J. Clin. Invest. 52, 337–341.

157. Goyal, R. K., Rattan, S., and Hersh, T. (1973) Comparison of the effects of prostaglandins E_1, E_2, and A_2, and of hypovolumic hypotension on the lower esophageal sphincter. Gastroenterology 65, 608–612.

158. Grbovíc, L., and Rodmanovíc, B. Z. (1978) A modulating role of prostaglandins in responses of guinea pig isolated ileum to various agonists. Arch. Int. Pharmacodyn. 235, 230–237.

159. Greenough, W. B., Pierce, N. F., Awqati, Q. A., and Carpenter, C. C. J. (1969) Stimulation of gut electrolyte secretion by prostaglandins, theophylline, and cholera toxin. J. Clin. Invest. 48, 32A.

160. Grmoljez, P. F., Kaminski, D. L., and Willman, V. L. (1975) The effect of prostaglandins on experimental paralytic ileus. Surg. Forum 26, 400–401.

161. Grubb, M. N., and Burks, T. F. (1976) Prostaglandins as modulators of intestinal motility. Clin. Res. 24, 12A.

162. Gryglewski, R. J., Panczenko, B., Korbut R., Grodzińska, L., and Ocetkiewicz, A. (1975) Corticosteroids inhibit prostaglandin release from perfused mesenteric blood vessels of rabbit and from perfused lungs of sensitized guinea pigs. Prostaglandins 10, 343–355.

163. Guth, P. H., Aures, D., and Paulsen, G. (1978) Topical aspirin + HCl lesions: Protection by prostaglandin and cimetidine. Gastroenterology 74, 1126.

164. Guth, P. H., Aures, D., and Paulsen, G. (1979) Topical aspirin plus HCl gastric lesions in the rat. Cytoprotective effect of prostaglandin, cimetidine and probanthine. Gastroenterology 76, 88–93.

165. Guth, P. H., Kauffman, G. L., Grossman, M. I., Carmichael, H. A., Nelson, L. M., and Russell, R. I. (1978) Cimetidine and prostaglandin prevent damage to gastric mucosa. Gastroenterology 75, 927–928.

166. Hahn, R. A., and Patil, P. N. (1972) Salivation induced by prostaglandin $F_{2\alpha}$ and modification of the response by atropine and physostigmine. Br. J. Pharmacol. 44, 527–533.

167. Hahn, R. A., and Patil, P. N. (1974) Further observations on the interaction of prostaglandin $F_{2\alpha}$ with cholinergic mechanisms in canine salivary glands. Eur. J. Pharmacol. 25, 279–286.

168. Håkanson, R., Liedberg, G., and Oscarson, J. (1973) Effects of prostaglandin E_1 on acid secretion, mucosal histamine content and histidine decarboxylase activity in rat stomach. Br. J. Pharmacol. 47, 498–503.

169. Hamberg, M., Hedqvist, P., Strandberg, K., Svensson, J., and Samuelsson, B. (1975) Prostaglandin endoperoxides. IV. Effects on smooth muscle. Life Sci. 16, 451–462.

170. Haroda, Y., and Katori, M. (1974) Fundamental studies on the superfusion technique for bioassay of prostaglandins. Jpn. J. Pharmacol. 24 (Suppl.), 31.

171. Hart, S. L. (1974) The actions of prostaglandins E_2 and $F_{2\alpha}$ on human foetal intestine. Br. J. Pharmacol. 50, 159–160.

172. Hedqvist, P. (1974) Restriction of transmitter release from adrenergic transmissions and their role in cardiovascular system. Pol. J. Pharmacol. Pharm. 26, 119–125.

173. Heintze, K., Leinesser, W., Petersen, U., and Heidenreich, O. (1975) Triphasic effect of prostaglandins E_1, E_2, and $F_{2\alpha}$ on the fluid transport of isolated gall-bladder of guinea pigs. Prostaglandins 9, 309–322.

174. Heisler, S. (1973) Effect of various prostaglandins and serotonin on protein secretion from rat exocrine pancreas. Experientia 29, 1234–1235.

175. Herman, A. G., Eckenfels, A., Ferreira, S. H. and Vane, J. R. (1972) Relationship between tone of isolated smooth muscle preparations and production of prostaglandins. Fifth International Congress on Pharmacology, San Francisco, p. 100 (Abstr.).

176. Hinsdale, J. G., Engel, J. J., and Wilson, D. E. (1974) Prostaglandin E in peptic ulcer disease. Prostaglandins 6, 495–500.

177. Holmes, S. W., Horton, E. W., and Main, I. H. M. (1963) The effect of prostaglandin E_1 on responses of smooth muscle to catecholamines, angiotensin and vasopressin. Br. J. Pharmacol. 21, 538–543.

178. Hong, E. (1974) Differential pattern of activity of some prostaglandins in diverse superfused tissues. Prostaglandins 10, 213–220.

179. Hong, E., and Lopez, C. (1977) Influence of the route of administration of prostaglandin E_1 on rat gastric secretion. Prostaglandins 13, 691–696.

180. Horton, E. W. (1963) Action of prostaglandin E_1 on tissues which respond to bradykinin. Nature (London) 200, 892–893.

181. Horton, E. W., and Jones, R. L. (1969) Prostaglandins A_1, A_2 and 19-hydroxy A_1; Their actions on smooth muscle and their inactivation on passage through the pulmonary and hepatic vascular beds. Br. J. Pharmacol. 37, 705–722.

182. Horton, E. W., and Jones, R. L. (1974) Biological activity of prostaglandin D_2 on smooth muscle. Br. J. Pharmacol. 52, 110P–111P.

183. Horton, E. W., and Main, I. H. M. (1963) A comparison of the biological activities of four prostaglandins. Br. J. Pharmacol. 21, 182–189.

184. Horton, E. W., and Main, I. H. M. (1965) A comparison of the actions of prostaglandins $F_{2\alpha}$ and E_1 on smooth muscle. Br. J. Pharmacol. 24, 470–476.

185. Horton, E. W., Main, I. H. M., Thompson, C. J., and Wright, P. M. (1968) Effect of orally administered prostaglandin E_1 on gastric secretion and intestine motility in man. Gut 9, 655–658.

186. Hoult, J. R. S., and Moore, P. K. (1978) Sulphasalazine is a potent inhibitor of prostaglandin 15-hydroxydehydrogenase: Possible basis for therapeutic action in ulcerative colitis. Br. J. Pharmacol. 64, 6–8.

187. Houvenaghel, A., and Wechsung, E. (1977) Influence of prostaglandins on blood flow through the superior mesenteric artery in the pig. Arch. Int. Pharmacodyn. 230, 332–334.

188. Hukovic, S., Zuizdic, E., and Radivojević, M. (1975) Effect of prostaglandins applied on mucosal of serosal side on contractions of isolated organs induced by nerve stimulations. Sixth International Congress on Pharmacology, 158, 352 (Abstr.).

189. Hunt, R. H., Dilawari, J. B., and Misiewicz, J. J. (1975) The effect of intravenous prostaglandin $F_{2\alpha}$ and E_2 on the motility of the sigmoid colon. Gut 16, 47–49.

190. Ihasz, M., Koiss, I., Nemeth, E. P., Folly, G., and Papp, M. (1976) Action of caerulein, glucagon, or prostaglandin E_1 on the motility of intestinal villi. Eur. J. Physiol. 364, 301–304.

191. Illes, P., and Knoll, J. (1975) Specific desensitization to PGE_1 and PGE_2 in guinea-pig ileum; Evidence for a common receptor site. Pharmacol. Res. Commun. 7, 37–47.

192. Illes, P., Vizi, S. E., and Knoll, J. (1976) Effect of prostaglandin E_1 on adrenergic transmission in isolated organs. Acta Physiol. Acad. Sci. Hung. 47, 191.

193. Impicciatore, M., Bertaccini, G., and Usardi, M. M. (1976) Effect of a new synthetic prostaglandin on acid gastric secretion in different laboratory animals. In: B. Samuelsson and R. Paoletti (eds.), Advances in Prostaglandin and Thromboxane Research, Vol. 2, Raven Press, New York, p. 945.

194. Ippoliti, A. F., Isenberg, J. I., Maxwell, V., and Walsh, J. H. (1976) The effect of 16,16-dimethyl prostaglandin E_2 on meal-stimulated gastric secretion and serum gastrin in duodenal ulcer patients. Gastroenterology 70, 488–491.

195. Ishii, T., Shimo, Y., and Sakanobori, N. (1977) Effects of PGE and indomethacin on the release of 3H-NA in guinea-pig *Taenia coli*. Jpn. J. Smooth Muscle Res. 13, 300–301.

196. Ishizawa, M., and Migazaki, E. (1973) Actions of prostaglandins on gastrointestinal motility. Sapporo Med. J. 42, 366–373.

197. Ishizawa, M., and Migazaki, E. (1975) Effect of prostaglandin $F_{2\alpha}$ on propulsive activity of the isolated segmental colon of the guinea pig. Prostaglandins 10, 759–768.

198. Ishizawa, M., Sato, K., Kinoshita, H., and Wada, T. (1970) Effects of prostaglandin on gastric secretion and on the gastrointestinal smooth muscle. Gastroenterol. Jpn. 5, 320.

199. Iwatsuki, K., Furuta, Y., and Hashimoto, K. (1973) Effect of prostaglandin $F_{2\alpha}$ on the secretion of pancreatic juice induced by secretin and by dopamine. Experientia 29, 319–320.

200. Jackson, D. M., Malor, R., Chesher, G. B., Starmer, G. A., Welburn, P. J., and Bailey, R. (1976) The interaction between prostaglandin E_1 and Δ^9-tetrahydrocannabinol on intestinal motility and on the abdominal constriction response in the mouse. Psychopharmacology 47, 187–193.

201. Jacobson, E. D. (1970) Comparison of prostaglandin E_1 and norepinephrine on the gastric mucosal circulation. Proc. Soc. Exp. Biol. Med. 133, 516–519.

202. Jacobson, E. D., Chaudhury, T. K. and Thompson, W. J. (1976) Mechanism of gastric mucosal cytoprotection by prostaglandins. Gastroenterology 70, 897.

203. Jacques, R. (1977) Inhibitory effect of methionine- and leucine-enkephalin on contractions of the guinea-pig ileum. Experientia 33, 374–375.

204. Johansson, C., and Ekelund, K. (1977) Effect of 16,16-dimethyl prostaglandin E_2 on the integrated response to a meal. In: H. L. Duthie (ed.), Gastrointestinal Motility in Health and Disease, University Park Press, Baltimore, pp. 195–204.

205. Johansson, C., Kollberg, B., Nordeman, R., and Bergström, S. (1979) Mucosal protection by prostaglandin E_2. Lancet 1, 317.

206. Johnson, D. G., Fujimoto, W. Y., and Williams, R. H. (1973) Enhanced release of insulin by prostaglandins in isolated pancreatic islets. Diabetes 22, 658–663.

207. Johnson, D. G., Thompson, W. J., and Williams, R. H. (1973) Stimulation of adenyl cyclase from isolated pancreatic islets by prostaglandins. Fed. Proc. 32, 3293.

208. Kadlec, O., Masek, K., and Seferna, I. (1974) A modulating role of prostaglandins in contractions of the guinea-pig ileum. Br. J. Pharmacol. 51, 565–570.

209. Kadlec, O., Masek, K., and Seferna, I. (1974) The role of prostaglandin E_2 in the contraction of neuromuscular preparation of the guinea-pig ileum. Physiol. Bohemoslov. 23, 353.

210. Kadlec, O., Masek, K., and Seferna, I. (1978) Modulation by prostaglandins of the release of acetylcholine and noradrenalin in guinea-pig isolated ileum. J. Pharmacol. Exp. Ther. 205, 635–645.

211. Kamikawa, Y., Serizawa, K., and Shimo, Y. (1977) Some possibilities for prostaglandin mediation in the contractile response to ATP of the guinea-pig digestive tract. Eur. J. Pharmacol. 45, 199–203.

212. Kaminski, D. L., Deshpande, Y. G., and Ruwart, M. J. (1977) The effect of prostaglandin $F_{2\alpha}$ on canine hepatic bile flow and biliary cyclic AMP secretion. J. Surg. Res. 22, 545–553.

213. Kaminski, D. L., Ruwart, M. J., and Deshpande, Y. G. (1977) The role of cyclic AMP in canine bile flow. Physiologist 20, 49.

214. Kaminski, D. L., Ruwart, M. J., and Deshpande, Y. G. (1977) The role of cyclic AMP in canine bile salt stimulated bile flow. Gastroenterology 72, 1077.

215. Kaminski, D. L., Ruwart, M. J., and Deshpande, Y. G. (1979) The effects of synthetic prostaglandin analogues on canine hepatic bile flow. Prostaglandins 18, 73–82.

216. Kaminski, D. L., Ruwart, M. J., and Willman, V. L. (1975) The effect of prostaglandin A_1 and E_1 on canine hepatic bile flow. J. Surg. Res. 18, 391–397.

217. Karim, S. M. M., Carter, D. C., Bhana, D., and Ganesan, P. A. (1973) Effect of orally administered prostaglandin E_2 and its 15-methyl analogues on gastric secretion. Br. Med. J. 1, 143–146.

218. Karim, S. M. M., Carter, D. C., Bhana, D., and Ganesan, P. A. (1973) Effect of orally and intravenously administered prostaglandin 15(R)-15 methyl E_2 on gastric secretion in man. Adv. Biosci. 9, 255–264.

219. Karim, S. M. M., Carter, D. C., Bhana, D., and Ganesan, P. A. (1973) Inhibition of basel and pentagastrin induced gastric acid secretion in man with prostaglandin 16,16-dimethyl E_2 methyl ester. Int. Res. Commun. Syst. Med. Sci. March 1973.

220. Karim, S. M. M., Carter, D. C., Bhana, D., and Ganesan, P. A. (1973) The effect of orally and intravenously administered prostaglandin 16,16-dimethyl E_2 methyl ester on human gastric acid secretion. Prostaglandins 4, 71–83.

221. Karim, S. M. M., and Fung, W. P. (1975) Effect of 15(R)-15 methyl prostaglandin E_2 on gastric secretion and a preliminary study on the healing of gastric ulcers in man. Int. Res. Commun. Syst. Med. Sci. 3, 348.

222. Karim, S. M. M., and Fung, W. P. (1976) Effects of some naturally occurring prostaglandins and synthetic analogs on gastric secretion and ulcer healing in man. In: B. Samuelsson, R. Paoletti (eds.), Advances in Prostaglandin and Thromboxane Research, Vol. 2, Raven Press, New York, p. 529.

223. Kauffman, G. L., and Grossman, M. I. (1978) Prostaglandin and cimetidine inhibit antral ulcers produced by parenteral salicylates. Gastroenterology 74, 1049.

224. Kauffman, G. L., and Grossman, M. I. (1978) Prostaglandin and cimetidine inhibit the formation of ulcers produced by parenteral salicylates. Gastroenterology 75, 1099–1102.

225. Kauffman, G. L., Whittle, B. J. R., Aures, D., and Grossman, M. I. (1978) Effects of prostacyclin and a stable analogue on gastric acid secretion and mucosal blood flow in unanesthetized dogs. Clin. Res. 26, 662A.

226. Kawarada, Y., Lambek, J., and Matsumoto, T. (1975) Pathophysiology of stress ulcer and its prevention. II. Prostaglandin E_1 and microcirculatory responses in stress ulcer. Am. J. Surg. 129, 217–222.

227. Kent, T. H., Cardelli, R. M., and Stamler, F. W. (1969) Small intestinal ulcers and intestinal flora in rats given indomethacin. Am. J. Pathol. 54, 237.

228. Kenyon, G. S., Ansell, I. F., and Carter, D. C. (1978) Methylated analogues of prostaglandin E_2 and the gastric mucosal barrier, Prostaglandins 15, 779–794.

229. Khairallah, P. A., Page, I. H., and Turker, R. K. (1969) Some properties of prostaglandin E_1 action on muscle. Arch. Int. Pharmacodyn. 169, 328–341.

230. Kimberg, D. V., Field, M., Johnson, J., Henderson, A., and Gerhon, E. (1971) Stimulation of intestinal mucosal adenyl cyclase by cholera enterotoxin and prostaglandins. J. Clin. Invest. 50, 1218.

231. Knapp, H. R., Oelz, O. and Oates, J. A. (1977) Effects of hyperosmolarity on prostaglandin release by the rat stomach in vitro. Fed. Proc. 36, 1020.

232. Knapp, H. R., Oelz, O., Sweetman, B. J., and Oates, J. A. (1978) Synthesis and metabolism of prostaglandins E_2, $F_{2\alpha}$ and D_2 by the rat gastrointestinal tract. Stimulation by a hypertonic environment in vitro. Prostaglandins 15, 751–757.

233. Konturek, S. J. (1976) Drug-induced inhibition of gastric secretion. Scand. J. Gastroenterol. 11 (Suppl. 42), 101–111.

234. Konturek, S. J. (1978) Effect of orally administered 15(R)-15-methyl prostaglandin E_2 and/or an anticholinergic drug on meal-induced gastric acid secretion and serum gastrin level in man. Gastroenterology 74, 1129.

235. Konturek, S. J. (1978) Prostaglandins and gastrointestinal secretion and motility. In: M. Grossman, V. Speranza, N. Basso, and E. Lezoche (eds.), Gastrointestinal Hormones and Pathology of the Digestive System, Plenum Press, New York, London, pp. 297–307.

236. Konturek, S. J., Bowman, J., Lancaster, C., Hanchar, A. J., and Robert, A. (1979) Cytoprotection of the canine gastric mucosa by prostacyclin: Possible mediation by increased mucosal blood flow. Gastroenterology 76, 1173.

237. Konturek, S. J., Hanchar, A. J., Nezamis, J. E., and Robert, A. (1979) Comparison of prostacyclin (PGI_2) and prostaglandin E_2 (PGE_2) on gastric secretory and serum gastric responses to a meal, pentagastrin and histamine. Gastroenterology 76, 1173.

237a. Konturek, S. J., Lancaster, C., Hanchar, A. J., Nezamis, J. E., and Robert, A. (1979) The influence of prostacyclin on gastric mucosal blood flow in resting and stimulated canine stomach. Gastroenterology 76, 1173.

238. Konturek, S. J., Kwiecien, N., Swierczek, J., and Oleksy, J. (1977) Effect of methylated PGE_2 analogs given orally on pancreatic response to secretin in man. Am. J. Dig. Dis. 22, 16–19.

239. Konturek, S. J., Kwiecien, N., Swierczek, J., Oleksy, J., Sito, E., and Robert, A. (1976) Comparison of methylated prostaglandin E_2 analogues given orally in the inhibition of gastric responses to pentagastrin and peptone meal in man. Gastroenterology 70, 683–687.

240. Konturek, S. J., Mikos, E., Pawlik, W., and Walus, K. (1979) Direct inhibition of gastric secretion and mucosal blood flow by arachidonic acid. J. Physiol. 286, 15–28.

241. Konturek, S. J., Radecki, T., Demitrescu, T., Kwiecien, K., Pucher, A., and Robert, A. (1974) Effect of synthetic 15-methyl analog of prostaglandin E_2 on gastric secretion and peptic ulcer formation. J. Lab. Clin. Med. 84, 716–725.

242. Konturek, S. J., Tasler, J., Jaworek, J., and Cieszkowski, M. (1980) Effect of prostacyclin on pancreatic secretion in dogs. In: B. Samuelsson, P. W. Ramwell, R. Paoletti (eds.), Advances in Prostaglandin and Thromboxane Research, Vol. 8, Raven Press, New York, pp. 1561–1568.

243. Konturek, S. J., Walus, K., and Pawlik, W. (1978) Comparison of prostaglandin I_2 and E_2 on gastric acid secretion and mucosal blood flow. Gastroenterology 74, 1130.

244. Koppanyi, T., and Maling, H. M. (1972) The effects of pretreatment with reserpine, α-methyl-p-tyrosine, or prostaglandin E_1 on adrenergic salivation. Proc. Soc. Exp. Biol. Med. 140, 787–793.

245. Kormano, M., and Katevuo, K. (1975) Intravenous prostaglandin and the gallbladder. Lancet 1, 797–798.

246. Kovatsis, A., Dozi-Vassiliades, J., Tsoukali, H., and Kotsaki-Kovatsi, V. (1974) Antagonistic action between PGE_1, and $PGF_{1\alpha}$ and AMP, ATP. Arzneim.-Forsch. 24, 83–85.

247. Kovatsis, A., Kovatsi-Kotsaki, V., Elezaglou, B., and Kounenis, G. (1976) Physiological antagonism between PGE_2, and PGA_1, $PGF_{1\alpha}$ and NADP, β-NAD on isolated rabbit jejunum. Arzneim.-Forsch. 26, 1997–1999.

248. Kovatsis, A., Kotsaki-Kovatsi, V., Tsoukali-Papadopoulou, H., and Elezoglou, V. (1974) Physiological antagonism between prostaglandins A_1, A_2 and AMP, ATP on isolated rabbit jejunum. J. Pharm. Belg. 29, 573–578.

249. Kowalewski, K., and Kolodej, A. (1974) Effect of prostaglandin-E_2 on gastric circulation of totally isolated ex vivo canine stomach. Pharmacology 11, 85–94.

250. Kowalewski, K., and Kolodej, A. (1975) Effect of prostaglandin-E_2 on myoelectrical and mechanical activity of totally isolated, ex-vivo-perfused, canine stomach. Pharmacology 13, 325–339.

251. Kowalewski, K., and Kolodej, A. (1978) Effect of 16,16-dimethyl prostaglandin E₂ given intra-arterially or intra-gastrically, on acid secretion by canine stomachs perfused *ex vivo*. Prostaglandins 15, 901–906.

252. Krarup, N., Larsen, J. A., and Munck, A. (1975) Choleretic effect of prostaglandin PGE₁ and PGE₂ in cats. Digestion 12, 272–273.

253. Kruidinier, J., Tao, P., and Wilson, D. E. (1978) The role of prostaglandins in lower esophageal sphincter pressure in man. Clin. Res. 26, 663A.

254. Laekeman, G. M., and Herman, A. G. (1978) Release of prostaglandin-like material by various agonists from the guinea-pig lung and intestine. Arch. Int. Pharmacodyn. 236, 307–309.

255. Laekeman, G. M., Herman, A. G., and VanBeek, H. A. (1977) Restoration of the hyoscine-induced inhibition of the twitch and tetanic contractions of the electrically stimulated guinea-pig ileum. J. Pharmacol. 8, 555–556.

256. Lancaster, C., and Robert A. (1978) Intestinal lesions produced by prednisolone: Prevention (cytoprotection) by 16,16-dimethyl prostaglandin E₂. Am. J. Physiol. 235, E703–E708.

257. Landgraf, R., and Landgraf-Leurs, M. M. C. (1979) The prostaglandin system and insulin release. Studies with the isolated perfused rat pancreas. Prostaglandins 17, 599–613.

258. Lauterburg, B., Paumgartner, G., and Preisig, R. (1975) Prostaglandin-induced choleresis in the rat. Experientia 31, 1191–1193.

259. Lee, Y. H., and Bianchi, R. G. (1972) The antisecretory and antiulcer activity of a prostaglandin analog, SC-24665, in experimental animals. Proceedings of the Fifth International Congress on Pharmacology, San Francisco, p. 136 (Abstr.).

260. Lee, Y. H., Cheng, W. D., Bianchi, R. G., Mollison, K., and Hansen, J. (1973) Effects of oral administration of PGE₂ on gastric secretion and experimental peptic ulcerations. Prostaglandins 3, 29–45.

261. Lefèbvre, P. J. and Luyckx, A. S. (1972) Effect of prostaglandin PGE₁ on blood flow and insulin output of dog pancreas in situ. Diabetes 21 (Suppl. 1), 369.

262. Lefèbvre, P. J., and Luyckx, A. S. (1973) Stimulation of insulin secretion after prostaglandin PGE₁ in the anesthetized dog. Biochem. Pharmacol. 22, 1773–1779.

263. Lemberg, A., Wikinski, R., Izurieta, E. M., Halperin, H., Paglione, A. M., De-Neuman, P., and Jauregui, H. (1971) Effects of prostaglandin E₁ and norepinephrine on glucose and lipid metabolism in isolated perfused rat liver. Biochim. Biophys. Acta 248, 198–204.

264. Levine, R. (1971) Effect of prostaglandins and cyclic AMP on gastric secretion. Ann. NY Acad. Sci. 180, 336–337.

265. Levine, R. A. (1973) The role of cyclic AMP and prostaglandins in hepatic and gastrointestinal functions. In: R. H. Kahn and W. E. M. Lands (eds.), Prostaglandins and Cyclic AMP, Academic Press, New York, pp. 75–117.

266. Levine, R. A., Schwartzel, E. H. Jr., Randall, P. A., and Bachman, S. (1978) Failure of prostaglandins E₁ and E₂ to alter canine gastric mucosal cyclic nucleotides. Gastroenterology 74, 1131.

267. Leyssac, P. P., Bukhave, K., and Frederiksen, O. (1974) Inhibitory effect of prostaglandins on isosmotic fluid transport by rabbit gall-bladder in vitro, and its modification by blockade of endogenous PGE-biosynthesis with indomethacin. Acta Physiol. Scand. 92, 496–507.

268. Lippmann, W. (1971) Inhibition of gastric acid secretion in the rat by synthetic prostaglandin analogues. Ann. NY Acad. Sci. 180, 332–335.

269. Lipshutz, W. H., Gaskins, R. D., and Lukash, W. M. (1974) Hypogastrinemia in patients with lower esophageal sphincter incompetence. Gastroenterology 67, 423–427.

270. Luderer, J. R., Demers, L. M., Bonnem, E. M., Saleem, A., and Jeffries, G. H. (1977) Elevated prostaglandin E in idiopathic intestinal pseudo-obstruction. New Engl. J. Med. 295, 1179.

271. Magerlein, B. J., DuCharme, D. W., Magee, W. E., Miller, W. L., Robert, A., and Weeks, J. R. (1973) Synthesis and biological properties of 16-alkylprostaglandins. Prostaglandins 4, 143–145.

272. Magerlein, B. J., and Miller, W. L. (1975) 16-Fluoroprostaglandins. Prostaglandins 9, 527–529.

273. Maher, J. W., Hollenbeck, J. I., Crandall, V., McGuigan, J., and Woodward, E. R. (1978) Prostaglandin E_2 effect on lower esophageal sphincter pressure and serum gastrin. J. Surg. Res. 24, 87–91.

274. Main, I. H. M. (1969) Effects of prostaglandin E_2 (PGE_2) on the output of histamine and acid in rat gastric secretion induced by pentagastrin or histamine. Br. J. Pharmacol. 36, 214P–215P.

275. Main, I. H. M., and Pearce, J. B. (1978) Differential inhibition by PGE_1, PGE_2 and endoperoxide analogue U46619 of secretion from the rat isolated gastric mucosa stimulated by histamine, pentagastrin and methacholine. Br. J. Pharmacol. 64, 423P–424P.

276. Main, I. H. M., and Whittle, B. J. R. (1972) Effects of prostaglandin E_2 on rat gastric mucosal blood flow, as determined by ^{14}C-aniline clearance. Br. J. Pharmacol. 44, 331P–332P.

277. Main, I. H. M., and Whittle, B. J. R. (1972) Effects of prostaglandins of the E and A series on rat gastric mucosal blood flow as determined by ^{14}C-aniline clearance. Fifth International Congress on Pharmacology, San Francisco, p. 145 (Abstr.).

278. Main, I. H. M., and Whittle, B. J. R. (1973) The effects of E and A prostaglandins on gastric mucosal blood flow and acid secretion in the rat. Br. J. Pharmacol. 49, 428–436.

279. Main, I. H. M., and Whittle, B. J. R. (1973) The relationship between rat gastric mucosal blood flow and acid secretion during oral or intravenous administration of prostaglandins and dibutryl cyclic AMP. Adv. Biosci. 9, 271–275.

280. Main, I. H. M., and Whittle, B. J. R. (1974) Methyl analogs of prostaglandin E_2 and gastrointestinal function in the rat. Br. J. Pharmacol. 52, 113P.

281. Main, I. H. M., and Whittle, B. J. R. (1974) Prostaglandin E_2 and the stimulation of rat gastric acid secretion by dibutryl cyclic 3′,5′-AMP. Eur. J. Pharmacol. 26, 204–211.

282. Maling, H. M., Williams, M. A., and Koppani, T. (1972) Salivation in mice as an index of adrenergic activity. I. Salivation and temperature responses to D-amphetamine and other sialogogues and the effects of adrenergic blocking agents. Arch. Int. Pharmacodyn. 199, 318–332.

283. Mann, N. S. (1975) Prevention of bile-induced acute erosive gastritis by prostaglandin E_2, Maalox and cholestyramine. Gastroenterology 68, 946.

284. Mao, C. C., Shanbour, L. L., Hodgins, D. S., and Jacobson, E. D. (1972) Cyclic adenosine-3′,5′-monophosphate (cyclic AMP) and secretion in the canine stomach. Gastroenterology 63, 427.

285. Masek, K., and Kadlec, O. (1976) The effect of prostaglandins of the E type on peripheral and central release of the neurotransmitters. In: B. Samuelsson and R. Paoletti (eds.), Advances in Prostaglandin and Thromboxane Research, Vol. 2, Raven Press, New York, pp. 841–842.

286. Matuchansky, C., and Bernier, J. J. (1971) Effects of prostaglandin E_1 on net and unidirectional movements of water and electrolytes across jejunal mucosa in man. Gut 12, 854.

287. Matuchansky, C., and Bernier, J. J. (1973) Effect of prostaglandin E_1 on glucose, water, and electrolyte absorption in the human jejunum. Gastroenterology 64, 1111.

288. McCallum, R. W., Ippoliti, A. F., and Sturdevant, R. A. L. (1975) Effect of oral 16,16-dimethyl prostaglandin E_2 (PGE_2) on the lower esophageal sphincter in man. Gastroenterology 68, 949.

289. Micossi, P., Pontiroli, A. E., Baron, S. H., Tamayo, R. C., Lengel, F., Bevilacqua, M., Raggi, U., Norbiato, G., and Foà, P. P. (1978) Aspirin stimulates insulin and glucagon secretion and increase glucose tolerance in normal and diabetic subjects. Diabetes 27, 1196–1204.

290. Mihas, A. A., Gibson, R. G., and Hirschowitz, B. I. (1976) Inhibition of gastric secretion in the dog by 16,16-dimethyl prostaglandin E_2. Am. J. Physiol. 230, 351–356.

291. Miller, T. A., and Jacobson, E. D. (1979) Gastrointestinal cytoprotection by prostaglandins. Gut 20, 75–87.

292. Miller, T. A., Henagan, J., and Robert, A. (1980) Effect of 16,16-dimethyl prostaglandin E_2 on resting and histamine-stimulated canine gastric mucosal blood flow. Dig. Dis. Sci., 25, 561–567.

293. Miller, W. L., Weeks, J. R. Lauderdale, J. W., and Kirton, K. T. (1975) Biological activities of 17-phenyl-18,19,20-trinorprostaglandins. Prostaglandins 9, 9–18.

294. Milton-Thompson, G. J., Billings, J. A., Cummings, J. H., Newman, A., and Misiewicz, J. J. (1973) The effect of circulating prostaglandin $F_{2\alpha}$ on the function of the human small intestine. Rend. Rom. Gastroenterol. 5, 139.

295. Misiewicz, J. J., Waller, S. L., Kiley, N., and Horton, E. W. (1969) Effect of oral prostaglandin E_1 on intestinal transit in man. Lancet I, 648–651.

296. Miyazaki, Y. (1968) Isolation of prostaglandin E-like substances from the mucous membrane layer of large intestine of pig. Sapporo Med. J. 34, 141.

297. Miyazaki, Y., Ishizawa, M., Sunano, S., Syuto, B., and Sakagami, T. (1967) Stimulating action of prostaglandin on the rabbit duodenal muscle. In: S. Bergström and B. Samuelsson (eds.). Prostaglandins: Proceedings of the Second Nobel Symposium, Almqvist and Wiksell, Stockholm, pp. 277–281.

298. Molina, E., Zoppia, L., and Sianesi, M. (1976) Effect of some natural prostaglandins on motility of the human gastrointestinal tract in vitro. Farmaco 31, 865–870.

299. Moncada, S., Mugridge, K. G., and Whittle, B. J. R. (1977) The differential response of a novel bioassay tissue, the rabbit transverse stomach-strip, to prostacyclin (PGI_2) and other prostaglandins. Br. J. Pharmacol. 61, 415P.

300. Moncada, S., Mullane, K. M., and Vane, J. R. (1979) Prostacyclin-release by bradykinin in vivo. Br. J. Pharmacol. 66, 96P–97P.

301. Moncada, S., Salmon, J. A., Vane, J. R., and Whittle, B. J. R. (1977) Formation of prostacyclin (PGI_2) and its product, 6-oxo-$PGF_{1\alpha}$ by the gastric mucosa of several species. J. Physiol. 275, 4P–5P.

302. Morita, A., Ishibashi, C., and Kobayashi, S. (1977) Effects of prostaglandin derivatives on the digestive system. 2. Antiulcer effects of prostaglandin E_2. Jpn. J. Pharmacol. 27 (Suppl.), 130P.

303. Morton, L. K. M., Saverymuttu, S. M., and Wood, J. R. (1974) Inhibition by prostaglandins of fluid transport in the isolated gallbladder of the guinea pig. Br. J. Pharmacol. 50, 460P.

304. Mukhopadhyay, A., Rattan, S., and Goyal, R. K. (1973) Esophageal response to prostaglandin E_1 (PGE_1) infusion. Clin. Res. 21, 52.

305. Mukhopadhyay, A., Rattan, S., and Goyal, R. K. (1975) Effect of prostaglandin E_2 on esophageal motility in man. J. Appl. Physiol. 39, 479–481.

306. Mukhopadhyay, A. K., Weisbrodt, N. W., Copeland, E. D., and Johnson, L. R. (1974) Effect of prostaglandin E_2 infusion on patterns of intestinal myoelectric activity. Gastroenterology 66, 752.

307. Nagy, L., Mozsik, G., Tarnok, F., Poth, I., Szalai, M., and Javor, T. (1977) Alterations in gastric secretion and serum gastrin level in pylorus-ligated and antrectomized rats after prostaglandin E_2 treatment. Acta Physiol. Acad. Sci. Hung. 49, 327–328.

308. Nagy, L., Mozsik, G., Tarnok, F., Szalai, M., Poth, I., and Javor, T. (1978) Interrelationships between the gastric secretory responses, prostaglandin E_2 inhibition and serum level of immunoreactive gastrin in pylorus-ligated and antrectomized rats. Pharmacology 16, 135–141.

309. Nakaji, N. T., Charters, A. C., Guillemin, R. C. L., and Orloff, M. J. (1976) Inhibition of gastric secretion by somatostatin. Gastroenterology 70, 989.

310. Nakamura, N., Shiozaki, S., Kojima, T., Shimizu, M., and Tanaka, M. (1977) Effects of caerulein on intestinal motility. Folia Pharmacol. Jpn. 73, 743–756.

311. Nakano, J., McCloy, R. E., Gin, A., and Nakano, S. K. (1975) Effect of prostaglandins E_1, E_2, and $F_{2\alpha}$, and pentagastrin on the gallbladder pressure in dogs. Eur. J. Pharmacol. 30, 107–112.

312. Nezamis, J. E., Robert, A., and Stowe, D. F. (1971) Inhibition by prostaglandin E_1 of gastric secretion in the dog. J. Physiol. 218, 369–383.

313. Newman, A., DeMoraes-Filho, J. P. P., Philippakos, D., and Misiewicz, J. J. (1975) The effect of intravenous infusions of prostaglandins E_2 and $F_{2\alpha}$ on human gastric function. Gut 16, 272–276.

314. Nilsson, F., and Ohrn, P. G. (1974) Duodeno-gastric reflux after administration of prostaglandin $F_{2\alpha}$. Studies of gastro-intestinal propulsion in the rat. Int. Res. Commun. Serv. 2, 1558.

315. Nompleggi, D., Myers, L., Castell, D. O., and Dubois, A. (1978) A prostaglandin E_2 analog increases gastric emptying. Clin. Res. 26, 323A.

316. Nompleggi, D., Myers, L., Castell, D. O., and Dubois, A. (1978) Do prostaglandins play a physiological role in gastric emptying and gastric secretion? Clin. Res. 26, 614A.

317. Nompleggi, D., Myers, L., Castell, D. O., and Dubois, A. (1979) A prostaglandin $F_{2\alpha}$ analog increases gastric emptying. Clin. Res. 27, 633A.

318. Nompleggi, D., Myers, L., Castell, D. O., and Dubois, A. (1979) Do endogenous prostaglandins play a role in gastric emptying and gastric secretion? Clin. Res. 27, 269A.

319. Nompleggi, D., Myers, L., Ramwell, P., Castell, D. O., and Dubois, A. (1980) PGE$_2$ involvement in the regulation of gastric emptying. In: B. Samuelsson, P. W. Ramwell, R. Paoletti (eds.), Advances in Prostaglandin and Thromboxane Research, Vol. 8, Raven Press, New York, pp. 1587–1588.

320. Nylander, B., and Andersson, S. (1974) Gastric secretory inhibition induced by three methyl analogs of prostaglandin E_2 administered intragastrically to man. Scand. J. Gastroenterol. 9, 751–758.

321. Nylander, B., and Andersson, S. (1975) Effect of two methylated prostaglandin E_2 analogs on gastroduodenal pressure in man. Scand. J. Gastroenterol. 10, 91–95.

322. Nylander, B., and Mattsson, O. (1975) Effect of 16,16-dimethyl PGE$_2$ on gastric emptying of a barium food test meal in man. Scand. J. Gastroenterol. 10, 289–292.

323. Nylander, B., Robert, A., and Andersson, S. (1974) Gastric secretory inhibition by certain methyl analogs of prostaglandin E_2 following intestinal administration in man. Scand. J. Gastroenterol. 9, 759–762.

324. Ohashi, S., Ohmuro, S., Sugawara, I., Kuwata, K., and Okamoto, E. (1973) Effects of prostaglandin E_1 on canine gastrointestinal motility in vivo and human isolated smooth muscle in vitro. Jpn. J. Smooth Muscle Res. 9, 69–77.

325. Ouji, A. (1974) The mechanism and action of prostaglandin $F_{2\alpha}$ on the smooth muscle of guinea-pig Taenia coli. Jpn. J. Pharmacol. 24, 575–582.

326. Ozi, A., Kato, M., and Hagibara, Y. (1973) The action of PGF$_{2\alpha}$ on the smooth muscle of the intestine. Jpn. Pharmacol. Soc. Abstr. (Kanto Reg. Meet.) 48, 26.

327. Pace-Asciak, C., Morawska, K., Coceani, F., and Wolfe, L. S. (1968) The biosynthesis of prostaglandin E_2 and $F_{2\alpha}$ in homogenates of the rat stomach. In: P. W. Ramwell and J. E. Shaw (eds.), Prostaglandin Symposium of the Worcester Foundation for Experimental Biology, Interscience, New York, pp. 371–378.

328. Pace-Asciak, C. R., and Nashat, M. (1977) Mechanistic studies on the biosynthesis of 6-keto-prostaglandin. Biochim. Biophys. Acta 487, 495–507.

329. Pace-Asciak, C., and Wolfe, L. S. (1971) A novel prostaglandin derivative formed from arachidonic acid by rat stomach homogenates. Biochemistry 10, 3857–3864.

330. Paustian, P. W., Gottlieb, A. J., Ritchie, E., Chapnick, B. M., Hyman, A. L., and Kadowitz, P. J. (1978) The effects of prostaglandin D_2 infusion on the feline intestinal vascular bed. Clin. Res. 26, 10A.

331. Pek, S., Tai, T.-Y., Elster, A., and Fajans, S. S. (1975) Stimulation by prostaglandin E_2 of glucagon and insulin release from isolated rat pancreas. Prostaglandins 10, 493–502.

332. Perrier, C. V., and Laster, L. (1970) Adenyl cyclase activity of guinea pig gastric mucosa: Stimulation by histamine and prostaglandins. J. Clin. Invest. 49, 73A.

333. Persson, N.-A., and Hedqvist, P. (1973) Reduced intestinal muscular response to adrenergic nerve stimulation after the administration of prostaglandins. Acta Physiol. Scand. (Suppl. 396), 108.

334. Peskar, B. M. (1977) On the synthesis of prostaglandins by human gastric mucosa and its modification by drugs. Biochim. Biophys. Acta 487, 307–314.

335. Peterson, W., Feldman, M., Taylor, I., and Brewer, M. (1979) The effect of 15(R)-15-methyl prostaglandin E_2 on meal-stimulated gastric acid secretion, serum gastrin, and pancreatic polypeptide in duodenal ulcer patients. Dig. Dis. Sci. 24, 381–384.

336. Petkov, V., and Radomirov, R. (1978) Influence of indomethacin and aspirin on the contractile effects of prostaglandin $F_{2\alpha}$($PGF_{2\alpha}$) at different Ca^{++} concentrations (experiments on guinea-pig ileum). Acta Physiol. Pharmacol. Bulg. 3, 18–23.

337. Petkov, V., Radomirov, R., Petkov, O., and Todorov, S. (1978) The character of the antagonism by polyphloretin phosphate of contractions to prostaglandins E_1 and $F_{2\alpha}$ in guinea-pig ileum. J. Pharm. Pharmacol. 30, 491–494.

338. Phair, R. D., Rago, N. S., Lands, W. E. M., and Pek, S. (1978) Role of endogenous prostaglandins (PGs) in insulin and glucagon responses to fatty acids (FAs). Fed. Proc. 38, 878.

339. Pierce, N. F., Carpenter, C. C. J., Elliott, H. J., and Greenough, W. B. (1971) Effects of prostaglandins, theophylline, and cholera exotoxin upon transmucosal water and electrolyte movement in the canine jejunum. Gastroenterology 60, 22.

340. Radmanovic, B. Z. (1972) Effect of prostaglandin E_1 on the peristaltic activity of the guinea-pig isolated ileum. Arch. Int. Pharmacodyn. 200, 396–404.

341. Ramwell, P. W., Shaw, J. E., Corey, E. J., and Andersen, N. (1969) Biological activity of synthetic prostaglandins. Nature (London) 221, 1251–1253.

342. Rashid, S. (1971) The release of prostaglandin from the oesophagus and the stomach of the frog. J. Pharm. Pharmacol. 23, 456–457.

343. Rattan, S., and Goyal, R. K. (1980) Effects of indomethacin and prostaglandin E_1 on the lower esophageal sphincter function. In: J. Christensen (ed.), Gastrointestinal Motility. Proceedings of the Seventh International Symposium, Raven Press, New York, pp. 292–306.

344. Rattan, S., Hersh, T., and Goyal, R. K. (1971) Effects of prostaglandins on the lower esophageal sphincter. Clin. Res. 19, 660.

345. Rattan, S., Hersh, T., and Goyal, R. K. (1972) Effect of prostaglandin $F_{2\alpha}$ and gastrin pentapeptide on the lower esophageal sphincter. Proc. Soc. Exp. Biol. Med. 141, 573–575.

346. Robert, A. (1968) Antisecretory property of prostaglandins. In: P. W. Ramwell and J. E. Shaw (eds.), Prostaglandin Symposium of the Worcester Foundation for Experimental Biology, Interscience, New York, pp. 47–54.

347. Robert, A. (1971) Duodenal ulcers in the rat: Production and prevention. In: C. J. Pfeiffer (ed.), Peptic Ulcer, Munksgaard, Copenhagen, pp. 21–23.

348. Robert, A. (1974) Effects of prostaglandins on the stomach and the intestine. Prostaglandins 6, 523–532.

349. Robert, A. (1975) An intestinal disease produced experimentally by a prostaglandin deficiency. Gastroenterology 69, 1045–1047.

350. Robert, A. (1976) Antisecretory, antiulcer, cytoprotective and diarrheogenic properties of prostaglandins. In: B. Samuelsson and R. Paoletti (eds.), Advances in Prostaglandin and Thromboxane Research, Vol. 2, Raven Press, New York, pp. 507–520.

351. Robert, A. (1979) Cytoprotection by prostaglandins. Gastroenterology 77, 761–767.

352. Robert, A., Hanchar, A. J., and Lancaster, C. (1978) Antisecretory and cytoprotective effects of prostacyclin (PGI₂). Fed. Proc. 37, 460.

353. Robert, A., Hanchar, A. J., Lancaster, C., and Nezamis, J. E. (1979) Prostacyclin (PGI₂) and PGD₂ prevent enteropooling and diarrhea caused by prostaglandins and cholera toxin. Fed. Proc. 38, 1239.

353a. Robert, A., Hanchar, A. J., Lancaster, C., and Nezamis, J. E. (1979) Prostacyclin inhibits enteropooling and diarrhea. In: J. R. Vane and S. Bergström (eds.), Prostacyclin. Raven Press, New York, pp. 147–158.

354. Robert, A., Hanchar, A. J., Nezamis, J. E., and Lancaster, C. (1979) Cytoprotection against acidified aspirin: Comparison of prostaglandin, cimetidine and probanthine. Gastroenterology 76, 1227.

355. Robert, A., Lancaster, C., Nezamis, J. E., and Badalamenti, J. N. (1973) A gastric antisecretory and antiulcer prostaglandin with oral and long-acting activity. Gastroenterology 64, 790.

356. Robert, A., and Magerlein, B. J. (1973) 15-Methyl PGE₂ and 16,16-dimethyl PGE₂: Potent inhibitors of gastric secretion. Adv. Biosci. 9, 247–253.

357. Robert, A., Nezamis, J. E., and Lancaster, C. (1975) Duodenal ulcers produced by nonsteroidal anti-inflammatory compounds plus bile duct ligation. Fed. Proc. 34, 442.

358. Robert, A., Nezamis, J. E., and Lancaster, C. (1975) Duodenal ulcers produced in rats by propionitrile: Factors inhibiting and aggravating such ulcers. Toxicol. Appl. Pharmacol. 31, 201–207.

359. Robert, A., Nezamis, J. E., and Lancaster, C. (1976) Effect of 16,16-dimethyl PGE₂ on gastric emptying. In: B. Samuelsson and R. Paoletti (eds.), Advances in Prostaglandin and Thromboxane Research, Vol. 2, Raven Press, New York, p. 946.

360. Robert, A., Nezamis, J. E., Lancaster, C., and Badalamenti, J. N. (1975) Cysteamine-induced duodenal ulcers: A new model to test antiulcer agents. Digestion 11, 199–214.

361. Robert, A., Nezamis, J. E., Lancaster, C., and Hanchar, A. J. (1977) Gastric cytoprotective property of prostaglandins. Gastroenterology 72, 1121.

362. Robert, A., Nezamis, J. E., Lancaster, C., and Hanchar, A. J. (1979) Cytoprotection by prostaglandins in rats: Prevention of gastric necrosis produced by alcohol, HCl, NaOH, hypertonic NaCl, and thermal injury. Gastroenterology 77, 433–443.

363. Robert, A., Nezamis, J. E., Lancaster, C., Hanchar, A. J., and Klepper, M. S. (1976) Enteropooling assay: A test for diarrhea produced by prostaglandins. Prostaglandins 11, 809–828.

364. Robert, A., Nezamis, J. E., and Phillips, J. P. (1967) Inhibition of gastric secretion by prostaglandins. Am. J. Dig. Dis. 12, 1073–1076.

365. Robert, A., Nezamis, J. E., and Phillips, J. P. (1968) Effect of prostaglandin E₁ on gastric secretion and ulcer formation in the rat. Gastroenterology 55, 481–487.

366. Robert, A., Nylander, B., and Andersson, S. (1974) Marked inhibition of gastric secretion by two prostaglandin analogs given orally to man. Life Sci. 14, 533–538.

367. Robert, A., Phillips, J. P., and Nezamis, J. E. (1968) Inhibition by prostaglandin E₁ of gastric secretion in the dog. Gastroenterology 54, 1263.

368. Robert, A., Schultz, J. R., Nezamis, J. E., and Lancaster, C. (1976) Gastric antisecretory and antiulcer properties of PGE₂, 15-methyl PGE₂, and 16,16-dimethyl PGE₂. Intravenous, oral and intrajejunal administration. Gastroenterology 70, 359–370.

369. Robert, A., and Standish, W. L. (1973) Production of duodenal ulcers, in rats, with one injection of histamine. Fed. Proc. 32, 322.

370. Robert, A., Stowe, D. F., and Nezamis, J. E. (1971) Prevention of duodenal ulcers by administration of prostaglandin E₂ (PGE₂). Scand. J. Gastroenterol. 6, 303–305.

371. Robert, A., and Yankee, E. W. (1975) Gastric antisecretory effect of 15(R)-15-methyl PGE₂, methyl ester and of 15(S)-15-methyl PGE₂, methyl ester. Proc. Soc. Exp. Biol. Med. 148, 1155–1158.

372. Robertson, R. P. (1973) Inhibition of insulin secretion by prostaglandin (PG)E_1 independent of hypotensive or alpha adrenergic effects. Diabetes 22, 305.

373. Robertson, R. P., and Chen, M. (1977) A role for prostaglandin E in defective insulin secretion and carbohydrate intolerance in diabetes mellitus. J. Clin. Invest. 60, 747–753.

374. Robertson, R. P., Gavareski, D. J., Porte, D., and Bierman, E. L. (1973) Prostaglandin E_1: Inhibition of glucose-induced insulin secretion in dogs. Clin. Res. 21, 219.

375. Robertson, R. P., Gavareski, D. J., Porte, D., and Bierman, E. L. (1974) Inhibition of in vivo insulin secretion by prostaglandin E_1. J. Clin. Invest. 54, 310–315.

376. Rodrigo, L. R., Pozo, F., Marin, B., and Schiaffini, O. (1976) Serum and bile modifications in the guinea-pig following chronic treatment with PGE_1 and PGE_2. Experientia 32, 1604–1605.

377. Rosenberg, J., Robert, A., Gonda, M., Dreiling, D. A., and Rudick, J. (1974) Synthetic prostaglandin analog and pancreatic secretion. Gastroenterology 66, 767.

378. Rossini, A. A., Lee, J. B., and Frawley, T. F. (1971) An unpredictable lack of effect of prostaglandins on insulin release in isolated rat islets. Diabetes (Suppl. 1), 20, 374.

379. Rudick, J., Gonda, M., Dreiling, D. A., and Janowitz, H. D. (1971) Effects of prostaglandin E_1 on pancreatic exocrine function. Gastroenterology 60, 272–278.

379a. Ruppin, H., Person, B., Robert, A., and Domschke, W. (1979) Gastric cytoprotection by prostaglandins (PG): Possible mediation by mucus secretion. Physiologist 22, 110.

380. Ruwart, M. J., Kaminski, D. L., and Jellinek, M. (1977) Evidence for additional mediator in prostaglandin-induced choleresis. Prostaglandins 14, 975–982.

381. Ruwart, M. J., Klepper, M. S., and Rush, B. D. (1978) The beneficial effects of prostaglandins in post-operative ileus. Gastroenterology 74, 1088.

382. Ruwart, M. J., Klepper, M. S., and Rush, B. D. (1979) Carbachol stimulation of gastrointestinal transit in the postoperative ileus rat. J. Surg. Res. 26, 18–26.

383. Ruwart, M. J., Klepper, M. S., and Rush, B. D. (1980) Mechanism of stimulation of gastrointestinal propulsion in postoperative ileus rats by 16,16-dimethyl PGE_2. In: B. Samuelsson, P. Ramwell and R. Paoletti (eds.); Advances in Prostaglandin and Thromboxane Research, Vol. 8, Raven Press, New York, pp. 1603–1607.

384. Ruwart, M. J., Klepper, M. S., and Rush, B. D. (1979) Regulation of gastric emptying, small intestinal transit and colonic transit in the rat. Gastroenterology 76, 1232.

385. Rybicka, J., and Gibinski, K. (1978) Methyl-prostaglandin E_2 analogues for healing of gastroduodenal ulcers. Scand. J. Gastroenterol. 13, 155–159.

386. Saccà, L., and Perez, G. (1976) Influence of prostaglandins on plasma glucagon levels in the rat. Metabolism 25, 127–130.

387. Saccà, L., Perez, G., Rengo, F., Pascucci, I., and Condorelli, M. (1975) Reduction of circulating insulin levels during the infusion of different prostaglandins in the rat. Acta Endocrinol. 79, 266–274.

388. Saccà, L., Rengo, F., Chiariello, M., and Condorelli, M. (1973) Glucose intolerance and impaired insulin secretion by prostaglandin A_1 in fasting anesthetized dogs. Endocrinology 92, 31–34.

389. Sakato, M., and Shimo, Y. (1976) Possible role of prostaglandin E_1 on adrenergic neurotransmission in the guinea-pig Taenia coli. Eur. J. Pharmacol. 40, 209–214.

390. Sakaki, H., Teraki, Y., and Tsunoo, S. (1974) Effect of prostaglandins on the sphincter of Oddi and the duodenal muscle of rabbits. Jpn. J. Pharmacol. 24 (Suppl.), 30.

391. Sanders, K. M. (1978) Endogenous prostaglandin E and contractile activity of isolated ileal smooth muscle. Am. J. Physiol. 234, E209–E212.

392. Sanders, K. M., and Ross, G. (1978) Effects of endogenous prostaglandin E on intestinal motility. Am. J. Physiol. 234, E204–E208.

393. Sanders, K. M., and Szurszewski, J. H. (1980) Endogenous prostaglandins and control of gastric motility. In: J. Christensen (ed.), Gastrointestinal Motility. Proceedings of the Seventh International Symposium, Raven Press, New York, pp. 232–234.

394. Sanger, G. J., and Watt, A. J. (1976) A postsynaptic action of prostaglandin E_1 on sympathetic responses in guinea-pig ileum. Br. J. Pharmacol. 58, 290P–291P.

395. Sanger, G. J., and Watt, A. J. (1978) The effect of PGE_1 on peristalsis and on perivascular nerve inhibition of peristaltic activity in guinea-pig isolated ileum. J. Pharm. Pharmacol. 30, 726–765.

396. Saunders, R. N., and Moser, C. A. (1972) Changes in vascular resistance induced by prostaglandins E_2 and $F_{2\alpha}$ in the isolated rat pancreas. Arch. Int. Pharmacodyn. 197, 86–92.

397. Schmidt, E., Bruch, H. P., Laven, R., and Hockerts, T. (1978) Modulation of the prostaglandin-induced intestinal motility in humans through the transmitters of vegetative nervous system. Eur. Surg. Res. 10, 329–335.

398. Scholes, G. B., Eley, K. G., and Bennett, A. (1968) Effect of prostaglandins on intestinal motility. Gut 9, 726.

399. Schuster, M. M., and Vanasin, B. (1971) Alteration of smooth muscle electrical and motor activity by prostaglandins. J. Clin. Invest. 50, 83a.

400. Scratcherd, T., and Case, R. M. (1973) The action of cyclic AMP, methyl xanthines and some prostaglandins on pancreatic, exocrine secretion. In: S. Andersson (ed.), Frontiers in Gastrointestinal Research, Almqvist and Wiksell, Stockholm, pp. 191–202.

401. Sharon, P., Ligumsky, M., Rachmilewitz, D., and Zor, U. (1978) Role of prostaglandins in ulcerative colitis: Enhanced production during active disease and inhibition by sulfasalazine. Gastroenterology 75, 638–640.

402. Shaw, J. E., and Ramwell, P. W. (1968) Inhibition of gastric secretion in rats by prostaglandin E_1. In: P. W. Ramwell and J. E. Shaw (eds.), Prostaglandin Symposium of the Worcester Foundation for Experimental Biology, Interscience, New York, pp. 55–66.

403. Shaw, J. E., and Urquhart, J. (1972) Parameters of the control of acid secretion in the isolated blood-perfused stomach. J. Physiol. 226, 107P–108P.

404. Shea-Donohue, P. T., Myers, L., Castell, D. O., and Dubois, A. (1980) Effect of prostacyclin on gastric emptying and secretion in rhesus monkey. In: B. Samuelsson, P. Ramwell, and R. Paoletti (eds.), Advances in Prostaglandin and Thromboxane Research, Vol. 8, Raven Press, New York, pp. 1557–1558.

405. Shearin, N. L., and Pancoe, W. L. (1976) Effect of prostaglandin E_1 on rat gastric motility and cyclic nucleotide content. Experientia 32, 1553–1554.

406. Shehadeh, Z., Price, W. E., and Jacobson, E. D. (1969) Effects of vasoactive agents on intestinal blood flow and motility in the dog. Am. J. Physiol. 216, 386–392.

407. Simon, B., and Kather, H. (1978) Unterschiedliche Wirkungsmechanismen zweier neuer saeuresekretionshemmender Medikamente—cimetidin und Prostglandine. Med. Welt 29, 1182–1183.

408. Sinar, D. R., Charles, L., Fletcher, R., and Castell, D. O. (1979) Prostaglandin E_1 decreases lower esophageal sphincter (LES) pressure: A possible explanation for LES hypotension with esophagitis. Clin. Res. 27, 580A.

409. Sinar, D. R., Fletcher, R., and Castell, D. O. (1979) Differences in the effect of arterial or venous prostaglandins E_1, E_2, or I_2 on lower esophageal sphincter pressure. Clin. Res. 27, 271A.

410. Sinzinger, H., Silberbaver, K., and Seyfried, H. (1979) Rectal mucosa prostacyclin formation in ulcerative colitis. Lancet 1, 444.

411. Smejkal, V. (1969) On the action of prostaglandin E_1 on smooth muscle of the digestive system. Cesk. Gastroenterol. Vyz. 23, 32–35.

412. Sokoloff, J., and Berk, R. N. (1973) The effect of prostaglandin E_2 on bile flow and biliary excretion of iopanoic acid. Invest. Radiol. 8, 9–12.

413. Soll, A. H., (1977) Secretagogue stimulation of O_2 consumption and ^{14}C-aminopyrine (AP) uptake by enriched canine parietal cells. Gastroenterology 72, 1166.

414. Soll, A. H. (1978) Prostaglandin inhibition of histamine-stimulated aminopyrine uptake and cyclic AMP generation by isolated canine parietal cells. Gastroenterology 72, 1146.

415. Soll, A. H., and Wollin, A. (1977) The effects of histamine (H), prostaglandin E_2 (PGE$_2$), and secretin (S) on cyclic AMP in separated canine fundic mucosal cells. Gastroenterology 72, 1166.

416. Sorensen, H. R., Boesby, S., and Pedersen, S. A. (1974) Effect of prostaglandin E_1 on resting gastroesophageal sphincter pressure in normal human subjects. Acta Pharmacol. Toxicol. 35, 54.

417. Sorensen, H. R., Boesby, S., and Pedersen, S. A. (1974) The effect of prostaglandin E_1 on resting gastroesophageal sphincter pressure in normal human subjects. Scand. J. Gastroenterol. 9 (Suppl. 27), 29.

418. Spellacy, W. N., Buhi, W. C., and Holsinger, K. K. (1971) The effect of prostaglandin $F_{2\alpha}$ and E_2 on blood glucose and plasma insulin levels during pregnancy. Am. J. Obstet. Gynecol. 111, 239–243.

419. Spenney, J. G. (1979) Prostaglandin-15-hydroxy-dehydrogenase and Δ^{13}-reductase: Differential content on rabbit fundic and antral mucosa and muscle. Gastroenterology 76, 1254.

420. Spenney, J. G. (1979) Prostaglandin metabolism in fundic and antral gastric mucosa: Differential content of 15-hydroxy prostaglandin dehydrogenase (PGDH). Fed. Proc. 38, 884.

421. Spławiński, J. A., Nies, A. S., Sweetman, B., and Oates, J. A. (1973) The effects of arachidonic acid, prostaglandin E_2 and prostaglandin $F_{2\alpha}$ on the longitudinal stomach strip of the rat. J. Pharmacol. Exp. Ther. 187, 501–510.

422. Stasiewicz, J., Szalaj, W., and Gabyelewicz, A. (1974) The study of guinea pig gallbladder reactivity after PGE$_1$ stimulation. Pol. J. Pharmacol. Pharm. 26, 249–252.

423. Strand, J. C., Miller, M. P., and McGiff, J. C. (1973) Comparison of the biological activities of prostaglandin E_2 methyl ester (15S) with prostaglandin E_2 (PGE$_2$). Fed. Proc. 32, 787.

424. Summers, R. W., Kent, T. H., and Osborne, J. W. (1970) Effects of drugs, ileal obstruction, and irradiation on rat gastrointestinal propulsion. Gastroenterology 59, 731–739.

425. Szalaj, W., Gabryelewicz, A., and Stasiewicz, J. (1975) Effect of prostaglandin E_1 on the reactivity of rat colon, including the role of the adrenergic system. Mater. Med. Pol. 7, 99–101.

426. Taira, N., Narimatsu, A., and Himori, N. (1976) Mode of actions of prostaglandins E_2, $F_{1\alpha}$ and $F_{2\alpha}$ in the dog salivary gland. In: J. Toumisto and M. K. Paasonen (eds.), Proceedings of the Sixth International Congress of Pharmacology, Pergamon Press, New York, p. 159.

427. Taira, N., Narimatsu, A., and Satoh, S. (1975) Differential block by 1-hyoscyamine of the salivary and vascular responses of the dog mandibular gland to prostaglandin $F_{2\alpha}$. Life Sci. 17, 1869–1876.

428. Taira, N., and Satoh, S. (1973) Prostaglandin $F_{2\alpha}$ as a potent excitant of the parasympathetic postganglionic neurons of the dog salivary gland. Life Sci. 13, 501–506.

429. Taira, N., and Satoh, S. (1974) Differential effects of tetrodotoxin on the sialogenous and vasodilator actions of prostaglandin E_2 in the dog salivary gland. Life Sci. 15, 987–993.

430. Takai, M., and Yagasaki, O. (1976) Effect of prostaglandin E_1 on the acetylcholine release from the mesenteric plexus of the guinea pig ileum. Jpn. J. Pharmacol. 26, 146P.

431. Tao, P., Wilson, D. E., and Scruggs, W. (1978) Comparative effects of a prostaglandin endoperoxide analogue and prostaglandin E_2 on canine gastric secretion. Clin. Res. 26, 666A.

432. Tepperman, B. L., Miller, T. A., and Johnson, L. R. (1978) Effect of 16,16-dimethyl prostaglandin E_2 on ethanol-induced damage to canine oxyntic mucosa. Gastroenterology 75, 1061–1065.

433. Thompson, W. J., and Jacobson, E. D. (1977) Comparison of the effects of secretory stimulants and inhibitors on gastric mucosal adenylyl cyclases of various species. Proc. Soc. Exp. Biol. Med. 154, 377–381.

434. Thornell, E., Jansson, R., Kral, J. G., and Svanvik, J. (1979) Inhibition of prostaglandin synthesis as a treatment for biliary pain. Lancet 1, 584.

435. Tonnesen, M. G., Jubiz, W., Moore, J. G., and Frailey, J. (1974) Circadian variation of prostaglandin E(PGE) production in human gastric juice. Am. J. Dig. Dis. 19, 644–648.

436. Torok, T., Vizi, S. E., and Knoll, J. (1976) Study of the smooth muscle depolarizing action of PGE by the sucrose gap method. Acta Physiol. Acad. Sci. Hung. 47, 263.

437. Türker, R. K., and Özer, A. (1970) The effect of prostaglandin E_1 and bradykinin on normal and depolarized isolated duodenum of the rat. Agents Actions 1, 124–127.

438. Türker, R. K., and Onur, R. (1971) Effect of prostaglandin E_1 on intestinal motility of the cat. Arch. Int. Physiol. Biochim. 79, 535–543.

439. Ubatuba, F. B. (1973) The use of hamster stomach in vitro as an assay preparation for prostaglandins. Br. J. Pharmacol. 49, 662–666.

440. Usardi, M. M., Ceserani, R., Doria, G., Gandolfi, C., and Turba, C. (1974) Prostaglandins VII: 8–12 Diisoprostaglandins: Synthesis and biological activities. Pharm. Res. Can. 6, 437–444.

441. Vanasin, B., Greenough, W., and Schuster, M. M. (1970) Effect of prostaglandin (PG) on electrical and motor activity of isolated colonic muscle. Gastroenterology 58, 1004.

442. Vance, J. E., Buchanan, K. D., and Williams, R. H. (1971) Glucagon and insulin release. Diabetes 20, 78–82.

443. Vane, J. R. (1971) Inhibition of prostaglandin synthesis as a mechanism of action for aspirin-like drugs. Nature (London) New Biol. 231, 232–235.

444. Vapaatalo, H., Parantainen, J., Metsae Ketelae, T., and Keyrilaeinen, K. (1978) Effects of polyunsaturated fatty acids on gastric secretion in rats. Arch. Pharmacol. 302 (Suppl.), R46.

445. Villaneuva, R., Hinds, L., Katz, R. L., and Eakins, K. E. (1972) The effect of polyphloretin phosphate on some smooth muscle actions of prostaglandins in the cat. J. Pharmacol. Exp. Ther. 180, 78–85.

446. Vogt, W., Suzuki, T., and Babilli, S. (1966) Prostaglandins in SRS-C and in darmstoff preparation from frog intestinal dialysates. Mem. Soc. Endocrinol. 14, 137–142.

447. Vural, H., and Baysal, F. (1972) Effects of some prostaglandins on the isolated gallbladder of guinea pigs. Ankara Univ. Tip. Fak. Mecm. 25, 5–11.

448. Vural, H., Baysal, F., and Kocak, N. (1972) Prostaglandins and the human appendix. Diyarbakiv Tip. Fak. Derg. 1, 149–154.

449. Wada, T., and Ishizawa, M. (1970) Effects of prostaglandin on the function of the gastric secretion. Jpn. J. Clin. Med. 28, 2465–2468.

450. Wada, T., and Ishizawa, M. (1970) Fundamental and clinical studies on the effects of prostaglandins on the alimentary canal. Proc. Soc. Gerontol. Okayama City, pp. 22–23.

451. Watson, L. C., Miller, T. A., Rayford, P. L., and Thompson, J. C. (1976) Effect of prostaglandin E_1 on plasma secretion and pancreatic exocrine function in dogs. Surg. Forum 27, 426–427.

452. Wax, J., Cling, W. A., Vamer, P., Bass, P., and Winder, C. F. (1970) Relationship of the enterohepatic cycle to ulcerogenesis in the rat small bowel with flufenamic acid. Gastroenterology 58, 772–780.

453. Way, L., and Durbin, R. P. (1969) Inhibition of gastric acid secretion in vitro by prostaglandin E_1. Nature (London) 221, 874–875.

454. Weeks, J. R., Schultz, J. R., and Brown, W. E. (1968) Evaluation of smooth muscle bioassays for prostaglandins E_1 and $F_{2\alpha}$. J. Appl. Physiol. 25, 783–785.

455. Weeks, J. R., Sekhar, N. C., and Ducharme, D. W. (1969) Relative activity of prostaglandins E_1, A_1, E_2 and A_2 on lipolysis, platelet aggregation, smooth muscle and the cardiovascular system. J. Pharm. Pharmacol. 21, 103–108.

456. Whittle, B. J. R. (1972) Studies on the mode of action of cyclic 3'5'-AMP and prostaglandin E_2 on rat gastric acid secretion and mucosal blood flow. Br. J. Pharmacol. 46, 546P–547P.

457. Whittle, B. J. R. (1976) Gastric antisecretory and antiulcer activity of prostaglandin E_2 methyl analogs. In: B. Samuelsson and R. Paoletti (eds.), Advances in Prostaglandin and Thromboxane Research, Vol. 2, Raven Press, New York, p. 948.

458. Whittle, B. J. R. (1977) Mechanisms underlying gastric mucosal damage induced by indomethacin and bile-salts, and the actions of prostaglandins. Br. J. Pharmacol. 60, 455–460.

459. Whittle, B. J. R., Boughton Smith, N. K., Moncada, S., and Vane, J. R. (1978) Actions of prostacyclin (PGI_2) and its product, 6-oxo-$PGF_{1\alpha}$ on the rat gastric mucosa in vivo and in vitro. Prostaglandins 15, 955–967.

460. Whittle, B. J. R., Mugridge, K. G., and Moncada, S. (1979) Use of rabbit transverse stomach-strip to identify the assay prostacyclin, PGA_2, PGD_2 and other prostaglandins. Eur. J. Pharmacol. 53, 167–172.

461. Willis, A. L., Davison, P., and Ramwell, P. W. (1974) Inhibition of intestinal tone, motility and prostaglandin biosynthesis by 5,8,11,14-eicosatetraynoic acid (TYA). Prostaglandins 5, 355–368.

462. Wilson, D. E., Chang, I. W., Paulsrud, J., and Holland, G. (1978) The effects of 11-methyl-16,16-dimethyl prostaglandin E_2 on canine gastric acid secretion. Prostaglandins 16, 121–126.

463. Wilson, D. E., Chang, I. W., and Raiser, M. (1977) Efficacy of a new prostaglandin analog on gastric secretion. Gastroenterology 72, 1150.

464. Wilson, D. E., and Levine, R. A. (1969) Decreased canine gastric mucosal blood flow induced by prostaglandin E_1. A mechanism for its inhibitory effect on gastric secretion. Gastroenterology 56, 1268.

465. Wilson, D. E., and Levine, R. A. (1970) Inhibition of hepatic glucose utilization by prostaglandin E_1 (PGE_1). Clin. Res. 18, 468.

466. Wilson, D. E., and Levine, R. A. (1972) The effect of prostaglandin E_1 on canine gastric acid secretion and gastric mucosal blood flow. Am. J. Dig. Dis. 17, 527–532.

467. Wilson, D. E., Phillips, C., and Levine, R. A. (1970) Inhibition of gastric secretion in man by prostaglandin A_1 (PGA_1). Gastroenterology 58, 1007.

468. Wilson, D. E., Phillips, C., and Levine, R. A. (1971) Inhibition of gastric secretion in man by prostaglandin A_1. Gastroenterology 61, 201–206.

469. Wilson, D. E., Quertermus, J., Raiser, M., Curran, J., and Robert, A. (1976) Inhibition of stimulated gastric secretion by an orally administered prostaglandin capsule: A study in normal men. Ann. Intern. Med. 84, 688–691.

470. Wilson, D. E., Winnan, G., Quertermus, J., and Tao, P. (1975) Effects of an orally administered prostaglandin analogue (16,16-dimethyl prostaglandin E_2) on human gastric secretion. Gastroenterology 69, 607–611.

471. Wilson, D. E., and Winter, S. L. (1978) The effects of 11-methyl-16-,16-dimethyl prostaglandin E_2 on gastric acid secretion in man. Prostaglandins 16, 127–133.

472. Wolfe, L. S., Coceani, F., and Pace-Asciak, C. (1967) Brain prostaglandins and studies of the action of prostaglandins on the isolated rat stomach. In: S. Bergström and B. Samuelsson (eds.), Prostaglandins, Almqvist and Wiksell, Stockholm, pp. 265–275.

473. Wollin, A., Code, C. F., and Dousa, T. P. (1974) Evidence for separate histamine and prostaglandin sensitive adenylate cyclases (AC) in guinea pig gastric mucosa (GM). Clin. Res. 22, 606A.

474. Yagasaki, O., Matsuyama, S., and Takai, M. (1974) The release of prostaglandins from the passively distended wall of guinea pig intestine. Jpn. J. Pharmacol. 24 (Suppl.), 31.

475. Yagasaki, O., Suzuki, H., and Sohji, Y. (1978) Effects of loperamide on acetylcholine and prostaglandin release from isolated guinea pig ileum. Jpn. J. Pharmacol. 28, 873–882.

476. Yamasuchi, T., Hitzig, B., and Coburn, R. F. (1976) Endogenous prostaglandin in guinea pig *Taenia coli*. Am. J. Physiol. 230, 149–157.

477. Yanagi, Y. (1978) Inhibition of prostaglandin biosynthesis in rat small intestine by SL-573. Biochem. Pharmacol. 27, 723–728.

478. Yankee, E. W., Axen, U., and Bundy, G. L. (1974) Total synthesis of 15-methyl-prostaglandins. J. Am. Chem. Soc. 96, 5865–5876.

479. Yankee, E. W., and Bundy, G. L. (1972) 15(S)-15-Methylprostaglandins. J. Am. Chem. Soc. 94, 3651–3652.

480. Zamecnik, A. M., Cerskus, J., Stoessl, A. L., Barnett, A. J., and McDonald, J. W. D. (1977) Synthesis of thromboxane B_2 and prostaglandins by bovine gastric mucosal microsomes. Prostaglandins 14, 819–827.

481. Zoretic, P. A., Soja, P., and Shiah, T. (1978) Synthesis and gastric antisecretory properties of an 8-aza- and a 10-oxa-8,12-secoprostaglandin. J. Med. Chem. 21, 1330–1332.

482. Zséli, J., Vizi, E. S., and Knoll, J. (1978) Effect of PGE_1 and indomethacin (IND) on cholecystokinin induced contraction of the guinea pig ileum. Acta Physiol. Acad. Sci. Hung. 51, 222–223.

PETER A. KOT, M.D.
THOMAS M. FITZPATRICK, Ph.D.

CARDIOVASCULAR ACTIONS OF PROSTAGLANDIN PRECURSORS AND SELECTED PROSTANOIC COMPOUNDS

INTRODUCTION

In 1930 Kurzrok and Lieb [88] reported that human semen added to human uterine muscle strips induced either contraction or relaxation of uterine muscle. The active agents were dialyzable through a collodion membrane, and the presence of spermatozoa was not essential for the reaction to occur. The age of the seminal specimen influenced whether relaxation or contraction of uterine muscle occurred, suggesting formation of several substances that produce opposite effects.

Several years later Goldblatt [58] tested the effects of human seminal fluid and extracts of seminal fluid on the arterial blood pressure of cats and rabbits. Relatively small amounts of seminal fluid or its components produced profound decreases in arterial blood pressure that lasted as long as 30–45 minutes. Neither heart rate nor force of contraction of isolated perfused frog's heart was altered by the seminal fluid or its extract.

In 1937 von Euler [40] demonstrated that the biologically active substance extracted from the human prostate had acidic properties and, like human seminal fluid, had a marked depressor action on the blood pres-

From the Department of Physiology and Biophysics, Georgetown University Schools of Medicine and Dentistry, Washington, D.C.

sure of the rabbit, cat, and dog. A substance extracted from the vesicular gland of the sheep, which von Euler called vesiglandin, possessed similar vasoactive properties. Neither substance greatly affected the mammalian heart. Vesiglandin and prostaglandin were thought to be two distinct substances because vesiglandin was less stable in acids and alkalis than prostaglandin and had only weak effects on the isolated intestine of the rabbit or guinea pig.

By the late 1950s the molecular structure of several prostaglandins had been determined by Bergström and his colleagues. It was established that the prostaglandins are 20-carbon carboxylic acids, synthesized from specific polyunsaturated fatty acids. The precursor fatty acids from which the prostaglandins are formed are dihomo-γ-linolenic acid, arachidonic acid and eicosapentaenoic acid (Fig. 1).

Although prostaglandins have a multiplicity of biologic actions that affect nearly every organ system of the body, this chapter is confined to a discussion of the actions of the precursor fatty acids and selected prostanoic compounds on the circulatory system. Cardiovascular actions of prostaglandins of the A, E, and F series have been well documented in a wide spectrum of animals species. In general, the PGEs, PGAs, and PGFs have positive chronotropic and inotropic effects on the heart. PGAs and PGEs decrease arterial blood pressure in animals, although species variations do exist. PGFs are usually vasoconstrictors and consequently produce a rise in systemic arterial pressure. Malik and McGiff [97] and Bergström and his colleagues [13] have written extensive reviews of the cardiovascular actions of the prostaglandins E, A, and F and their derivatives, as well as their specific actions on individual regional circulations.

FIGURE 1. Structural configuration of the fatty acid precursors to the monoenoic, bisenoic, and trienoic prostaglandins.

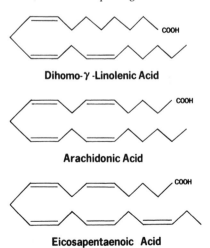

Dihomo-γ-Linolenic Acid

Arachidonic Acid

Eicosapentaenoic Acid

During the past five to six years attention has been focused on the precursors of the prostaglandins and particularly the cascade of compounds subsequently shown to be generated from arachidonic acid. The products of the arachidonic acid cascade possess potent cardiovascular actions and may play an important role in the regulation of the circulatory system in both physiologic and pathophysiologic states.

PROSTAGLANDIN PRECURSORS

Arachidonic Acid

Arachidonic acid is the most important precursor fatty acid from the biologic viewpoint. The source of arachidonic acid is the phospholipid component of most cell membranes. Upon release and enzymatic conversion, a number of biologically active compounds are formed from arachidonic acid, as shown in Fig. 2.

CARDIAC ACTIONS

Studies on the cardiac effects of arachidonic acid are limited, and the reported effects are quite variable. Belford [11] reported that arachidonic acid increases the force of contraction of the heart in the intact rat.

In isolated spontaneously beating guinea pig atria, arachidonic acid

FIGURE 2. Cascade of the possible vasoactive metabolites of arachidonic acid.

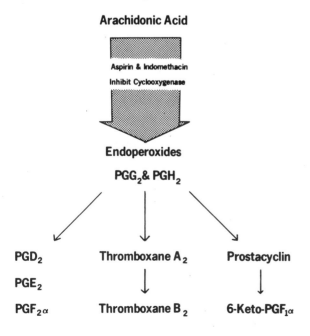

induced a marked positive chronotropic action but only a small positive inotropic effect [17]. Both the chronotropic and inotropic effects were dose dependent. However, the inotropic effect was shown to be dependent on heart rate. When heart rate frequency was kept constant by electrical pacing, the small inotropic action of arachidonic acid was eliminated. Neither catecholamine depletion nor β-adrenergic blockade with pindolol modified the chronotropic action of arachidonic acid. Tachyphylaxis to the positive inotropic effect of arachidonic acid was noted with repeated applications. Of interest was the observation that indomethacin and aspirin did not block the positive chronotropic action of arachidonic acid. This raised the possibility that the positive chronotropic effect of arachidonic acid is mediated by a nonprostaglandin substance or peroxides formed from arachidonic acid.

In the anesthetized dog with an intact circulation, arachidonic acid produced variable effects on myocardial contractile force [86]. When arachidonic acid increased myocardial contractile force, the increase always occurred during the maximum decrease in systemic arterial pressure. This suggested that the increase in myocardial contractile force was a reflex response secondary to the fall in systemic arterial pressure. Ganglion blockade eliminated the positive inotropic effect caused by arachidonic acid, indicating that the cardiac changes were due to enhanced cardiac sympathetic nerve activity mediated by baroreceptor reflexes.

However, very large doses of arachidonic acid (900 μg/kg, administered intravenously) elicited a small positive inotropic effect in the presence of ganglion blockade. Whether this represented a direct effect of arachidonic acid on the myocardium or increased conversion of arachidonic acid into intermediate products in sufficient quantity to elicit a cardiac effect was not determined.

The antiarrhythmic properties of arachidonic acid have been tested in rats [48] and cats [101]. Both arachidonic and linoleic acids possessed strong antiarrhythmic effects in the rat in comparison to linolenic and oleic acids. High doses of arachidonic acid were required to display its antiarrhythmic effects in comparison with the prostaglandins. Since indomethacin pretreatment interfered with the antiarrhythmic action of arachidonic acid, it appears that one of the derivatives of arachidonic acid is responsible for the antiarrhythmic action.

BLOOD PRESSURE EFFECTS

As part of a study on the pharmacologic actions of arachidonic acid, Jaques [74] reported that administration of arachidonic acid in a dose of 0.1 mg/kg produced a transient fall in arterial blood pressure in the cat that lasted 1–3 minutes. Atropine attenuated but did not suppress the hypotensive actions of arachidonic acid.

Ichikawa and Yamada [72] reported that both free and albumin-bound arachidonic acids produced a dose-dependent decrease in systemic arterial pressure in the rabbit and the dog. Both albumin-bound arachidonic acid and the free acid produced a similar hypotensive effect, suggesting that once arachidonic acid is released into the bloodstream, its biologic effects can be expressed.

These studies generated little interest in the cardiovascular actions of arachidonic acid until it was demonstrated in the 1960s that arachidonic acid was the precursor to the bisenoic series of prostaglandins.

In 1973 Larsson and Änggård [89] reported that arachidonate infused intraarterially in the rabbit produced a dose-dependent decrease in arterial blood pressure. When the animals were pretreated with indomethacin or 5,8,11,14-eicosatetraynoic acid (ETYA), subsequent infusion of arachidonate had no effect on blood pressure. Vasoactive substances generated from arachidonic acid were responsible for the hypotensive effect, since prior administration of these two prostaglandin synthesis inhibitors prevented the depressor response from occurring.

Cohen et al. [27] also reported that intravenous administration of arachidonic acid (10 mg/kg) produced a systemic hypotensive response and a reflex tachycardia in the spontaneously hypertensive rat. These responses were blocked by pretreatment of the animals with nonsteroidal antiinflammatory agents. Cohen et al. hypothesized that the depressor response observed following arachidonic acid administration was due to the generation of PGE_2, not to the arachidonic acid itself.

The hemodynamic mechanisms involved in the hypotensive response were not delineated at this point. In 1974 Silver and his colleagues [138] reported that arachidonic acid induced sudden death in rabbits when administered intravenously in a dose of 1.4 mg/kg. Histologic sections revealed numerous platelet aggregates in the microcirculation of the lung. Many of the aggregates completely obliterated the lumen of capillaries. A single dose of aspirin protected the animals from the lethal effects of arachidonic acid. This protective effect sometimes lasted for several days. Other fatty acids closely related to arachidonic acid had no effect at doses four times the LD_{50} of arachidonic acid.

Pulmonary platelet aggregates have been implicated by Pirkle and Carstens [125] as a cause of sudden death in some humans. They proposed that platelet aggregation may be mediated by prostaglandin endoperoxides generated from endogenous platelet arachidonic acid. Since mechanical occlusion of pulmonary vessels by platelet aggregates could markedly reduce pulmonary venous return to the left side of the circulation, the hypotensive response following arachidonic acid administration could be attributed to a reduction in cardiac output.

In 1974 our group [128] undertook a systematic study of the acute hemodynamic changes produced by the prostaglandin precursors in dogs. Acute intravenous injections of arachidonic acid (300 µg/kg) produced a profound drop in systemic arterial pressure from which recovery rapidly ensued. The onset of the drop in systemic arterial pressure did not occur for 15 seconds following administration into the inferior vena cava. In contrast, the onset of the decline in arterial pressure following administration of PGE_2 (5 µg/kg) through the same catheter was 4.5 seconds. The delay in the onset of action of arachidonic acid suggested that time was required for transformation of arachidonic acid into some prostaglandinlike substance with vasoactive properties. Arachidonic acid itself was shown not to be vasoactive: pretreatment of animals with acetylsalicylic acid completely blocked all responses to arachidonic acid administration. The duration of the hypotensive effect was approximately 5 minutes, and there was no evidence of tachyphylaxis to arachidonic acid at a dose of 300 µg/kg on repeated injections at 5-minute intervals for up to six doses. A widening of arterial pulse pressure was noted during the maximum drop in arterial blood pressure. Linoleic acid and oleic acid were administered intravenously in dogs in the same dose levels as arachidonic acid. Neither of these fatty acids produced any hemodynamic changes, indicating that the responses to arachidonic acid were not a nonspecific fatty acid effect.

To determine what mechanisms were responsible for the hypotensive action of arachidonic acid, anesthetized dogs were instrumented with electromagnetic flow probes on the ascending aorta as well as several other major vessels of the arterial circulation [44]. Acute changes in ascending aortic blood flow were monitored following bolus intravenous injections of arachidonic acid (300 µg/kg) in the dog (Fig. 3). Ascending aortic blood flow, which reflects left ventricular output minus coronary blood flow, remained at or above control values throughout the response. Mesenteric blood flow, which was simultaneously measured, was acutely sensitive to arachidonic acid and exhibited a biphasic response. Initially mesenteric blood flow transiently decreased and then

FIGURE 3. Changes in systemic arterial pressure (SAP), femoral flow (FF), aortic flow (AF), and mesenteric flow (MF) following a 300 µg/kg intravenous dose of arachidonic acid (AA).

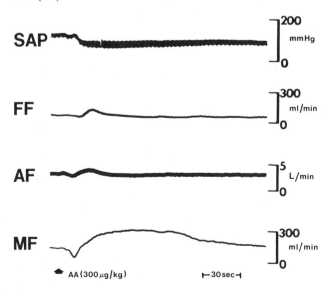

increased 87% above control values for the duration of the hypotensive response.

Ånggård and Larsson [4] employed a radioactive microsphere technique to study the effects of arachidonic acid on blood flow through different organs and tissues of the rabbit. They observed a marked increase in hepatic and gastric blood flow and a decrease in cutaneous and brachial muscle blood flow. Cardiac output was not simultaneously determined in this study.

The primary mechanism responsible for the systemic hypotensive action of exogenously administered arachidonic acid is a decrease in total peripheral vascular resistance. Since cardiac output remained at or above control value in the dog following arachidonic acid administration, significant mechanical occlusion of the pulmonary microcirculation by platelet aggregates did not occur. Otherwise, a reduction in cardiac output would be anticipated as a result of a decrease in pulmonary venous return to the left ventricle. Mousty and his colleagues [111] also concluded that platelet aggregation was not responsible for the cardiovascular actions of arachidonic acid.

Subsequent studies have demonstrated that vascular walls are capable of generating a vasodilator substance, prostacyclin (PGI_2), from prostaglandin endoperoxides or arachidonic acid [103]. The hemodynamic actions of prostacyclin, which are discussed at greater length later, closely mimic the hemodynamic changes induced by administration of arachidonic acid. Therefore, it is likely that the systemic hypotensive effects of arachidonic acid are due to the generation of prostacyclin.

REGIONAL CIRCULATIONS

Pulmonary Circulation. Arachidonic acid produces a pressor response in the blood-perfused lung lobe of the dog [70,160] and in the lungs of dogs with an intact circulation [70,141]. The pressor response is dose related and is a result of pulmonary vascular constriction, since flow through the lobe is kept constant. Pretreatment with aspirin completely eliminates the pressor response, indicating that conversion of arachidonic acid to one of its derivatives is required for its vascular action on the lung circulation. A number of other blocking agents, including phentolamine, propranolol, atropine, and cyproheptadine, did not modify the pulmonary pressor response to arachidonic acid.

Platelets and other cellular elements of blood are not essential for the pulmonary vascular response to arachidonic acid. Neither low molecular weight dextran nor physiologic saline solution, when used as the perfusion medium, attenuated the pulmonary pressor response to arachidonic acid. Indeed, Hyman and his colleagues [70] observed markedly enhanced responses to arachidonic acid in the lung circulation when either of these two perfusates was substituted for whole blood. In the same animal preparation, perfusion of the lung with dextran did not alter the response to PGE_2 or $PGF_{2\alpha}$. The enhanced pressor response to arachidonic acid, when using artificial perfusion media, may be related to the absence of protein binding of arachidonic acid. This hypothesis was supported by studies demonstrating that addition of albumin to the perfusion media decreased the response to arachidonic acid.

The action of arachidonic acid is also modified by alterations in the physiologic state of the animal. Hypoxia decreases the pulmonary vascular response to arachidonic acid, suggesting that conversion of arachidonic acid into other products may be altered in the hypoxic state.

The above-mentioned studies were performed using bolus injections of arachidonic acid. Formation of predominantly vasoconstrictor metabolites from arachidonic acid must have occurred during transit through the lung, accounting for the pressor response of this substance in the lung circulation. By the time the systemic circulation was reached, vasodilator substances were generated in sufficient quantity to produce the characteristic hypotensive effect.

In vitro studies of the effects of arachidonic acid on isolated strips of canine intrapulmonary arteries and veins differ from in vivo studies. Arachidonic acid relaxed isolated intrapulmonary arteries and had no significant effects on pulmonary veins [59]. Since both the in vivo and in vitro effects of arachidonic acid are inhibited by indomethacin, it is likely that conversion of arachidonic acid into different vasoactive substances occurs in the two situations.

On the other hand, slow intravenous infusion of arachidonic acid decreases pulmonary vascular resistance in the dog and cat [70]. Gerber and his colleagues [52] confirmed this finding by demonstrating that intravenous infusions of arachidonic acid reversed the pulmonary vasoconstriction produced by hypoxia. Arterial blood samples obtained during the arachidonic acid infusion contained both PGE_2 and 6-keto-$PGF_{1\alpha}$, which is the stable breakdown product of prostacyclin. Both PGE_2 and prostacyclin are pulmonary vasodilators and probably mediated the decrease in pulmonary vascular resistance under these circumstances.

Lung transit does not significantly modify the systemic hypotensive action of arachidonic acid [150]. A 100 µg/kg dose of arachidonic acid administered intravenously produced the same decrease in arterial pressure as an identical dose injected intraarterially. This suggests that the vasoactive products formed from arachidonic acid are not significantly degraded during transit through the lung.

Coronary Circulation. In the isolated rabbit heart, infusions of arachidonic acid produced a sustained decrease in coronary vascular resistance, which was accompanied by the generation of a prostaglandinlike substance [113].

Arachidonic acid relaxed isolated bovine, canine, and human coronary arteries [87]. The response of isolated coronary arteries to arachidonic acid is completely blocked by pretreatment with indomethacin, meclofenemate, or aspirin. When relaxation of isolated coronary arteries has been achieved by the administration of arachidonic acid, addition of indomethacin results in contraction of the vessel segment. The arachidonic acid is converted into an unstable vasodilating substance by coronary prostaglandin synthetase. The vasodilating substance is neither PGE_2 nor $PGF_{2\alpha}$, since both these compounds induce constriction of isolated coronary arteries.

When bovine coronary artery strips were incubated with 1-[^{14}C] arachidonic acid, a substance was generated with chromatographic properties identical to those of 6-keto-$PGF_{1\alpha}$ [126]. A similar prostaglandinlike material was released from the isolated perfused rabbit heart by infusion of exogenous arachidonate or following hormonal stimulation [73]. Since 6-keto-$PGF_{1\alpha}$ was inactive on coronary artery strips, it was postulated that a labile intermediate was formed in the enzymatic conversion of endoperoxides to 6-keto-$PGF_{1\alpha}$ and that this substance was responsible for coronary artery relaxation. The synthesis of this vasodilating substance in the heart is confined to the coronary vascular smooth muscle. Subsequent studies [30,31] demonstrated that prostacyclin was the metabolite of arachidonic acid that possessed coronary vasodilating properties. This conclusion was based on several observations: (1) prostacyclin is the only prostanoic substance that consistently relaxes coronary artery strips, and (2) the relaxing effect of sodium arachidonate on coronary artery strips is abolished by 15-hydroperoxy arachidonic acid, which is a specific inhibitor of prostacyclin synthetase.

Splanchnic Circulation. As previously discussed, arachidonic acid (300 µg/kg) produces a biphasic change in mesenteric blood flow in dogs with an intact circulation [44]. There is an initial transient decrease in mesenteric blood flow, followed by an increase in blood flow that persists throughout the remainder of the response.

However, when arachidonic acid is administered directly into the superior mesenteric artery in doses ranging from 0.1 to 1.0 mg, the initial transient decrease in blood flow was observed in only about one-half the animals [24]. The predominant effect was a prolonged increase in mesenteric blood flow. Since aortic pressure was not altered by the administration of arachidonic acid under these circumstances, the enhanced blood flow into this vascular bed was due to selective dilatation of the mesenteric vasculature. Indomethacin markedly reduced the vasodilator response in the mesenteric vascular bed produced by the direct administration of arachidonic acid. It is likely that the initial transient decrease in blood flow was due to the generation of vasoconstrictor products and the prolonged vasodilator response to the formation of prostacyclin or PGE_2. Dusting and his colleagues [33] also observed that arachidonic acid produced a dose-dependent vasodilatation in the mesenteric vascular bed of the dog.

Malik and his colleagues [98] investigated the effects of arachidonic acid on the vasoconstrictor responses to adrenergic stimuli of isolated perfused rabbit and rat mesenteric arteries. They observed that arachidonic acid reduced the vasoconstrictor responses to either injections of norepinephrine or sympathetic nerve stimulation in the rabbit but potentiated those responses in the rat. Since simultaneous infusion of indomethacin abolished this effect of arachidonic acid, it is presumed that the modulating effect of arachidonic acid on adrenergic transmission in mesenteric arteries is mediated by prostaglandins generated from arachidonic acid.

Bridenbaugh and his colleagues [18] investigated the effects of arachidonic acid infusions on superior mesenteric artery flow and mean arterial blood pressure in the dog during splanchnic artery occlusion shock and in sham animals. Arachidonic acid decreased superior mesenteric artery flow in the shock animals but not in the nonshock animals. The decrease in superior mesenteric artery flow in the shock animals was associated with a concomitant reduction in mean arterial pressure. These changes in mean arterial pressure did not occur in the nonshock animals. PGE_2 levels were dramatically increased in the shock animals receiving arachidonic acid in contrast to the PGE_2 concentrations measured in sham animals. The vasodilator effects of PGE_2 may be one of the factors contributing to the hypotensive state in the shock animals.

Musculocutaneous Circulation. The effects of arachidonic acid on the femoral vascular bed have been examined in dogs, although slightly different experimental techniques were employed. In the completely isolated hind limb preparation, sodium arachidonate produced a dose-dependent increase in limb perfusion pressure [43]. The limb vascular response to sodium arachidonate was not mediated by release of endogenous norepinephrine, since phentolamine administered prior to the sodium arachidonate did not modify the pressor response of the limb vasculature.

In a modified dog hind limb preparation, Dusting and his colleagues [33] found that sodium arachidonate produced a dose-dependent vasodilatation in the femoral vascular bed, which was markedly attenuated by pretreatment with indomethacin. No well-defined explanation for these opposite responses of the hind limb vasculature has been elucidated. However, varied doses and methods of administration of arachidonic acid could account for these differences.

Changes in forearm blood flow were measured by occlusion plethysmography in four healthy male volunteers before and during infusion of sodium arachidonate [156]. Forearm blood flow increased 400% during infusion of sodium arachidonate. However, the vasodilator effect was only partially attenuated by pretreatment with indomethacin.

Renal Circulation. Several studies in dogs have demonstrated that infusions of sodium arachidonate into one renal artery will increase blood flow in that kidney [14,146]. The alterations in renal blood flow produced by sodium arachidonate are associated with changes in electrolyte excretion. The increases in renal blood flow produced by sodium arachidonate were never as large as those produced by PGE_2.

In addition, the infusion of sodium arachidonate caused a redistribution of blood flow to the inner or juxtamedullary portion of the cortex

[22,90]. No changes in blood flow were noted in the outer cortical neph-rons. Pretreatment of animals with indomethacin abolished the effects of sodium arachidonate on renal blood flow. Indomethacin by itself diminished the relative perfusion of the juxtamedullary cortex, sug-gesting that endogenous production of prostaglandins is involved in the normal regulation of blood flow to this region of the renal cortex.

Urinary efflux of prostaglandins was increased by 50% during sodium arachidonate infusion into the renal artery. Most of the urinary pros-taglandins were PGE_2 and to a much lesser extent $PGF_{2\alpha}$.

Plasma renin activity is also augmented by infusion of sodium arach-idonate in the dog [14] and rabbit [91]. Likewise, enhanced renin release occurs when slices of rabbit renal cortex are incubated with sodium arachidonate [154]. These responses can be blocked by pretreating the animals with indomethacin. Therefore, stimulation of renin release by sodium arachidonate appears to be a direct effect of the prostaglandin system.

Dihomo-γ-Linolenic Acid

There are relatively few studies of the cardiovascular actions of dihomo-γ-linolenic acid (DGLA), the precursor of the monoenoic prostaglandins. It occurs in tissues in much smaller quantities than arachidonic acid and has not been intensively studied.

CARDIAC ACTIONS

In dogs DGLA (2.5 mg/kg) administered as an intravenous bolus injec-tion produced a consistent increase in myocardial contractile force [129]. The cardiac effects of DGLA were not altered by ganglionic blockade with hexamethonium chloride or by β-adrenergic blockade with prac-tolol. Pretreatment of the animals with aspirin markedly attenuated or completely abolished the cardiac effects of DGLA, indicating that the major positive inotropic action of DGLA is due to synthesis of a substance generated from DGLA.

BLOOD PRESSURE EFFECTS

DGLA produces a characteristic biphasic systemic arterial blood pressure response in the dog [129]. There is a transient decrease in arterial pres-sure with an onset approximately 4 seconds after intravenous admin-istration, followed by a second more profound, and longer lasting drop with an onset at about 15 seconds. The arterial pressure response was not qualitatively altered by either ganglionic or β-adrenergic blockade. Pretreatment with aspirin markedly attenuated or even abolished the blood pressure response, suggesting that conversion of DGLA into an-other substance was required for the vasodepressor action. Whether

DGLA produces similar hemodynamic effects in other species is unknown.

REGIONAL CIRCULATION (PULMONARY CIRCULATION)

In the canine isolated lung lobe preparation DGLA produces a dose-related increase in lobar perfusion pressure [161]. Since flow through the lobe was kept constant in this preparation, the rise in perfusion pressure reflects an increase in pulmonary vascular resistance. Similar dose-related increases in pulmonary vascular resistance following DGLA have been observed employing a modified isolated lung lobe preparation [71]. The elevation of pulmonary vascular resistance appears to be a result of constriction of lobar arteries and small intrapulmonary veins.

The pulmonary vascular actions of DGLA are blocked by pretreating with indomethacin and are augmented when the lobe is perfused with dextran instead of whole blood. Compared to arachidonic acid, DGLA was 8–10 times less potent as a pulmonary vasoconstrictor.

Eicosapentaenoic Acid

There are no specific hemodynamic effects of eicosapentaenoic acid (EPA), the precursor of the trienoic prostaglandins. Dyerberg and his colleagues [36] have shown that unlike arachidonic acid, EPA does not induce platelet aggregation in human platelet-rich plasma.

In our own laboratory [127] EPA was administered intravenously to dogs in varying dose levels. Very high doses of EPA (4 mg/kg) produced a transient decrease in systemic arterial pressure and a temporary elevation of pulmonary arterial pressure. The transient hemodynamic changes were similar to those produced by a comparable dose of linoleic acid (Fig. 4) but qualitatively and quantitatively different from the hemodynamic responses induced by a much lower dose of arachidonic acid.

FIGURE 4. Comparison of the changes in airway pressure (AIR), systemic arterial pressure (SAP), and pulmonary arterial pressure (PAP) in response to linoleic acid (LA), eicosapentaenoic acid (EPA), and arachidonic acid (AA). Doses and routes of administration are indicated in the upper portion of the tracings. Vertical lines indicate time of administration of each fatty acid.

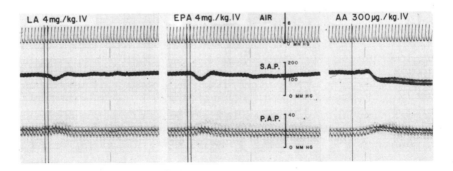

It appears that EPA is not biologically active on the circulation and that the transient hemodynamic changes induced by high doses of this unsaturated fatty acid represent nonspecific fatty acid effects.

SELECTED PROSTANOIC COMPOUNDS

Endoperoxide Intermediates

Cyclic endoperoxides, PGG_2 and PGH_2, are intermediate products formed from arachidonic acid by a microsomal fatty acid cyclooxygenase. Because of the rapid decomposition of these compounds at 37°C (half-life of about 5 minutes), it has been difficult to elucidate their specific actions on the systemic circulation. Several very stable synthetic analogues have been developed that closely resemble the naturally occurring endoperoxides in their molecular geometry.

Three of these analogues have been studied in the canine circulation. Two are cyclic ether endoperoxide analogues; (15S)-hydroxy-9α,11α-epoxymethano-prosta-5Z,13E-dienoic acid, referred to as U-44069 and (15S)-hydroxy-11α,9α-epoxymethano-prosta-5Z,13E-dienoic acid, referred to as U-46619 [19]. The other is an azo-endoperoxide analogue, (15S)-hydroxy-9α,11α-(azo)-prosta-5Z,13E-dienoic acid [28]. Because these compounds are stable, the analogues do not behave in exactly the same manner as the naturally occurring endoperoxides. However, the analogues have proved to be useful in providing information about the biologic actions of these natural endoperoxides on the cardiovascular system.

CARDIAC ACTIONS

PGG_2 and PGH_2. No specific studies of the cardiac actions of PGG_2 and PGH_2 have been reported. Instability of the naturally occurring endoperoxides, which degrade rapidly into other products, precludes specific assessment of the direct actions of these compounds on cardiac muscle.

Synthetic Analogues. In open-chest anesthetized dogs, myocardial contractile force was measured with a Walton-Brodie strain-gauge arch. Each of the three endoperoxide analogues had a direct positive inotropic action on the heart [130]. Ganglion blockade with hexamethonium chloride did not block the cardiac actions of the analogues. Similarly, pretreatment with indomethacin did not prevent the increase in myocardial contractile force produced by the synthetic endoperoxide analogues. Effects of these analogues on other indices of changes in myocardial contractility, such as left ventricular dp/dt, V_{max}, and ventricular function curves have not been investigated. All three endoperoxide analogues produced moderate reductions in heart rate during the pressor response. The decrease in heart rate was markedly attenuated or abolished in animals during ganglion blockade, suggesting that the reduction in heart rate was mediated by neurogenic reflexes.

BLOOD PRESSURE EFFECTS

PGG$_2$ and PGH$_2$. In the anesthetized guinea pig intravenous administration of PGG$_2$ and PGH$_2$ produces a triphasic arterial pressure response [61]. Initially there is a transient decrease in arterial pressure, followed by a brief rise and finally a prolonged reduction in pressure. The initial decrease and the subsequent short rise in systemic arterial pressure are attributed directly to the endoperoxides. The vasoconstrictor effects of the endoperoxides on the pulmonary circulation could restrict venous return to the left side of the circulation and reduce left ventricular output with a consequent reduction in arterial pressure. When the endoperoxides reach the systemic vasculature they induce vasoconstriction and an increase in systemic vascular resistance, which accounts for the temporary rise in arterial pressure. Eventual conversion of the endoperoxides into vasodilating substances is felt to be responsible for the prolonged reduction in pressure.

In the anesthetized cat, Hedqvist and his colleagues [63] did not observe the triphasic arterial blood pressure response. PGH$_2$, when administered intravenously in a dose of 5 µg/kg, was more effective as a vasodepressor agent than PGE$_2$. However, when administered intraarterially PGE$_2$ was as active a vasodepressor substance as PGH$_2$. Comparison of the arterial blood pressure responses to intraarterial and intravenous administration of PGG$_2$ and PGH$_2$ revealed no significant difference in the magnitude of the depressor response when administered by either route. This suggests that the endoperoxides or their active metabolites are not significantly degraded by the pulmonary circulation.

In the normotensive rat both PGG$_2$ and PGH$_2$ were found to be systemic hypotensive agents [5]. Both PGG$_2$ and PGH$_2$ were substantially less potent than PGE$_2$ when administered intraarterially. Comparison of the arterial blood pressure responses to intravenous and intraarterial administration of PGG$_2$ and PGH$_2$ indicated that PGG$_2$ was equally active by either route, but that PGH$_2$ was more active when given by the intravenous route. The enhanced hypotensive action of PGH$_2$ when given by the intravenous route could result from a combined action on the pulmonary circulation and the systemic circulation. If pulmonary vasoconstriction were of sufficient degree to restrict blood flow to the left heart and reduce cardiac output, the added effect of reduced systemic blood flow plus decreased total peripheral resistance would produce a greater depressor response.

In the canine circulation, PGH$_2$ produces a systemic depressor response [77]. In five animals, a 2-µg/kg dose of PGH$_2$ administered into a lobar artery reduced the mean aortic pressure from 106 to 86 mm Hg. The variability of arterial blood pressure responses to PGG$_2$ and PGH$_2$

observed in different species is difficult to reconcile. Several factors could contribute to the complex nature of the blood pressure responses. First, there may be differences in the sensitivity of the pulmonary and systemic vasculature to the naturally occurring endoperoxides in different species of animals. Second, the ability to convert PGG_2 and PGH_2 into vasoactive metabolites may vary from one species to another. Third, the rapidity with which PGG_2 and PGH_2 are converted into other active products and the route by which the substances are administered could bear on whether a vasoconstrictor or a vasodilator response is produced. Finally, the degree of vessel tone appears to influence the type of response produced by the endoperoxides. Employing direct microscopic visualization of arterioles in the hamster cheek pouch preparation, Lewis and his colleagues [92] reported that direct application of PGG_2 on arterioles having low vascular tone produced a brief vasoconstriction that reached a maximum between 30 and 60 seconds. When high tone in the arterioles was induced by continuous superfusion of norepinephrine, PGG_2 produced a small vasoconstriction followed by protracted vasodilatation.

Synthetic Analogues. All three of the endoperoxide analogues are predominantly systemic pressor agents in the dog [130]. This systemic pressor response is primarily the result of systemic vasoconstriction and is consistent with the ability of these compounds to contract strips of rabbit aorta [99] and helical strips of canine saphenous vein [57].

The epoxymethano analogues appear to be twice as potent systemic pressor agents as the azo analogue. Typically the arterial blood pressure response to intravenous administration of any of the analogues is a transient initial decrease in pressure followed by a sustained elevation that lasts 5–10 minutes. When systemic arterial pressure was recorded simultaneously with pulmonary arterial pressure, the transient decrease in systemic arterial pressure was coincident with the rise to peak pulmonary arterial pressure. This suggested that the intense pulmonary vasoconstriction probably restricted pulmonary venous return to the left heart and consequently reduced left ventricular output.

To determine the direct effects of the endoperoxide analogues on the systemic circulation, studies were performed in dogs during left ventricular bypass [1]. In this preparation, the systemic circulation is perfused with an extracorporeal pump and cardiac effects do not contribute to the changes in arterial blood pressure. The epoxymethano analogues produced an increase in systemic arterial pressure only, without the transient initial decrease in pressure observed in animals with an intact circulation. Therefore, the rise in systemic arterial pressure was due to an increase in systemic vascular resistance alone. These findings are consistent with the interpretation that a reduced cardiac output was responsible for the initial transient decrease in arterial pressure observed in animals with an intact circulation. The observations of Ginzel and his colleagues [56] provide additional supporting evidence for this conclusion. They administered endoperoxide analogues into different segments of the circulation. When administered into the right atrium, the analogues produced the expected initial transient decrease in arterial pressure. This transient decrease in pressure disappeared when the entire or a major portion of the analogues was administered either into the left atrium or by aerosolization, so that the pulmonary circulation was initially bypassed. These studies further suggest that the major site of pulmonary vasoconstriction exists in the precapillary vessels of the lung. A terminal decrease in arterial pressure was not observed in the bypass animals, suggesting that vasodilator substances are not generated from the endoperoxide analogues.

Other investigators [76,77] have also reported that endoperoxide analogues produce a dose-dependent systemic pressor response in the canine circulation. A significant increase in systemic vascular resistance, however, was observed only when the total dose of the PGH_2 analogue was 10 μg or greater.

In the cat, one of the epoxymethano analogues produced mixed systemic arterial pressure responses [63]. The most common response was the characteristic initial drop followed by a moderate rise in systemic arterial pressure. However, in some animals a pure depressor or pressor response was also observed.

REGIONAL CIRCULATION (PULMONARY CIRCULATION)

PGG_2 and PGH_2. In the intact cat intravenous administration of PGH_2 (5 μg) produced a rise in pulmonary artery pressure [63]. In the perfused canine lobar artery a bolus injection of 2 μg of PGH_2 resulted in a moderate but significant increase in lobar arterial pressure [77]. Since flow through the isolated lobe was kept constant, the increase in pulmonary vascular resistance resulted from constriction of both small pulmonary arteries and veins. Neither pretreatment with indomethacin nor substitution of dextran for whole blood in the perfused lobe altered the pulmonary pressor response. PGH_2 also produced marked contractile activity on isolated helical segments of canine intrapulmonary veins.

Synthetic Analogues. All three endoperoxide analogues were markedly vasoconstrictor in the canine pulmonary circulation, when injected intravenously [130]. During left ventricular bypass an intravenous injection of either of the two epoxymethano analogues results in a rapid rise in pulmonary artery pressure [1]. The duration of the pulmonary pressor response was longer than that produced by $PGF_{2\alpha}$, suggesting that degradation of the analogues was a slow process. The endoperoxide analogues were more potent pulmonary vasoconstrictors than $PGF_{2\alpha}$, with an order of potency of approximately 20 : 1. Constriction of both small intrapulmonary arteries and veins was responsible for the increase in pulmonary vascular resistance [76,77]. The effects of the endoperoxide analogues on the pulmonary vasculature were independent of alterations in bronchomotor tone, since similar pressor responses were obtained in ventilated and unventilated lobes.

CORONARY CIRCULATION

PGG$_2$ and PGH$_2$. Both endoperoxides produced an increase in tension of coronary artery strips removed from fresh porcine hearts [37]. The contractile response of the coronary artery strips was characterized by an initial small contraction followed by a slower rise in tension, which required several minutes to reach maximum tension. The PGG$_2$ and PGH$_2$ used in this study were synthesized from sheep seminal vesicular microsomes, and the structures and purity of the endoperoxides were confirmed by mass spectrometry and thin-layer chromatography, respectively.

Svensson and Hamberg [143] have also shown that PGH$_2$ contracts swine coronary artery but found its contractile effects to be two to 10 times less potent than that of thromboxane A$_2$.

Using isolated bovine and pig coronary artery strips, Needleman and his colleagues [116] demonstrated that PGG$_2$ or PGH$_2$ produced dose-dependent relaxation of the bovine coronary artery but contraction of the pig coronary artery. These opposite effects of endoperoxides on coronary artery strips from two different animal species are difficult to interpret. The endoperoxides are rapidly converted into substances that may be responsible for the relaxant effect observed in vascular smooth muscle. In vitro studies support this hypothesis, since the relaxing activity of endoperoxides is blocked with 15-hydroperoxy arachidonic acid, a substance that prevents the formation of prostacyclin, a known coronary vasodilating agent.

Synthetic Analogues. In the cat, U46619 and U44069 have been shown to be potent vasoconstrictors in the isolated perfused coronary circulation [120]. U46619 was more potent as a coronary vasoconstrictor than U44069, and both were significantly more potent as vasoconstrictors than PGH$_2$.

RENAL CIRCULATION

PGG$_2$ and PGH$_2$. No studies have been reported on the effects of PGG$_2$ and PGH$_2$ on the renal vascular bed. Whether endogenously produced endoperoxides play a functional role in regulation of the renal circulation is difficult to assess. The instability of these substances in vivo and their rapid conversion into a variety of active intermediate compounds may alter or mask the direct vascular action of the endoperoxides themselves. Consequently, clear-cut separation of the vascular effects of the endoperoxides from their generated products is nearly impossible.

Synthetic Analogues. Both epoxymethano endoperoxide analogues have been examined for their effects on the canine renal vascular bed [41]. When injected directly into the renal artery, both analogues caused dose-related decreases in renal blood flow. The $11\alpha,9\alpha$-epoxymethano isomer was approximately twice as potent as the $9\alpha,11\alpha$-epoxymethano analogue. No changes in aortic pressure occurred in the range of doses employed. Pretreatment with indomethacin had no influence on the renal blood flow changes induced by the analogues. α-Adrenergic blockage and blockade of angiotensin receptors did not affect the reductions in renal blood flow caused by the analogues. Thus, neither adrenergic nor renin-angiotensin mechanisms contribute to the renal vascular responses.

Although Gerber and his colleagues [53] observed similar renal vascular responses during infusion of a cyclic ether endoperoxide analogue in the dog, they found that the reduction in renal blood flow was potentiated by prior administration of indomethacin. Presumably indomethacin pretreatment inhibited the normal renal production of vasodilator prostaglandins, which would tend to attenuate the vasoconstrictor action of the endoperoxide analogue. However, no direct evidence was offered to support this hypothesis. The decrease in renal blood flow was not associated with a redistribution of intrarenal blood flow.

OTHER REGIONAL CIRCULATIONS

The vascular activity of PGG_2, PGH_2, and the synthetic endoperoxide analogues has been investigated in a number of other vascular beds. Ellis et al. [39] employed a cranial window technique in the cat to observe the responses of the pial arteries to direct application of PGG_2. Local application of PGG_2 induced a sustained dilatation of both the large and small pial arteries. Maximal effects were achieved 2–4 minutes after application. The sustained dilatation of the pial vessels was observed only with PGG_2, not with other prostaglandins tested, but no explanation for this unique property was offered.

Both epoxymethano endoperoxide analogues produce constriction of canine saphenous vein [57]. The potency of these analogues as venoconstrictors is several orders of magnitude greater than that of the primary prostaglandins.

Strips of lamb ductus arteriosus responded in an opposite manner to the naturally occurring endoperoxides and the synthetic endoperoxide analogues. Both PGG_2 and PGH_2 relaxed the ductus arteriosus at a low oxygen pressure [26]. The relaxation process was gradual and reached a plateau in 10–30 minutes. Basal tone was not reestablished in the ductal smooth muscle for a prolonged period. Unlike the natural endoperoxides, the synthetic analogues contracted the hypoxic ductus. These opposing effects again strongly suggest that the relaxant effect of the natural endoperoxides is not a result of their direct action, but probably occurs through their conversion to other compounds.

Prostaglandin D_2

Various prostaglandins are produced by either the spontaneous degradation of the cyclic endoperoxides or their conversion by the respective isomerase and/or reductase enzymes that are present in many tissues [118]. This conversion may occur via the prostaglandin D_2 (PGD_2) pathway rather than that of PGE_2 or $PGF_{2\alpha}$ [96]. Although structurally similar to PGE_2 [61], PGD_2 has a spectrum of activity that is distinct from both PGE_2 and $PGF_{2\alpha}$ [67]. However, little has been reported about the activity of PGD_2 on the circulatory system [96].

PGD_2 was initially considered to be an inert product of endoperoxide inactivation, since it failed to produce a response in either gerbil colon or rabbit aorta preparations and did not alter rat blood pressure [118]. Recently, several other smooth muscle preparations have proved to be highly responsive to PGD_2 [67,75]. Studies have been directed at the effects of exogenous PGD_2 on systemic arterial pressure [3], pulmonary [79], and renal vascular [15] responses.

CARDIAC ACTIONS

The effects of PGD_2 on heart rate and myocardial contractile force are inconsistent. These differences may be due to variations in anesthesia and surgical techniques employed.

PGD_2 increased heart rate in both the anesthetized and unanesthetized dog [153]. Intravenous administration of 10 μg/kg PGD_2 increased left ventricular dp/dt in chloralose-anesthetized dogs. However, these cardiac changes were transient and were considered to be a reflex response to the decreased systemic arterial pressure.

In open-chest dogs, anesthetized with sodium pentobarbital, PGD_2 had no effect on heart rate and decreased myocardial contractile force [3]. This negative inotropic action of PGD_2 persisted after ganglion blockade with hexamethonium chloride and during left ventricular bypass. Thus, in this preparation, the negative inotropic effect of PGD_2 appeared to be a direct effect on the heart, not the result of a reflex response or changes in preload or afterload.

In the isolated guinea pig heart, PGD_2 is a potent coronary constrictor. Concentrations of 10^{-6} M PGD_2 increased coronary vascular resistance sufficiently to decrease the amplitude of ventricular contraction [132]. Thus the negative inotropic response in the dog may be due in part to a decrease in coronary perfusion.

BLOOD PRESSURE EFFECTS

The hemodynamic actions of PGD_2 appear to be species specific [3]. These variations may, however, be due to differences in doses and route of administration [75].

In the nonpregnant ewe, doses as low as 10 ng/kg of PGD_2, administered into the descending aorta, produced an immediate rise in systemic arterial pressure. A similar rise in perfusion pressure was produced when PGD_2 was injected into the isolated hind limbs of these ewes [75]. Pharmacologic blockade of α-adrenergic receptors, sympathetic ganglia, and sympathetic neuroeffector transmitter failed to abolish this response. Thus, PGD_2 appears to directly increase peripheral resistance in the sheep by action on specific prostaglandin receptors in the arterial smooth muscle [75]. Similar results have been reported in the rabbit [67,75] and guinea pig [61].

Pregnancy modifies this pressor response to PGD_2 [96]. Near-term ewes become relatively insensitive to the pressor effects of exogenous PGD_2 [75]. In the pregnant rabbit, PGD_2 has a mild depressor effect [96].

In the dog, PGD_2 is consistently a systemic vasodepressor [3]. In the anesthetized, open-chest dog, a 5 μg/kg intravenous bolus injection of PGD_2 produced a 25% reduction in mean systemic arterial pressure [3]. In the closed-chest dog, the systemic response was somewhat reduced. Doses of 0.1–10 μg/kg produced a 5–20% decrease in blood pressure [153]. When infused intravenously at a rate of 1.0 μg/kg/min in the conscious instrumented dog, PGD_2 produced a 12% reduction in systemic arterial pressure. This depressor action of PGD_2 appears to be due to a direct vasodilating action on the peripheral vasculature [3], since PGD_2 (5 μg/kg) produced a 14% decrease in blood pressure during left ventricular bypass.

Some species are unresponsive to PGD_2. In the conscious baboon doses of 1 and 5 μg/kg had no effect on mean systemic arterial pressure [46].

REGIONAL CIRCULATIONS

Pulmonary Circulation. PGD_2 consistently produces an increase in pulmonary arterial pressure [79]. Constriction of intrapulmonary veins and the precapillary segments of the pulmonary vasculature are thought to be responsible for these changes in vascular resistance [141].

In the intact pentobarbital-anesthetized dog, doses of 3 and 10 μg produce increases in pulmonary vascular resistance of 47% and 91%, respectively [79]. In the closed-chest dog increases in pulmonary arterial pressure of 8–28% were produced by intravenous doses of 0.1–10 μg/kg. When PGD_2 was infused at the rate of 1.0 μg/kg/min in the unanesthetized dog there was a 30% increase in pulmonary arterial pressure [153]. Pulmonary constriction was even more pronounced in the open-chest dog. An intravenous dose of 5 μg/kg produced between a 65% and 70% increase in mean pulmonary arterial pressure in two separate studies [3,45].

Renal Circulation. In the kidney, PGD_2 is produced in substantial quantities when arachidonic acid is incubated with rat medulla [83], rabbit renal papilla [96], or dog kidney [41]. If significant amounts of PGD_2 are also produced in vivo, there may be a physiologic role for this prostaglandin in the kidney.

Dilatation of the renal vasculature and an increase in renal blood flow occurred during infusion of PGD_2 in the dog [15,41,50] and rabbit [96]. At low doses renal blood flow was enhanced in both inner and outer cortical regions [15,50]. However, higher concentrations produced a shift in the blood flow distribution toward the juxtamedullary nephrons [50].

Bolger et al. [15] suggested that PGD_2 is primarily involved in the control of renal hemodynamics only, since no changes in diuresis or natriuresis were observed in their study. On the other hand, Friesinger et al. [50] have obtained dose-related effects of PGD_2 on water and electrolyte excretion as well as changes in hemodynamic parameters. Explanation for this discrepancy is unclear, since the two preparations were very similar.

Uteroplacental Circulation. $PGF_{2\alpha}$ was once considered to be the chief product of arachidonic acid metabolism in the uterus. However, a study published in 1978 indicated that both PGD_2 and PGE_2 are also produced by uterine tissue, with PGD_2 actually being the major product [83].

When infused into the left ventricle of the near-term rabbit at a rate of 10 μg/kg/min the uterine vasculature dilated while the placental vasculature strongly constricted [96]. PGD_2 levels have not been assayed during the various stages of pregnancy and labor. However, if those concentrations correlated to the natural occurring events, endogenous PGD_2 may be a partial determinant of the normal uteroplacental blood flow in the pregnant animal.

Thromboxane A_2

Some platelet and vascular effects of the prostaglandin endoperoxides are thought to be due to their conversion to other active metabolic products [84]. Incubation of either arachidonic acid or PGH_2 with washed platelets leads to the formation of thromboxane A_2 [62], a very labile bicyclic compound with a biological half-life of about 30 seconds [144]. This compound induces irreversible platelet aggregation, releases serotonin from platelets [62], and is a significantly more potent contractor of rabbit aorta strips than the endoperoxide intermediates [115]. Thromboxane A_2 appears to be the major component of the previously described rabbit aorta constrictor substance [62] that is released from isolated guinea pig lungs during anaphylaxis or in the presence of other noxious stimuli [123].

Initially only platelets were considered to be capable of transforming endoperoxides into thromboxane A_2. However, lung tissue, spleen, kidney, leukocytes, umbilical arteries, brain, and carrageenan-induced granuloma have been demonstrated to contain sufficient isomerase enzyme to complete this conversion [131]. Because of the extreme instability of thromboxane A_2, indirect methods such as smooth muscle bioassay [64] and measurement of thromboxane B_2, a more stable metabolic product [131], are used to assess the relative quantities and effects of thromboxane A_2.

Thromboxane A_2 is generated experimentally by incubating arachidonic acid with a suspension of either human [114] or horse [21] platelets for 30 seconds at 37°C. The mixture is rapidly filtered and immediately added to the test organ [144]. Since this mixture contains other platelet products including ADP and its breakdown products [142], the biologic action of this filtrate must be viewed with a certain amount of caution.

CARDIAC ACTIONS

No specific studies of the cardiac action of thromboxane A_2 have been reported. This is due primarily to the instability of this compound.

BLOOD PRESSURE EFFECTS

Rabbit-aorta-constricting substance had been shown to contract all vascular tissues tested [115]. Likewise, thromboxane A_2 contracts rabbit aorta, human umbilical arteries [144], and swine coronary arteries [143]. Thromboxane A_2 also strongly contracts rabbit coeliac and mesenteric arteries, whereas the endoperoxides induce a prolonged relaxation that may be preceded by a contraction of short duration [21]. Thus, these vessels may be used as a bioassay to differentiate thromboxane A_2 from the endoperoxides. Thromboxane A_2 is a potent systemic pressor agent when administered intravenously to guinea pigs [144]. However, its major function appears to be that of a local vasoconstrictor in isolated vascular beds that have been in some way compromised [114].

REGIONAL CIRCULATION

Coronary Circulation. Thromboxane A_2 is the most potent coronary constrictor among the naturally occurring compounds studied thus far [120]. It ranges from 10 to 30 times more potent than endoperoxides, PGE_2, or $PGF_{2\alpha}$ in constricting isolated bovine [31], porcine [37,143], and feline [120] coronary arteries.

The synthesis of thromboxane A_2 has not been demonstrated in normal coronary arteries [126]. Therefore, thromboxane A_2 is probably not involved in the regulation of coronary vascular tone. However, any event that promotes platelet deposition might be accompanied by thromboxane A_2 synthesis, which would further enhance platelet aggregation and local vasospasm [112]. It is conceivable, therefore, that thromboxane A_2 may participate in the response to myocardial ischemia.

The thromboxane A_2 that is synthesized by human platelet microsomes contracts coronary vascular smooth muscle [37]. When injected into the left circumflex artery of 1–3-month-old puppies, thromboxane A_2 induced a decrease in coronary blood flow that is accompanied by increased platelet aggregation in the area perfused by that artery [151]. Thromboxane A_2 also produced a dose-dependent decrease in coronary artery blood flow in isolated guinea pig hearts [147]. Decreased left ventricular systolic pressure and left ventricular dp/dt were proportional to the decrease in coronary blood flow. Since thromboxane A_2 does not affect the contractile force of isolated papillary muscles, these changes appear to be due to variations in coronary blood flow [147]. When injected into the coronary arteries of rabbits, thromboxane A_2 (1.0 μg) induced acute myocardial ischemia as demonstrated by serial electrocardiographic and histologic changes [108]. Ellis et al. [37] hypothesized that platelet aggregation in areas of damaged endothelium results in release of thromboxane A_2, which caused constriction of the larger coronary arteries.

Renal Circulation. Thromboxane A_2 constricts the renal vasculature [110] and may play an important role in the regulation of renal vascular resistance and blood flow distribution within the kidney [109].

For example, chronic unilateral ureteral obstruction is characterized by an initial vasodilatory phase that is followed by a progressive fall in renal blood flow [107]. A potent vasoconstrictor substance of renal origin might explain such a phenomenon. Morrison et al. [110] have demonstrated that an isolated rabbit kidney with an obstructed ureter releases vasoactive substance following intraarterial infusions of either bradykinin, angiotensin II, arachidonic acid, or ATP. This compound contracts the rabbit aorta and has a short half-life (37 seconds). The ability of imidazole, a thromboxane synthetase inhibitor, to block the production of this substance suggests that it is thromboxane A_2.

PGE_2 is the primary product formed by incubating cortical and medullary microsomes with arachidonic acid in both the obstructed and unobstructed kidney. However, thromboxane B_2 is also found in microsomal preparations of the obstructed kidney. Thus, ureteral obstruction appears to alter the biosynthetic capabilities of the kidney. Increased thromboxane A_2 production in this situation may play an important role in diminishing total renal blood flow to the nonfunctioning kidney. In vivo studies are needed to clarify the significance of these findings.

Cerebral Circulation. Thromboxane A_2 appears to be the preferential product of arachidonic acid metabolism in brain tissue. Guinea pig and rat cerebral cortex produce five to six times more thromboxane B_2 than either PGE_2 or $PGF_{2\alpha}$ [162]. Thromboxane A_2 is also a potent contractor of cerebral artery strips. Bovine cerebral artery strips were three times more responsive to platelet-generated thromboxane A_2 than coronary arteries from the same animals [38]. Ellis et al. [38] have hypothesized that damage to cerebral endothelial cells, due to either trauma or platelet aggregation, will lead to an increased production of thromboxane A_2 and subsequent constriction of the associated cerebral arteries.

Thromboxane B_2

Thromboxane B_2, previously designated as PHD [62], was considered to be a stable, biologically inert product of thromboxane A_2 metabolism [84]. However, subsequent studies have shown that thromboxane B_2

increases airway pressure [49,152], constricts the pulmonary vasculature [49,78], and elevates systemic arterial pressure [49]. In light of the relative stability of thromboxane B_2, this compound may be responsible for at least a portion of the vascular smooth muscle action of thromboxane A_2.

CARDIAC ACTIONS

Although no specific studies of the cardiac actions of thromboxane B_2 have been reported, in the dog myocardial contractile force decreased by 11% following a 25-μg/kg dose of thromboxane B_2 [49]. Reasons for this change have not been investigated.

BLOOD PRESSURE EFFECTS

Thromboxane B_2 is active on the systemic vasculature [49]. It produces a moderate elevation of systemic arterial pressure. Intraarterial administration of 25 μg/kg produced a consistent elevation of systemic arterial pressure (10%). However, the effects on the systemic vasculature were inconsistent when thromboxane B_2 was administered intravenously.

REGIONAL CIRCULATION (PULMONARY CIRCULATION)

Thromboxane B_2 is less effective than $PGF_{2\alpha}$ in altering canine pulmonary mechanical function when administered either intravenously or by aerosol [152]. Airway pressure increases to a greater degree following intravenous than intraarterial administration of thromboxane B_2 [49]. This response is somewhat paradoxical, since bronchial smooth muscle is predominantly supplied by the systemic circulation. However, a substance such as thromboxane B_2, which causes acute elevations of pulmonary pressure when injected intravenously, may have direct access to bronchial smooth muscle via blood flow through bronchopulmonary anastomoses [85].

When injected directly into the pulmonary artery of the cat or dog in concentrations up to 3 μg/kg, thromboxane B_2 increased lobar arterial pressure in a dose-dependent manner up to 60% but had no effect on left atrial pressure [78]. In the intact dog high doses of thromboxane B_2 (25–50 μg/kg), administered either intravenously or intraarterially, also produced significant increases in pulmonary arterial pressure [49]. These responses are most likely due to constriction of intrapulmonary veins and upstream vessels [78].

Tachyphylaxis to thromboxane B_2 occurs in both the bronchial and the pulmonary vasculature. This may indicate saturation of binding sites, depletion of the catabolic enzymes in the lung, or generation of specific antagonists.

Prostacyclin

Prostacyclin is an unstable product of arachidonic acid metabolism that relaxes arterial smooth muscle strips and is the most potent inhibitor of platelet aggregation described thus far [35]. It appears to be the major product of arachidonic acid metabolism in all vascular beds. Microsomal enzymes in the vascular endothelial wall [104] convert prostaglandin endoperoxides PGG_2 and PGH_2 into prostacyclin. This enzyme conversion may be inhibited in vitro by 15-hydroperoxy arachidonic acid [20]. Prostacyclin is degraded nonenzymatically to a more stable product, 6-keto-$PGF_{1\alpha}$, which has been identified as the principal metabolite when coronary arteries are incubated with arachidonic acid [126].

CARDIAC ACTIONS

Instead of the reflex tachycardia that normally accompanies sudden decreases in systemic arterial pressure, prostacyclin produces a paradoxical bradycardia when administered by either intravenous or intracoronary injection [25,66]. A cardiac chemoreceptor reflex appears to be responsible for this decreased heart rate [25], since vagotomy reverses the bradycardia and intraarterial administration of prostacyclin produces the expected tachycardia [66]. Prostacyclin may also possess antiarrhythmic properties. It effectively counteracts aconitine-induced arrhythmias, although not to the same extent as PGE_2 or $PGF_{2\alpha}$ [102].

The inotropic actions of prostacyclin are less clearly defined. The isolated rabbit heart is unaffected by prostacyclin [82]. However, low concentrations of prostacyclin increase the contractile force of the isolated rat heart and higher concentrations decrease myocardial contractile force [82]. A similar dose-dependent relationship has been demonstrated in the intact dog [45]. These changes were eliminated when the left ventricle was bypassed, suggesting that in the intact circulation the changes in contractile force are due in part to variations in preload and/or afterload.

BLOOD PRESSURE EFFECTS

Prostacyclin produces a dose-dependent decrease in systemic arterial pressure when administered intravenously in rats, rabbits, dogs, and monkeys [6,8,47,133,155]. In one human study [145], comparable vasodepressor responses were produced when prostacyclin was administered intravenously or inhaled as an aerosol. Women appeared to be more sensitive to the depressor actions of prostacyclin than men.

The vasodepressor action of prostacyclin is due primarily to arteriolar vasodilatation of most peripheral vascular beds [7] and closely resembles the vascular response to arachidonic acid [45]. The vasodepressor response was significantly attenuated in dogs when the vagi were cut [66] or the heart was paced [25]. Therefore, part of the systemic depressor response to prostacyclin may be due to a reduction in cardiac output secondary to a decreased heart rate [66].

The magnitude of this systemic hypotensive response is similar whether prostacyclin is administered intravenously or intraarterially [7,122,150]. Thus, prostacyclin, unlike other prostaglandins [42], is not degraded during passage through the lungs [7,122,150,158]. When administered intravenously, prostacyclin is twice as potent as PGE_2 in the rabbit [8], approximately four to eight times more potent in the rat, and about 10 times more potent in the dog [45]. However, when administered into the ascending aorta, both PGE_1 and PGE_2 are slightly more potent than prostacyclin [6,54].

Arterial plasma concentrations of prostacyclin are higher than venous concentrations [105]. This difference may be due to either the release of prostacyclin from the pulmonary vasculature [60] or the more efficient production of prostacyclin by arteries than by veins [136,140].

It has been suggested that prostacyclin may be a circulating hormone [105] that participates in the regulation of vascular tone [122] and blood pressure [32]. Deficiencies in prostacyclin production and/or alterations in the responsiveness of the circulatory system to this substance may contribute to various cardiovascular disease states. For example, increased vascular tone and augmented vessel responsiveness to stimuli that are associated with hypertension might represent a deficiency of prostacyclin. Markov [100] demonstrated decreased prostacyclin biosynthesis in the lungs, hearts, and aortas of spontaneously hypertensive rats. On the other hand, Pace-Asciak et al. [122] have shown that spontaneously hypertensive rats have an increased capability to produce a prostacyclinlike compound. These hypertensive rats were also more responsive to exogenous prostacyclin. This has been interpreted as an adaptive response to increased catecholamine production characteristic of hypersensitive animals.

REGIONAL CIRCULATIONS

Pulmonary Circulation. Prostacyclin is the only product of arachidonic acid metabolism that produces a pulmonary vasodepressor response [7,35]. Prostacyclin produces a dose-dependent decrease in pulmonary vascular resistance in the dog [80], cat [68,69], monkey [68], and sheep [7]. However, it was found that pulmonary arterial pressures in humans [145] and in rhesus monkeys [47] were not affected by intravenous administration of prostacyclin. When arachidonic acid is infused intravenously in dogs, there is an increase in pulmonary production of prostacyclin [34] that is coincident with the decrease in pulmonary arterial pressure [35]. The magnitude of this pulmonary depressor response to prostacyclin depends in part on the resting tone of the vasculature. If pulmonary vascular resistance is increased by infusing a pulmonary vasoconstrictor such as an endoperoxide analogue (U-46619), the response to prostacyclin is augmented [68,69]. This may explain the lack of pulmonary vascular response to prostacyclin as reported in some earlier studies [47,145].

Cyclooxygenase synthetase inhibitors potentiate the pulmonary hypertension produced by hypoxia [35]. Therefore a vasodilator prostaglandin may be generated that partially offsets the expected increase in pulmonary pressure. Prostacyclin, which is the only known metabolite of arachidonic acid that decreases pulmonary arterial pressure [80], may be the active substance that maintains low pulmonary vascular resistance in both resting and stressed states.

Coronary Circulation. Prostacyclinlike substances are released into the coronary circulation following a wide variety of stimuli including hypoxia, nerve stimulation, and the administration of various humoral agents [31]. Inhibition of prostaglandin synthesis by the use of nonsteroidal antiinflammatory drugs causes an increase in coronary vascular tone [45]. Therefore, it has been proposed that prostaglandins participate in the regulation of coronary blood flow [31].

Administration of arachidonic acid into the coronary circulation of the dog causes vasodilatation [65] and decreased resistance in that vascular bed [113]. PGE_2, which was initially considered to be the active vasodilator metabolite of arachidonic acid [35], is not a potent vasodilator in the coronary circulation [113]. Therefore, arachidonic acid must be converted to some other vasodilating substance by coronary vessels [81]. Prostacyclin is the main prostaglandin released from isolated rat, rabbit, and guinea pig hearts [133] and invariably relaxes coronary artery strips [35]. Pretreatment of these hearts with 15-hydroperoxy arachidonic acid, a specific antagonist of prostacyclin synthetase [20], blocks the relaxation of bovine coronary artery strips induced by arachidonic acid. This relaxation of bovine coronary artery appears to be due predominantly to the intramural conversion of the endoperoxide intermediates to prostacyclin [35]. Therefore, prostacyclin may be the arachidonic acid metabolite that regulates local coronary vessel tone.

In isolated rabbit and guinea pig hearts, prostacyclin produced a significant decrease in coronary perfusion pressure [93,134], and a slight decrease in myocardial contractile force [93] with no consistent change in heart rate. In the intact rabbit heart prostacyclin can be produced from arachidonic acid, but not from the natural endoperoxide PGH_2. If, however, these endothelial linings are damaged, bolus injections of PGH_2 produce a decrease in perfusion pressure [117]. It appears that the endoperoxides are unable to penetrate the intact endothelial lining as a viable substrate to the site of prostacyclin synthesis, but the more soluble arachidonic acid can [139]. Thus coronary endothelial cells can produce prostacyclin directly from arachidonic acid [51] and need not rely on the endoperoxide produced by circulating platelets.

When infused at 0.5 mmole/kg/min for 5 hours in the cat, prostacyclin reduced myocardial oxygen demands, prevented lysosomal disruption, maintained the integrity of the myocardium, and inhibited the platelet aggregation that normally accompanies myocardial ischemic episodes [121]. Likewise, intracoronary administration of prostacyclin (1–10 μg) prevented total blockage of dog coronary arteries that were partially obstructed with platelet thrombi [2]. It has been proposed that atherosclerotic plaque contains certain hydroperoxy fatty acids that are known to inhibit prostacyclin synthesis [20]. Thus, the affected vessels would produce less prostacyclin and would become more susceptible to platelet aggregation and subsequent myocardial damage due to ischemia [29].

Splanchnic Circulation. The splanchnic vasculature is particularly sensitive to the vasodepressor metabolites of arachidonic acid [35]. Spiral strips of rabbit mesenteric and coeliac arteries relax in response to the natural endoperoxides [21]. Intravenous administration of higher concentrations of arachidonic acid and PGH_2 produce a biphasic response characterized by an initial transient decrease in mesenteric flow, followed by a longer lasting increase in flow [44,124]. In the unanesthetized dog, prostacyclin decreases resistance in all abdominal vascular beds except the pancreas. When treated with 15-hydroperoxy arachidonic acid isolated mesenteric arteries no longer synthesize prostacyclin and contract in response to the endoperoxides [35]. Prostacyclin is produced in significant quantities in the gastric mucosa [106] and increases gastric blood flow when administered into the superior mesenteric artery [23,55]. Thus, the initial decreased mesenteric flow is most likely due to the formation of endoperoxides, whereas the longer lasting decrease in mesenteric resistance is due to the intramural transformation of the endoperoxides into prostacyclin [106].

Renal Circulation. Prostaglandins may contribute to the regulation of renal blood flow, renin release, and salt and water excretion [137] through modification of renal hemodynamics [94]. Inhibition of prostaglandin synthetase results in increased renal vascular resistance [12] and decreased renal blood flow [148], with a shift in flow distribution to the outer cortex [12]. Administration of indomethacin also produces a decrease in plasma renin activity [51]. The prostaglandin synthetase complex is associated with different cellular elements, each capable of generating different prostanoic products [95].

PGE_2 is produced by the kidney [9,82,117,157], particularly by renal medullary microsomes [159], and was originally proposed as the principal intermediary of the renal prostaglandin system [10]. Exogenously administered PGE_2 dilates the renal vasculature of all species tested except the rat [9,10], in which it constricts the renal artery. Physiologically, PGE_2 may diffuse from the medullary interstitial cells into the blood and tubular fluid, affecting medullary blood flow and the transport of salt and water [94]. However, it seems highly unlikely that PGE_2 would affect the hemodynamic events taking place in the cortex [35].

Prostacyclin is the principal product of arachidonic acid metabolism [20,163] in the renal vasculature [9,20,163]. Interlobular and afferent arterioles have a high capacity to convert arachidonic acid to prostacyclin [149]. In addition, prostacyclin is the principal metabolite of PGH_2 in human and rabbit cortical microsomes [16,159]. Prostacyclin is a renal vasodilator in all species, including the rat [9,10], and can therefore be considered to be a potential inhibitor of renal vascular action of pressor hormones in all species [95].

The prostaglandin system also participates in the release of renin that results from renal artery hypotension [119]. Arachidonic acid evokes renin release. In addition, indomethacin blocks the increased renin production that normally accompanies clamping of the renal artery [119]. Unlike PGE_2, prostacyclin stimulates renin secretion in rabbit renal cortical slices [154,159]. In the dog at concentrations that do not affect systemic arterial pressure, prostacyclin significantly increases renin production [135]. Since prostacyclin is produced in the renal cortex and is capable of stimulating release of renin in both the intact kidney [135] and renal cortical slices [159], it is probably the cyclooxygenase metabolite of arachidonic acid that affects renin production [119].

CONCLUSION

We have reviewed present knowledge of the cardiovascular actions of the prostaglandin precursors and selected prostanoic derivatives that appear to be of biologic significance. The precursors themselves do not induce significant alterations in cardiac function or vascular dynamics. However, compounds that are derived from the precursors of the monoenoic and bisenoic prostaglandins are extremely active in the circulation and often have opposing actions. The majority of the intermediate compounds derived from the precursors are very labile substances because they are rapidly biotransformed into other active compounds or inactive end products. Consequently the cardiovascular responses are brief and often complex. In some instances the extremely short half-life of a substance precludes adequate characterization of its specific effects on the circulation. Analogues of some intermediates, such as the endoperoxides, have been synthesized. Although these stable synthetic compounds provide an opportunity for assessing their biologic actions on the circulation, their behavior is not identical to that of the naturally occurring compounds. A more precise analysis of the cardiovascular effects of each compound in the arachidonic acid pathway may result from the recent development of specific prostaglandin antagonists and the synthesis of enzyme inhibitors for the various steps in the arachidonic acid cascade. Further studies will be required to delineate the roles of these substances in the physiologic regulation of the circulation and their possible implications in pathophysiologic states.

REFERENCES

1. Alter, I., Kot, P. A., Ramwell, P. W., Rose, J. C. , and Shnider, M. R. (1977) Circulatory effects of prostaglandin endoperoxide analogues studied in the dog during left ventricular bypass. Br. J. Pharmacol. 61, 395–398.
2. Aiken, J. W., and Shebuski, R. J. (1979) Relative effectiveness of locally produced versus circulating prostacyclin (PGI$_2$) in preventing blockage of partially obstructed dog coronary arteries with platelet thrombi, Fed. Proc. 38, 419.
3. Angerio, A. D., Ramwell, P. W., Kot, P. A., and Rose, J. C. (1977) Cardiovascular responses to PGD$_2$ in the dog. Proc. Soc. Exp. Biol. Med. 156, 393–395.
4. Änggård, E., and Larsson, C. (1974) Stimulation and inhibition of prostaglandin biosynthesis: Opposite effects on blood pressure and intrarenal blood flow distribution. In: H. J. Robinson and J. R. Vane (eds.), Prostaglandin Synthetase Inhibitors, Raven Press, New York, pp. 311–316.
5. Armstrong, M., Boura, A. L. A., Hamberg, M., and Samuelsson, B. (1976) A comparison of the vasodepressor effects of the cyclic endoperoxides PGG$_2$ and PGH$_2$ with those of PGD$_2$ and PGE$_2$ in hypertensive and normotensive rats. Eur. J. Pharmacol. 39, 251–258.
6. Armstrong, J. M., Chapple, D., Dusting, G. J., Hughes, R., Moncada, S., and Vane,

J. R. (1977) Cardiovascular actions of prostacyclin (PGI$_2$) in chloralose anesthetized dogs. Br. J. Pharmacol. 61, 136P.

7. Armstrong, J. M., Dusting, G. J., Moncada, S., and Vane, J. R. (1978) Cardiovascular actions of PGI$_2$, a metabolite of AA which is synthesized by blood vessels. Circ. Res. 43 (Suppl.), I112–I119.

8. Armstrong, J. M., Lattimer, N., Moncada, S., and Vane, J. R. (1978) Comparison of the vasodepressor effects of prostacyclin and 6-oxa prostaglandin F$_{1\alpha}$ with those of prostaglandin E$_2$ in rats and rabbits. Br. J. Pharmacol. 62, 125–130.

9. Baer, P. G., and McGiff, J. R. (1979) Comparison of effects of prostaglandin E$_2$ and I$_2$ on rat renal vascular resistance. Eur. J. Pharmacol. 54, 359–363.

10. Baer, P. G., Kauker, M. L., and McGiff, J. R. (1979) Prostacyclin effects on renal hemodynamic and excretory function in the rat. J. Pharmacol. Exp. Ther. 208, 294–297.

11. Belford, J. (1970) Cardiotonic activity of arachidonic acid and other fatty acids. Fed. Proc. 29, 745.

12. Beilin, L. J., and Bhattacharya, J. (1977) The effect of prostaglandin synthesis inhibitors on renal blood flow distribution in conscious rabbits. J. Physiol. 269, 395–405.

13. Bergström, S., Carlson, L. A., and Weeks, J. R. (1968) The prostaglandins: A family of biologically active lipids. Pharmacol. Rev. 20, 1–48.

14. Bolger, P. M., Eisner, G. M., Ramwell, P. W., and Slotkoff, L. M. (1976) Effect of prostaglandin synthesis on renal function and renin in the dog. Nature (London) 259, 244–245.

15. Bolger, P. M., Eisner, G. M., Shea, P. T., Ramwell, P. W., and Slotkoff, L. M. (1977) Effects of PGD$_2$ on canine renal function. Nature (London) 267, 628–630.

16. Bolger, P. M. Eisner, G. M., Ramwell, P. W., Slotkoff, L. M., and Corey, E. J. (1978) Renal actions of prostacyclin. Nature (London) 271, 467–469.

17. Borbola, J., Susskand, K. Siess, M., and Szekeres, L. (1977) The effects of arachidonic acid in isolated atria of guinea pigs. Eur. J. Pharmacol. 41, 27–36.

18. Bridenbaugh, G. A., Flynn, J. T., and Lefer, A. M. (1976) Arachidonic acid in splanchnic artery occulsion shock. Am. J. Physiol. 231, 112–118.

19. Bundy, G. L. (1975) The synthesis of prostaglandin endoperoxide analogs, Tetrahedron Let. 24, 1957–1960.

20. Bunting, S., Gryglewski, R. M., Moncada, S., and Vane, J. R. (1976) Arterial walls generate from prostaglandin endoperoxides a substance (prostaglandin X) which relaxes strips of mesenteric and coeliac arteries and inhibits platelet aggregation. Prostaglandins 12, 897–913.

21. Bunting, S., Moncada, S., and Vane, J. R. (1976) The effects of prostaglandin endoperoxides and thromboxane A$_2$ on strips of rabbit coeliac artery and certain other smooth muscle preparations. Br. J. Pharmacol. 57, 462P–463P.

22. Chang, L. C. T., Spławiński, J. A., Oates, J. A., and Nies, A. S. (1975) Enhanced renal prostaglandin production in the dog. II. Effects on intrarenal hemodynamics. Circ. Res. 36, 204–207.

23. Chapnick, B. M., Feigen, L. P., Hyman, A. L., and Kadowitz, P. J. (1978) Vasodilator effects of prostacyclin in canine intestine. Fed. Proc. 37, 732.

24. Chapnick, B. M., Feigen, L. P., Hyman, A. L., and Kadowitz, P. J. (1978) Differential effects of prostaglandins in the mesenteric vascular bed. Am. J. Physiol. 235, H326–H332.

25. Chapple, D. J., Dusting, G. J., Hughes, R., and Vane, J. R. (1978) A vagal reflex contributes to the hypotensive effect of prostacyclin in anesthetized dogs. J. Physiol. 281, 43P–44P.

26. Coceani, F., Bishai, I., White, E., Bodach, E., and Olley, P. M. (1978) Action of prostaglandins, endoperoxides and thromboxanes on the lamb ductus arteriosus. Am. J. Physiol. 234, H117–H112.

27. Cohen, M., Sztokalo, J., and Hinsch, E. (1973) The antihypertensive action of arach-

idonic acid in the spontaneous hypertensive rat and its antagonism by anti-inflammatory agents. Life Sci. 13, 317–325.

28. Corey, E. J., Nicolaou, K. C., Machida, Y., Malmsten, C. L., and Samuelsson, B. (1975) Synthesis and biological properties of a 9,11-azo-prostanoid: Highly active biochemical mimic of prostaglandin endoperoxides. Proc. Natl. Acad. Sci. US 72, 3355–3358.

29. Dembińska-Kieć, A., Gryglewska, T., Zmuda, A., and Gryglewski, R. J. (1977) The generation of prostacyclin by arteries and by the coronary vascular bed is reduced in experimental atherosclerosis in rabbits. Prostaglandins 14, 1025–1034.

30. Dusting, G. J., Lattimer, N., Moncada, S., and Vane, J. R. (1977) Prostaglandin X, the vascular metabolite of arachidonic acid responsible for relaxation of bovine coronary artery strips. Br. J. Pharmacol. 59, 443P.

31. Dusting, G. J., Moncada, S., and Vane, J. R. (1977) Prostacyclin (PGX) is the endogenous metabolite responsible for relaxation of coronary arteries induced by arachidonic acid. Prostaglandins 13, 3–15.

32. Dusting, G. J., Moncada, S. Mullane, K. M., and Vane, J. R. (1978) Implications of prostacyclin generation for modulation of vascular tone. Clin. Sci. Mol. Med. 55, S195–S198.

33. Dusting, G. J., Moncada, S., and Vane, J. R. (1978) Vascular actions of arachidonic acid and its metabolites in perfused mesenteric and femoral beds of the dog. Eur. J. Pharmacol. 49, 65–72.

34. Dusting, G. J., Moncada, S., Mullane, K. M., and Vane, J. R. (1978) Biotransformation of arachidonic acid in the circulation of the dog. Br. J. Pharmacol. 63, 359P.

35. Dusting, G. J., Moncada, S., and Vane, J. R. (1979) Prostaglandins, their intermediates and precursors: Cardiovascular actions and regulatory role in normal and abnormal circulatory systems. Prog. Cardiovasc. Dis. 21, 405–430.

36. Dyerberg, J., Bang, H. O., Stoffersen, E., Moncada, S., and Vane, J. R. (1978) Eicosapentaenoic acid and prevention of thrombosis and atherosclerosis. Lancet 2 (8081), 117–119.

37. Ellis, E. F., Oelz, O., Roberts, L. J., Payne, N. A., Sweetman B. J., Nies, A. S., and Oates, J. A. (1976) Coronary arterial smooth muscle contraction by a substance released from platelets: Evidence that it is thromboxane A_2. Science 193, 1135–1137.

38. Ellis, E. F., Nies, A. S., and Oates, J. A. (1977) Cerebral arterial smooth muscle contraction by thromboxane A_2. Stroke 8, 480–483.

39. Ellis, E. F., Wei, E. P., and Kontos, H. A. (1979) Vasodilatation of cat cerebral arterioles by prostaglandins D_2, E_2, G_2 and I_2. Am. J. Physiol. 237, H381–H385.

40. Von Euler, U. S. (1937) On the specific vasodilating and plain muscle stimulating substances from accessory genital glands in man and certain animals (prostaglandin and vesiglandin). J. Physiol. 88, 213–234.

41. Feigen, L. P., Chapnick, B. M., Flemming, J. E., and Kadowitz, P. J. (1977) Renal vascular effects of endoperoxide analogs, prostaglandins, and arachidonic acid. Am. J. Physiol. 233, H573–H579.

42. Ferreira, S. H., and Vane, J. R. (1967) Prostaglandins: Their disappearance from and release into the circulation. Nature (London) 216, 868–873.

43. Fitzpatrick, T. M., Johnson, M., Kot, P. A., Ramwell, P. W., and Rose, J. C. (1977) Vasoconstrictor response to arachidonic acid in the isolated hind limb of the dog. Br. J. Pharmacol. 59, 269–273.

44. Fitzpatrick, T. M., Ramwell, P. W., Kot, P. A., and Rose, J. C. (1977) Effects of arachidonic acid on regional blood flow distribution in the intact dog. Fed. Proc. 36, 624.

45. Fitzpatrick, T.M., Alter, I., Corey, E. J., Ramwell, P. W., Rose, J. C., and Kot, P. A. (1978) Cardiovascular responses to PGI_2 (prostacyclin) in the dog. Circ. Res. 42, 192–194.

46. Fletcher, J. R., and Ramwell, P. W. (1977) Hemodynamic responses to PGD_2 in the awake baboon. Clin. Res. 25, 270A.

47. Fletcher, J. R., Corey, E. J., Saba, J. L., and Ramwell, P. W. (1977) Prostacyclin, a potent vasodepressor in primates. Prostaglandins 14, 1024.

48. Forster, W., Mentz, P., Blass, K. E., and Mest, H. J. (1976) Antiarrhythmic effects of arachidonic, linoleic, linolenic and oleic acid, and the influence of indomethacin and polyphloretin phosphate. In: B. Samuelsson and R. Paoletti (eds.), Advances in Prostaglandin and Thromboxane Research, Vol. 1, Raven Press, New York, pp. 433–438.

49. Friedman, L. S., Fitzpatrick, T. M., Bloom, M. F., Ramwell, P. W., Rose, J. C., and Kot, P. A. (1979) Cardiovascular and pulmonary effects of thromboxane B_2 in the dog. Circ. Res. 44, 748–751.

50. Friesinger, G. C., Oelz, O., Sweetman, B. J., Nies, A. S., and Data, J. L. (1978) Prostaglandin D_2, another renal prostaglandin? Prostaglandins 15, 969–981.

51. Frölich, J. C., Hollifield, J. W., Dormois, J. C., Frölich, B. L., Seyberth, H., Michelakis, A. M., and Oates, J. A. (1976) Suppression of plasma renin activity by indomethacin in man. Circ. Res. 39, 447–452.

52. Gerber, J. G., Volkel, N., Nies, A. S., Kadowitz, P. J., McMurtry, I., and Reeves, J. T. (1978) Pulmonary vasodilatation during hypoxia with infusion of arachidonic acid. Physiologist 21, 43.

53. Gerber, J. G., Ellis, E., Hollifield, J., and Nies, A. S. (1979) Effect of prostaglandin endoperoxide analogue on canine renal function, hemodynamics and renin release. Eur. J. Pharmacol. 53, 239–246.

54. Gerkens, J. F., Friesinger, G. C., Branch, R. A., Shand, D. G., and Gerber, J. G. (1978) A comparison of the pulmonary, renal and hepatic extractions of $PGF_{2\alpha}$ and PGE_2 - PGI_2, a potent circulating hormone. Life Sci. 22, 1837–1842.

55. Gerkens, J. F., Gerber, J. G., Shand, D. G., and Branch, R. A. (1978) Effect of PGI_2, PGE_2 and 6-keto-$PGF_{1\alpha}$ on canine gastric blood flow and acid secretion. Prostaglandins 16, 815–823.

56. Ginzel, K. H., Morrison, M. A., Baker, D. G., Coleridge, H. M., and Coleridge, J. C. G. (1978) Stimulation of afferent vagal endings in the intrapulmonary airways by prostaglandin endoperoxide analogues. Prostaglandins 15, 131–138.

57. Goldberg, M. R., Hebert, V. S., and Kadowitz, P. J. (1977) Effects of prostaglandins and endoperoxide analogs on canine saphenous vein. Am. J. Physiol. 233, H361–H368.

58. Goldblatt, M. W., (1935) Properties of human seminal plasma. J. Physiol. 84, 208–218.

59. Gruetter, C. A., McNamara, D. B., Hyman, A. L., and Kadowitz, P. J. (1978) Contractile responses of intrapulmonary vessels from three species to arachidonic acid and an epoxymethano analog of PGH_2. Can. J. Physiol. Pharmacol. 56, 206–215.

60. Gryglewski, R. J., Korbut, R., and Ocetkiewicz, A. (1978) Generation of prostacyclin by lungs in vivo and its release into arterial circulation. Nature (London) 273, 765–767.

61. Hamberg, M., Hedqvist, P., Strandberg, K., Svensson, J., and Samuelsson, B. (1975) Prostaglandin endoperoxides, IV. Effects on smooth muscle. Life Sci. 16, 451–462.

62. Hamberg, M., Svensson, J., and Samuelsson, B. (1975) Thromboxanes: A new group of biologically active compounds derived from prostaglandin endoperoxides. Proc. Natl. Acad. Sci. (US) 72, 2994–2998.

63. Hedqvist, P., Strandberg, K., and Hamberg, M. (1978) Bronchial and cardiovascular actions of prostaglandin endoperoxides and an endoperoxide analogue. Acta Physiol. Scand. 103, 299–307.

64. Hempker, D. P., and Aiken, J. W. (1979) Rat aortic strip as a bioassay tissue for thromboxane A_2 and rabbit aorta contracting substance (RCS) released from guinea pig lung by bradykinin or anaphylaxis. Prostaglandins 17, 239–248.

65. Hintze, T. H., and Kaley, G. (1977) Prostaglandins and the control of blood flow in the canine myocardium. Circ. Res. 40, 313–320.

66. Hintze, T., Kaley, G., Martin, E. G., and Messina, E. J. (1978) PGI_2 induced bradycardia in the dog. Prostaglandins 15, 712.

67. Horton, E. W., and Jones, R. L. (1974) Biological activity of prostaglandin D₂ on smooth muscle. Br. J. Pharmacol. 52, 110P–111P.

68. Hyman, A.L., Chapnick, B. M., Kadowitz, P.J., Lands, W. E. M., Crawford, C.G., Fried, J., and Barton, J. (1977) Unusual pulmonary vasodilatory activity of 13, 14-dihydro prostacyclin methyl ester: Comparison with endoperoxides and other prostanoids. Proc. Natl. Acad. Sci. (US) 74, 5711–5715.

69. Hyman, A.L., Chapnick, B. M., Nelson, P. K., and Spannhake, E. W., and Kadowitz, P. J. (1978) Pulmonary vascular effects of prostacyclin in the cat. Fed. Proc. 37, 731.

70. Hyman, A. L., Mathe, A. A., Leslie, C. A., Matthews, C. C., Bennett, J. T., Spannhake, E. W., and Kadowitz, P. J. (1978) Modification of pulmonary vascular responses to arachidonic acid by alterations in physiologic state. J. Pharmacol. Exp. Ther. 207, 388–401.

71. Hyman, A. L., Spannhake, E. W., Chapnick, B. M., McNamara, D. B., Mathe, A. A., and Kadowitz, P. J. (1978) Effect of dihomo-γ-linolenic acid on the pulmonary vascular bed. Am. J. Physiol. 234,, H133–H138.

72. Ichikawa, S., and Yamada, J. (1962) Biological actions of free and albumin-bound arachidonic acid. Am. J. Physiol. 203, 681–684.

73. Isakson, P. C., Raz, A., Denny, S. E., Pure, E., and Needleman, P. (1977) A novel prostaglandin is the major product of arachidonic acid metabolism in rabbit heart. Proc. Natl. Acad. Sci. (US) 74, 101–105.

74. Jaques, R. (1959) Arachidonic acid, an unsaturated fatty acid which produces slow contractions of smooth muscle and causes pain. Pharmacological and biochemical characterization of its mode of action. Helv. Physiol. Pharmacol. Acta 17, 255–267.

75. Jones, R. L. (1976) Cardiovascular actions of prostaglandins D and E in the sheep. Evidence for two distinct receptors. In: B. Samuelsson and R. Paoletti (eds.), Advances in Prostaglandin and Thromboxane Research, Vol. 1, Raven Press, New York, pp. 221–230.

76. Kadowitz, P. J., and Hyman, A. L. (1977) Influence of a prostaglandin endoperoxide analogue on the canine pulmonary vascular bed. Circ. Res. 40, 282–287.

77. Kadowitz, P. J., Gruetler, C. A., McNamara, D. B., Gorman, R. R., Spannhake, E. W., and Hyman, A. L. (1977) Comparative effects of endoperoxide PGH₂ and an analog on the pulmonary vascular bed. J. Appl. Physiol. 42, 953–958.

78. Kadowitz, P. J., Hyman, A. L., and Spannhake, E. W. (1977) Effect of thromboxane B₂ on the pulmonary vascular bed. Fed. Proc. 36, 403.

79. Kadowitz, P. J., Spannhake, E. W., Greenberg, S., Feigen, L. P., and Hyman, A. L. (1977) Comparative effects of arachidonic acid, bisenoic prostaglandins, and an endoperoxide analog on the canine pulmonary vascular bed. Can. J. Physiol. Pharmacol. 55, 1369–1377.

80. Kadowitz, P. J., Chapnick, B. M., Feigen, L. P., Hyman, A. L., Nelson P.K., and Spannhake, E. W. (1978) Pulmonary and systemic vasodilator effects of the newly discovered prostaglandin, PGI₂. J. Appl. Physiol. 45, 408–413.

81. Kalkarni, P. S., Roberts, R., and Needleman, P. (1976) Paradoxical endogenous synthesis of a coronary dilating substance from arachidonate. Prostaglandins 12, 337–353.

82. Karmazyn, M., Horrobin, D. F., Manku, M. S., Cunnane, S. C., Karmali R. A., Ally, A. I., Morgan, R. O., Nicolaou, K. C., and Barnette, W. E. (1978) Effects of prostacyclin on perfusion pressure, electrical activity and force of contraction in isolated rat and rabbit hearts. Life Sci. 22, 2079–2086.

83. Katori, M., Harada, Y., Yamashita, Y., and Ishibashi, M. (1978) Release of PGD₂ as a major product from isolated rat pregnant uterus. Prostaglandins 15, 697.

84. Kolata, G. B. (1975) Thromboxanes: The power behind the prostaglandins? Science 190, 770–771, 812.

85. Kot, P. A., Rose, J. C., Ramwell, P. W., Fitzpatrick, T. M., Bloom, M. F., and Friedman, L. S. (1980) Modification of the cardiovascular actions of prostaglandins by thromboxane B₂. In: B. Samuelsson, P. W. Ramwell, and R. Paoletti (eds.), Advances in

Prostaglandin and Thromboxane Research, Vol. 7, Raven Press, New York, pp. 679–682.

86. Kot, P. A., Johnson, M., Ramwell, P. W., and Rose, J. C. (1975) Effects of ganglionic and β-adrenergic blockade on cardiovascular responses to the bisenoic prostaglandins and their precursor arachidonic acid. Proc. Soc. Exp. Biol. Med. 149, 953–957.

87. Kulkarni, P. S., Roberts, R., and Needleman, P. (1976) Paradoxical endogenous synthesis of a coronary vasodilating substance from arachidonate. Prostaglandins 12, 337–353.

88. Kurzrok, R., and Lieb, C. C. (1930) Biochemical studies of human semen. II. The action of semen on the human uterus. Proc. Soc. Exp. Biol. Med. 28, 268–272.

89. Larsson, C., and Änggård, E. (1973) Arachidonic acid lowers and indomethacin increases the blood pressure of the rabbit. J. Pharm. Pharmacol. 25, 653–655.

90. Larsson, C., and Änggård, E. (1974) Increased juxtamedullary blood flow on stimulation of intrarenal prostaglandin biosynthesis. Eur. J. Pharmacol. 25, 326–334.

91. Larsson, C., Weber, P., and Änggård, E. (1974) Arachidonic acid increases and indomethacin decreases plasma renin activity in the rabbit. Eur. J. Pharmacol. 28, 391–394.

92. Lewis, G. P., Westwick, J., and Williams, T. J. (1977) Microvascular responses produced by the prostaglandin endoperoxide PGG_2 in vivo. Br. J. Pharmacol., 59, 442P.

93. Link, H. B., Rosen, R., and Schror, K. (1978) Prostacyclin: A potent coronary dilating agent in rat isolated heart. J. Physiol. 284, 106P–107P.

94. McGiff, J. R., and Itskovitz, H. D. (1973) Prostaglandins and the kidney. Circ. Res. 33, 479–488.

95. McGiff, J. C., and Wong, P. Y.-K. (1979) Compartmentalization of prostaglandins and prostacyclin within the kidney: Implications for renal function. Fed. Proc. 38, 89–93.

96. McLaughlin, M. K., Phernetton, T. M., and Rankin, J. H. G. (1979) PGD_2 effects on the rabbit utero-placental circulation. Proc. Soc. Exp. Biol. Med. 162, 187–190.

97. Malik, K. U., and McGiff, J. C. (1976) Cardiovascular actions of prostaglandins. In: S. M. M. Karim (ed.), Prostaglandins: Physiological, Pharmacological and Pathological Aspects, University Park Press, Baltimore, pp. 103–200.

98. Malik, K. U., Ryan, P., and McGiff, J. C. (1976) Modification by prostaglandins E_1 and E_2, indomethacin and arachidonic acid of the vasoconstrictor responses of the isolated perfused rabbit and rat mesenteric arteries to adrenergic stimuli. Circ. Res. 39, 163–168.

99. Malmsten, C. (1976) Some biological effects of prostaglandin endoperoxide analogs. Life Sci. 18, 169–176.

100. Markov, C. M. (1978) Role of prostaglandins in the pathogenesis of hypertension. Clin. Sci. Mol. Med. 55, S207–S210.

101. Mest, H. J., and Forster, W. (1973) Evidence for antiarrhythmic efficiency of arachidonic and linoleic acid—Preliminary results. Prostaglandins 4, 751–753.

102. Mest, H. J., and Forster, W. (1978) The antiarrhythmic action of prostacyclin (PGI_2) on aconitine induced arrhythmias in rats. Acta Biol. Med. Ger. 37, 827–828.

103. Moncada, S., Gryglewski, R., Bunting, S., and Vane, J. R. (1976) An enzyme isolated from arteries transforms prostaglandin endoperoxides to an unstable substance that inhibits platelet aggregation. Nature (London), 263, 663–665.

104. Moncada, S., Gryglewski, R. J., Bunting, S., and Vane, J. R. (1976) A lipid peroxide inhibits the enzyme in blood vessel microsomes that generates from prostaglandin endoperoxides the substance (prostaglandin X) which prevents platelet aggregation. Prostaglandins 12, 715–737.

105. Moncada, S., Korbut, R., Bunting, S., and Vane, J. R. (1978) Prostacyclin is a circulating hormone. Nature (London) 273, 767–768.

106. Moncada, S., Salmon, J. A., Vane, J. R., and Whittle, B. J. R. (1978) Formation of prostacyclin and its product 6-oxa-$PGF_{1\alpha}$ by gastric mucosa of several species. J. Physiol. 275, 4P–5P.

107. Moody, T. E., Vaughn, E. D., and Gillenwater, J. Y. (1975) Relationship between renal blood flow and ureteral pressure during 18 hours of total unilateral occlusion: Implication for changing sites of renal resistance. Invest. Urol. 13, 246–251.

108. Morooka, S., Kobayash, M., Takahashi, T., Takashima, Y., Sakamoto, M., and Shimamoto, T. (1979) Experimental ischemic heart disease. Effects of synthetic thromboxane A_2. Exp. Mol. Pathol. 30, 449–457.

109. Morrison, A. R., Nishikawa, K., and Needleman, P. (1977) Unmasking of thromboxane A_2 synthesis by ureteral obstruction in the rabbit kidney. Nature (London) 267, 259–260.

110. Morrison, A. R., Nishikawa, K., and Needleman, P. (1978) Thromboxane A_2 biosynthesis in the ureter obstructed isolated perfused kidney of the rabbit. J. Pharmacol. Exp. Ther. 205, 1–8.

111. Mousty, J. C., Juchmes-Ferir, A., and Damas, J. (1977) Activation de l'acide arachidonique. Arch. Int. Physiol. Biochim. 85, 377–379.

112. Needleman, P., and Kaley, G. (1978) Cardiac and coronary prostaglandin synthesis and function. New Engl. J. Med. 298, 1122–1128.

113. Needleman, P., Marshall, G. R., and Sobel, B. E. (1975) Hormone interactions in the isolated rabbit heart: Synthesis and coronary vasomotor effects of prostaglandins, angiotensin and bradykinin. Circ. Res. 37, 802–808.

114. Needleman, P., Minkes, M., and Raz, A. (1976) Thromboxanes: Selective biosynthesis and distinct biological properties. Science 193, 163–165.

115. Needleman, P., Moncada, S., Bunting, S., Vane, J. R., Hamberg, M., and Samuelsson, B. (1976) Identification of an enzyme in platelet microsomes which generates thromboxane A_2 from prostaglandin endoperoxides. Nature (London) 261, 558–560.

116. Needleman, P., Kulkarni, P. S., and Raz, A. (1977) Coronary tone modulation: Formation and actions of prostaglandins, endoperoxides and thromboxanes. Science 195, 409–412.

117. Needleman, P., Bronson, S. D., Wyche, A., Sivakoff, M., and Nicolaou, K. C., (1978) Cardiac and renal prostaglandin I_2. Biosynthesis and biological effects in isolated perfused rabbit tissues. J. Clin. Invest. 61, 839–849.

118. Nugteren, D. H., and Hazelhof, E. (1973) Isolation and properties of intermediates in prostaglandin biosynthesis. Biochim. Biophys. Acta 326, 448–461.

119. Oates, J. A., Whorton, A. R., Gerkens, J. F., Branch, R. A., Hollifield, J. W., and Frölich, J. C. (1979) The participation of prostaglandins in the control of renin release. Fed. Proc. 38, 72–74.

120. Ogletree, M. L., Smith, J. B., and Lefer, A. M. (1978) Actions of prostaglandins on isolated perfused cat coronary arteries. Am. J. Physiol. 235, H400-H406.

121. Ogletree, M. L., Smith, J. B., Nicolaou, K. C., and Lefer, A. M. (1978) Beneficial action of prostacyclin (PGI$_2$) in myocardial ischemia. Fed. Proc. 37, 566.

122. Pace-Asciak, C. R., Carrara, M. C., Rangaraj, G., and Nicolaou, K. C. (1978) Enhanced formation of PGI$_2$, a potent hypotensive substance by aortic ring and homogenates of spontaneous hypertensive rats. Prostaglandins 15, 1005–1012.

123. Palmer, M. A., Piper, P. J., and Vane J. R. (1973) Release of rabbit aorta contracting substance (RCS) and prostaglandins induced by chemical or mechanical stimulation of guinea pig lungs. Br. J. Pharmacol. 49, 226–242.

124. Paustian, P. W., Chapnick, B. M., Feigen, L. P., Hyman, A. L., and Kadowitz, P. J. (1977) Effects of 13, 14-dihydroprostacyclin methyl ester on the feline intestinal vascular bed. Prostaglandins 14, 1141–1152.

125. Pirkle, H., and Carstens, P. (1974) Pulmonary platelet aggregates associated with sudden death in man. Science 185, 1062–1064.

126. Raz, A., Isakson, P. C., Minkes, M. S., and Needleman, P. (1977) Characterization of a novel metabolic pathway of arachidonate in coronary arteries which generates a potent endogenous coronary vasodilator. J. Biol. Chem. 252, 1123–1126.

127. Rose, J. C., and Kot, P. A. (1977) Cardiovascular responses to the prostaglandin precursors. In: P. W. Ramwell (ed.), The Prostaglandins, Vol. 3, Plenum Press, New York, pp. 135–144.

128. Rose, J. C., Johnson, M., Ramwell, P. W., and Kot, P. A. (1974) Effects of arachidonic acid on systemic arterial pressure, myocardial contractility and platelets in the dog. Proc. Soc. Exp. Biol. Med. 147, 652–655.

129. Rose, J. C., Johnson, M., Ramwell, P. W., and Kot, P. A. (1975) Cardiovascular and platelet responses in the dog to the monoenoic prostaglandin precursor dihomo-γ-linolenic acid. Proc. Soc. Exp. Biol. Med. 148, 1252–1256.

130. Rose, J. C., Kot, P. A., Ramwell, P. W., Doykos, M., and O'Neill, W. P. (1976) Cardiovascular responses to three endoperoxide analogs in the dog. Proc. Soc. Exp. Biol. Med. 153, 209–212.

131. Samuelsson, B., Folco, G., Grandström, E., Kindahl, H., and Malmsten, C. (1978) Prostaglandins and thromboxanes: Biochemical and physiological considerations. In: F. Coceani and P. M. Olley (eds.), Advances in Prostaglandin and Thromboxane Research, Vol. 4, Raven Press, New York, pp. 1–25.

132. Schror, K. (1978) PGD_2—A potent coronary vasoconstricting agent in the guinea pig isolated heart. Naunyn-Schmiedebergs Arch. Pharmakol. 302, 61–62.

133. Scholkens, B. A., and Weithmann, U. (1978) Pharmacological action of prostacyclin (PGI_2). Naunyn-Schmiedebergs Arch. Pharmakol. 302, R28.

134. Schror, K., and Moncada, S. (1979) Effects of prostacyclin on coronary circulation, heart rate and myocardial contractile force in isolated hearts of guinea pig and rabbit—Comparison with prostaglandin E_2. Prostaglandins 17, 367–373.

135. Seymour, A. A., Davis, J. O., Freeman, R. H., Stephens, G. A., DeForrest, J. M., Rowe, B. P., and Williams, G. M. (1979) Prostaglandin I_2 and D_2 stimulate renin secretion from filtering and non-filtering canine kidneys. Fed. Proc. 38, 893.

136. Silberbauer, K., Sinzinger, H., and Winter, M. (1978) Prostacyclin production by vascular smooth muscle cells. Lancet 1(8078), 1356–1357.

137. Silberbauer, K., Sinzinger, H., and Winter, M. (1979) Prostacyclin activity in rat kidney stimulated by angiotensin II. Br. J. Exp. Pathol. 60, 38–44.

138. Silver, M. J., Hoch, W., Kocsis, J. J., Ingerman, C. M., and Smith, J. B. (1974) Arachidonic acid causes sudden death in rabbits. Science 183, 1085–1087.

139. Sivakoff, M., Pure, E., and Needleman, P. (1979) Prostaglandins and the heart. Fed. Proc. 38, 78–82.

140. Skidgel, R. A., and Printz, M. P. (1978) PGI_2 production by rat blood vessels: Diminished prostacyclin formation in veins compared to arteries. Prostaglandins 16, 1–16.

141. Spannhake, E. W., Lemen, R. J., Wegmann, M. J., Hyman, A. L., and Kadowitz, P. J. (1978) Effects of arachidonic acid and prostaglandins on lung function in the intact dog. J. Appl. Physiol. 44, 397–405.

142. Svensson, J., and Fredholm, B. B. (1977) Vasoconstrictor effect of thromboxane A_2. Acta Physiol. Scand. 101, 366–368.

143. Svensson, J., and Hamberg, M. (1976) Thromboxane A_2 and prostaglandin H_2: Potent stimulators of the swine coronary artery. Prostaglandins 12, 943–950.

144. Svensson, J., Strandberg, K., Tuvemo, T., and Hamberg, N. (1977) Thromboxane A_2: Effects on airway and vascular smooth muscle. Prostaglandins 14, 425–436.

145. Szczeklik, A., Gryglewski, R. J., Niżankowska, E., Niżankowski, R., and Musiał, J. (1978) Pulmonary and anti-platelet effects of intravenous and inhaled prostacyclin in man. Prostaglandins 16, 651–660.

146. Tannenbaum, J., Spławiński, J. A., Oates, J. A., and Nies, A. S. (1978) Enhanced renal prostaglandin production in the dog. 1. Effects on renal function. Circ. Res. 36, 197–203.

147. Terashita, Z., Fukji, H., Nishikawa, K., Hirata, M., and Kikuchi, S., (1978) Coronary

vasospastic action of TXA$_2$ in isolated working guinea pig hearts. Eur. J. Pharmacol. 53, 49–56.

148. Terragno, N. A., Terragno, D. A., and McGiff, J. R. (1977) Contribution of prostaglandins to the renal circulation in conscious anesthetized and laparotomized dogs. Circ. Res. 40, 590–595.

149. Terragno, N. A., McGiff, J. R., and Terragno, A., (1978) Prostacyclin (PGI$_2$) production by renal blood vessels. Relationship to an endogenous prostaglandin synthesis inhibitor (EPSI). Clin. Res. 26, 545A.

150. Waldman, H. M., Alter, I., Kot, P. A., Rose, J. C., and Ramwell, P. W. (1978) Effect of lung transit on systemic depressor responses to arachidonic acid and prostacyclin in dogs. J. Pharmacol. Exp. Ther. 204, 289–293.

151. Wang, H. H., Kulkarni, P. S., and Eakins, K. E. (1978) Effects of prostaglandins (PGIs) and thromboxane A$_2$ (TXA$_2$) on the coronary circulation of adult and puppy dogs. Fed. Proc. 37, 731.

152. Wasserman, M. A., and Griffin, R. L. (1977) Thromboxane B$_2$—Comparative bronchoactivity in experimental systems. Eur. J. Pharmacol. 46, 303–313.

153. Wasserman, M. A., DuCharme, D. W., Griffin, R. L., DeGaaf, G. L., and Robinson, F. G. (1977) Bronchopulmonary and cardiovascular effects of prostaglandin D$_2$ in the dog. Prostaglandins 13, 255–269.

154. Weber, P. C., Larsson, C., Änggård, E., Hamberg, M., Corey, E. J., Nicolaou, K. C., and Samuelsson, B. (1976) Stimulation of renin release from rabbit renal cortex by arachidonic acid and prostaglandin endoperoxides. Circ. Res. 39, 868–874.

155. Weeks, J. R. (1978) The general pharmacology of prostacyclin PGI$_2$ (PGX): A new prostaglandin especially active on the cardiovascular system. Acta Biol. Med. Ger. 37, 707–714.

156. Wennmalm, Å.(1977) Vasodilatory action of arachidonic acid in humans following indomethacin treatment. Prostaglandins 13, 809–810.

157. Whittaker, N., Bunting, S., Salmon, J., Moncada, S., Vane, J. R., Johnson, R. A., Morton, D. R., Kinner, J. H., Gorman, R. R., McGuire, J. C., and Sun, F. F. (1976) The chemical structure of prostaglandin X (prostacyclin). Prostaglandins 12, 915–928.

158. Whittle, B. J. R., Moncada, S., and Vane, J. R. (1978) Some actions of prostacyclin (PGI$_2$) on the cardiovascular system and gastric microvasculature. Acta Biol. Med. Ger. 37, 5–6.

159. Whorton, A. R., Smigel, M., Oates, J. A., and Frölich, J. C. (1978) Regional differences in prostacyclin formation by the kidney. Prostacyclin is a major prostaglandin of renal cortex. Biochim. Biophys. Acta 529, 176–180.

160. Wicks, T. C., Rose, J. C., Johnson, M., Ramwell, P. W., and Kot, P. A. (1976) Vascular responses to arachidonic acid in the perfused canine lung. Circ. Res. 38, 167–171.

161. Wicks, T. C., Ramwell, P. W., Rose, J. C., and Kot, P. A. (1977) Vascular responses to the monoenoic prostaglandin precursor dihomo-γ-linolenic acid in the perfused canine lung. J. Pharmacol. Exp. Ther. 201, 417–420.

162. Wolfe, L. S., Rostworowski, K., and Marion, J. (1976) Endogenous formation of the prostacyclin endoperoxide metabolite, thromboxane B$_2$, by brain tissue. Biochem. Biophys. Res. Commun. 70, 907–913.

163. Wong, P. Y.-K., Sun, F. F., and McGiff, J. C. (1978) Metabolism of prostacyclin in blood vessels. J. Biol. Chem. 253, 5555–5557.

M. BYGDEMAN, M.D.

A. GILLESPIE, M.D.

PROSTAGLANDINS IN HUMAN REPRODUCTION

INTRODUCTION

Among the different prostaglandin compounds isolated and identified from human tissues, it is mainly prostaglandin E_2 and $F_{2\alpha}$ that have been implicated in the physiological regulation of different events in the reproductive organs in the human (e.g. male fertility, ovulation, the life span of the corpus luteum, tubal contractility, and nonpregnant and pregnant uterine contractility). Although prostacyclin and thromboxane A_2 seem to be present in reproductive tissues, the physiological involvement of these compounds in reproductive processes is largely unknown.

The modification or stimulation of reproductive events by exogenous prostaglandins has been a major area of research. As a result, prostaglandins and inhibitors of their biosynthesis have found practical application, especially on indications related to the stimulatory effect of prostaglandins on human myometrium.

From the Department of Obstetrics and Gynecology, Karolinska Institutet, Stockholm, Sweden, and the Department of Obstetrics and Gynecology, University of Adelaide, Queen Victoria Hospital, Adelaide, South Australia, Australia.

MALE GENITAL TRACT

Prostaglandins in Seminal Fluid

The existence of a substance or group of substances with smooth muscle stimulating and vasodepressive properties was first described in extracts of human semen, prostate, and seminal vesicle [61,176–178]. The active principle was given the name prostaglandin by von Euler. It was soon realized that semen was the richest natural source of prostaglandin, and seminal extracts were used for many of the early experiments on the properties of prostaglandins.

Initially human seminal fluid was found to contain considerable amounts of several classical prostaglandins (e.g. PGE_1, PGE_2, PGE_3, $PGF_{1\alpha}$, and $PGF_{2\alpha}$) [148]. Later the existence of eight more prostaglandins was reported: A_1, A_2, B_1, B_2, and their four 19-hydroxylated equivalents [72], and thereafter 19-hydroxy PGE_1 and 19-hydroxy PGE_2 [93,164] and 19-hydroxy $PGF_{1\alpha}$ and 19-hydroxy $PGF_{2\alpha}$ [165].

Today most evidence indicates that the PGA and PGB compounds as well as their 19-hydroxy derivatives are largely artifactual, since they are found only after incubation or storage, not in fresh frozen semen [43,94]. Small concentrations may, however, occur naturally, the compounds being formed by the degradation of the PGEs or even perhaps directly from the endoperoxide precursors prior to ejaculation.

Very recently evidence was presented for the existence of a group of 8-iso-prostaglandins, 8-iso-PGE_1, 8-iso-PGE_2, 8-iso-$PGF_{1\alpha}$, 8-iso-$PGF_{2\alpha}$, and the four corresponding 19-hydroxy prostaglandins [163]. Other minor prostaglandin components may also be identified in the future.

Of all human tissues and secretions examined, the seminal plasma possesses the highest concentration of prostaglandins. Quantitatively the 19-hydroxy PGEs are the most important. On the average, seminal fluid from normal men contains about 270 μg total 19-hydroxy PGE per milliliter and 60 μg PGE per milliliter. The total 19-hydroxy PGF amounts to approximately 20 μg/ml and PGF 2–8 μg/ml (Table 1). A normal ejaculate of 3 ml will thus contain over 1 mg of prostaglandin.

Significant amounts of prostaglandins have also been identified in several subhuman primates, sheep, and goat [26,55,116]. The relation between the different compounds varies considerably, however. Masturbation samples from chimpanzees, rhesus, and stump-tailed macaques contained 19-hydroxy PGE levels of 390–780 μg/ml with only one-fifth that amount of 19-hydroxy PGE_2 and 5 μg/ml of PGE. These high levels of 19-hydroxy PGE_1 indicate that the substance vesiglandin, which von Euler isolated from monkey semen, was 19-hydroxy PGE_1.

Eliasson [55] attempted to identify the tissue source of human seminal prostaglandins by measuring prostaglandins in split ejaculates. He reported that prostaglandin was liberated in the same fraction as fructose, and thus human seminal prostaglandins would appear to arise from the seminal vesicles. Hamberg [71] has also shown that human seminal vesicles have the capacity to biosynthesize prostaglandins. However, at least two studies have shown no relation between the concentration of

TABLE 1. Prostaglandin Present in Human Seminal Fluid from Fertile Men

Compound	Number of men	Mean ± SD (µg/ml)	Reference
PGE_1	6	25.0 ± 4.7	30
PGE_2		23.0 ± 5.8	30
PGE_3		5.5 ± 1.8	30
$PGF_{1\alpha}$		3.6 ± 1.7	30
$PGF_{2\alpha}$		4.4 ± 2.0	30
PGE	29	54.4 ± 22.1	24
PGE	23	63.2 ± 35.5	18
PGE	22	73.2 ± 71.6	166
PGF		2.1 ± 1.8	166
19-Hydroxy PGE		267 ± 240	166
19-Hydroxy PGF		18.3 ± 14.1	166

PGE and fructose in whole ejaculates from apparently healthy men or men in infertile marriages [23,48]. There are several possible reasons for the discrepancy. Seminal PGEs may not be synthesized exclusively at seminal vesicle levels; the production sites and production mechanisms may be differential, as well as the regulation of the biosynthesis. On the other hand, the seminal vesicles appear to be the preferential site of seminal 19-hydroxy PGE production, since a close correlation has been reported for 19-hydroxy PGE and fructose in men in whom these prostaglandins were low [42].

At present little is known about the factors involved in the control of the secretion of prostaglandins in the seminal fluid and accessory sex organs of the male. The studies of Sturde [158,159] indicate that seminal prostaglandin levels are regulated by androgens. In a more recent study the effect of testosterone on different prostaglandins in hypogonadel men [155] was studied. During treatment the concentration of 19-hydroxy PGE_1 and 19-hydroxy PGE_2 increased significantly, while the concentration of PGE_1 and PGE_2 remained unchanged, indicating that the endogenous production of various prostaglandin compounds is subject to different forms of regulation.

Prostaglandins and Male Fertility

The high concentration of prostaglandins in the seminal fluid of man as compared with most tissues and body fluids has led to the logical assumption that these compounds are intimately involved in reproductive processes. Asplund [6] and Hawkins and Labrum [76] observed a relationship between seminal prostaglandins and number of children. Averaged data indicate that men whose wives had more than 0.5 conception per year had significantly higher levels of seminal prostaglandins than men with wives having no conceptions. The authors concluded that there was a positive relation between the concentration of prostaglandins in the semen and the ability of the couple to effect conception.

These early results based on bioassays have later been confirmed by quantitative chemical methods. Human males who were infertile for no apparent reason possessed significantly lower concentrations of seminal prostaglandin, especially E prostaglandins, than men of normal fertility [18,24,41]. Bygdeman et al. [24] showed that seminal fluid from fertile men contained about 55 µg of total E prostaglandin per milliliter, an amount that was significantly higher than the corresponding value (18 µg/ml) in semen of men from infertile marriages where no other abnormalities could be detected. The relation between 19-hydroxy PGE or 19-hydroxy PGF concentrations and fertility is not known. Evidence for a correlation between fertility and seminal prostaglandin concentration has also been found in sheep. Following artificial insemination, the fertility of the rams increased by more than 15% if PGE_2 and $PGF_{2\alpha}$ were added to the diluted ram semen in amounts comparable with the total amounts of prostaglandins in one ejaculate [50].

The precise mechanism by which seminal prostaglandins influence fertility is unknown. In fact, the correlation need not to be one of cause and effect; the infertility could be due to some other factor that also produced low prostaglandin levels in semen. However, it has been suggested that prostaglandins in human seminal fluid could influence fertility in several ways. Prostaglandins could act on the male to influence fertility by regulating for example, sperm physiology, steroidogenesis, and the activity of sex accessory tissue and smooth muscles. The seminal prostaglandins could also act on the female to enhance the likelihood of fertilization.

Most of the available information does not indicate any correlation between the concentration of prostaglandins in semen with sperm function. Sperm motility is not dependent on or related to the concentration of seminal prostaglandins. It also seems that at least classical prostaglandins have no direct effect on sperm metabolism and function [34]. It must be remembered, however, that the failure to observe effects of prostaglandins on ejaculated sperm could partially be due to the following conditions: the spermatozoa have already been exposed to the prostaglandins in the seminal plasma during ejaculation, and this primary exposure might have reduced the response to prostaglandins subsequently added.

In contrast to PGEs, 19-hydroxy PGEs have a marked inhibitory action on sperm respiration. When 19-hydroxy PGEs were tested on washed ejaculated human spermatozoa, a lowered production of labeled carbon dioxide from [^{14}C]fructose was also observed [115].

Von Euler [178] suggested that prostaglandins might be involved in the contractile events of ejaculation, since the epididymis, vas deferens, and seminal vesicles contain smooth muscle and prostaglandins have a potent action on such tissue. This suggestion has been reinforced more recently by the finding that prostaglandins can influence neurotransmission in the sex accessory tissues of the male. Hedqvist and von Euler [78] measured the contractile response of the vas deferens of several laboratory animals to noradrenalin and nerve stimulation in the absence and presence of varying concentrations of PGE_1, PGE_2, and $PGF_{2\alpha}$. PGE_1 and PGE_2 potentiated noradrenalin-induced smooth muscle contractile responses of the isolated guinea pig vas deferens and seminal vesicles; PGE_1 was effective in concentrations from 0.2 to 200 ng/ml. However, the contractile response of the vas deferens to postganglionic nerve stimulation was inhibited by low doses of PGE_1 and potentiated by high doses.

The authors speculate that the ability of prostaglandin to modulate neurotransmission in vas deferens and seminal vesicles could have importance in regulating contractile function of the sex accessory organs.

It is possible that changes in uterine contractility during intercourse may facilitate sperm transport. During sexual stimulation there is a marked increase in uterine activity that changes to inhibition following female orgasm. A pressure gradient between the vagina and the uterus may be the result favoring a passive sperm transport. These changes in uterine and vaginal contractility might be caused by seminal prostaglandins, but experimental evidence to support this assumption is still lacking in the human. Evidence that PGE_1, PGE_2, or $PGF_{2\alpha}$ enhances sperm migration, hence fertilization have, however, been provided in experiments in rabbits [38,156].

As described elsewhere in more detail, both PGEs and PGFs generally have a stimulatory effect on human uterine contractility following intravenous, intrauterine, and vaginal administration. For both compounds the threshold dose following intrauterine administration is at the microgram level [132]. However, at least for PGE_2 and $PGF_{2\alpha}$ uterine sensitivity was markedly decreased at midcycle. Prostaglandin E_2 (0.5–1.0 mg), given intravaginally to women, results in increased uterine activity [80]. The effect of 19-hydroxy PGE and 19-hydroxy PGF on human uterine contractility in vivo is not known. The potency of 19-hydroxy PGE_2, which stimulates the contractility of the pregnant monkey uterus, is approximately one-third of that of PGE_2. 19-Hydroxy PGF is significantly less active.

The amount of PGE compounds present in a single ejaculate (approximately 100–200 µg) is less than the vaginal dose required to induce an apparent uterine response. However, an effect on uterine contractility is still possible, since during intercourse uterine reactivity to prostaglandins may be increased because of different hormonal and nervous stimuli associated with sexual stimulation, and the vaginal absorption may be enhanced by local changes in the vaginal mucosa.

In addition, the importance of 19-hydroxy compounds that are present in milligram amounts in the ejaculate is unknown. Both stimulation and inhibition of uterine contractility following vaginal administration of seminal fluid have been reported [56,107]. However, in these early studies the semen may not have been handled in a way that prohibited the conversion of 19-hydroxy PGEs to 19-hydroxy PGA and 19-hydroxy PGB compounds.

FEMALE GENITAL TRACT

Ovarian Function

The ovulatory process includes the sequential events of ovum maturation, follicular rupture, and development of corpus luteum. The prostaglandins appear to be deeply involved in these processes in subprimates, but their role in corresponding events in the human remains to be established [120]. In general, PGE_2 mimics the effect of luteinizing hormone (LH) on isolated follicles from laboratory animals.

FOLLICULAR RUPTURE

Investigations from a number of laboratories have indicated that PGE_2 and $PGF_{2\alpha}$ are involved in the normal process of ovulation in the rat and rabbit [5,129]. Ovulation is initiated by a cyclic surge of LH secretion from the pituitary induced by LH releasing hormone (RH). Three processes will take place in the responding follicle: the resumption of the nuclear maturation division of the oocyte, a steroidogenic shift from estrogen to progesterone production, and follicular rupture. Inhibition of prostaglandin synthesis by the systemic or local administration of inhibitors (e.g., indomethacin or aspirin) has been shown to block ovulation in the rat and rabbit [5,186]. Since this block could not be overcome by LH, but could be reversed by administration of exogenous prostaglandins, the prostaglandin involvement appeared to be on the ovarian level. However, treatment with indomethacin does not seem to prevent other follicular responses to LH (Table 2).

An increasing concentration in follicular fluid of $PGF_{2\alpha}$ and PGE_2 in response to the ovulatory surge of LH in the rat and rabbit with some preponderance of PGE over PGF has been demonstrated [119].

An increase was not found in follicles that failed to ovulate. These increases could be prevented by systemic or intrafollicular administration

TABLE 2. Effects of Prostaglandins in Follicular Function in Laboratory Animals

Prostaglandins may modulate	Prostaglandins obligatory
↓	↓
Ovum maturation	Follicular rupture
Activation of adenylate cyclase	
Steroidogenesis	
Luteinization	

Modified from Lindner et al. (123).

of indomethacin [5]. Available data in the rabbit indicate that both PGE_2 and $PGF_{2\alpha}$ are mainly produced by granulosa cells [40].

The precise mechanism of prostaglandin in follicular rupture is unknown. It has been suggested that follicular rupture involves an enzymatic weakening of the follicular wall [11], and prostaglandins might be involved in the activation, release, or synthesis of an ovulatory enzyme [137]. Prostaglandin could also act by influencing smooth muscle contractions, which have a proposed role in ovulation. $PGF_{2\alpha}$ stimulated ovarian contractility in subprimates and primates, including man, has been demonstrated [44]. There is also evidence for the existence of rhythmic contractions of the follicle wall that increase in frequency and amplitude in response to $PGF_{2\alpha}$ [173].

The role of prostaglandins in follicular rupture in the human is unknown. The effect on ovulation of one biosynthesis inhibitor, aspirin, has been studied in the human. Basal body temperature and LH levels in urine, plasma progesterone, and cervical mucus were followed during a control and treatment cycle. No effects on the parameters mentioned above indicating inhibition of ovulation were observed. Laparotomy was performed in the secretory phase to exclude an entrapped ovum and follicular luteinization [39]. The lack of effect of aspirin makes it doubtful that prostaglandins are involved in follicular rupture in the human. Trials with more specific and effective inhibitors of PG synthetase are, however, necessary before final conclusions can be reached.

LUTEOLYSIS

The importance of the uterus in controlling the length of the estrous cycle was first recognized more than 50 years ago. Since that time the uterus has been shown to control the life span of the functional corpus luteum in many species including the sheep, cow, horse, pig, pseudo-pregnant rat, rabbit, and hamster [86].

There is considerable evidence to support the concept that $PGF_{2\alpha}$ is the uterine factor responsible for luteolysis. Endogenous administration of $PGF_{2\alpha}$ unquestionably causes luteolysis in many subprimate species in vivo. Increasing levels of $PGF_{2\alpha}$ toward the end of the estrous cycle just before luteal regression have also been established in several animals. Frequent sampling has shown a pulsatile release of $PGF_{2\alpha}$. The frequency of the peaks increases as the end of the luteal phase is reached [117]. Moreover, administration of $PGF_{2\alpha}$ into the uterine vein in doses equivalent to the measured levels could induce premature luteal regression.

The very rapid inactivation of circulating prostaglandins seems to exclude a systemic route of supply and to favor a local mechanism for direct transfer of $PGF_{2\alpha}$ from the uterus to the adjacent ovary. The intimate anatomic relationships between the utero-ovarian vein and the ovarian artery and the prolongation of the life span of the corpus luteum merely by separating these structures support this assumption [133]. The uterine prostaglandins then appear to exert their luteolytic action in the manner of classical hormones. This concept seems plausible because the postulated pathway shunts the lungs, where prostaglandins are subject to rapid biological degradation.

Although it is not clear how $PGF_{2\alpha}$ induces luteal regression, several possible mechanisms have been suggested. For example, the vasoactive properties of $PGF_{2\alpha}$ may cause a constriction of the blood flow to the ovary. Indeed, a significant decrease in blood flow to the corpus luteum in association with its regression has been demonstrated, but this reduced blood flow is probably an effect rather than a cause of the luteolysis. Preliminary results on ovarian blood flow in rat indicate a positive correlation between luteal blood flow and progesterone production (Jansson et al., personal communication). This is in agreement with previous observations in the sheep of a dramatic drop in ovarian blood flow at the time of functional luteolysis. A redistribution of the blood flow within the ovary has been reported to be one of the consequences of in vivo administration of $PGF_{2\alpha}$ [87], but it remains to be established whether this change is of significance for the luteolytic effect of $PGF_{2\alpha}$ or whether the drop in flow is merely the result of a structural disintegration of the vasculature of the corpus luteum.

It has also been suggested that $PGF_{2\alpha}$ affects the number of available LH receptors in the corpus luteum [83], but this change may be expressed too late to account for the prompt decline in luteal progesterone secretion [8]. Lindner et al. [123] have implied that $PGF_{2\alpha}$ exerts its luteolytic action not by an independent action on the luteal cell, but by interfering with the action of LH. This view conforms to the general concept that prostaglandins act chiefly as modulators of the action of other hormones.

The effect of $PGF_{2\alpha}$ administration on the functional performance of the human corpus luteum has been investigated in several studies. Hillier et al. [85] reported a reduced progesterone output after infusion of 12.5–205 μg/min of $PGF_{2\alpha}$ in the late luteal phase of the menstrual cycle. No effect was observed in patients treated during the early luteal phase of the cycle. Vaginal spotting occurred following infusion, but the menstrual cycle was not shortened. A transient fall in progesterone concentration was also observed by Wentz and Jones [179] during intravenous infusion of 50 μg/min $PGF_{2\alpha}$. However, in most of the studies published, no significant fall in plasma progesterone could be detected [89,184].

Even the intrauterine route of administration seems ineffective. Lyneham et al. [127] administered $PGF_{2\alpha}$ into the uterus via a Foley catheter over a 12-hour period to eight healthy volunteers. The amount of $PGF_{2\alpha}$ infused varied between 500 and 2000 μg every second hour for six doses. There was no evidence of luteolysis in any patient, although vaginal bleeding of varying duration occurred in all women within 36 hours of administration of $PGF_{2\alpha}$.

It may be concluded that $PGF_{2\alpha}$ administered systemically or locally into the uterus during the menstrual cycle is not luteolytic or only weakly so. However, $PGF_{2\alpha}$ is rapidly broken down in the lung and liver, and only a small amount may reach the corpus luteum. The experimental conditions could well be insufficient for the induction of functional luteolysis.

To overcome this weakness in the experimental design, Lyneham et al. [127] recently studied the effect of the administration of $PGF_{2\alpha}$ directly into the corpus luteum. These investigators performed laparoscopy in five patients during the secretory phase and injected various amounts of $PGF_{2\alpha}$ into the corpora lutea. Doses of 100 µg of $PGF_{2\alpha}$ had no effect on peripheral plasma progesterone levels or uterine bleeding. However, an injection of 500 or 1000 µg produced a rapid and profound fall in plasma progesterone level coinciding with the onset of uterine bleeding. The plasma levels of progesterone returned to normal luteal levels for 3 days despite the continued bleeding, and then fell again.

Since $PGF_{2\alpha}$ is metabolized rapidly in vivo, interest has been directed toward the development of metabolically resistant analogues with a high affinity for the human corpus luteum. Studies by Hammarström et al. [75] have suggested that 17-phenyl $PGF_{2\alpha}$ and 15-methyl $PGF_{2\alpha}$ have a very high affinity for the $PGF_{2\alpha}$ receptors. These compounds are also protected from rapid metabolic degradation. The effect of these two analogues on human corpus luteum function has recently been investigated [118]. Intravenous infusion of both compounds during 2 consecutive days in the secretory phase of the menstrual cycle did lower serum progesterone, but only transiently. The menstrual cycle was also slightly shortened in some of the cases.

Both the studies just cited indicate that if a high PG concentration in the corpus luteum is obtained, the effect on the peripheral plasma concentration will be influenced more markedly but the corpus luteum still will not regress. Obviously, long-term infusion of $PGF_{2\alpha}$ into the ovarian artery would determine beyond doubt whether $PGF_{2\alpha}$ is luteolytic in humans. Ethical considerations have prohibited such studies.

Recent studies in women [9] have demonstrated a close anatomical relationship between the tortuous ovarian artery and the utero-ovarian vein. The vascular arrangement is very similar to that found in the sheep. If ^{85}Kr was infused into the utero-ovarian vein in women undergoing hysterectomy, an increase of radioactivity was recorded in the ovary in five out of eight cases. Radioactivity in the control ovary showed no increase in one of the two women in whom the radioactivity of both ovaries was measured. The results indicate that a local transfer of gas from the ovarian branch of the uterine vein into the adjacent ovary, which may be due to a countercurrent exchange mechanism between the vessels of the human uterine adnexa similar to that demonstrated in the sheep, could take place also in the human [10].

An interesting observation is that human chorionic gonadotropin (HCG) stimulated the formation of cyclic AMP in incubated fresh human corpus luteum up to at least 10 days of age. Moderate concentrations of $PGF_{2\alpha}$ concentrations (0.1–1.0 µg/ml) caused no or only a slight inhibition of cyclic AMP formation but inhibited strongly the stimulating action of HCG [74b].

Specific receptors for $PGF_{2\alpha}$ have also been identified in human corpus luteum. Although, as described above, there are several similarities between animal data and human results concerning the role of $PGF_{2\alpha}$ in the regulation of the life span of the corpus luteum, at least one fundamental difference exists: hysterectomy does not influence the cyclic events of the human ovary. Nor did Kindahl et al. find any increase in circulating levels of 15-keto-13,14-dihydro $PG_{2\alpha}$ during the luteal phase [117] (Fig. 1). Powell and co-workers [141] have suggested that the human corpus luteum is insensitive to the luteolytic action of exogenous $PGF_{2\alpha}$ because the compound is synthesized locally in the ovary and $PGF_{2\alpha}$ produced in the ovary plays a role in the regulation of the life span of the corpus luteum.

In the human the maintenance of pregnancy depends on a functional corpus luteum until approximately the seventh week of pregnancy calculated from the last menstrual period [48]. During this early stage of gestation, administration of appropriate doses of $PGF_{2\alpha}$ in humans will result in an abortion in almost all cases [28,46].

There are several possible mechanisms by which prostaglandin may act. The compounds may have a direct luteolytic effect in early pregnancy, or they may stimulate intensive uterine contractions, resulting in the expulsion of the conceptus without directly influencing the functional performance of the corpus luteum.

It is generally agreed that intravenous, intrauterine, or vaginal administration of effective doses of $PGF_{2\alpha}$ or prostaglandin analogues during early pregnancy is associated with a significant decrease of the plasma progesterone concentration in peripheral plasma 4–6 hours after the initiation of treatment. The treatment also results in an intensive stimulation of uterine contractility, which significantly precedes the decline in progesterone [28,46,184]. It is therefore likely that the abortifacient effect of prostaglandins in the human is mainly due to induced uterine contractility. The fall in plasma progesterone probably reflects a disruption of the implanted ovum rather than a primary luteolytic effect of the compound. The secondary removal of the possible luteolytic support of the conceptus may also be an important factor in the fall of plasma progesterone levels.

Nonpregnant Uterus

The effect of prostaglandins on the contractility of the human nonpregnant uterus has attracted interest for many years. Initially attention was aroused by the possible importance of prostaglandins in human fertility. Today interest is also stimulated by the possibility that endogenous prostaglandins are of importance in the regulation of both normal and abnormal uterine activity, especially during menstruation.

EFFECT OF PROSTAGLANDINS ON UTERINE CONTRACTILITY

The first reports on the action of prostaglandins on the nonpregnant myometrium were based on in vitro studies. These studies showed that PGE compounds generally inhibited and PGF compounds stimulated the contractility of human myometrial strips [19].

The effect in vivo on human uterine contractility differs to some extent

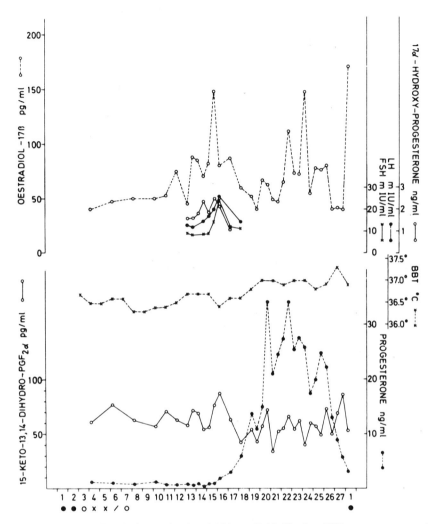

FIGURE 1. Peripheral plasma levels of 15-keto-13,14-dihydro- PGF$_{2\alpha}$ progesterone, luteinizing hormone (LH), follicle-stimulating hormone (FSH), estradiol, and 17β- and 17α-hydroxy progesterone in one human female. Basal body temperature (BBT) was measured every morning: menstrual bleeding symbolized by solid circles, very scant; open circles, scant; diagonal, moderate; and crosses, strong. (From Kindahl et al. [117], by permission.)

from that observed in vitro. Intravenous injection of PGE and PGF compounds in effective doses regularly result in an elevation of uterine tonus. An increase in frequency and amplitude of the contractions can also be observed in many instances [44,102,146]. The threshold dose of a single intravenous injection is approximately 20 μg of PGE$_1$ or PGE$_2$ and about 50 μg of PGF$_{2\alpha}$. Continuous intravenous infusion of PGF$_{2\alpha}$ or PGE$_2$ over a period of several hours induces a contractility pattern with contractions of high amplitude, similar to that observed during menstruation [146].

The effect of other prostaglandins (e.g., thromboxane and prostacyclin) on the contractility pattern of the human uterus remains to be studied.

Oral administration of 1.0 mg of PGE$_2$ in tablet form in most cases also results in a stimulation of uterine activity during both the proliferative and secretory phases of the menstrual cycle. It is noteworthy that an inhibitory response to oral administration of PGE$_2$ during the first days of menstrual bleeding has been reported [22].

Following systemic administration, only a small and possibly variable amount may reach the uterus because of the rapid metabolic degradation of the compounds in lung and liver. More precise information on the sensitivity of the myometrium to prostaglandins may therefore be obtained if the compounds are administered locally into the uterus. From the end of menstruation until approximately 4 days before ovulation, intrauterine instillation of small amounts of either PGE$_2$ or PGF$_{2\alpha}$ generally results in stimulation of uterine contractility. The effect can be characterized by a gradual rise in uterine tonus accompanied by increased amplitude of contractions. No evidence of inhibition is observed. As little as 1 µg of either compound usually effects a response, and stimulation is sustained or more pronounced if larger doses are administered [130–132,171,172].

In contrast to the stimulatory response of the preovulatory uterus, higher doses of PGE$_2$ or PGF$_{2\alpha}$ at about the time of ovulation induce little change in the typical low amplitude, high frequency pattern. An inhibition has been reported when the dose of PGE$_2$ is increased further to 100 or 200 µg, and this may have importance in passive sperm transport [172].

In the latter part of the secretory phase locally administered PGE$_2$ or PGF$_{2\alpha}$ normally results in stimulation of uterine contractility, whereas during menstrual bleeding inhibition following PGE$_2$ instillation has been reported [132]. Uterine contractility is inhibited by small amounts (1–5 µg) of PGE$_2$ and more strongly depressed by larger doses (40 µg). PGF$_{2\alpha}$, on the other hand, stimulates uterine contractility even during menstruation.

REGULATION OF UTERINE CONTRACTILITY

The nonpregnant human uterus exhibits a characteristic general pattern of spontaneous activity that varies during the different phases of the menstrual cycle. In midcycle the contractility is characterized by frequent contractions of low amplitude, whereas during menstruation low frequency contractions with high amplitude are typical. It has been supposed that the variation in ovarian hormone production plays an important role in the regulation of uterine activity. There are, however, many reasons to believe that endogenous prostaglandins are also involved.

Both PGE_2 and $PGF_{2\alpha}$ are present in human endometrium, and several studies indicate an increased synthesis as menstruation approaches [37,125,144]. At least in animals, the synthesis is stimulated by estradiol acting together with progesterone [142]. Administration of indomethacin diminishes uterine contractility not only in dysmenorrhoic but also in healthy women [126]. At least during late secretory phase and during menstruation, the concentration in the endometrium of endogenous $PGF_{2\alpha}$ seems to be high enough to cause stimulation of uterine contractility, keeping in mind that at this time 1–4 µg of $PGF_{2\alpha}$ administered into the uterine cavity has an obvious effect. Although in many animals $PGF_{2\alpha}$ produced by the endometrium regulates the life span of the corpus luteum, in the human it may be of importance in maintaining uterine tone and spontaneous motility.

PRIMARY DYSMENORRHEA

A pathological uterine contractility pattern is observed during dysmenorrhea. The existence of a high tonus level (> 50 mm Hg) between contractions and high amplitudes of the concentrations has been emphasized. The local endometrial blood flow decreases during the contractions. The decrease is most pronounced during contractions of high amplitude and long duration and without periods of proper relaxation in between. The combination of a long-lasting ischemia and hypercontractility is considered to be responsible for the menstrual pain [1]. Several studies utilizing gas chromatography–mass spectrometry measurements of the endometrium, and radioimmunoassay of jet wash specimens and menstrual blood flow have demonstrated several times higher levels of $PGF_{2\alpha}$ in women suffering from dysmenorrhea than in normal volunteers [37,125,144]. An increased concentration of the metabolite 15-keto-13,14-dihydro-$PGF_{2\alpha}$ in peripheral blood during dysmenorrhea has also been reported (Fig. 2) [125]. Treatment with prostaglandin biosynthesis inhibitors produced a rapid change of the contractility pattern with a decrease in basal tonus, and in low amplitude and frequency of the contractions, accompanied by complete pain relief in many dysmenorrheic patients [47,126]. Administration of either oral contraceptives or indomethacin resulted in normalization of the elevated plasma levels of 15-keto-13,14-dihydro-$PGF_{2\alpha}$ [125]. The rapid effect of prostaglandin biosynthesis inhibitors on uterine contractility that was demonstrated (1–2 hours) probably reflects the immediate inhibition of the enhanced synthesis of prostaglandins and supports the idea that premenstrual storage of increased amounts of prostaglandins is of minor importance in the development of uterine hypercontractility.

Data available today strongly suggest that an increased concentration of $PGF_{2\alpha}$ is an important part of the pathophysiology of primary dysmenorrhea. Since, however, prostaglandin levels are not elevated in all patients with primary dysmenorrhea, the PG theory cannot explain the myometrial hyperactivity in all cases. Furthermore, other uterine stimulants may well act via final prostaglandin release.

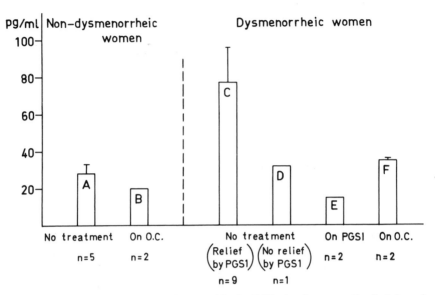

FIGURE 2. Concentration of 15-keto-13,14-dihydro-$PGF_{2\alpha}$ in plasma on the first day of menstruation: OC = oral contraceptives; PGSI = prostaglandin synthetase inhibitors; n = number of patients. (From Lundström and Gréen [125] by permission.)

UTERINE BLEEDING

As described above, prostaglandins are produced by the endometrium in increasing amounts as the time of menstruation approaches. The physiological significance of this circumstance was discussed in relation to uterine contractility, but the increased production may also be of importance for the regulation of uterine bleeding. Administration of classical prostaglandins (PGE_2 or $PGF_{2\alpha}$) to nonpregnant women will induce bleeding. The bleeding is believed to result from strong uterine contractions [184]. The most recent support for a role of prostaglandins in the monthly shedding of the endometrium is derived from observations that menstrual blood loss can be significantly reduced by the administration of prostaglandin biosynthesis inhibitors [4,49].

Several authors have suggested that dysfunctional and organic bleeding, and bleeding induced by intrauterine devices (IUDs) are associated with overproduction of E and F prostaglandins (for references, see Topozada [170]). Recently, both $PGF_{2\alpha}$ and PGE_2 were measured by radioimmunoassay in endometrial tissue obtained at different phases of the menstrual cycle from 17 women with dysfunctional menorrhagia, and the results were compared with levels in 12 eumenorrhoic women. Subjects with menorrhagia had significantly higher concentrations of PGE_2 in the premenstrual phase compared with women with a normal loss [77]. Administration of prostaglandin biosynthesis inhibitors to patients with an IUD was also found to reduce significantly the mean blood loss during two menstrual periods in comparison with two pre- and two posttreatment cycles. Although these observations suggest that prostaglandins may have a role in the menstrual process, the substances chiefly involved and the mechanisms by which this local action is exerted remain to be identified.

Studies performed so far have evaluated mainly the role of classical prostaglandins. It is well known, however, that the endoperoxide intermediates PGG_2 and PGH_2, as well as thromboxane A_2 and prostacyclin, which are all formed from arachidonic acid, have profound effects on platelet aggregation, on clot formation, and on vascular tonus; thus certainly they also have the capacity to be involved in the regulation of menstrual bleeding.

Pregnant Uterus

EFFECT OF PROSTAGLANDINS ON CONTRACTILITY

One of the first observations on the effects of the prostaglandins was that they influence the activity of human myometrium. The first experiments were with whole or crude extracts of seminal plasma known to contain high levels of a mixture of prostaglandins; overall, a relaxing effect on human nonpregnant myometrium was observed [19]. A difference in the effect on the prostaglandins was also observed, depending on whether the myometrium was from a pregnant or a nonpregnant woman [19]. In general, prostaglandins of the E and F series show the most marked effect on pregnant myometrium, namely, stimulation. Early work [27] concentrated on assessing threshold dose administered by bolus injection. This approach established that E prostaglandins were about 10 times more active than F prostaglandins in stimulating pregnant myometrium and that the prostaglandins were able to stimulate the human pregnant uterus at early stages of gestation. Thus these substances differ from the best known oxytocic, oxytocin, which has very little oxytocic activity in the first and second trimester. The threshold dose experiments also indicated that the myometrial sensitivity increases in the third trimester, becoming maximal near term. These facts have played a large part in determining the therapeutic uses of oxytocin and prostaglandin, as discussed later.

INTERACTIONS WITH OXYTOCIN

Enhancement of Myometrial Response to Oxytocin by Prostaglandin. In 1966 Pickles et al. [139] described a phenomenon, which they named "enhancement," whereby the rat myometrial response to oxytocin was markedly increased, for periods of up to 90 minutes, after exposure to ketonic prostaglandins. The essence of the enhancement response is that the increased response to oxytocin occurs after the exposure to the prostaglandin has ceased. This phenomenon has been described for human pregnant myometrium both in vitro [15] and in vivo [60]. Prostaglandins of the F series do not cause enhancement.

Potentiation of Myometrial Response to Oxytocin and Prostaglandins. When pregnant rat myometrium is exposed to oxytocin and PGE or PGF, a potentiation of the stimulatory myometrial response occurs and the amplitude of contractile response elicited by the prostaglandin and oxytocin together is greater than the sum of the amplitudes of contractile responses elicited by the two stimulants administered separately [139]. In contrast to enhancement, both the E and F prostaglandins exhibit potentiation when administered concurrently with oxytocin. Potentiation of human myometrial response has been described in vitro [151] and in vivo [60].

Whether the gestational-dependent differences in myometrial sensitivity to oxytocin and prostaglandins and enhancement or potentiation of myometrial response to oxytocin by prostaglandins have a physiological role is not yet clear.

OCCURRENCE OF ENDOGENOUS PROSTAGLANDINS IN LABOR

There is now an abundance of evidence in the domestic animals investigated that a surge of prostaglandin production by intrauterine tissues precedes the onset of parturition [169]. This phenomenon has not been demonstrated in the human, and there has not yet been a clear demonstration of a change in prostaglandin synthesis before the onset of uterine contractions in the human female. There is, however, much circumstantial evidence to implicate the prostaglandins in human parturition.

Peripheral Blood Levels of Prostaglandins in Pregnancy. There are numerous reports of measurement of levels of prostaglandins in blood during pregnancy in the human. Results are varied and contradictory. Some reports [14,36,69,79,175] have indicated that blood levels in the third trimester are the same as in nonpregnant women. Levels in the midtrimester have been reported as maximal [69] or minimal [79]. The measured range covered by the articles cited is enormous and varies from levels of about 30 to nearly 2000 pg/ml.

In general, higher levels have been found in labor than in the antenatal period [14,32,79,97], but there is not agreement about changes in concentration during labor, since PGF levels have been variously reported as highest in the first stage [14,17] and highest at delivery [39,97]. An increase in PGF concentration with the progress of labor has been reported by some authors [14,17,32,97], but this effect has not been found by others [16,64,84]. The levels of PGE in plasma [81,95,140] have not been studied as extensively as PGF levels, and any correlation between plasma levels of PGE, gestation, and labor is not possible.

Much of the variation in results reported by the authors cited above is due either to assay methodology or to release of $PGF_{2\alpha}$ (and also PGE_2)

from platelets during collection or subsequent handling of the blood sample, or autoxidation of precursor fatty acids. This circumstance, plus the known short half-life (< 1 minute [62,73]) of the primary prostaglandins, makes it apparent that many measurements of levels of prostaglandins in plasma have given little information about endogenous production of prostaglandins in the whole body, let alone in the uterus.

Recent work—undertaken with great care to minimize the generation or prostaglandins by collecting the blood into ice cold tubes containing acetylsalicylic acid and ethylenediaminetetraacetic acid, using highly specific and sensitive radioimmunoassay techniques, and avoiding sampling within 1 hour of cervical assessment—failed to show any statistically significant difference between plasma levels of PGE and PGF in late pregnancy, early labor, and late labor [135]. The concentrations measured (in the order of 5 pg/ml for PGE and 8 pg/ml for PGF) were in the range expected on the basis of prostaglandin infusion studies with measurement by gas-liquid chromatography–mass spectrometry methods [7]. A significant rise in levels of 13,14-dihydro-15-keto-prostaglandin F in peripheral plasma occurred with the onset of labor. This substance, the principal metabolite of PGF, has a longer half-life (8 minutes) than the primary prostaglandins and is now considered to be the compound of choice to monitor as a measure of PGF production [64].

Thus it would seem that the validity of much of the early work in assessing levels of prostaglandins in peripheral circulation throughout pregnancy and labor is in doubt. Even with the most accurate methods of assay and care to avoid generation of prostaglandins during collection, no change in peripheral levels of the primary prostaglandins has been shown to occur with the onset of labor. Despite this, the levels of a major metabolite do increase, indicating that there is an increase in prostaglandin metabolism with the onset of labor in the human [64,135].

Several authors have measured prostaglandin levels in blood from the uterine vein on the assumption that such readings may better reflect the endogenous intrauterine production. No difference in prostaglandin levels in uterine venous plasma and peripheral plasma was reported by one group [140], whereas another group found higher levels in uterine venous plasma than in peripheral plasma [90]. A study [108] of uterine venous prostaglandin levels before and after labor showed higher levels after labor than before.

Amniotic Fluid and Prostaglandin Content. The difficulties associated with the generation of prostaglandins in plasma, due to the trauma of collection of blood, are not present in studies of amniotic fluid, which does not show significant synthesis or catabolism of the prostaglandins. Many workers have examined amniotic fluid, at various gestations and in labor. Large interstudy variations in concentrations have been reported, but in general it has been found that amniotic fluid concentrations in early and midpregnancy are lower than near term [51,82,90, 109,147] and that levels during labor are higher than before labor [51,82,84,91,100,109,112,147]. Furthermore, some authors have found that the concentrations of PGF [51,109] and PGE [51,112] increase progressively during the course of labor.

Thus it would seem that there is an accumulation of PGE and PGF in the amniotic fluid during labor in the human and that this results from an increase in the intrauterine production of prostaglandins E and F during labor. The increase may well be a result of an increase in substrate availability as the concentration of free arachidonic acid in liquor increases from before labor to established labor [110,128]. On the other hand, no statistically significant relationship was observed between concentrations of arachidonic acid and PGF and its metabolite [110]. Further evidence for an increase in prostaglandin synthesis during labor comes from measurements of the chief metabolite, 13,14-dihydro-15-keto-$F_{2\alpha}$, in liquor during labor, where a significant increase was demonstrated [111].

Prostaglandin Levels in the Umbilical Circulation. Levels of prostaglandins in umbilical arterial and venous plasma have been measured by several investigators [35,45,140]. No consistent arteriovenous difference has been demonstrated, and it is not likely that these measurements will reflect the true levels in the fetus because at the time of sampling (at delivery), closure of the umbilical vessels is occurring and this process itself is thought to result from generation of prostaglandins locally. In one study where care was taken at blood collection to minimize generation of prostaglandins, an arteriovenous excess for PGE but not PGF or 13,14-dihydro-15-keto-PGF was demonstrated [134].

Prostaglandin Metabolism and Synthesis in the Uterus. Arachidonic acid in its free form is the obligatory precursor for the synthesis of PGE_2 and $PGF_{2\alpha}$ via the "prostaglandin synthetase" group of enzymes. Fatty acids are not usually found in large amounts in the free form but are stored by incorporation into phospholipids.

Arachidonic acid accounts for about 20% of the total fatty acid content of the glycerophospholipids of chorioamnion and decidua. By comparison, the arachidonic acid content of parietal peritoneum near term, is only 0.4% [151]. The significance of this difference in arachidonic acid concentration is not clear. However, since the arachidonic acid content of fetal membranes has been estimated as 50–60 mg and since only 25–35 μg/24 hours of $PGF_{2\alpha}$ is formed during the course of labor [70], the membranes may hold potential precursor for much greater prostaglandin production than is thought necessary for labor [151]. That this "precursor storage" is a function of the membrane is suggested by the demonstration of a slight decrease in the arachidonic acid content of fetal membranes obtained after labor compared with the content of membranes obtained before labor [151].

The incorporation of the fatty acids, arachidonic, and palmitic acids into amnion phospholipids has been studied in vitro [152]. Palmitic acid is a saturated fatty acid and is not a precursor for prostaglandin synthesis. Both fatty acids were incorporated readily into amnion phospholipids. Of the arachidonic acid incorporated, most was into lecithin (53%) and phosphatidylethanolamine (27%), and this distribution corresponds to the concentrations of these phospholipids in human amnion at term [143]. The palmitic acid was incorporated mainly into lecithin (70%) and less into phosphatidylethanolamine (11%). Lecithin in amnion at term contains 36% palmitic acid and only 8% arachidonic acid. Since these concentrations are not in the same ratio as the incorporation rates of palmitic (70%) and arachidonic acids (53%), a high turnover rate of arachidonic acid is suggested. These studies also showed that arachidonic acid incorporation by membranes before labor was 33% less than by membranes after labor [152].

If membrane arachidonic acid is to be a precursor for prostaglandin synthesis, a means of liberating it from the phospholipids must be present. Arachidonic acid is usually incorporated into glycerophospholipids in the 2-acyl position; hence a phospholipase A_2 is required for liberation of the arachidonic acid. Human chorioamnion has been shown to contain a high level of phospholipase A_2 activity [151], and this enzyme is also present in decidua [151]. The greatest enzyme activity occurs in amnion and decidua, with much less in chorion and almost none in myometrium [65]. No difference in activity has been shown with the onset of labor, but evidence that the enzyme is active at that time is found in the demonstration of an eightfold increase in amniotic fluid arachidonic acid from before labor to established labor [128], the increase during labor being correlated with cervical dilatation [110]. Most workers favor a lysosomal origin for the phospholipase A_2, the lysosomal site being either the decidua [2,67,68,151] or the fetal membranes [151,154].

Fetal membranes have been examined for their ability to metabolize prostaglandins. High rates of both synthesis and degradation of prostaglandins were demonstrated in chorion, with very little metabolism occurring in the amnion [113]. Biosynthesis of the prostaglandins has also been demonstrated in umbilical cord [93] and decidua [160]. The significance of these in vitro findings in relation to the events occurring in labor in utero is not clear.

Thus it seems that the prostaglandins play a role in parturition in the human. The fetal membranes contain high levels of prostaglandin precursors and the enzymes necessary to release them. The juxtaposition of membranes, decidua, and myometrium is ideal for a local action of synthesized prostaglandin. Once myometrial activity is initiated, local microtrauma may promote further local prostaglandin synthesis and increased uterine contractions. With dilatation of the cervix, the reflex release of oxytocin from the posterior pituitary is thought to occur. The released oxytocin may in turn act synergistically with the synthesized prostaglandin to allow the evolution of the myometrial activity of labor. The stimulus to the commencement of this progressive activity originates in the fetus in domestic animals [169]; the role of the human fetus has not yet been demonstrated.

Fallopian Tubes

The effect of exogenous prostaglandins on tubal motility in vivo and in vitro has been studied in several animal species. Generally PGE compounds inhibit spontaneous contractions of the fallopian tube; whereas PGF compounds stimulate tubal contractility. It has been suggested that prostaglandins may play a physiological role in ovum transport, and that the oviductal response to prostaglandin depends on the endocrine status of the animal. The sensitivity of the tubes to the stimulating compound $PGF_{2\alpha}$ increases at ovulation. Progesterone increases the responsiveness to the inhibitory effect of PGE_2 and decreases the stimulatory effect of $PGF_{2\alpha}$. The specific binding of $PGF_{2\alpha}$ and PGE_2 to tubal tissue also agrees with the pattern of egg transport [157].

There are reasons to believe that prostaglandins also possess important functions in the control of smooth muscle activity in the human fallopian tube. Both PGE and PGF compounds have been shown by histoimmunological techniques to occur in high concentrations in human tubal mucosa [138].

EFFECT OF PROSTAGLANDINS ON TUBAL CONTRACTILITY

Early in vitro studies by Sandberg et al. [149,150] indicated that the human oviduct is extremely sensitive to both PGE and PGF compounds. PGE_1 and PGE_2 increase the tonus of longitudinal muscle strips from the proximal portion and relax those from the distal segment of the human fallopian tubes. The F compounds invariably induce a stimulatory response.

Recently a series of studies on spontaneous motility and reactivity to different prostaglandins of the different muscle layers of the human fallopian tube has been published. The spontaneous contractility of muscle strips dissected from the outer longitudinal and the inner circular muscle layers at the ampullary-isthmic junction was recorded. It was found that the amplitude and the duration of individual contractions are similar during various phases of the menstrual cycle, whereas the frequency of contractions is significantly increased during the periovulatory period in both muscle layers. It was concluded from these studies that endogenous estrogens stimulate human oviductal contractility, whereas endogenous progesterone has a depressive action on tubal activity [122]. Pretreatment with a blocker of endogenous prostaglandin synthesis abolishes the spontaneous contractile activity of the human oviduct in vitro in a concentration-dependent manner [33].

The effect of different prostaglandins on the different muscle layers of the oviduct is complex. In general, however, prostaglandins of the E type inhibit the spontaneous activity in the circulating musculature and increase contractile activity in the longitudinal layer, whereas $PGF_{2\alpha}$ causes marked stimulation on both layers [33,121,183]. $PGF_{2\alpha}$ was found to reduce the tissue cyclic AMP levels concomitantly with its stimulatory effect on contractility and PGE_2 to increase the cyclic AMP content in the circular layer, as well as inhibiting myogenic activity.

In vivo, either intravenous injection or instillation of $PGF_{2\alpha}$ into the tubal lumen stimulates tubal contractility, and PGE_2 administered by the same routes inhibits it [44].

REGULATION OF TUBAL CONTRACTILITY

A relation between the adrenergic system and prostaglandins has been shown for a number of tissues. It is possible that the hormonal control of tubal contractility in the human is mediated both by autonomic nervous mechanisms and by local synthesis of prostaglandins.

The physiological role of endogenous prostaglandins in the fallopian tube in relation to fertilization and ovum transport is largely unexplored. It seems probable, however, that the prostaglandins may participate in the highly intricate regulation of these mechanisms.

CLINICAL APPLICATIONS

Considering all the possible physiological functions of different prostaglandins, it is not surprising that a variety of clinical applications have been suggested. So far, however, prostaglandins are used routinely only on indications related to their stimulating effects on human myometrium.

Termination of Pregnancy

Termination of pregnancy by induced abortion is practiced all over the world. Although new, more effective, and more acceptable contraceptive methods have been introduced, therapeutic abortion does not seem to have lost its importance as a means of fertility control.

Considerable efforts have been made and also are desirable in the future to improve the abortion technology. Further improvements in terms of minimizing complications, increasing effectiveness, technical ease of performance, and convenience, and reducing costs are still possible to achieve. This is especially true for second-trimester abortion, where the techniques in current use result in significantly higher maternal morbidity and mortality in comparison with first-trimester abortion.

SECOND TRIMESTER

Extra- or intraamniotic administration of $PGF_{2\alpha}$ and PGE_2 for termination of second-trimester pregnancy has been used on a routine basis since 1974. Several effective and well-tolerated dose schedules have been developed (Table 3). If the extraamniotic route is used, two-hourly doses of 750 μg of $PGF_{2\alpha}$ or 200 μg of PGE_2 are instilled via a Foley catheter introduced through the cervical canal. A success rate between 85% and 95% within 36 hours has been reported [20,58]. Instillation of prostaglandins into the extraamniotic space produces adequate myometrial

TABLE 3. Approximate Doses of Prostaglandin for Termination of
Second-Trimester Pregnancy

Route of administration	Compound		
	$PGF_{2\alpha}$	PGE_2	15(S)15-1 Methyl $PGF_{2\alpha}$
Intravenous	~ 100 mg (50–100 μg/min)	~ 10 mg (5–10 μg/min)	~ 5 mg (2.5 μg/min)
Extraamniotic	~ 5 mg (~ 9 × 0.75 mg)	~ 1–2 mg (~ 9 × 0.25 mg)	~ 1 mg (once)
Intraamniotic	40–50 mg (once)	5–10 mg (once)	2.5 mg (once)
Vaginal suppositories	—	60–80 mg (3 or 4 × 20 mg)	3.0 mg* (once)
Intramuscular	—	—	2.0 mg (6 × 0.3 mg)

*Methyl ester.

stimulation, while maintaining low plasma levels of the drugs. Interruption of pregnancy by extraamniotic administration of PGE_2 or $PGF_{2\alpha}$ can be accomplished with total doses 10–20 times lower than are required by the intravenous route; consequently, systemic side effects are markedly reduced.

Intraamniotic administration is mainly used after the fifteenth week of pregnancy, when the amniotic cavity is more easily punctured. Several different dose schedules have been suggested for intraamniotic administration of $PGF_{2\alpha}$. Among these are 25 mg repeated after 6 hours, or a single dose of 40 or 50 mg. Reinstillation of 20–40 mg of $PGF_{2\alpha}$ has been given after 24–48 hours if required, depending on the patient's response.

Several multicenter studies organized by the World Health Organization [180,181] have shown that a single intraamniotic dose of 50 mg of $PGF_{2\alpha}$ is as effective as a 25-mg dose of $PGF_{2\alpha}$ repeated after 6 hours (86.6% and 85.6%, respectively), but superior to 40 mg (80.5%). Side effects and complications are generally of the same magnitude for the three dose schedules used.

Two studies randomly comparing intraamniotic administration of hypertonic saline with $PGF_{2\alpha}$ given by the same route have been published [53,180]. The studies show that intraamniotic administration of $PGF_{2\alpha}$ is more effective than unaugmented hypertonic saline. $PGF_{2\alpha}$ is also easier to administer, since the volume to be injected (8–10 ml) is much smaller than that of hypertonic saline (200 ml).

For a number of hypothetical reasons intraamniotic $PGF_{2\alpha}$ may also be less dangerous than saline: (1) hypernatremia is not a risk, (2) inadvertent intravascular or intraperitoneal injection of $PGF_{2\alpha}$ appears to be less dangerous because $PGF_{2\alpha}$ is rapidly metabolized, (3) there is less tissue damage from inappropriate administration of $PGF_{2\alpha}$, and (4) consumptive coagulopathies appear to be less frequent with $PGF_{2\alpha}$ (for references, see Brenner and Berger [13]).

Although as abortifacients the prostaglandins thus may be regarded as safer than saline infusion, comparative studies indicate that in practice, when both methods are used by skilled physicians, there are few differences in complication rates. The frequency of gastrointestinal side effects is higher following $PGF_{2\alpha}$ therapy and possibly also cervical laceration or cervical vaginal fistula, especially if prostaglandin therapy is augmented with intravenous oxytocin administration when there are still significant amounts of intraamniotic $PGF_{2\alpha}$ stimulating the uterus [96].

The most important advantage of prostaglandin in comparison with hypertonic saline and other compounds presently in use for termination of second-trimester pregnancy is, however, that during recent years analogues have been developed that are suitable for noninvasive administration.

Some of the major complications associated with second-trimester abortion are due to inadvertent injections of the compound. If the vaginal or the intramuscular route is used, such complications can be avoided. The simplicity of the treatment will also facilitate large abortion programs in countries that do not have enough trained medical personnel. The noninvasive routes offer the additional advantage that the treatment is equally useful during the early and the latter parts of the second trimester. Delaying the abortion from thirteenth to fifteenth week of pregnancy to after the fifteenth week, when intraamniotic puncture can be performed, is therefore not necessary.

Promising results have been reported for intramuscular injection of 16-phenoxy-ω-tetranor-PGE_2 methyl sulfonylamide, and for vaginal administration of 16,16-dimethyl-trans-Δ^2-PGE_1 methyl ester and 9-deoxo-16,16-dimethyl-9-methylene PGE_2. These analogues appear to be at least as effective as the classical prostaglandins, and the frequency of gastrointestinal side effects is significantly reduced [25,99].

PREOPERATIVE CERVICAL DILATATION

It is generally agreed that the frequency of complications with vacuum aspiration or dilatation and curettage increases with increasing gestational age [52]. Some of these complications (e.g. cervical dilatation and uterine perforation) are directly related to the mechanical dilatation that is necessary for the procedure, especially during the latter part of the first trimester and during the early part of the second trimester. Grimes et al. [66] have reported that if dilatation and curettage is performed after the twelfth week of gestation, cervical injury is twice as frequent and uterine perforation more than six times as frequent as it is with the saline infusion technique.

Other complications (e.g. hemorrhage and incomplete evacuation of the conceptus) may possibly be related to an insufficient or difficult dilatation. The increasing concern about the effects of cervical injuries on long-term reproductive behavior has also focused clinicians' interest on methods producing a gradual cervical dilatation [182]. Several studies show that pretreatment with prostaglandin analogues (e.g. 15-methyl $PGF_{2\alpha}$ methyl ester, 16,16-dimethyl PGE_2 or its p-benzaldehyde semi-carbazone ester, 16-phenoxy-tetranor-PGE_2 methyl sulfonylamide, or 9-deoxo-16,16-dimethyl-9-methylene PGE_2) is an effective therapy to achieve gradual dilatation of the cervix [12,21,59,88,105].

The pretreatment changes the surgical evacuation of the uterus to a simple and more uneventful procedure, even in nulliparous women. In comparison with mechanical dilatation, the risk for operative and post-operative complications is significantly reduced. The drawbacks of the procedure are mainly long pretreatment time, uterine contractions that sometimes are painful, and the occurrence of gastrointestinal side effects.

MENSTRUAL REGULATION

Vacuum aspiration is an effective and safe method for termination of pregnancy during the first trimester. During very early pregnancy it is possible to use a flaccid polyethylene catheter that can be introduced through the cervical canal without dilatation. Nevertheless, skill and training are needed to obtain a high degree of efficacy and a low frequency of complications.

The development of nonsurgical alternatives that are generally applicable and suitable for self-administration is therefore highly warranted, especially in view of the increased number of first-trimester abortions. The recent finding that prostaglandins of the E and F types have the ability to stimulate powerful uterine contractions and to produce abortion not only during second trimester but also in early pregnancy is therefore a significant breakthrough [46,98,136]. If the treatment is restricted to the first three weeks following the first missed menstrual period, the frequency of complete abortion will be high or in the order of 95%. The clinical importance of the finding is, however, dependent on the possibility of prostaglandin treatment to compete with the surgical procedure. Initial experience has been disappointing in that respect, since classical prostaglandins were found to be suitable only following intrauterine administration, and premedication was necessary to limit the frequency of side effects [46,91,136]. However, the availability of prostaglandin analogues has changed the situation. Some of these substances are more active and better tolerated than the classical compounds when administered in therapeutically effective amounts by noninvasive routes.

Successful results of menstrual regulation by treatment with prostaglandin analogues have been reported following intrauterine and vaginal administration. The analogues that seem to be most suitable for intrauterine administration are 15-methyl PGE_2, 15-methyl $PGF_{2\alpha}$ methyl ester, 16-phenoxy-tetranor-PGE_2 methyl sulfonylamide, and 16,16-dimethyl-trans-Δ^2-PGE_1 methyl ester [103,104,161,185], and for vaginal administration, 15-methyl $PGF_{2\alpha}$ methyl ester, 16,16-dimethyl PGE_2, and

16,16-dimethyl-trans-Δ^2-PGE$_1$ methyl ester [28,29,63,74a,106,124,162]. For intrauterine treatment a single injection is used, whereas for vaginal treatment both repeated and single administrations are tried.

ABNORMAL PREGNANCY

The termination of abnormal pregnancy, the occurrence of hydatiform mole, and missed abortion have been gynecological problems for a long time. Surgical evacuation of the uterus is sometimes associated with serious complications. Oxytocin administration is often insufficient to induce effective uterine contractility. Intraamniotic prostaglandin administration is not suitable, and although intravenous infusion or extraamniotic administration of classical prostaglandins may be used, this is by no means an optimal therapy. Noninvasive administration is preferable, and PGE$_2$ vaginal suppositories for this purpose are available in only a few countries. Clinical trials have shown that even better alternatives are intramuscular injections of 17-phenoxy-tetranor-PGE$_2$ methyl sulfonylamide, vaginal administration of 15-methyl PGF$_{2\alpha}$ methyl ester, or single extraamniotic injection of dihomo-15-methyl PGF$_{2\alpha}$ methyl ester [101].

Induction of Labor

The first report on the clinical application of a prostaglandin goes back to 1968, when Karim described the use of PGF$_{2\alpha}$ for labor induction [97]. During the past few years intravenous administration of PGE$_2$ or PGF$_{2\alpha}$ has become an alternative to oxytocin for labor induction. The initial recommended dose for PGE$_2$ is 0.1–0.2 μg/min, and for PGF$_{2\alpha}$ it is 1.0–2.0 μg/min. The dose level is progressively stepped up with intervals of 30–60 minutes until there is adequate myometrial stimulation, or up to 1–2 μg/min for PGE$_2$ or 10–20 μg/min for PGF$_{2\alpha}$. Induction combining amniotomy with intravenous infusion of PGE$_2$ or PGF$_{2\alpha}$ has effected delivery within 24 hours in nearly all women treated [3,167]. Side effects (mainly vomiting, diarrhea, and transient venous erythema) may occur, but are usually of minor severity and do not require interruption of drug administration [3].

In comparative studies, PGE$_2$, PGF$_{2\alpha}$, and oxytocin appear to be equally effective in patients with favorable prognosis for induction. The prostaglandins are slightly superior for complicated inductions and in pregnancies complicated by fetal death or anencephaly. The margin of effective dose is somewhat narrower for prostaglandins, and the frequency of gastrointestinal side effects is commoner with PGF$_{2\alpha}$ [167].

PGE$_2$ may also be administered by the oral route in contrast to oral PGF$_{2\alpha}$, which causes an unacceptably high rate of gastrointestinal side effects. A commonly used dose schedule is one initial dose of 0.5 mg increased to 1.0 or 1.5 mg with intervals of 30–60 minutes [54,168]. Oral PGE$_2$ administration and intravenous infusion of oxytocin, if combined with early amniotomy, seem to be equally effective [114,145]. This method is generally well accepted by patients. The main advantage is the ease and simplicity of the treatment. Complications are rare, particularly in multiparous patients with good prospects of inducibility.

Cervical Ripening

The possibility of ripening the cervix at or near term is an important new therapeutic possibility for prostaglandins. An unripe cervix in late pregnancy is a bad prognostic sign, especially in the primigravida. If labor has to be induced, it may be protracted and difficult. Although the cervix ripens if given time, few, if any, obstetrical indications for delivery diminish with the passage of time. The normal mechanism by which the cervix ripens before effacement and dilatation during labor is still unknown. Experimental data suggest that prostaglandins, possibly together with placental hormones, have a physiological role [57].

Prostaglandins, mainly PGE_2, have been administered orally, vaginally, into the cervical canal, or into the extraamniotic space in clinical trials. Data indicate that extraamniotic or intracervical administration of 0.5 mg of PGE_2 in gel form is more effective than other routes of administration. If cervical ripening is obtained, reduced fetal and maternal complications rates will result [31,174]. The disadvantages of the therapy at present are the risk associated with the introduction of an extraamniotic catheter and lack of stable prostaglandin preparations available for routine clinical use.

REFERENCES

1. Åkerlund, M., Andersson, K. E., and Ingemarsson., I. (1976) Effect of terbutaline on myometrial activity, uterine blood flow and lower abdominal pain in women with primary dysmenorrhea. Br. J. Obstet. Gynaecol. 83, 673–680.
2. Akesson, B. (1975) Occurrence of phospholipase A_1 and A_2 in human decidua. Prostaglandins 9, 667–673.
3. Amy, J. J., and Thiery, M. (1979) Induction of labour with prostaglandins. In: S. M. M. Karim (ed.), Practical Applications of Prostaglandins and Their Synthesis Inhibitors, MTP Press, Lancaster, pp. 437–446.
4. Anderson, A. B. M., Haynes, P. P., Guilleband, J., and Turnbull, A. C. (1976) Reduction of menstrual blood loss by prostaglandin synthetase inhibitors. Lancet 1, 774–776.
5. Armstrong, D. T., Grinwich, D. L., Moon, Y. S., and Zamecnik, J. (1974) Inhibition of ovulation in rabbits by intrafollicular injection of indomethacin and prostaglandin F antiserum. Life Sci. 14, 129–140.
6. Asplund, J. A. (1947) A quantitative determination of the content of contractive substances in human sperm and their significance for the motility and vitality of the spermatozoa. Acta Physiol. Scand. 13, 103–108.
7. Béguin, F. M., Bygdeman, M., Gréen, K., Samuelsson, B., Toppozada, M., and Wiqvist, N. (1972) Analysis of prostaglandin $F_{2\alpha}$ and metabolites in blood during constant intravenous infusion of prostaglandin $F_{2\alpha}$ in the human female. Acta Physiol. Scand. 86, 430–432.
8. Behrman, H. R., and Hichens, M. (1976) Rapid block of gonadotropin uptake by corpora lutea in vivo induced by prostaglandin $F_{2\alpha}$. Prostaglandins 12, 83–95.

9. Bendz, A. (1977) The anatomical basis for a possible countercurrent exchange mechanism in the human adnex. Prostaglandins 13, 355–362.

10. Bendz, A., Einer-Jensen, N., Lundgren, O., and Jansson, P. O. (1979) Exchange of krypton-85 between the blood vessels of the human uterine adnexa. J. Reprod. Fertil. 57, 137–142.

11. Bjersing, L. (1977) In: E. S. E. Hafez (ed.), Human Ovulation: Mechanisms, Detection and Regulation, Elsevier, Amsterdam, pp. 149–159.

12. Borell, U., Bygdeman, M., Leader, A., Lundström, V., and Martin, J. N. (1976) Successful first trimester abortion with 15(S)15-methyl prostaglandin $F_{2\alpha}$ methyl ester vaginal suppositories. Contraception 13, 87–93.

13. Brenner, W. E., and Berger, G. S. (1978) Pharmacologic methods of inducing midtrimester abortion: Risks and benefits. In: J. J. Sciarra, G. I. Zatuchni, and J. J. Speidel (eds.), Risks, Benefits, and Controversies in Fertility Control, Harper & Row, New York, pp. 292–321.

14. Brummer, H. C. (1971) Interaction of E prostaglandins and syntocinon on the pregnant human myometrium. J. Obstet. Gynaecol. Br. Commonw. 78, 305–309.

15. Brummer, H. C. (1972) Serum $PGF_{2\alpha}$ levels during late pregnancy, labour and the puerperium. Prostaglandins 2, 185–194.

16. Brummer, H. C. (1973) Serum $PGF_{2\alpha}$ levels during human pregnancy. Prostaglandins 3, 3–5.

17. Brummer, H. C., and Craft, I. L. (1973) Prostaglandin $F_{2\alpha}$ and labour. Acta Obstet. Gynecol. Scand. 52, 273–275.

18. Brummer, H. C., and Gillespie, A. (1972) Seminal prostaglandins and fertility. Clin. Endocrinol. 1, 363–368.

19. Bygdeman, M. (1964) The effect of different prostaglandins on the motility of the human myometrium. Acta Physiol. Scand. (Suppl.) 242, 1–78.

20. Bygdeman, M., Béguin, F., Toppozada, M., and Wiqvist, N. (1973) Intrauterine administration of prostaglandin $F_{2\alpha}$ for induction of abortion. Adv. Biosci. 9, 525–531.

21. Bygdeman, M., Borell, U., Leader, A., Lundström, V., Martin, J. N., Jr., Eneroth, P., and Gréen, K. (1976) Induction of first and second trimester abortion by vaginal administration of 15-methyl $PGF_{2\alpha}$ methyl ester. In: B. Samuelsson and R. Paoletti (eds.), Advances in Prostaglandin and Thromboxane Research, Vol. 2, Raven Press, New York, pp. 693–704.

22. Bygdeman, M., Bremme, K., Gillespie, A., and Lundström, V. (1979) Effects of the prostaglandins on the uterus. Acta Obstet. Gynecol. Scand. (Suppl.) 87, 33–38.

23. Bygdeman, M., and Eliasson, R. (1969) Distribution of prostaglandins, fructose and acid phosphatase in human seminal plasma. Andrologie 1, 5–10.

24. Bygdeman, M., Fredricsson, B., Svanborg, K., and Samuelsson, B. (1970) The relation between fertility and prostaglandin content of seminal fluid in man. Fertil. Steril. 26, 622–629.

25. Bygdeman, M., Gréen, K., Bergström, S., Bundy, G., and Kimball, F. (1979) New prostaglandin E_2 analogues for pregnancy termination. Lancet 1, 1136–1137.

26. Bygdeman, M., and Holmberg, O. (1966) Isolation and identification of prostaglandins from ram seminal plasma. Acta Chem. Scand. 20, 2308–2310.

27. Bygdeman, M., Kwon, S. U., Mukherjee, T., Roth-Brandel, U., and Wiqvist, N. (1970) Effects of PGF compounds on contractility of human pregnant uterus. Am. J. Obstet. Gynecol. 106, 567–572.

28. Bygdeman, M., Martin, J. N., Leader, A., Lundström, V., Ramadan, M., Eneroth, P., and Gréen, K. (1976) Outpatient postconceptional fertility control with vaginally administered 15(S)15-methyl $PGF_{2\alpha}$ methyl ester. Am. J. Obstet. Gynecol. 124, 495–498.

29. Bygdeman, M., Martin, J. N., Leader, A., Lundström, V., Ramadan, M., Eneroth, P., and Gréen, K. (1976) Early pregnancy interruption by 15(S)15-methyl $PGF_{2\alpha}$ methyl ester. Obstet. Gynecol. 48, 221–224.

30. Bygdeman, M., and Samuelsson, B. (1966) Analyses of prostaglandins in human semen. Prostaglandins and related factors. Clin. Chem. Acta 13, 465–474.

31. Calder, A. A. (1979) Prostaglandins for pre-induction cervical ripening. In: S. M. M. Karim (ed.), Practical Applications of Prostaglandins and Their Synthesis Inhibitors, MTB Press, Lancaster, pp. 301–318.

32. Caldwell, B. V., Burnstein, S., Brock, W. A., and Speroff, L. (1971) Radioimmunoassay of the F prostaglandin. J. Clin. Endocrinol. 33, 171–175.

33. Cashetto, S., Lindblom, B., Wiqvist, N., and Wilhelmsson, L. (1979) Prostaglandins and the contractile function of the human oviductal ampulla. Gynecol. Obstet. Invest. 10, 212–220.

34. Cenedella, R. J. (1975) Prostaglandins and male reproductive physiology. In: J. A. Thomas and R. L. Singbal (eds.), Advances in Sex Hormone Research, Vol. 1, University Park Press, Baltimore, pp. 325–358.

35. Challis, J. R. G., Osathanondh, R., Ryan, K. J., and Tulchinsky, D. (1974) Maternal and fetal plasma prostaglandin levels at vaginal delivery and Caesarean section. Prostaglandins 6, 281–288.

36. Challis, J. R. G., and Tulchinsky, D. (1974) A comparison between the concentration of prostaglandin F in human plasma and serum. Prostaglandins 5, 27–31.

37. Chan, W. Y., and Hill, J. C. (1978) Determination of menstrual prostaglandin levels in nondysmenorrhoic and dysmenorrhoic subjects. Prostaglandins 15, 365–375.

38. Chang, M. C., Hunt, D. M., and Polge, C. (1973) Effects of prostaglandins on sperm and egg transport in the rabbit. Adv. Biosci. 9, 805–810.

39. Chaudhuri, C., and Elder, M. G. (1975) Lack of evidence for inhibition of ovulation by aspirin in women. Prostaglandins 11, 727–735.

40. Clark, M. R., Triebwasser, W. F., Marsh, J. M., and Lemaire, W. J. (1978) Prostaglandins in ovulation. Ann. Biol. Anim. Biochim. Biophys. 18, 427–434.

41. Collier, J. G., Flower, R. L., and Stanton, S. L. (1975) Seminal prostaglandins in infertile men. Fertil. Steril. 26, 868–871.

42. Conte, D., Laguzzi, G., Giovenco, P., Dondero, F., and Isidori, A. (1979) Relationship between seminal PGE and 19-OH-PGE and fructose in man. Prostaglandins 17, 135–139.

43. Cooper, J., and Kelly, R. W. (1975) The measurement of E and 19-hydroxy E prostaglandins in human seminal fluid. Prostaglandins 10, 507–514.

44. Coutinho, E. M., and Maia, M. S. (1971) The contractile response of the human uterus, fallopian tubes and ovary to prostaglandins in vivo. Fertil. Steril. 22, 539–543.

45. Craft, I. L., Scrivener, R., and Dewhurst, C. J. (1973) Prostaglandin $F_{2\alpha}$ levels in the maternal and fetal circulations in late pregnancy. J. Obstet. Gynaecol. Br. Commonw. 80, 616–618.

46. Csapo, A. I. (1976) Prostaglandin impact. In: B. Samuelsson and R. Paoletti (eds.), Advances in Prostaglandin and Thromboxane Research, Vol. 2, Raven Press, New York, pp. 705–718.

47. Csapo, A. J., Pulkkinen, M. O., and Hentzl, M. R. (1977) The effect of naproxen sodium on the intrauterine pressure and menstrual pain of dysmenorrhoic patients. Prostaglandins 13, 193–199.

48. Csapo, A. J., Pulkkinen, M., and Wiest, W. G. (1973) The effect of luteectomy and progesterone replacement therapy in early pregnant patients. Am. J. Obstet. Gynecol. 115, 759–765.

49. Damarawy, H., and Toppozada, M. (1976) Control of bleeding due to IUDs by a prostaglandin biosynthesis inhibitor. IRCS Med. Sci. 4, 5.

50. Dimov, V., and Georgiev, G. (1977) Ram semen prostaglandin concentration and its effect on fertility. J. Anim. Sci. 44, 1050–1054.

51. Dray, F., and Frydman, R. (1976) Primary prostaglandins in amniotic fluid in pregnancy and spontaneous labour. Am. J. Obstet. Gynecol. 126, 13–19.

52. Edelman, D. A., Brenner, W. E., and Berger, G. S. (1974) The effectiveness and complications of abortion by dilatation and vacuum aspiration versus dilatation and rigid metal curettage. Am. J. Obstet. Gynecol. 119, 473–481.

53. Edelman, D. A., Brenner, W. E., Mehta, A. C., Philips, F. S., Bhatt, R. V., and Bhiwandiwala, P. (1976) A comparative study of intraamniotic saline and two prostaglandin $F_{2\alpha}$ dose schedules for midtrimester abortion. Am. J. Obstet. Gynecol. 125, 188–195.

54. Elder, M. G., and Stone, M. (1974) Induction of labour by low amniotomy and oral administration of a solution compared with a table of prostaglandin E_2. Prostaglandins 6, 427–432.

55. Eliasson, R. (1959) Studies on prostaglandins. Acta Physiol. Scand. 45 (Suppl. 158), 1–73.

56. Eliasson, R., and Posse, N. (1960) The effect of prostaglandin on the nonpregnant human uterus in vivo. Acta Obstet. Gynecol. Scand. 39, 112–126.

57. Ellwood, D. A., Mitchell, M. D., Andersson, A., and Turnbull, A. C. (1979) Oestrogens, prostaglandins and cervical ripening. Lancet 1, 376–377.

58. Embrey, M. P., Hillier, K., and Mahendran, P. (1973) Termination of pregnancy by extraamniotic prostaglandins and the synergistic effect of oxytocin. Adv. Biosci. 9, 507–513.

59. Ganguli, A. C., Gréen, K., and Bygdeman, M. (1977) Preoperative dilatation of the cervix by single vaginal administration of 15-methyl $PGF_{2\alpha}$ methyl ester. Prostaglandins 14, 779–784.

60. Gillespie, A. (1972) Prostaglandin-oxytocin enhancement and potentiation and their clinical application. Br. Med. J. 1, 150–152.

61. Goldblatt, M. W. (1933) A depressor substance in seminal fluid. J. Soc. Chem. Ind. 52, 1056–1057.

62. Granström, E. (1972) On the metabolism of prostaglandin $F_{2\alpha}$ in female subjects. Eur. J. Biochem. 27, 462–469.

63. Gréen, K. Bygdeman, M., and Bremme, K. (1978) Interruption of early first trimester pregnancy by single vaginal administration of 15-methyl $PGF_{2\alpha}$ methyl ester. Contraception 18, 541–550.

64. Gréen, K., Bygdeman, M., Toppozada, M., and Wiqvist, N. (1974) The role of prostaglandin $F_{2\alpha}$ in human parturition. Endogenous plasma levels of 15-keto-13,14-dihydro-prostaglandin $F_{2\alpha}$ during labor. Am. J. Obstet. Gynecol. 120, 25–31.

65. Grieves, S. A., and Liggins, G. C. (1976) Phospholipase A activity in human and ovine uterine tissues. Prostaglandins 12, 229–241.

66. Grimes, D. A., Schulz, K. F., Cates, W., and Tyler, C. W. (1977) Midtrimester abortion by dilatation and evacuation. New Engl. J. Med. 296, 1141–1145.

67. Gustavii, B. (1972) Labour: A delayed menstruation? Lancet 2, 1149–1150.

68. Gustavii, B. (1975) Release of lysosomal acid phosphatase into the cytoplasm of decidual cells before the onset of labour in humans. Br. J. Obstet. Gynaecol. 82, 177–181.

69. Gutiernez-Cernosek, R. M., Zuckerman, J., and Levine, L. (1972) Prostaglandin $F_{2\alpha}$ in sera during human pregnancy. Prostaglandins 1, 331–337.

70. Hamberg, M. (1974) Quantitative studies on prostaglandin synthesis in man. II. Excretion of the major urinary metabolite of prostaglandins $F_{1\alpha}$ and $F_{2\alpha}$ during pregnancy. Life Sci. 14, 247–252.

71. Hamberg, M. (1976) Biosynthesis of prostaglandin E_1 by human seminal vesicles. Lipids 11, 249–250.

72. Hamberg, M., and Samuelsson, B. (1966) Prostaglandins in human seminal plasma. J. Biol. Chem. 241, 257–263.

73. Hamberg, M., and Samuelsson, B. (1971) On the metabolism of prostaglandins E_1 and E_2 in man. J. Biol. Chem. 246, 6713–6721.

74. Hamberger, L., Nilsson, L., Björn-Rasmussen, E., Atterfeldt, P., and Wiqvist, N.

(1978) Early abortion by vaginal prostaglandin suppositories. Contraception 17, 183–194.

74a.Hamberger, L., Nilsson, L., Dennefors, B., Kahn, I., and Sjögren, A. (1979) Cyclic AMP formation of isolated human corpora lutea in response to HCG-interference by $PGF_{2\alpha}$. Prostaglandins 17, 615–621.

75. Hammarström, S., Powell, W. S., Kylden, U., and Samuelsson, B. (1976) Some properties of a prostaglandin $F_{2\alpha}$ receptor in corpora lutea. In: B. Samuelsson and R. Paoletti (eds.), Advances in Prostaglandin and Thromboxane Research, Vol. 2, Raven Press, New York, pp. 235–246.

76. Hawkins, O. F., and Labrum, A. H. (1961) Semen prostaglandin levels in 50 patients attending a fertility clinic. Acta Physiol. Scand. 13, 1–10.

77. Haynes, P. F., Flint, A. P. F., Anderson, A. B. M., and Turnbull, A. C. (1978) Studies on the role of prostaglandins in human menstruation. Br. J. Obstet. Gynaecol. 85, 78–82.

78. Hedqvist, P., and von Euler, U. A. (1972) Prostaglandin induced neurotransmission failure in the field stimulated isolated vas deferens. Neuropharmacology 11, 177–187.

79. Hennam, J. F., Johnson, D. A., Newton, J. R., and Collins, W. P. (1974) Radioimmunoassay of prostaglandin $F_{2\alpha}$ in peripheral venous plasma from men and women. Prostaglandins 5, 531–541.

80. Henzl, M. R., Noriega, A., Aznar, R., Ortega, E., and Segre, E. (1972) The uterine effects of vaginally administered prostaglandin E_2. Prostaglandins 1, 205–215.

81. Hertelendy, F., Woods, R., and Joffe, B. M. (1973) Prostaglandin E levels in peripheral blood during labour. Prostaglandins 3, 223–227.

82. Hibbard, B. M., Sharma, S. C., Fitzpatrick, R. J., and Hamlett, J. D. (1974) Prostaglandin $F_{2\alpha}$ concentrations in amniotic fluid in late pregnancy. J. Obstet. Gynaecol. Br. Commonw. 81, 35–38.

83. Hichens, M., Grinwich, O. L., and Behrman, H. R. (1974) $PGF_{2\alpha}$ induced loss of corpus luteum gonadotropin receptors. Prostaglandins 7, 449–458.

84. Hillier, K., Calder, A. A., and Embrey, M. P. (1974) Concentration of prostaglandin $F_{2\alpha}$ in amniotic fluid and plasma in spontaneous and induced labour. J. Obstet. Gynaecol. Br. Commonw. 81, 257–263.

85. Hillier, K., Dutton, A., Corker, C. S., Singer, A., and Embrey, M. P. (1972) Plasma steroid and luteinizing hormone levels during prostaglandin $F_{2\alpha}$ administration in luteal phase of the menstrual cycle. Br. Med. J. 4, 333–336.

86. Horton, E. W., and Poyser, N. L. (1976) Uterine luteolytic hormone. A physiological role for prostaglandin $F_{2\alpha}$. Physiol. Rev. 56, 595–651.

87. Jansson, P. O., Albrecht, I., and Ahren, K. (1975) Effects of prostaglandin $F_{2\alpha}$ on ovarian blood flow and vascular resistance in the pseudopregnant rabbit. Acta Endocrinol. (Copenhagen) 79, 337–347.

88. Jerve, F., and Fylling, P. (1978) Therapeutic abortion: The 1975 report from Ullevaal Hospital. Acta Obstet. Gynecol. Scand. 57, 237–240.

89. Jewelewícz, R., Cantor, B., Dyrenfurth, I., Warren, M. P., and van de Wiele, R. L. (1972) Intravenous infusion of prostaglandin $F_{2\alpha}$ in the midluteal phase of the normal human menstrual cycle. Prostaglandins 1, 443–451.

90. Johnson, D. A., Manning, P. A., Henman, J. F., Newton, J. R., and Collins, W. P. (1975) The concentration of prostaglandin $F_{2\alpha}$ in maternal plasma, foetal plasma and amniotic fluid during pregnancy in women. Acta Endocrinol. (Copenhagen) 79, 589–597.

91. Jones, J. R., Gentile, G. P., Kemmann, E. K., and Soriero, A. A. (1975) Intrauterine instillation of prostaglandin $F_{2\alpha}$ in early pregnancy. Prostaglandins 9, 881–892.

92. Jonsson, C. E., Tuvemo, T., and Hamberg, M. (1976) Prostaglandin biosynthesis in the human umbilical cord. Biol. Neonate 29, 162–170.

93. Jonsson, H. T., Middleditch, B. S., and Desiderio, D. H. (1975) Prostaglandins in human seminal fluid. Two novel compounds. Science 187, 1093–1094.

94. Jonsson, M. T., Middleditch, B. S., Scheznayder, M. A., and Desiderio, D. M. (1976) 11,15,19-Trihydroxy-9-ketoprost-13-enoic acid and 11,15,19-trihydroxy-9-ketoprost-5,13-dienoic acid in human seminal fluid. J. Lipid Res. 17, 1–6.

95. Jubiz, W., Frailey, J., Child, C., and Bartholomew, K. (1972) Physiological role of the prostaglandins of the E (PGE), F (PGF) and AB (PGAB) groups. Estimation by radioimmunoassay in unextracted human plasma. Prostaglandins 2, 471–487.

96. Kajanoja, P., Jungner, G., Widholm, O., Karjalainen, O., and Seppälä, M. (1974) Rupture of the cervix in prostaglandin abortion. Br. J. Obstet. Gynaecol. 81, 242–244.

97. Karim, S. M. M. (1968) Appearence of prostaglandin $F_{2\alpha}$ in human blood during labour. Br. Med. J. 4, 618–621.

98. Karim, S. M. M. (1976) Singapore experience with prostaglandin. Routine use and recent advances. In: S. M. M. Karim (ed.), Obstetrical and Gynecological Uses of Prostaglandins, Vol. 1, MTP Press, Lancaster, pp. 127–154.

99. Karim, S. M. M., Choo, H. T., Lim, A. L., Eyo, K. C., and Ratnam, S. S. (1978) Termination of second trimester pregnancy with intramuscular administration of 16-phenoxy-ω-17,18,19,20-tetranor-PGE$_2$ methyl sulphonylamide. Contraception 15, 1063–1068.

100. Karim, S. M. M., and Devlin, J. (1967) Prostaglandin content of amniotic fluid during pregnancy and labour. J. Obstet. Gynaecol. Br. Commonw. 74, 230–234.

101. Karim, S. M. M., Ng, S. C., and Ratnam, S. S. (1979) Termination of abnormal intrauterine pregnancy with prostaglandins. In: S. M. M. Karim (ed.), Practical Applications of Prostaglandins and Their Synthesis Inhibitors, MTP Press, Lancaster, pp. 319–374.

102. Karim, S. M. M., Hillier, K., Somers, K., and Trussel, R. R. (1971) The effects of prostaglandin E$_2$ and F$_{2\alpha}$ administered by different routes on uterine activity and the cardiovascular system in pregnant and nonpregnant women. Br. J. Obstet. Gynaecol. 78, 172–179.

103. Karim, S. M. M., Rao, N., Ratnam, S. S., Prasad, R. N. V., Wong, Y. M., and Ilancheran, A, (1977) Termination of early pregnancy with 16-phenoxy-ω-17,18,19,20-tetranor-PGE$_2$ methyl sulphonylamide. Contraception 16, 377–381.

104. Karim, S. M. M., and Ratnam, S. S. (1976) Termination of pregnancy with prostaglandin analogues. In: B. Samuelsson and R. Paoletti (eds.), Advances in Prostaglandin and Thromboxane Research, Vol. 2, Raven Press, New York, pp. 727–736.

105. Karim, S. M. M., and Ratnam, S. S. (1977) Newer aspects of practical applications in obstetrics and gynecology. In: N. Kharasch and J. Fried (eds.), Biochemical Aspects of Prostaglandins and Thromboxanes, Academic Press, New York, pp. 115–132.

106. Karim, S. M. M., Ratnam, S. S., and Ilancheran, A. (1977) Menstrual induction with vaginal administration of 16,16-dimethyl-trans-Δ^2-PGE$_1$ methyl ester. Prostaglandins 14, 615–616.

107. Karlsson, S. (1959) The influence of seminal fluid on the motility of the nonpregnant human uterus. Acta Obstet. Gynecol. Scand. 38, 503–521.

108. Keirse, M. J. N. C., and Flint, A. P. F. (unpublished data) Quoted in: F. Coceani and P. M. Olley (eds.), Advances in Prostaglandin and Thromboxane Research, Vol. 4, Raven Press, New York, p. 90.

109. Keirse, M. J. N. C., Flint, A. P. F., and Turnbull, A. C. (1974) F Prostaglandins in amniotic fluid during pregnancy and labour. J. Obstet. Gynaecol. Br. Commonw. 81, 131–135.

110. Keirse, M. J. N. C., Hicks, B. R., Mitchell, M. D., and Turnbull, A. C. (1977) Increase in the prostaglandin precursor, arachidonic acid, in amniotic fluid, during spontaneous labour. Br. J. Obstet. Gynaecol. 84, 937–940.

111. Keirse, M. J. N. C., Mitchell, M. D., and Turnbull, A. C. (1977) Changes in prostaglandin F and 13, 14-dihydro-15-keto prostaglandin F concentrations in amniotic fluid at the onset of and during labour. Br. J. Obstet. Gynaecol. 84, 743–746.

112. Keirse, M. J. N. C., and Turnbull, A. C. (1973) E Prostaglandins in amniotic fluid during late pregnancy and labour. J. Obstet. Gynaecol. Br. Commonw. 80, 970–973.

113. Keirse, M. J. N. C., and Turnbull, A. C. (1976) The fetal membranes as a possible source of amniotic fluid prostaglandins. Br. J. Obstet. Gynaecol. 83, 146–151.

114. Kelly, J., Flynn, H. M., and Bertrand, F. V. (1973) A comparison of oral prostaglandin E_2 and intravenous syntocinon in the induction of labour. Br. J. Obstet. Gynecol. 80, 923–926.

115. Kelly, R. W. (1977) Effect of seminal prostaglandins on the metabolism of human spermatozoa. J. Reprod. Fertil. 50, 219–222.

116. Kelly, R. W., Taylor, P. L., Hearn, J. P., Short, R. V., Martin, D. E., and Marston, J. H. (1976) 19-Hydroxy prostaglandin E as a major component of the semen of primates. Nature (London) 260, 544–545.

117. Kindahl, H., Granström, E., Edqvist, L. E., and Eneroth, P. (1976) Prostaglandin levels in peripheral plasma during the reproductive cycle. In: B. Samuelsson and R. Paoletti (eds.), Advances in Prostaglandin and Thromboxane Research, Vol. 2, Raven Press, New York, pp. 667–671.

118. Leader, A., Bygdeman, M., Eneroth, P., Martin, N. J., Jr., and Wiqvist, N. (1976) The effect of infusion with two analogues of prostaglandin $F_{2\alpha}$ on corpus luteum function. In: B. Samuelsson and R. Paoletti (eds.), Advances in Prostaglandin and Thromboxane Research, Vol. 2, Raven Press, New York, pp. 679–685.

119. Lemaire, W. J., Leidner, R., and Marsh, J. M. (1975) Pre- and postovulatory changes in the concentration of prostaglandins in rat Graafian follicles. Prostaglandins 9, 221–229.

120. Lemaire, W. J., and Marsh, J. M. (1975) Interrelationship between prostaglandin, cyclic AMP and steroids in ovulation. J. Reprod. Fertil. (Suppl.) 22, 53–74.

121. Lindblom, B., Hamberger, L., and Wiqvist, N. (1978) Differential contractile effects of prostaglandins E and F on the isolated circular and longitudinal smooth muscle of the human oviduct. Fertil. Steril. 30, 553–558.

122. Lindblom, B., Hamberger, L., and Ljung, B. (1980) Contractile patterns of isolated oviductal smooth muscle under different hormonal conditions. Fertil. Steril. 33, 283–287.

123. Lindner, H. R., Zor, U., Kohen, F., Bauminger, S., Amesterdam, A., Lahao, M., and Salomon, Y. (1980) Significance of prostaglandins in the regulation of cyclic events in the ovary and uterus. In: B. Samuelsson, P. W. Ramwell, and R. Paoletti (eds.), Advances in Prostaglandin and Thromboxane Research, Vol. 8, Raven Press, New York, pp. 1371–1390.

124. Lundström, V., Bygdeman, M., Fotiou, S., Gréen, K., and Kinoshita, K. (1977) Abortion in early pregnancy by vaginal administration of 16,16-dimethyl PGE_2 in comparison with vacuum aspiration. Contraception 16, 167–173.

125. Lundström, V., and Gréen, K. (1978) Endogenous levels of prostaglandin $F_{2\alpha}$ and its main metabolites in plasma and endometrium of normal and dysmenorrhoic women. Am. J. Obstet. Gynecol. 130, 640–646.

126. Lundström, V., Gréen, K., and Wiqvist, N. (1976) Prostaglandins, indomethacin and dysmenorrhea. Prostaglandins 11, 893–904.

127. Lyneham, R. C., Korda, A. R., Shutt, O. A., Smith, I. D., and Sherman, R. P. (1975) The effect of intrauterine prostaglandin $F_{2\alpha}$ on corpus luteum function in the human. Prostaglandins 9, 431–442.

128. MacDonald, P. C., Schultz, F. M., Duenhoelter, J. J., Gant, N. F., Jimenez, J. M., Pritchard, J. A., Porter, J. C., and Johnston, J. M. (1974) Initiation of human parturition. I. Mechanism of action of arachidonic acid. Obstet. Gynecol. 44, 629–636.

129. Marsh, J. M., Jang, N. S. T., and Lemaire, W. J. (1974) Prostaglandin synthesis in rabbit Graafian follicles in vitro. Effect of luteinizing hormone and cyclic AMP. Prostaglandins 7, 269–283.

130. Martin, J. N., Jr., and Bygdeman, M. (1975) The effect of locally administered $PGF_{2\alpha}$ on the contractility of the nonpregnant human uterus in vivo. Prostaglandins 9, 245–253.

131. Martin, J. N., Jr., and Bygdeman, M. (1975) The effect of locally administered PGE_2 on the contractility of nonpregnant human uterus in vivo. Prostaglandins 10, 253–265.

132. Martin, J. N., Jr., Bygdeman, M., and Eneroth, P. (1978) The influence of locally administered prostaglandin E_2 and $F_{2\alpha}$ on uterine motility in the intact nonpregnant human uterus. Acta Obstet. Gynecol. Scand. 57, 141–147.

133. McCracken, J. A., Barcikowski, B., Carlson, J. C., Gréen, K., and Samuelsson, B. (1973) The physiological role of prostaglandin $F_{2\alpha}$ in corpus luteum regression. Adv. Biosci. 9, 599–624.

134. Mitchell, M. D., Brunt, J., Bibby, J., Flint, A. P. F., Anderson, A. B. M., and Turnbull, A. C. (1978) Prostaglandin in the human umbilical circulation at birth. Br. J. Obstet. Gynaecol. 85, 114–118.

135. Mitchell, M. D., Flint, A. P., Bibby, J., Brunt, J., Arnold, J. M., Anderson, A. B. M., and Turnbull, A. C. (1978) Plasma concentrations of prostaglandins during late human pregnancy: Influence of normal and preterm labour. J. Clin. Endocrinol. Metab. 46, 947–951.

136. Mocsary, P., and Csapo, A. I. (1975) Menstrual induction with $PGF_{2\alpha}$ and PGE_2. Prostaglandins 10, 545–547.

137. Morales, T. I., Woessner, J. F., Howell, D. S., Marsh, J. M., and Lemaire, W. J. (1978) A microassay for the direct demonstration of collagenolytic activity in Graafian follicles of the rat. Biochim. Biophys. Acta 524, 428–434.

138. Ogra, S. S., Kirton, K. T., Tomasi, T. B., Jr., and Lippes, J. (1974) Prostaglandins in the human fallopian tube. Fertil. Steril. 25, 250–255.

139. Pickles, J. R., Hall, W. J., Clegg, P. C., and Sullivan, T. J. (1966) Some experiments on the mechanisms of action of prostaglandins on the guinea pig and rat myometrium. Mem. Soc. Endocrinol. 14, 89–103.

140. Pokoly, T. B., and Jordan, J. C. (1975) Relation of steroids and prostaglandin at vaginal delivery and Caesarean section. Obstet. Gynecol. 46, 577–580.

141. Powell, W. S., Hammarström, S., Samuelsson, B., and Sjöberg, B. (1974) Prostaglandin $F_{2\alpha}$ receptor in human corpora lutea. Lancet 1, 1120.

142. Poyser, N. L. (1978) Hormonal control of prostaglandin synthesis in reproductive processes. Pol. J. Pharmacol. Pharm. 30, 171–181.

143. Pritchard, E. T., Armstrong, W. D., and Wilt, J. C. (1968) Examination of lipids from amnion, chorion and vernix. Am. J. Obstet. Gynecol. 100, 289.

144. Pulkkinen, M. O., Henzl, M. R., and Csapo, A. J. (1978) The effect of naproxen sodium on the prostaglandin concentrations of menstrual blood and uterine jet washings in dysmenorrhoic women. Prostaglandins 15, 543–550.

145. Ratnam, S. S., Khew, K. S., Chen, C., and Lim, T. C. (1974) Oral prostaglandin E_2 in induction of labour. Aust. NZ. J. Obstet. Gynecol. 14, 26–30.

146. Roth-Brandel, U., Bygdeman, M., and Wiqvist, N. (1970) Effect of intravenous administration of prostaglandin E_1 and $F_{2\alpha}$ on the contractility of the nonpregnant human uterus in vivo. Acta Obstet. Gynecol. Scand. (Suppl.) 5, 19–25.

147. Salmon, J. A., and Amy, J. J. (1973) Levels of prostaglandin $F_{2\alpha}$ in amniotic fluid during pregnancy and labour. Prostaglandins 4, 523–533.

148. Samuelsson, B. (1963) Isolation and identification of prostaglandins from human seminal plasma. J. Biol. Chem. 238, 3229–3234.

149. Sandberg, F., Ingelman-Sundberg, A., and Rydén, G. (1964) The effect of prostaglandin E_2 and E_3 on the human uterus and fallopian tubes in vitro. Acta Obstet. Gynecol. Scand. 43, 95–102.

150. Sandberg, F., Ingelman-Sundberg, A., and Rydén, G. (1965) The effect of prostaglandin $F_{1\alpha}$, $F_{1\beta}$, $F_{2\alpha}$ and $F_{2\beta}$ on the human uterus and fallopian tubes in vitro. Acta Obstet. Gynecol. Scand. 44, 585–594.

151. Schultz, F. M., Schwarz, B. F., MacDonald, P. C., and Johnston, J. M. (1975) Initiation

of human parturition. II. Identification of phospholipase A in fetal chorioamnion and uterine decidua. Am. J. Obstet. Gynecol. 123, 650–653.

152. Schwartz, A. L., Forster, C. S., Smith, P. A., and Liggins, G. C. (1977) Human amnion metabolism. II. Incorporation of fatty acids into tissue phospholipids in vitro. Am. J. Obstet. Gynecol. 127, 475–481.

153. Schwarz, B. E., Schultz, F. M., MacDonald, P. C., and Johnston, J. M. (1975) Initiation of parturition. III. Fetal membrane content of prostaglandin E_2 and $F_{2\alpha}$ precursor. Obstet. Gynecol. 46, 564–568.

154. Schwarz, B. E., Schultz, F. M., MacDonald, P. C., and Johnston, J. M. (1976) Initiation of human parturition. IV. Demonstration of phospholipase A_2 in the lysosomes of human fetal membranes. Am. J. Obstet. Gynecol. 125, 1089–1091.

155. Skakkebaeck, N. E., Kelly, R. W., and Cocker, C. S. (1976) Prostaglandin concentrations in the semen of hypogonadal men during treatment with testosterone. J. Reprod. Fertil. 47, 119–121.

156. Spilman, C. H., Finn, A. E., and Norland, J. F. (1973) Effect of prostaglandins on sperm transport and fertilization in the rabbit. Prostaglandins 4, 57–64.

157. Spilman, C. H., and Harper, M. J. K. (1975) Effects of prostaglandins on oviductal motility and egg transport. Gynecol. Invest. 6, 186–205.

158. Sturde, H. C. (1971) The effect of antiandrogen cyproterone on the ejaculum of young men, including sperm prostaglandins. Arch. Dermatol. Forsch. 241, 86–95.

159. Sturde, H. C. (1971) Behaviour of sperm prostaglandins under therapy with androgen. Arzneim.-Forsch. 21, 1302–1307.

160. Sykes, J. A. C., Williams, K. I., and Rogers, A. F. (1975) Prostaglandin production and metabolism by homogenates of pregnant human deciduum and myometrium. J. Endocrinol. 64, 18–19.

161. Tagaki, S., Sakata, H., Yoshida, T., Nakazawa, S., Fuji, T. K., Tominaga, Y., Iwasa, Y., Ninagawa, T., Hiroshima, T., Tomida, Y., Itoh, K., and Matsukawa, R. (1977) Termination of very early pregnancy by ONO-802, 16,16-dimethyl-trans-Δ^2-PGE_1 methyl ester. Prostaglandins 14, 791–798.

162. Tagaki, S., Sakata, H., Yoshida, T., Den, K., Fuji, T. K., Ameniya, H., and Tomita, M. (1978) Termination of early pregnancy by ONO-802 (16,16-dimethyl-trans-Δ^2-PGE_1 methyl ester). Prostaglandins 15, 913–919.

163. Taylor, P. L. (1979) The 8-iso prostaglandins: Evidence for eight components in human semen. Prostaglandins 17, 259–267.

164. Taylor, P. L., and Kelly, R. W. (1974) 19-Hydroxylated E prostaglandins as the major prostaglandins of human semen. Nature (London) 250, 665–667.

165. Taylor, P. L., and Kelly, R. W. (1975) The occurrence of 19-hydroxy F prostaglandins in human semem. FEBS Lett. 57, 22–25.

166. Templeton, A. A., Cooper, I., and Kelly, R. W. (1978) Prostaglandin concentrations in the semen of fertile men. J. Reprod. Fertil. 52, 147–150.

167. Thiery, M., and Amy, J. J. (1977) Spontaneous and induced labour. Two roles for the prostaglandins. Obstet. Gynecol. Ann. 6, 127–175.

168. Thiery, M., Yo Le Sian, A., de Hemptienne, D., Derom, R., Martens, G., van Kets, H., and Amy, J. J. (1974) Induction of labour with prostaglandin E_2 tablets. Br. J. Obstet. Gynaecol. 81, 303–306.

169. Thorburn, G. D., Challis, J. R. C., and Currie, W. B. (1977) Control of parturition in domestic animals. Biol. Reprod. 16, 18–27.

170. Toppozada, M. (1979) Prostaglandins and their synthesis inhibitors in dysfunctional uterine bleeding. In: S. M. M. Karim (ed.), Practical Applications of Prostaglandins and Their Synthesis Inhibitors, MTP Press, Lancaster, pp. 237–265.

171. Toppozada, M., Graafar, A., and Shaala, S. (1974) In vivo inhibition of the human nonpregnant uterus by prostaglandin E_2. Prostaglandins 8, 401–410.

172. Toppozada, M., Graafar, A., Shaala, S., and Osman, M. (1975) The relaxant property

of local prostaglandin E_2 on the nonpregnant uterus—A cycle response. Prostaglandins 9, 475–486.

173. Tsang, B. K., Ainsworth, L., Downey, B. R., and Armstrong, D. T. (1975) Preovulatory changes in cyclic AMP and prostaglandin concentrations in follicular fluid of gilts. Prostaglandins 17, 141–148.

174. Ulmsten, U., and Wingerup, L. (1979) Cervical ripening induced by prostaglandin E_2 in viscous gel. Acta Obstet. Gynecol. Scand. Suppl. 84, 1–21.

175. Van Orden, D. E., and Farley, D. D. (1973) Prostaglandin $F_{2\alpha}$ radioimmunoassay utilizing polyethylene glycol separation technique. Prostaglandins 4, 215–233.

176. von Euler, U. S. (1934) Zur Kenntnis der pharmakologischen Wirkungen Nativsekreten und extrakter mannlicher accessorischer Geschlechtsdrüsen. Arch. Exp. Pathol. Pharmakol. 175, 78–84.

177. von Euler, U. S. (1935) The specific blood pressure lowering substance in human prostate and seminal vesicle secretions. Klin. Wochenschr. 14, 1182–1183.

178. von Euler, U. S. (1936) On the specific vasodilating and plain muscle stimulating substances from accessory genital glands in man and certain animals (prostaglandin and vesiglandin). J. Physiol. 88, 213–234.

179. Wentz, A. C., and Jones, G. S. (1973) Transient luteolytic effect of prostaglandin $F_{2\alpha}$ in the human. Obstet. Gynecol. 42, 172–181.

180. WHO Task Force on Prostaglandins for Fertility Regulation (1976) Comparison of intraamniotic prostaglandin $F_{2\alpha}$ and hypertonic saline for induction of second trimester abortion. Br. Med. J. 2, 1373–1376.

181. WHO Task Force on Prostaglandins for Fertility Regulation (1977) Comparison of single intraamniotic injections of 15-methyl prostaglandin $F_{2\alpha}$ and prostaglandin $F_{2\alpha}$ for termination of second trimester pregnancy. An international multicentre study. Am. J. Obstet. Gynecol. 129, 601–606.

182. WHO Task Force on Sequele of Abortion (1979) Gestation, birth weight and spontaneous abortion in pregnancy after induced abortion. Lancet 1, 142–145.

183. Wilhelmsson, L., Lindblom, B., and Wiqvist, N. (1979) The human uterotubal junction: Contractile patterns of different smooth muscle layers and the influence of prostaglandin E_2, prostaglandin $F_{2\alpha}$ and prostaglandin I_2 in vitro. Fertil. Steril. 32, 303–307.

184. Wiqvist, N., Bygdeman, M., and Kirton, K. T. (1971) Nonsteroidal antifertility agents in the female. In: E. Diczfalusy and U. Borell (eds.), Nobel Symposium No. 15, Wiley, New York, pp. 137–155.

185. Ylikorkala, O., Kirkinen, P., Jouppila, P., and Järvinen, P. A. (1975) Intrauterine injection of 15(S)15-methyl prostaglandin $F_{2\alpha}$ for termination of early pregnancy in out-patients. Prostaglandins 10, 333–341.

186. Zor, U., and Lamprecht, S. A. (1977) Mechanism of prostaglandin action in endocrine glands. In: G. Litwack (ed.), Biochemical Actions of Hormones. Academic Press, New York, pp. 85–133.

AHMAD A. ATTALLAH, Ph.D.

JAMES B. LEE, M.D.

PROSTAGLANDINS, RENAL FUNCTION, AND BLOOD PRESSURE REGULATION

INTRODUCTION

The discovery, isolation, and identification of the renomedullary pros-taglandins (PGs) some 15 years ago [162,163] stemmed from the result of investigations into the so-called antihypertensive-endocrine function of the kidney. According to this theory, certain states of hypertension may not be caused solely by prohypertensive vasoconstricting factors (renin-angiotensin-aldosterone and adrenergic activity), but may be the result of an absolute or relative deficiency of renal antihypertensive vasodilating factors that allow prohypertensive factors to act unopposed. The isolation and identification of renomedullary PGE_2 and PGA_2 was the first evidence of the presence of a new lipid class of vasodilatory compounds in the renal medulla, providing biochemical support for the renal antihypertensive-endocrine hypothesis. The additional presence of the venoconstrictor $PGF_{2\alpha}$ in the renal medulla was also detected. These early investigations were undertaken without knowledge of the existence of the seminal vesicle PGs, for which the literature was then in an embryonic stage. Later prostaglandin research differed in that PGs were detected in most biological tissues following a direct search for

From the Hypertension Program Unit, Department of Medicine, Erie County Medical Center, State University of New York at Buffalo, Buffalo, New York their presence. Hypotheses were subsequently formulated to attempt to define a physiological role for the PGs in any given biological system. In contrast to these investigations, where even today the PGs may aptly be described as "fats in quest of a function," the discovery of the vasodilating PGs in the kidney was in conformation with preexisting renal antihypertensive theorem.

Following the identification of the renal PGs, it soon became evident, however, that the renal PGs not only affected blood pressure but had notable effects on renal blood flow, sodium homeostasis, water excretion, the renin-angiotensin system, the sympathetic nervous system, and the kinins. A voluminous literature accumulated, and approximately 3000 publications on this topic have appeared since the discovery of the renal prostaglandins in 1961. Therefore, due to space limitations, the cited bibliography is arbitrarily selective and important aspects of the renal PGs such as their interaction with the central and adrenergic nervous system, their effects on the micro- and regional circulations, and their action on cardiac muscle have been omitted. Certain of these cardiovascular PG actions are treated in detail in the chapter by Kot and Fitzpatrick in this volume.

BIOSYNTHESIS AND METABOLISM

In general, the biosynthetic and metabolic pathways of PG synthesis in the kidney are almost identical to those outlined by Hall and Behrman (this volume). However, there are certain important differences in renal PG production and degradation rates, particularly with regard to the regional distribution of synthetic and metabolizing PG enzymes, which form the basis of this discussion.

The renal prostaglandins are synthesized primarily by the renal medulla, although a definite capacity for PG synthesis exists in the cortex. Studies utilizing incubations with sheep seminal vesicles revealed that the principal precursor for prostaglandin production is arachidonic acid esterified to phospholipid which, following its release by phospholipase, is transformed into the unstable endoperoxide intermediates PGG_2 and PGH_2 by PG cyclooxygenase (PG synthetase) and to 12-hydroperoxy-arachidonic acid (HPETE) by PG lipoxygenase [44,45,119,205]. The unstable HPETE is converted to the stable 12-hydroxyarachidonic acid (HETE) in platelets and lung. Figure 1 summarizes the biosynthetic pathways of the PGs; for details, see Hall and Behrman (this volume).

It is now known that the intermediates PGG_2 and PGH_2 have important biological activities of their own and may be transformed not only into PGE_2, $PGF_{2\alpha}$, and PGD_2 but also, via other pathways, into the potent platelet aggregating and vasoconstrictor thromboxane A_2 [120] and the platelet inhibiting and vasodilating PGI_2 [190,191,220]. The major inactive metabolite of thromboxane A_2 is thromboxane B_2, whereas the unstable PGI_2 readily hydrates to the stable metabolite 6-keto-$PGF_{1\alpha}$ [219,220]. The latter compound is metabolized by β- and ω-oxidation in

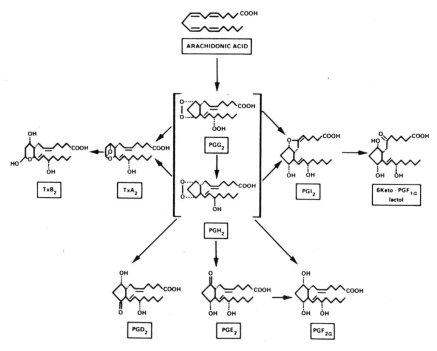

FIGURE 1. Metabolic pathways of PG and thromboxane biosynthesis from arachidonic acid.

the kidney to dinor-6-keto-PGF$_{1\alpha}$ and dinor-ω-1 hydroxy-6-keto-PGF$_{1\alpha}$, which appear in the urine [220]. In the whole animal, Sun and Taylor [266] have shown that PGI$_2$ is also metabolized by the rat to at least seven additional metabolites of 6-keto-PGF$_{1\alpha}$ and 15-keto-PGI$_2$. The thromboxane pathway predominates in platelets [249,250], but can be unmasked in the kidney by ureteral obstruction [193], whereas the PGI$_2$ pathway predominates in fetal vessels [273] and adult vascular endothelium [291].

The details of PG biosynthesis are provided in a recent review by Morrison and Needleman [194].

The thromboxane-PGI$_2$ interactions between platelets and vascular endothelium have received a great deal of attention recently, since it has been postulated that PGI$_2$ is the active factor normally preventing platelet deposition in vascular tissue. Since PGI$_2$ is produced in and dilates the coronary vasculature of most species (but not the pig [80]), and since it is inhibited by acetylsalicylic [283] and lipid peroxides [191], it has been postulated that a deficiency in its synthesis could be a major factor underlying atherosclerosis in general and human coronary vasoconstriction and thrombosis in particular [81,237; see Gryglewski, this volume] by allowing thromboxane A$_2$, a powerful vasoconstrictor and platelet aggregating compound [201], to act unopposed. To date, however, there is no convincing evidence that this is, in fact, a pathophysiological role for either thromboxanes or PGI_2.

The precise metabolic pathways for renal prostaglandin synthesis, particularly PGI_2 and thromboxane A_2, are less clearly understood and have only recently been receiving widespread attention. Rather conclusive evidence has been produced that the primary sites of renomedullary prostaglandin production are the interstitial cells and the collecting duct cells of the renal papilla [39,64,315], where the major prostaglandin produced is PGE_2 [4,117,163], with lesser amounts of PGD_2 [95], $PGF_{2\alpha}$ [163], and possibly PGA_2 [163] (see below). In the hydronephrotic rabbit kidney, PG synthesis was detected in the thin limbs of Henle as well as the cortical and medullary collecting tubules [259]. PG synthesis has also been demonstrated in isolated glomeruli [121] with synthesis of PGE_2 and $PGF_{2\alpha}$ predominating over much smaller amounts of PGD_2, 6-keto-$PGF_{1\alpha}$, and thromboxane B_2. Recently, however, Grenier and Smith [112] have shown that homogenates of isolated rabbit collecting duct cell have a significant capacity to synthesize 6-keto-$PGF_{1\alpha}$, the stable metabolite of PGI_2, exceeding even rates of PGE_2 production at low medium arachidonate levels (12 mm). The highest capacity for PG synthesis is therefore observed in the renal medulla, which is regionally dissociated from the highest rate of PG metabolism, seen in the renal cortex [154]. Utilizing PGH_2 as substrate, it was shown that the renal medulla possessed the highest activity of PG endoperoxide isomerase [225], which apparently is located in the endoplasmic reticulum [40]. PGE synthesis and cyclic AMP production in rat renal papilla are enhanced at high oxygen tension [262,307], are inhibited by indomethacin and antioxidants [306], and are unaffected by oxidative phosphorylation inhibitors [123], suggesting that oxygen can regulate PG production in this area of the kidney known to normally exhibit a very low pO_2 ($\sim$ 30 mm Hg). It is of interest in this regard that hypertonic media also stimulate production of PGE_2, $PGF_{2\alpha}$, and PGD_2 in rat renal papilla [308]; this hyperosmotic condition, like low oxygen tension, approaches a physiological state known to exist in vivo in this unique tissue.

Although renal PGE_2 synthesis is inhibited by the PG synthetase inhibitor indomethacin [100,209], both indomethacin and probenecid also markedly inhibit the active transport of PGE_2 from tubular fluid to lumen [37,238], suggesting that PGE_2 might normally be transported by the classical organic acid pathway known to exist in the cortex but not the medulla. However, Rosenblatt et al. [245] have shown in the anesthetized dog that although probenecid administration abolished [³H]PGE secretion, indomethacin failed to alter [³H]PGE secretion at concentrations where there was an 80% reduction of endogenous urinary PGE excretion rate ($U_{PGE}V$), suggesting that the component of $U_{PGE}V$ secondary to organic acid transport may be quantitatively minor. Further studies will be necessary to resolve this extremely important effect of indomethacin on PGE organic acid transport. Although it appears that a major portion of urinary PGE_2 is renal in origin [98] and that the site of entry may be the loop of Henle [298], much additional investigation is necessary to determine the precise disposition and transport of renomedullary PGs once they have been synthesized by the renal collecting duct and/or interstitial cells. This is underscored by the significant contribution of seminal vesicle PGE_2 to total urinary PGE_2 in the male. Once released, PGs are transported in human blood bound to albumin [236], with less polar compounds such as PGA bound to a greater extent (90%) than more polar compounds such PGE_2 (45%) and $PGF_{2\alpha}$ (18%). Furthermore, it has been recently shown [17] that therapeutic doses of aspirin markedly decrease the ratio of bound to free PGA and PGE in human sera, similar to the effects of aspirin on glucocorticoid and thyroxin binding. Thus, in addition to inhibition of PG synthesis, nonsteroidal antiinflammatory agents have important effects of PG binding in blood, the significance of which is not clear.

Although the renal cortex is primarily the site of metabolism of PGs, a significant capacity for synthesis exists [154], and an enzyme specific for $PGF_{2\alpha}$ synthesis has been observed in rabbit renal cortex [233]. Utilizing an immunofluorescent procedure, Smith and Bell [258] detected PG cyclooxygenase activity in endothelial cells of cortical arteries and arterioles and in cortical collecting duct cells. Furthermore, the enzyme was detected in epithelial and mesangial cells of the glomerulus, leading these authors to conclude that cortical arteriolar PG synthesis is responsible for the effects of PGs on renal blood flow. Indeed, Whorton et al. [297] detected substantial amounts of 6-keto-$PGF_{1\alpha}$, the metabolite of PGI_2, in rabbit renal cortex in vitro, and Needleman et al. [198] demonstrated the capacity of the perfused rabbit kidney to produce PGI_2, although the major end product of the endogenous arachidonic acid cascade appeared to be PGE_2. These important observations may help resolve a difficult problem, namely, how PGs believed originally to be synthesized in medulla only traverse to the arterial resistance bed of the cortex, where they have their major hemodynamic and renin-releasing actions. In summary, PGE_2 appears to be the major product of renal tubular and interstitial cell synthesis, whereas PGI_2 (as measured by its metabolite 6-keto-$PGF_{1\alpha}$) seems to be the major compound produced by the renal vascular cells.

The PGE and PGF compounds are metabolized in a single passage through the lungs [87] by 15-hydroxy prostaglandin dehydrogenase (15-PGDH) and 15-keto-13,14-dihydroreductase (13-PGR) into the less polar biologically inactive metabolites 15-keto PGs and 15-keto-13,14-dihydro PGs, respectively [9,10,87] (see Figure 7, Hall and Behrman this volume). A third enzyme apparently catalyzes the conversion of 15-keto-13,14-dihydro PGs to the biologically active 13,14-dihydro PGEs or PGFs. Similar pathways exist in other tissues with particularly high concentrations of 15-PGDH and 15-PGR in the renal cortex [8]. The former enzyme has been resolved into NAD^+- and $NADP^+$-dependent components [165]. The conversion of $PGF_{2\alpha}$ to these three nonpolar metabolites by the

100,000-g supernates of whole kidney homogenates has been described by Hoult and Moore [130]. By ω-oxidation, PGE and PGF may also be converted to the more polar dinor and tetranor compounds that appear in the urine.

A fourth enzyme, PGE-9-keto reductase, has been reported in renal cortex [138,166]. Since its activity is enhanced by sodium chloride [288], this enzyme may be involved in the ability of the kidney to excrete a salt load. Conversely, a renal enzyme that oxidizes PGF to PGE has been reported [166], although its significance remains unknown.

Unlike PGE and PGF, PGA and PGI selectively escape degradation by the lungs [82] and could thus function as circulating antihypertensive "hormones" in the classical sense. Indeed, PGI_2 not only is not metabolized by the lung but is spontaneously released from the lung [114,115], which has led to the hypothesis that this endocrinelike phenomenon may have a circulating antihypertensive role and function in preventing platelet thrombi in arterial segments of the circulation.

RENAL HEMODYNAMICS AND SODIUM HOMEOSTASIS

Renal Blood Flow

In general the effect of PGs on renal function have been studied with regard to exogenous administration, stimulation of endogenous synthesis, inhibition of endogenous synthesis, and interactions of all the above with other non-PG renal and extrarenal vasoactive factors.

EXOGENOUS EFFECTS

A voluminous early literature demonstrates that administration of $PGE_{1,2}$, $PGA_{1,2}$, and more recently PGH_2 [84], PGD_2 [43,83], and PGI_2 (but not $6\text{-keto-PGF}_{1\alpha}$) are potent renal vasodilators, all producing an increase in urine flow and sodium excretion [42,55]. With respect to PGD_2, some investigators found urine flow and sodium excretion to be unchanged [43], while others [95] observed an increase in sodium and water excretion when renal blood flow rose. The major intracellular site appears to be the juxtamedullary region [55]. Despite these observations, it is generally accepted that little physiological information accrues from such studies, since PGs that are exogenously administered may not act at sites normally utilized by PGs synthesized within the renal medulla.

STIMULATION OF SYNTHESIS

An increase in deep cortical and inner medullary blood flow accompanied by an enhanced production of PGE_2 has been noted following administration of the PG precursor arachidonic acid [55,155,157,270]. The rise in renal blood flow was largely the result of a redistribution of blood to inner cortex and papilla and was accompanied by natriuresis; both effects were inhibited by indomethacin. Gerber et al. [103] found similar effects, except for natriuresis, in nonfiltering dog kidney, suggesting that the intrarenal action of PGs is not the result of their transport from medulla to cortex but is the effect of enhanced synthesis of PGs produced locally in the cortex. It would appear that arachidonic acid and PG endoperoxides increase renal blood flow by virtue of their conversion to PGs, since stable PG endoperoxides that are not converted to other compounds produce renal vasoconstriction in anesthetized dogs [104]. In fact, the renal vasodilatory effects of the prostaglandin cascade may require conversion of PGE_2 to the metabolite 13,14-dihydro-PGE_2, which is more potent than PGE_2 itself in producing elevations in renal blood flow [105].

In addition to precursor administration, increased PGE production with accelerated renal blood flow and natriuresis can also be produced by diuretics such as ethacrynic acid, bumetanide, or furosemide [213, 300,301]. These effects are inhibited by indomethacin [299], suggesting that arachidonic acid conversion to renal PGs may mediate the response to diuretics. Interestingly, with bumetanide there is an increase in kidney volume and subcapsular pressure accompanied by a rise in urinary PGE and kinin excretion [211]. Subsequently, there was normalization of subcapsular pressure, together with a fall in PGE but with continued elevation in volume and kinin excretion, both of which were inhibited by indomethacin. Thus there may be important interactions with PGs and kinins in the mechanism of diuretic action.

INHIBITION OF SYNTHESIS

Administration of meclofenamate or indomethacin to the anesthetized animal results in a decrease in renal blood flow accompanied by a fall in renal PGE production [7,147,172,218,281], which is the result primarily of a decrease in inner cortical blood flow [132,147], suggesting that renomedullary PG release and transport to inner cortex supports basal renal blood flow. However, this phenomenon was not observed in the conscious animal [268,274]; thus renal PGs may function importantly to offset ischemic vasoconstricting renal stimuli such as sympathetic stimuli (anesthesia, surgery, stress, etc.), but do not mediate basal renal blood flow. This is supported by the recent studies of Zimmerman, Mommsen, and Kraft, who demonstrated in the conscious dog in high renin states (low salt diet, following furosemide and one- and two-clip Goldblatt hypertension) that indomethacin and meclofenamate markedly reduced renal blood flow but not in normotensive sodium-depleted animals [310]. In contrast, in the conscious rat, indomethacin is without effect on renal blood flow, but in acutely saline loaded rats it results in a decreased renal blood flow, which is primarily outer cortical in origin [78], revealing yet another important species variable affecting PG synthesis and renal blood flow.

INTERACTIONS WITH VASOACTIVE COMPOUNDS

Infusion of angiotensin II or norepinephrine, renal nerve stimulation, renal ischemia, or hemorrhagic hypothesion results in a decrease in renal blood flow (and usually glomerular filtration rate) coincident with a rise in renal venous PGE [70,122,177,184]. The renal vasoconstrictor effects of these manipulations were augmented by indomethacin and inhibited by PGE administration [173,494], suggesting that renal PGE responds to renal vasoconstricting stimuli involving both the renin-angiotensin system and the sympathetic nervous system by an accelerated synthesis and release to the cortex, where physiological antagonism of the effects of angiotensin II and norepinephrine may occur as a major compensatory intrarenal response to ischemic stimuli. Noradrenaline and vasopressin result in comparable rises in released PGE in perfused kidneys, and the effects of both hormones are inhibited by indomethacin; therefore it is believed that the release of PGEs during intrarenal vasoconstriction is not mediated by specific α-adrenergic receptors [30].

Interestingly, renal PGE release is also enhanced by the vasodilator bradykinin [186]. Since kinins formed intrarenally also release PGE [197], it is possible that certain of the vasodilatory effects of this peptide are mediated by renal PGE. On the other hand, Olsen [212] found that bradykinin infusion, during mannitol diuresis in the anesthetized dog, increased urinary PG renal blood flow, subcapsular pressure, renal volume, and sodium excretion, effects that were essentially unchanged by prior treatment with indomethacin, producing unmeasurable urinary PG values. This suggests that vasodilation induced by bradykinin is independent of released PGs and supports the concept that bradykinin releases PGs by direct activation of phospholipase [11,135,152].

PATHOLOGICAL CONSIDERATIONS

With the notable exception of bradykinin, it appears that multiple stimuli that produce initial renal vasoconstriction result in a compensatory release of vasodilating PGs. It is now also clear that in pathological renal states that are also associated with intrarenal vasoconstriction (acute and chronic renal failure), a similar phenomenon obtains. In animals, prior administration of PGE_2 does not obviate the fall in inulin clearance in the nephrotoxic model of acute renal failure (uranyl nitrate), but does in the vasoconstrictor model (norepinephrine infusion) [183]. Furthermore, in human chronic renal failure secondary to lupus erythematosus, urinary immunoreactive PGE (iPGE) is high and falls subsequent to aspirin treatment, a decrease associated with an 18% fall in creatinine clearance and a 14% fall in inulin clearance [143]. Similar observations have been made with PG synthesis inhibition in patients with renal vasoconstriction associated with cirrhosis with ascites [312]. Thus it would appear that intrarenal PGs are important compensatory determinants of renal blood flow, tending to offset not only physiological effects causing intrarenal vasoconstriction, but also pathological events leading to reductions in renal blood flow and glomerular filtration.

Sodium Excretion

The highly controversial role of prostaglandins in the renal handling of sodium involves a host of factors, including alterations in intrarenal hemodynamics, physical factors, natriuretic "hormone," vasopressin, oxytocin, calcitonin, glucagon, kallikrein, and aldosterone.

Since the studies to be cited are conflicting and at times irreconcilable, an attempt has been made to present this material in a way that reflects the different aspects from which PGs and sodium excretion have been studied: exogenous administration, endogenous release, PG synthesis inhibition, and the effects in vivo of alterations of sodium intake.

EXOGENOUS ADMINISTRATION

In vivo experiments in man and animals have clearly shown that exogenous prostaglandins of the A,D,E, and I series are natriuretic when infused intravenously or into the renal artery at rates that did not lower blood pressure [42,54,99,113,127,160,164,278]. In most animal studies, PG administration resulted in an increase in renal blood flow while glomerular filtration rate (GFR) remained unchanged [54,99,278]. As previously noted, PG-induced elevation in renal blood flow and natriuresis may be mediated at least in part by the kinins, since the elevation in sodium excretion following PGE_1 administration in vivo was accompanied by an increase in urinary kallikrein [188]. The specificity and physiological significance of administration of exogenous prostaglandins in vivo is questionable, both because many other renal vasodilators such as acetylcholine produce almost identical effects [54,181] and because it is unclear whether exogenous PGs reach tubular sites normally occurring with endogenously released PGs.

In addition to a hemodynamic mechanism for PG-induced natriuresis, a direct effect of PG on sodium transport has been proposed by several investigators [54,99,113,124]. In in vitro studies, PGE_1 increased transmembrane sodium transport in toad bladder and isolated frog skin [25,170], whereas PGE_2 has been shown to decrease sodium transport in isolated collecting ducts of rabbits [131]. Some reports, however, have failed to show a direct effect of either PGE_1, $PGF_{2\alpha}$, or PGA_2 on isolated perfused ascending limbs, collecting tubules, or rabbit renal slices [73,90], although micropuncture studies have revealed that there is a significant decrease in net sodium efflux in nephron segments at or beyond the late proximal tubule, suggesting a direct inhibitory tubular effect of PGs [139,264].

ENDOGENOUS EFFECTS OF PROSTAGLANDINS

To obviate the disadvantages associated with exogenous PG administration, Tannenbaum et al. [270] infused the PG precursor arachidonic acid to stimulate endogenous prostaglandin synthesis and release. Unlike the effects of exogenous PGs, arachidonic acid did not produce large changes in renal blood flow, whereas similar effects were observed when sodium excretion was increased, actions that could be abolished by PG synthesis inhibition. Similar effects were observed by Chang et al. [55] and Bolger et al. [41].

In addition to PG precursors, loop diuretics such as furosemide and ethacrynic acid appear to increase endogenous PG synthesis and/or decrease endogenous PG metabolism. In man, endogenous stimulation of circulating arachidonic acid (probably systemically stimulated) was found after furosemide administration [290]. This occurred in conjunction with increases in plasma renin activity, urinary $PGF_{2\alpha}$, and sodium excretion. The elevation in arachidonic acid, PRA, and urinary $PGF_{2\alpha}$ could be inhibited by indomethacin, although furosemide-induced natriuresis persisted. This suggests that the increase in urinary sodium output induced by furosemide is not mediated by prostaglandins. These findings are in contrast to the results obtained by Oliw et al. [208], who found that pretreatment of rabbits with indomethacin reduced the effect of furosemide on electrolyte excretion by more than 80%. These results, together with the observation that in the anesthetized animal and the conscious human, indomethacin also inhibits furosemide-induced increases in renal blood flow [148,228,299], support the possibility that the increased sodium output seen after furosemide administration is the result of increased blood flow, which could be mediated by the increased renal prostaglandin release that is known to occur during furosemide and chorazanil administration [214,300]. The reason for the conflicting and opposite results reported with furosemide and the PGs by various investigators is obscure but is discussed in greater detail below.

PROSTAGLANDIN SYNTHESIS INHIBITION

Since the evidence for direct effects of prostaglandins on sodium transport is inconclusive, efforts have been made to study the problem indirectly through inhibition of endogenous prostaglandin synthesis. In essential fatty acid deficiency (and presumably PG deficiency), the ability of the rat kidney to excrete an acute salt load appears to be diminished [246], suggesting a possible physiological natriuretic function for the renal PGs.

In the conscious dog undergoing water diuresis, Kirschenbaum and Stein [145] showed that meclofenamate as well as RO 20-5720 (two PG synthesis inhibitors) increased sodium excretion. Furthermore, in anesthetized dogs during volume expansion with Ringer's solution, no effect on sodium output was observed after PG synthesis inhibition, despite a fall in renal blood flow and renal venous PGE material [146]. This suggests that under certain circumstances the renal PGs are not natriuretic and in fact may act in an antinatriuretic fashion that is not yet clear. Kirschenbaum [144] also investigated the natriuresis observed during administration of such renal vasodilators as acetylcholine and bradykinin; it was demonstrated that this effect is not mediated by prostaglandins by pointing out that there was no difference in urinary sodium output with these agents, with or without PG synthesis inhibition.

In contrast to the aforementioned studies, Fejes-Toth et al. [85] found that PG inhibition in conscious dogs is accompanied by an enhanced vasopressin-induced antinatriuresis. Altsheler et al. [5], also using unanesthetized dogs, observed no changes in sodium excretion after PG synthesis inhibition during water diuresis. In addition, these investigators observed antinatriuresis after saline administration and in dogs with a reduced renal mass following PG synthesis inhibition, observations that again cannot be reconciled with the results of Kirschenbaum et al. [144,145]. Düsing et al. [77,79] and Feldman et al. [86] showed similar results during acute salt loading in extracellular volume expansion or in adrenalectomized animals, respectively. In man, Frölich et al. [96] and Donker et al. [69] observed marked sodium retention after indomethacin administration. However, Patak et al. [228] and Rumpf et al. [248] found no effect of indomethacin under similar conditions. The conflicting results obtained by these different investigators, which cannot be explained at the moment, are probably attributable to the level of consciousness, the preexisting state of sodium balance, or the type of volume expansion utilized.

ALTERATIONS IN SODIUM INTAKE

Another approach utilized to explore the possible interaction between prostaglandins and renal sodium is the measurement of urinary, venous, or tissue prostaglandins during conditions of varying sodium intake. In man, current evidence favors an antinatriuretic role of circulatory or intrarenal prostaglandins in normotensive man, since (1) plasma PGA rises in concert with renin and aldosterone during states of volume depletion such as sodium restriction [232,319] or following hemodialysis [136], and (2) infusion of PGA results in a rise in plasma renin and aldosterone in normotensive man [109], suggesting that volume depletion may lead to increased renal PG production, resulting in turn in renin release and subsequent aldosterone-mediated antinatriuresis. In contrast to these results is the finding that PGA and PGE increase in renal venous blood following saline infusion in the renal artery of man [227] and dog [271].

A similar confusing situation exists for the presence of urinary PGs during salt loading. Scherer et al. [251] and Weber et al. [289] found a decrease in urinary PGE_2 after saline infusion in rabbits, with no effect on $PGF_{2\alpha}$. Davila et al. [65] reported that both urinary PGE_2 and $PGF_{2\alpha}$ decreased during salt loading. By contrast, low sodium intake resulted in significant increase in urinary PGE_2 and $PGF_{2\alpha}$. Under similar experimental conditions, however, Lifschitz et al. [168] did not find any significant changes in PGE_2 concentration in the urine.

Attallah et al. [16] observed an increase in iPGA in outer rabbit renal medulla and a decrease in papillary iPGA during chronic salt loading in the rabbit, effects that were inhibited by indomethacin. Tobian et al. [275], however, found an increase in PGE-like material in the whole kidney of rats on a low salt diet and a corresponding decrease on high salt intakes. More recently in in vitro experiments, Danon et al. [62] demonstrated that hypertonicity (induced by sodium chloride in the media) stimulates PGE_2, $PGF_{2\alpha}$ and PGD_2 output in homogenates of rat renal papilla.

Thus, there are conflicting and at times irreconcilable data implicating the renal PGs as natriuretic or antinatriuretic factors. Therefore, studies were undertaken in our laboratories to investigate the urinary excretion of PGE_2, the concentration of PGE_2 in cortex, outer medulla, and papilla, and the biosynthesis of PGE_2 during chronic alterations in sodium intake in conscious rabbits by a combined in vivo–in vitro approach [262]. In these studies, mean urinary PGE_2 excretion, during a 10-day observation period, was increased significantly in animals on low sodium when compared to normal or high sodium intakes. The effect of sodium intake on de novo PGE_2 biosynthesis calculated as the difference between total in vitro PGE_2 production and initial content on low, normal, and high sodium intakes is shown in Figure 2. It is evident that papillary PGE_2 biosynthesis rose significantly on low salt intake. There was no difference in PGE_2 biosynthesis between rabbits on normal salt and high salt intake. A similar pattern was observed with outer medullary PGE_2 biosynthesis, which also displayed an inverse correlation with sodium intake. The greatest effect was observed between normal salt and low salt diet, with only a slight decrease between normal salt and high salt diet. Cortical PGE_2 synthesis, however, did not rise significantly on low salt intake when compared to normal salt intake but did fall on high salt intake.

These studies of altered dietary sodium intake revealed that in renal papillary, outer medullary, and to a much lesser extent cortical tissue,

FIGURE 2. Renal de novo PGE_2 biosynthesis at low, normal, and high sodium chloride intakes. Each value represents the mean ± standard error of nine observations. (From Ref. 262 with permission of the publisher.

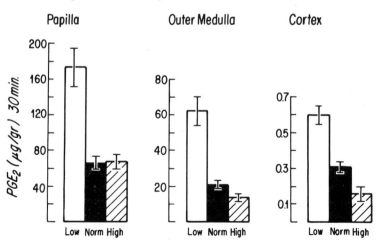

PGE$_2$ biosynthesis is markedly and significantly increased in vitro in animals that have been volume depleted by sodium restriction in vivo. In this regard, it should be emphasized that it is not possible to distinguish whether the increased PGE$_2$ biosynthesis during low sodium intake is the result of sodium depletion per se or of the associated decrease in extracellular fluid volume. The mechanism of the rise in outer medullary and papillary PGE$_2$ is unclear. Numerous stimuli are known to enhance renal PGE$_2$ production both in vivo and in vitro, including vasopressin, angiotensin, norepinephrine, sympathetic nervous stimulation, hyperosmolality, potassium depletion, and bradykinin. Vasopressin activation of renal PGE$_2$ production appears unlikely during volume depletion, since Share et al. [257] and Brennan et al. [49] observed unchanged peripheral vasopressin plasma levels during marked sodium restriction in human subjects and in dogs, respectively. Although it is impossible to exclude the many other multifactorial stimuli that might participate in PGE$_2$ synthesis stimulation, the major known humoral system, which unequivocally rises with PGE$_2$ during volume depletion, is the renin-angiotensin axis. Although PGE$_2$ stimulates renin release and might be functioning in this fashion in the present experiments, it is also possible that its enhanced synthesis is mediated by the rise in angiotensin that occurs during sodium restriction. This is supported by our recent finding on the effect of Sar[1]-Ile[8]-angiotensin II, an angiotensin II antagonist, on urinary PGE$_2$ and PGF$_{2\alpha}$ excretion in rabbits maintained on low sodium diets (Fig. 3). Both urinary PGE$_2$ and PGF$_{2\alpha}$ excretion declined markedly with the angiotensin II blocker at a time when plasma renin showed a fivefold rise.

The significance of the rise in renal PGE$_2$ biosynthesis during volume depletion secondary to low sodium intake is unclear. A natriuretic role for PGE$_2$ has long been postulated on the following basis: (1) PGE$_2$ given exogenously produces an increase in renal blood flow and natriuresis, (2) inhibition of PGE$_2$ biosynthesis by indomethacin under certain conditions results in sodium retention and a decrease in renal blood flow, and (3) micropuncture studies reveal that PGE$_2$ inhibits chloride transport in the thick ascending limb. However, one major criticism of these studies is that when prostaglandin is administered exogenously, the effects may not represent those of endogenously produced prostaglandins, which may act at different renal sites. Although a natriuretic role for the renal PGs had been postulated for years, there is relatively recent evidence that PGs and PG precursors stimulate renin release, that plasma and urinary PGs rise during salt depletion, and that prostaglandin synthesis inhibition results in decreased renin release and natriuresis under certain conditions. Thus an antinatriuretic role is suggested for these compounds through stimulation of renin release with subsequent angiotensin-mediated aldosterone production and sodium retention.

The alternate interpretation of the significance of the increase in PGE$_2$ biosynthesis is that during volume depletion there may be an initial reduction of renal blood flow, resulting in an increased synthesis and release of renal PGE$_2$ that functions to maintain renal blood flow and

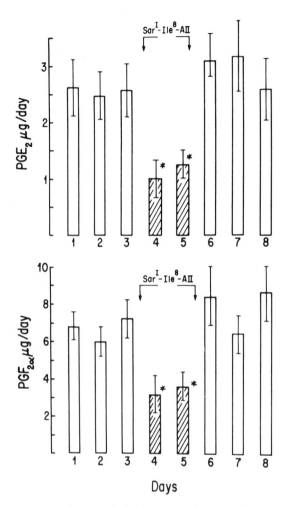

FIGURE 3. Effect of Sar[1]-Ile[8]-angiotensin II on urinary prostaglandins excretion in animals on low salt intake (* $p < 0.001$).

urine formation by offsetting the mitigating effect on renal blood flow of the maximally stimulated renin-angiotensin-aldosterone axis. Additional studies will be necessary to precisely establish the significance of the increased PGE_2 synthesis and release observed during volume depletion observed during volume depletion secondary to dietary sodium restriction.

DIURETICS

It has been proposed that the mechanisms by which the loop diuretics lower blood pressure, induce salt and water loss, and augment renal blood flow and renin release are at least partly mediated by prostaglandins. To test this hypothesis, two experimental approaches have been employed. One is to investigate the effect of diuretics on PG synthesis and metabolism. The second, more indirect, approach involves the influence of PG synthesis inhibitors on the pharmacological profile of the diuretics.

Effects of Diuretics on Prostaglandin Synthesis and Metabolism. Although the data concerning the second approach are conflicting, almost all studies in which PG excretion was evaluated after diuretic administration clearly show a striking rise in renal PGs. Originally observed in dog renal venous blood after a single injection of furosemide and ethacrynic acid [300,301], this effect was subsequently documented in animals and man by several groups. In most of these investigations, furosemide was shown to markedly enhance urinary PG excretion. Figure 4 illustrates a typical effect of furosemide on urinary PGE_2 excretion, with and without indomethacin. Furosemide alone significantly increased U_{PGE_2} by 10 minutes, and this volume declined to control values within 50 minutes. Furosemide plus indomethacin at 2 mg/kg reduced furosemide-induced $U_{PGE_2}V$, while indomethacin at 10 mg/kg eliminated the furosemide effect. The $U_{PGE_2}V$, 50 minutes following furosemide, with or without indomethacin, returned to values not significantly different from control. The elevation in urinary excretion of PGs is not only restricted to the loop diuretics but has been observed with clonidine

FIGURE 4. Effect of furosemide and indomethacin on rabbit urinary PGE_2 excretion. Each value represents the mean ± standard error of six observations.

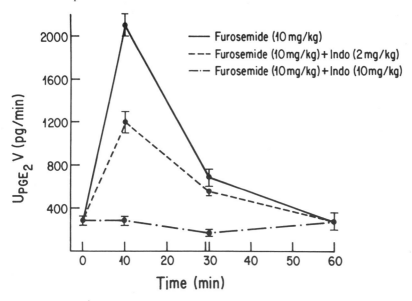

[210] and chlorazanil [214]. On the other hand, in one study, chloro-thiazide or benzolamide did not alter $U_{PGE_2}V$ [229].

One of the explanations for the rise in urinary PGs with the loop diuretics is that these compounds inhibit PG metabolism, since 15-hy-droxy PGDH and 9-keto-reductase have been shown to be inhibited by furosemide in vitro [231,263]. Another explanation for the rise in urinary PGs might be direct or indirect stimulation of PG synthesis by the loop diuretics. Recent studies [18,21] have, in fact, shown an increase in de novo papillary PGE_2 biosynthesis by 12.5 minutes following furosemide administration; a decline to control levels followed within 60 minutes of the furosemide. De novo cortical PGE_2 biosynthesis was not altered significantly by furosemide. One possible explanation for the enhanced papillary synthesis is that there may be an increased availability of the PG substrate arachidonic acid following furosemide administration [290].

Effects of Prostaglandin Synthesis Inhibition on the Pharmacologic Actions of Diuretics. Although most diuretics investigated appear to increase the urinary excretion of PGs, the role of PG in the renal response to these drugs is as yet unclear. In some studies aspirinlike drugs totally or partially blunt the natriuretic response to diuretics, but PG synthesis inhibition in other studies failed to modify the action of the same di-uretics. The reasons for such discrepancies remain unclear.

Effects on Blood Pressure. The vasodepressor properties of furosemide were shown to be blocked when this drug was given simultaneously with indomethacin in normotensive and hypertensive man [228]. These find-ings are also supported by studies by Lopez-Ovejero et al. [174], who demonstrated that indomethacin blunts or even reverses the antihyper-tensive effects of chlorthalidone, hydrochlorothiazide, and propranolol. The mechanisms by which indomethacin interferes with the blood pres-sure lowering effects of these drugs however, remains unknown.

Effects on Renal Blood Flow. Most of the published studies showed that the increase in renal blood flow induced with the loop diuretics was inhibited with indomethacin [23,64,299]. Similarly, the ability of these diuretics to alter blood flow distribution within the kidney was reduced. These findings strongly suggest that PGs may mediate the dilation of the renal vasculature produced by diuretics and contribute to the natri-uresis by reallocating flow within the kidney.

Effects on Renin Release. It has long been known that diuretic therapy induces the release of renin, which in turn produces angiotensin II and aldosterone. The mechanism by which this stimulation occurs is not believed to involve volume depletion, but it may be related to the macula densa and the renal baroreceptor system. It is well accepted that furo-semide increases and indomethacin decreases plasma renin activity, and the combination of the two drugs results in an intermediate response [96,97,228,247]. The mechanism by which indomethacin reduces renin release appears to be unrelated to changes in sodium balance [97] or to interference with the tubular secretion of furosemide; however it may be a direct effect or an indirect action through PG synthesis inhibition.

Figure 5 illustrates the effect of furosemide alone and in the presence of indomethacin on plasma renin activity (PRA). Following furosemide alone, PRA rose markedly and remained significantly elevated by 60 minutes following furosemide. In contrast to the modest effect of indomethacin at 2 mg/kg on $U_{PGE_2}V$ (Fig. 4), indomethacin at 2 mg almost eliminated the furosemide-induced rise in PRA to values not significantly different from those in the presence of 10 mg/kg indomethacin at all time intervals.

From the data of Figure 5 and previous reports, it can be concluded that furosemide increases and indomethacin decreases PRA. However additional PG-independent mechanisms may be involved in the action of furosemide on renin release, as suggested by the foregoing in vivo studies and recent in vitro studies by Desaulles and Schwartz [67], which demonstrated a lack of effect of indomethacin on furosemide-induced rise in renin release by rat kidney slices.

Effects on Salt and Water Loss. Although the use of diuretics in combination with PG synthesis has clarified some aspects of the role of PGs in urine formation, the various experimental preparations and methodologies utilized have yielded conflicting interpretations and conclusions. Thus, in several studies in man [97,228] indomethacin alone

FIGURE 5. Effect of furosemide and indomethacin on plasma renin activity in the rabbit. (AI = angiotensin I) Each value represents the mean ± standard error of five observations.

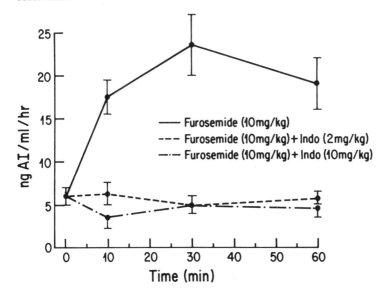

caused little sodium retention, but significantly reduced the natriuretic and diuretic activity of furosemide. In one study [174], the antinatriuretic actions of indomethacin could be reversed only by combined use of spironolactone and furosemide. Neither of these two agents was effective alone in the presence of indomethacin. In patients with impaired renal function, aspirin was also shown to interfere with the natriuretic response to furosemide [143]. However, in other studies in normal man [31,252], aspirinlike drugs were without influence on furosemide-induced natriuresis. Some studies in animals [32,148,208] demonstrated an antagonism between PG synthesis inhibitors and several diuretics, but others [31,290] revealed no such opposing effects.

Figure 6 illustrates the effect of furosemide administration with and without indomethacin on urinary salt and water excretion in conscious rabbits [21]: $U_{Na}V$ rose to a maximum at 10 minutes, declining to control values by 50 minutes. Significant enhancement of the furosemide effect on $U_{Na}V$ was observed in the presence of 2 mg/kg indomethacin, whereas at 10 mg/kg indomethacin significantly reduced furosemide-stimulated natriuresis. UV as shown on the right of Figure 6 paralleled $U_{Na}V$. Thus, furosemide-induced salt and water loss was markedly enhanced with the low dose of indomethacin and significantly decreased at a higher dose of the PG synthesis inhibition.

In an attempt to explain these observations, we also studied the effect

FIGURE 6. Effect of furosemide and indomethacin on rabbit urinary sodium and water excretion. Each value represents the mean ± standard error of six observations.

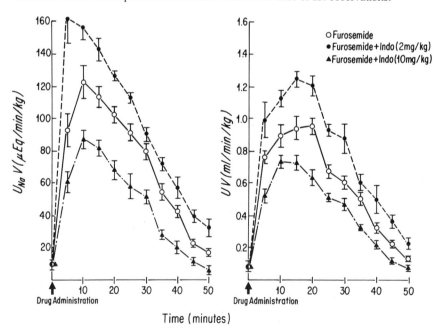

of various doses of indomethacin administered in vivo on in vitro PGE_2 biosynthesis, by renal cortical and papillary slices [21]. The studies show that indomethacin resulted in a dose-dependent inhibition in renal PGE_2 biosynthesis, exhibiting a regional pattern, with cortical inhibition being more profound than that of papilla. This may be the result of a greater cortical than papillary blood flow distribution; as well as the presence of an organic acid transport mechanism in cortical cells that at any given dose might lead to a higher indomethacin concentration in the cortex. Thus low doses of indomethacin, which primarily affect the renal cortical region, may enhance furosemide-induced natriuresis by decreasing the production of a cortical antinatriuretic factor such as angiotensin II, since indomethacin also reduces cortical renin release and angiotensin II formation [287]. On the other hand, high doses of indomethacin, which inhibit renal papillary as well as cortical PGE_2 production, may reduce furosemide-induced natriuresis, possibly by decreasing the production of a papillary natriuretic factor. This natriuretic factor could be a prostaglandin, since as shown in Figure 4, PGE_2 production was enhanced by furosemide.

In conclusion, recent studies have shown that the loop diuretics increase PG release, possibly via stimulation of synthesis and/or inhibition of metabolism. Under certain conditions, PG synthesis inhibition can interfere with the response to diuretic therapy. The degree of antagonism appears, however, to be related to the dose of the PG synthesis inhibitor, the state of sodium balance, the renin-angiotensin axis, and renal hemodynamics. Interestingly, all patients with essential hypertension, nephrotic syndrome, or impaired kidney function show a decreased response to diuretic therapy when the latter is combined with PG synthesis inhibitors. At present, this reaction has important clinical implications in the management of hypertensive and edematous states requiring diuretic therapy in the presence of such conditions as rheumatoid arthritis and gout, for which nonsteroidal antiinflammatory treatment is necessary.

WATER EXCRETION

Interaction with Vasopressin

Since the renomedullary collecting duct has a high capacity for PGE_2 synthesis, a possible role for PGE_2 in the regulation of water excretion has been explored in detail. Original studies revealed that PGE_1 inhibits vasopressin but not cyclic AMP water movement in the toad bladder and isolated collecting duct cell, suggesting an inhibitory effect on vasopressin-stimulated adenyl cyclase [110,217]. This is supported by the finding that PGE mediates the decrease in 3′,5′-cyclic AMP in the isolated collecting duct tubule [110], toad bladder [170], and renal medulla [28,182]. Furthermore, in in vivo studies, inhibition of PG biosynthesis with aspirin, indomethacin, or meclofenamate results in a marked enhancement of vasopressin-stimulated water reabsorption and maximal

U_{osm} in the rat, dog, and man [6,36,175]. The mechanism of action of the sulfonylureas, known to enhance vasopressin-induced water movement, also appears to involve inhibition of PGE synthesis in the toad bladder [317]. Interestingly, vasopressin in turn stimulates PGE biosynthesis in the toad bladder [316], rabbit interstitial cell tissue cultures [315], and medullary slices [137], an effect abrogated by phospholipase inhibition [315] and associated with decreased water permeability response to vasopressin. This suggests that water permeability may be inhibited by PGE synthesized in response to vasopressin—a possible physiological negative feedback system. In this connection Zusman et al. [318] showed that in the toad bladder, adrenal steroids with predominantly glucocorticoid effects inhibited vasopressin-stimulated PGE biosynthesis that was associated with enhanced vasopressin-stimulated water movement, suggesting that at least part of the mechanism of the increase in vasopressin-induced water movement by adrenal steroids lies in PG synthesis inhibition. In support of the concept that PGs antagonize vasopressin-mediated water reabsorption, Walker et al. [285] and Dunn et al. [72] reported an 80% decrease in urinary PGE_2 excretion in Brattleboro homozygous diabetes insipidus rats when compared to Long Evans controls. Furthermore, these authors demonstrated an increase in PGE_2 excretion in the diabetes insipidus rats upon treatment with vasopressin.

In summary, PGs appear to have a role in attenuating the action of vasopressin by inhibition of adenyl cyclase or modulation of medullary blood flow and interstitial tonicity.

Potassium and the Renal Concentrating Defect

The most consistently observed alteration in renal function during chronic hypokalemia is the loss of maximal urinary concentrating ability [254]. Since prostaglandins antagonize vasopressin stimulation of adenyl cyclase and water permeability in experimental animals [110,217], are increased in the urine of dogs with experimental hypokalemia [101], are stimulated by low-medium potassium in vitro in renal medullary interstitial cells in culture [313] and in renal medullary slices [76], and are elevated in the urine of hypokalemic patients with Bartter's syndrome [107], it has been hypothesized that the polyuria of potassium deficiency is mediated by enhanced renal synthesis of prostaglandins.

Although PG synthesis inhibition was originally reported to correct the hypokalemia, alkalosis, hyperreninemia, and decreased sensitivity to angiotensin II in Bartter's syndrome, further studies with chronic indomethacin therapy revealed that there was not full correction of the hypokalemia and that renal potassium loss continued at a time when renin and aldosterone were normal [47], suggesting that potassium loss could be the cause, not the result, of the hyperaldosteronism. In addition, although Galvez et al. [101] reported in preliminary studies that indomethacin corrected the defect in maximal urinary concentration in six potassium-depleted dogs, further studies in 28 animals failed to confirm this: there was no improvement in concentration following 3 days of indomethacin despite a significant reduction in PGE excretion [88]. Furthermore, Hood and Dunn [125] failed to observe a change in urinary PGE_2 during 2 weeks of potassium depletion despite the onset of polyuria. These studies thus suggest that PG synthesis and excretion is either enhanced or unchanged under relatively acute potassium depletion.

To assess the effect of chronic dietary potassium restriction on renal PG production, Attallah et al. [20] and Beck and Shaw [29] recently tested the hypothesis that renal PG may mediate the renal functional defects of potassium depletion in rabbits and rats, respectively. After 3 weeks of potassium restriction, urinary PGE_2 excretion was significantly lower in the hypokalemic rabbits and rats when compared to normal control. Figure 7 demonstrates that in the rabbit, reduction in urinary PGE_2 was evident only after the twentieth day on the potassium-restricted diet. This delayed response may explain the failure of previous investigations to note an effect of potassium on PG excretion [125]. In support of the urinary findings, renal tissue PGE_2 was markedly lower in hypokalemic animals when compared to normal controls (Table 1). It is evident that de novo papillary, medullary, and cortical PGE_2 biosynthesis decreased significantly in animals on low potassium intake.

In summary, chronic potassium depletion is associated with a decrease in renal PGE_2 biosynthesis, not an increase—a finding that does not

FIGURE 7. Effect of dietary potassium restriction on rabbit daily urinary PGE_2 excretion. Each value represents the mean ± standard error of six observations. (From Ref. 20 with permission of the publisher.)

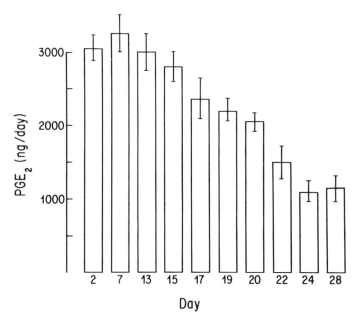

TABLE 1. Effect of Dietary Potassium on de Novo Renal PGE_2 Biosynthesis in Rabbit

	Normal K^+	p	Low K^+
Papilla	20.2 ± 2.0	< 0.005	12.1 ± 1.2
Outer medulla	8.73 ± 1.69	< 0.025	3.70 ± 0.73
Cortex	0.057 ± 0.009	< 0.005	0.024 ± 0.005

Note: Results expressed as micrograms per gram per half-hour. Each value represents the mean $\pm$ SE of 24 experiments. De novo synthesis was calculated as the difference between total PGE_2 production in vitro and initial slice PGE_2 concentration.
Source: From Attallah et al. [20], with permission of the publisher.

support the hypothesis that PGE_2 mediates the renal concentrating defect of potassium nephropathy.

PROSTAGLANDINS AND THE RENIN-ANGIOTENSIN AXIS

One of the most intensively studied areas in renal PG research is the interaction of PGs with the renin–angiotensin II–aldosterone axis. On the one hand, PGA_1, PGD_2, PGE_2, and PGI_2 have been shown to result in renin release, but on the other hand angiotensin II is a potent stimulator of PG synthesis, indicating a positive feedback interplay between the renin and prostaglandin axes. This discussion summarizes what is known regarding these effects and how these interactions may affect sodium and water homeostasis and blood regulation.

Prostaglandins and Renin Release

In addition to the extensively investigated mechanisms of renin release in the kidney cortex, prostaglandins and their precursors have also been implicated as important stimulators of renal renin release. The studies that show a prostaglandin-renin interaction were performed in vivo in man and both in vivo and in vitro in animals. Therefore, the effects of PGs on renin are discussed in terms of the action of PG administration in vivo, PG synthesis inhibition in vivo, and PG administration in vitro.

IN VIVO PROSTAGLANDIN ADMINISTRATION

The early results in which PGs were infused provided conflicting data on renin release. Vander [278] did not find any change in renin release after infusion of PGE_1 and PGE_2 into the renal artery of dogs. However, Werning et al. [294] observed a significant rise in plasma renin activity (PRA) coincident with natriuresis and diuresis upon infusion of higher rates of PGE_1 in the aorta of dogs. The discrepancy in the results of these two studies appears to be related to differences in PG dosage. The results of Werning et al. were confirmed by Yun et al. [304] in anesthetized dogs, which showed an increase in renal renin secretion rate following PGE_1 and PGE_2 infusion into the renal artery of filtering kidneys. In nonfiltering kidneys, PGE_2 resulted in an increase in renin release [305]. In these studies, $PGF_{2\alpha}$ was without effect. More recently, Gerber et al. [102] showed in the dog that PGI_2 administration also results in enhanced renin release.

The renin release in the denervated nonfiltering unnephrectomized kidney caused by PGI_2 and PGE_2 [255,305] suggests that the action of PGs is not mediated by the sympathetic nervous system, or by changes in sodium concentration at the macula densa. Whether PG-induced renin release is mediated by the renal baroreceptor mechanism or by a direct action on the juxtaglomerular apparatus is unknown: some studies show an inhibition by indomethacin of the increase in renin following reduction of renal perfusion pressure [35,63], and other studies report the opposite [256]. The most likely compounds among the renal prostaglandins for releasing renin are PGE_2 and PGI_2; some studies show a similar capability for PGD_2 [255], and others revealed no PGD_2 effect [102].

Since exogenous administration of PGs may be unphysiological in the sense that any observed actions may result from effects of infused PGs at sites not normally reached by endogenously produced PGs, a more physiological approach was pursued by utilization of the PG precursor arachidonic acid as a substrate for stimulating renin release by enhancement of endogenous PG biosynthesis. It was observed that increased PRA occurred in the vena cava of rats and rabbits following infusion of arachidonic acid in the aorta [156,286]. No natriuresis followed the renin release that was stimulated by arachidonic acid, suggesting that the increase in renin secretion results from factors other than changes in sodium concentration at the macula densa. Bolger et al. [41] observed similar changes in the filtering dog kidney, although a significant natriuresis occurred. The effect of arachidonic acid in releasing renin was also observed in the nonfiltering dog kidney by Data et al. [63]. In humans, the effect of PGA_1 infusion on plasma renin activity was studied by Golub et al. [109] and Carr [53], with the former investigators observing a rise in PRA and the latter detecting no effect. These contradictory reports have yet to be reconciled.

In summary, it seems reasonable to conclude at the present time that exogenous PGs and PG precursors have a definite stimulatory effect on renal cortical renin release that is partly a direct effect of PGs on the macula densa cells. Although PGs have the capacity to stimulate renin release when administered exogenously, there is no evidence that endogenously produced prostaglandins normally exert this effect under appropriate physiological stimuli.

IN VIVO PROSTAGLANDIN SYNTHESIS INHIBITION

Basal PRA decreases in normotensive rabbits after administration of indomethacin [156]. Similar effects were found by Patak et al. [228] in normal and hypertensive man without any change in urine volume and sodium output, observations also noted by other investigators [96,247]. In animals and humans, furosemide-stimulated renin release is inhibited by indomethacin [69,96,247]. PG synthesis inhibition also decreased the elevated PRA present in orthostasis [247], in renovascular hypertensive rabbits [241], and in rabbits following hemorrhage [243]. More recently, significant decreases in PRA and blood pressure were observed by Stahl et al. [261] in rats on a low sodium diet receiving indomethacin. However, in man on a low sodium intake, indomethacin inhibited the elevated levels of renin only in the presence of β-adrenergic blockade [97]. This, together with the apparent failure of indomethacin to inhibit the increased renin response to isoproteranol [35,256], suggests that PG-mediated renin release during low sodium intake may be the result of activation of β-adrenergic pathways, which predominates even during PG synthetase inhibition.

The results of PG synthesis inhibition have not yielded definitive information on a physiological role for renal PGs in renin release. It is possible that indomethacin itself directly inhibits renin release as well as acting through PG synthesis inhibition. Clarification of the involvement of PGs and renin release will probably have to await more physiologically oriented studies.

IN VITRO PROSTAGLANDIN ADMINISTRATION
AND SYNTHESIS INHIBITION

In 1976 Dew and Michelakis [68] showed that addition of PGE_2 to rabbit renal cortical cell suspensions caused a rise in renin release, whereas $PGF_{2\alpha}$ resulted in a decrease. Contradictory results were obtained by Weber et al. [287], who could not find a stimulation of renin release following incubation of rabbit renal cortical slices with PGE_2. In this study, arachidonic acid was shown to be the most potent renin stimulator, suggesting that PG synthesis stimulation by arachidonic acid increases renin release by PG endoperoxides. At a concentration of 5×10^6 M, PGI_2 also has been shown to stimulate renin release from cortical slices [296] with a linear time response over a 30-minute period; 6-keto-$PGF_{1\alpha}$ was without effect. Based on these results, it has been speculated that PGI_2 may be the major PG responsible for cortical renin release [296], since 17.8% of PGs produced by rabbit renal cortical microsomes are 6-keto-$PGF_{1\alpha}$ [297]. However, this hypothesis needs much further exploration, since it is known that PGI_2 is inactivated after 7–11 minutes at 25°C [266], and it is difficult to reconcile this with the facts that the action of PGI_2 on renin release is maximal at 30 minutes and that its metabolite 6-keto-$PGF_{1\alpha}$ had no effect on renin release. In addition, 60% of the cortical PGs formed were $PGF_{2\alpha}$, a compound known to inhibit renin release [287].

Angiotensin II and Prostaglandin Synthesis

McGiff et al. [184] originally found that infusion of angiotensin II into the renal artery of dogs led to an initial decrease in renal blood flow followed by a return to control despite continued infusion of angiotensin

II. The tachyphylactic effect was accompanied by increased PG-like material in the renal venous blood. Both the tachyphylaxis and PG-like release were inhibited by indomethacin, leading to speculation that the increase in PGE-like material acts as a regulator of renal blood flow to offset the vasoconstricting effects of angiotensin II. Infusion of angiotensin II in man also leads to an increase in urinary PGE_2 excretion [98]. In vitro experiments with rat renal papillary slices [61] and interstitial cell tissue cultures [315] also have shown that angiotensin II increases PGE release.

Since angiotensin II stimulates PG release, and since situations leading to an increase in the renin-angiotensin axis (low sodium diet, renal nerve stimulation, renal ischemia, norepinephrine, diuretic therapy) are associated with a concomitant rise in renal PG production, the following question arises: Are these increases in PG release mediated by angiotensin II? Needleman et al. [199] observed a fall in PG release following administration of certain angiotensin II antagonists. In contrast, in in vivo studies inhibition of angiotensin II generation with the converting enzyme inhibitors SQ 20881 [134] and SQ 14225 [215] or blockade with saralasin [207,265] failed to produce a change in PGE release.

Recently however, Attallah et al. [19] observed a marked decrease in de novo in vitro PGE_2 biosynthesis by slices of rabbit renal cortex, outer medulla, and papilla from rabbits on a low (but not high) sodium diet following chronic in vivo administration of the angiotensin II blocker Sar^1-Ile^8-angiotensin II (Fig. 3). This was accompanied by a significant reduction in urinary PGE_2 excretion. Utilizing this combined in vivo–in vitro approach, Attallah et al. [22] also showed a marked inhibitory effect on PGE_2 synthesis, with angiotensin converting enzyme inhibition by SQ 20881 and SQ 14225. Furthermore, the rise in de novo in vitro PGE_2 synthesis by rabbit papillary slices following the administration of furosemide in vivo was completely abolished by prior administration of saralasin [18].

These investigators provide the first evidence that the increase in PG synthesis during either low sodium diet or loop diuretic therapy may be mediated by a primary increase in the renin–angiotensin II axis. The only other explanation would be that angiotensin-converting enzyme inhibitors and blockers directly inhibit PG synthesis in an action similar to that of indomethacin. At present, there is no evidence in support of this hypothesis.

Physiological Aspects

The only physiological role of an interplay between the renin–angiotensin II–aldosterone axis and the prostaglandin system at the present appears to be related to renal-adrenal function during volume depletion resulting from dietary sodium restriction. Figure 8 summarizes a hypothetical schema involving renin and the PGs in the renal adaptation to sodium deprivation. Since renin increases in the presence of PG synthesis inhibition in the human on a low salt diet, and since this

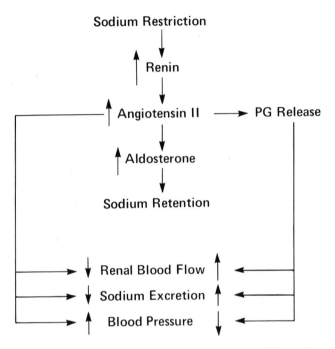

FIGURE 8. Hypothetical schema of the interaction of the renin-angiotensin-aldosterone axis and PG in the renal adaptation to dietary sodium restriction. [From J. B. Lee, Prostaglandin and the renin angiotensin axis. Clin. Nephrol. 14, 159–163 (1980).]

rise is blocked by propanolol [97], it would appear that during sodium restriction PGs do not stimulate renin production but rather the β-adrenergic nervous system prevails to bring about the elevation in renin release. This in turn results ultimately in generation of angiotensin II, which has at least three actions.

First, it is widely accepted that angiotensin II results in an enhanced adrenal production of aldosterone, which acts on the kidney to result in appropriate sodium retention. Since angiotensin II is known to stimulate PGE production in vivo and since angiotensin-converting enzyme inhibition and angiotensin blockade in vivo markedly reduce PGE$_2$ biosynthesis in vitro [19], a second important action of the increase in angiotensin II during sodium deprivation may be to stimulate PGE$_2$ synthesis. This is supported by the results of Stahl et al. [262], who have shown that sodium deprivation in vivo in the rabbit results in stimulation of de novo PGE$_2$ biosynthesis in vitro.

A third effect of angiotensin is to produce renal (and sytemic) vasoconstriction, leading to an elevation in blood pressure that is associated with a reduction in renal blood flow and sodium excretion. However, during sodium restriction, blood pressure does not rise, but in fact remains the same or in the case of many hypertensive patients declines significantly. It is possible therefore that the rise in PG production during salt restriction offsets these actions of angiotensin II resulting in normotension and maintenance of basal renal blood flow and sodium excretion. Much additional investigation will be necessary, however, to document this possible role for PGs during sodium restriction.

In summary, the renin–angiotensin II–aldosterone axis acts in concert with the prostaglandin system: both rise during stimuli, which tends to reduce renal blood flow (partial renal artery occlusion, renal nerve stimulation, hemorrhage, sodium restriction, etc.). Although PGs are known to be capable of stimulating renin release, current evidence suggests that at least under conditions of sodium restriction, angiotensin II leads to a rise in PG synthesis.

PROSTAGLANDINS AND THE
KALLIKREIN-KININ SYSTEM

The first indication of a relationship between the kinins and the renal prostaglandins was the observation that bradykinin (but not eledoisen) released PGE-like compounds when infused in the renal artery [186]. It is believed that PG release by the kinins is accomplished through stimulation of phospholipase deacylation, since inhibition of phospholipase A_2 by mepacrine results in a decrease in release of both arachidonic acid and prostaglandin by rabbit renal interstitial cells [314], and since mepacrine also inhibits PG synthesis stimulated by bradykinin but not arachidonic acid [280].

The mechanism by which kinins cause systemic blood pressure lowering and peripheral arteriolar dilation is believed to be mediated at least in part by prostaglandins, since PG synthesis inhibition by nonsteroidal antiinflammatory agents attenuates the magnitude and/or duration of the hypotensive effect of bradykinin [58,279] as well as the vasodilatory effect of the latter in isolated kidney preparations and in the coronary artery [185,198]. The kinins have also been reported to involve PGs in their action on renal function. Although PGE_2 is the major PG released by the kinins in the kidney [198], thromboxane A_2 can also be produced in the perfused kidney when the ipsilateral ureter is ligated [193]. Both bradykinin and PGE_2 blunt adrenergically induced renal vasoconstriction by sympathetic nerve stimulation or norepinephrine [176,178], a phenomenon that is reversed by PG synthesis inhibition [178]. This suggests that renal PGE_2 mediates the action of bradykinin in adrenergic regulation of renal blood flow. The effect of bradykinin to increase renal blood flow and produce natriuresis and diuresis is also thought to be mediated by PGE_2 (and possibly PGI_2), since these vasodilatory and saliuretic effects are partially inhibited by indomethacin in situ [185]. In vivo, however, PG synthesis inhibition does not affect bradykinin stimulation of renal blood flow [56], although a significant reduction in bradykinin-induced natriuresis and renal PG production occurs [38]. Measurement of urinary kallikrein during varying sodium intakes have been conflicting. In man, Margolius et al. found a significant rise during low sodium intake, a condition also associated with a rise in renin activity and urinary PGE_2 [179]. In spontaneously hypertensive rats and dogs with unilateral renal artery occlusion, there is a decrease in urinary kallikrein [140,141]. This effect has also been observed in humans with essential hypertension [180]. By contrast, during mineralcorticoid excess in animals [141], and in humans with hypertension secondary to aldosteronomas [180], there is a significant increase in the urinary excretion of kallikrein, suggesting that mineralocorticoids may be a major determinant of renal kinin production.

In summary, many of the renal effects of the kinins as well as their extrarenal antihypertensive actions are currently thought to be mediated by enhanced PG synthesis by release of arachidonic acid. Much additional work is necessary, however, to determine the pathophysiological significance of these kinin-prostaglandin interactions.

BARTTER'S SYNDROME

Characterized by hyperplasia of the juxtaglomerular apparatus, hyperreninemia, hyperaldosteronism, hypokalemic alkalosis, and normal blood pressure [27], Bartter's syndrome is also associated with elevated plasma and urinary PGs. All these symptoms can be reversed by aspirin, indomethacin, and similar drugs [89,142,171,203,204,282], suggesting that an increase in renal PG production is a basic cause of this syndrome, leading to the clinical picture of primary aldosteronism with a normal blood pressure. However, the failure of chronic indomethacin treatment to fully arrest the hypokalemia and renal potassium loss at a time when renin and aldosterone are normal [47] suggests that potassium loss could be the cause of the hyperaldosteronism, not the result. Recently, Gill and Bartter [106] postulated a prostaglandin-independent defect in distal chloride reabsorption as a possible primary cause of this syndrome, since maximal free water clearance was low in association with a high clearance of chloride, both of which were normal in patients with hypokalemia, hyperreninemia, and hyperaldosteronism secondary to psychogenic vomiting. Hypokalemia in Bartter's syndrome was postulated to arise from a decrease in distal potassium reabsorption at the site of active chloride transport, or from increased potassium secretion resulting from an enhanced distal tubular flow.

Recently elevated urinary kallikrein was reported in Bartter's syndrome and, like the increased PRA and PGE, decreased with indomethacin [116]. Furthermore, Vinci et al. [284] observed high plasma bradykinin and urinary kallikrein with low urinary kinins in these patients with hyperreninemia and elevated immunoreactive urinary PGE_1. Treatment with indomethacin or ibuprofen normalized the kinins, renin, and PGs. However, it seems unlikely that the increase in PGs and kallikrein is the primary abnormality in this syndrome; rather, it may be related to a defect in distal chloride transport [26]. The vascular unresponsiveness to infused angiotensin II observed in Bartter's syndrome has been attributed to elevated vascular PGs [235] and/or increased plasma bradykinin [26].

BLOOD PRESSURE REGULATION

Exogenous Administration

NORMOTENSIVE ANIMALS AND MAN

A voluminous literature shows that PGE_2 and PGA_2 lower blood pressure by peripheral arteriolar dilation in normotensive animals, in animals with experimental hypertension, and in the case of PGA_2 and PGA_1, in humans with essential hypertension. More recently it has been shown that PGI_2 has peripheral vasodilating and blood pressure lowering properties [42,82,216], while thromboxane A_2 is a potent vasoconstrictor [118,267]. It is unclear whether normal blood pressure regulation is influenced by intrarenal PG synthesis with actions locally within the kidney or by elaboration of a circulating PG. Furthermore, findings suggesting localized PGE_2 and PGI_2 synthesis [108,190,272,276] by peripheral vascular tissue have supported a local circulatory role, with interaction of PGs and other vasoactive components released into the microcirculation.

Fitzpatrick et al. [92] have shown that PGI_2 lowers blood pressure by peripheral vasodilation, being 10 times more active than PGE_2 or PGD_2. Furthermore, unlike the latter compounds, PGI_2 did not increase pulmonary artery pressure or decrease myocardial contractile force. These investigators suggest that, of all the prostaglandins, PGI_2 most closely resembles the vasodepressor actions of arachidonic acid in the dog. Armstrong et al. [14] observed similar phenomena in rats and rabbits, PGI_2 being 2–4.8 times a more potent hypotensive agent than PGE_2. 6-Keto-$PGF_{1\alpha}$, the stable metabolite of PGI_2, was essentially without effect on blood pressure. Since stable endoperoxides of PGs have been shown to be powerful vasoconstrictors [244] and since PGE_2 has opposite effects to arachidonic acid and PGI_2, both of which relax bovine coronary artery strips [151,200], Armstrong et al., [13] concluded that PGI_2, not PGE_2, is the main end product of arachidonic acid that is responsible for the hypotensive effect of arachidonic acid. According to this theory PGI_2 formed locally in arterioles throughout the body is a major vasodepressor system, and a deficiency of PGI_2, not PGE_2, may contribute to hypertensive disease. Despite the attractiveness of this hypothesis, much additional investigation is needed to confirm the theory, especially with regard to the role of the kidney in the expression of the antihypertensive endocrine function, which is not accounted for in this postulation. Finally, it is important to note that although the existence of PGA has been questioned, the recently described hypotensive properties of PGI_2

are almost identical to those originally shown for renal PGAs and their 13,14-dihydro metabolites [15,160,162].

Infusion of PGE_1 into normotensive man results in a reflex tachycardia accompanied by facial flushing, headache, abdominal cramps, and diarrhea [33,34,206]. Relatively few additional studies have been done in the humans because of these side effects. PGA infusions into normotensive man are not accompanied by such side effects. There is again a reflex tachycardia, with unchanged blood pressure [51,192], but natriuretic or diuretic effects are absent.

PATIENTS WITH ESSENTIAL HYPERTENSION

In hypertensive man, PGA_2 (medullin) was originally infused at an intravenous rate of 380 μg/min and a fall in blood pressure from 180/105 to 165/95 mm Hg was observed. This was accompanied by a vasoreceptor-mediated increase in heart rate and cardiac output, thus the mechanism of hypotension was by peripheral arteriolar dilation [160]. Subsequently, PGA_1 was extensively studied in approximately 30 subjects with essential hypertension [52,164,295]. At intravenous infusion rates between 0.5 and 5 μg/kg/min, there was an initial marked increase in renal blood flow, renin secretion, and sodium, potassium, and water excretion at a time when blood pressure remained elevated. However, this transient natriuresis fell to control preinfusion levels when blood pressure dropped from hypertensive (205/115 mm Hg) to normotensive levels (140/90 mm Hg), again through a peripheral vasodilating effect. Similar results were reported for PGA_2 in essential hypertension [127] and in human renovascular hypertension [150], although the principal effect in the latter study was a rise in renal venous renin without change in blood pressure. PGA_1 was without effect on blood pressure, however, when given to essential hypertensive subjects who had been volume depleted with furosemide [149], suggesting that the latter compound might produce a rise in endogenous PGs, which could account for the significant blunting of the natriuretic and blood pressure responses to PGA_1 during sodium depletion.

In summary, exogenous administration of PGA, PGD, PGE, and PGI lowers blood pressure in animals by peripheral arteriolar dilation. In hypertensive man, PGA exhibits complex actions involving transient initial increase in renal blood flow and natriuresis leading to a 10% decrease in plasma volume. This is accompanied by a secondary peripheral vasodilation and fall in blood pressure associated with a reflex increase in heart rate and a return of the elevated renal blood flow and sodium excretion to preinfusion control values. Thus PGA produces normotension with "normal" renal blood flow and sodium excretion by a complex and intricate interplay involving renal resistance, sodium and water homeostasis, peripheral resistance, plasma volume, renin secretion, and indirectly, cardiac output and the adrenergic baroreceptor system, all factors known to be intimately woven into the mosaic of human essential hypertension.

Prostaglandin Synthesis Inhibition

Although indomethacin and meclofenamate result in an acute rise in blood pressure in the anesthetized animal [66,153,172,304], with enhanced vascular reactivity to norepinephrine, nerve stimulation, and angiotensin [4,91], no effect was observed in the unanesthetized animal [167,195,241,310], suggesting that the renal prostaglandins do not support basal systemic blood pressure. In this regard, it is of interest that indomethacin abolishes the tachyphylactic response to angiotensin [184], while the administration of angiotensin antagonists inhibits the effect of indomethacin [189]. All this evidence underscores the importance of prior enhancement of renal prohypertensive systems leading to adaptive depressor responses of the prostaglandins.

In man, the blood pressure response to indomethacin is variable: some reports reveal elevations in blood pressure [228,292] and others no effect [96,202]. The lack of blood pressure rise in some of these studies may reflect the decrease in both prohypertensive activity (renin-angiotensin) and antihypertensive activity (PGs) that is caused by indomethacin. Since the antihypertensive action of propranolol is abolished by indomethacin in patients with essential hypertension [75], one of the many mechanisms proposed for the action of propranolol may involve release of PGs.

Prostaglandin Synthesis Stimulation

Agents that stimulate renal PG synthesis associated with a fall in blood pressure include the precursor arachidonic acid in animals [59,153] and man [293], bradykinin [186], and the loop diuretics furosemide, bumetanide, and ethacrynic acid [24,213,300,301]. In this connection, it is of interest that furosemide reduces left atrial pressure in hypervolemic dogs made anuric by ureteral ligation [46]. This effect is inhibited by indomethacin, thus implicating the renal (or possible extrarenal) PGs as important mediators of the nondiuretic direct vasodilating action of furosemide.

Experimental Hypertension

Numerous studies have shown arachidonic acid, PGE, and PGA to be antihypertensive in rats with renovascular or spontaneous hypertension. Similar antihypertensive effects were noted in the sodium-volume-induced hypertensive rats transplanted with tissue cultures of renomedullary interstitial cells [196]. In rats with renovascular hypertension, indomethacin or meclofenamate either produces no effect [187] or aggravates preexisting hypertension [234,253], particularly if renal blood flow is initially decreased [242]. Resolution of the conflicting effects of prostaglandin synthesis inhibition in renovascular hypertension has at least partially been achieved by Zimmerman [309], who observed no change in renal vascular resistance, renal blood flow, or blood pressure in conscious dogs, administered meclofenamate following the establishment of two-kidney Goldblatt hypertension. In the anesthetized dog, however, meclofenamate produced a significant fall in renal blood flow and rise in renal resistance, although the elevated blood pressure remained unaffected. Thus it is important to carefully consider the state of the experimental model (anesthesia, sodium balance, volume, sympathetic nervous system, renin-angiotensin, etc.) before interpreting the presence or absence of prostaglandin synthesis inhibition effects, which apparently depend critically on the status of such variables. Measurements of PG and PG synthesis in this animal model have been conflicting [133,234].

An increased synthesis and/or decreased metabolism of PGA, PGE, and PGF has been observed in the spontaneously hypertensive rat (SHR) [12,71,104,169,221,240]. In the Wistar-Okamoto rat, 9-hydroxy-PGDH was decreased [3], whereas 15-hydroxy-PGDH was low in the New Zealand strain [12]. A decrease in pulmonary inactivation of PGE_2 and $PGF_{2\alpha}$ has also been reported in the New Zealand strain [158]. Recently PGI_2 has also been found to be elaborated from aortic rings and homogenates from the SHR in enhanced concentration when compared to normals [224]. Since PGI_2 is three to four times as active as PGE_2 in lowering blood pressure in this preparation [223], it is a good candidate for a naturally occurring, systemic antihypertensive agent. When the enhanced PG synthesis is inhibited by indomethacin in the SHR, there is a significant aggravation of the elevated blood pressure [167]. These findings suggest that a deficiency of PGs does not underlie the hypertension of the SHR but that there is an increased elaboration of PGs in response to whatever is the initiating stimulus to this hypertensive state.

Although a role for prostaglandins or neutral lipids has been suggested for other forms of experimental hypertension (DOCA, "postsalt," post-Goldblatt, angiotensin-salt, and renoprival hypertension), their role in these hypertensive models remains unclear. Recently, Rioux et al. [239] observed increased synthesis and release of PG-like material from aortic strips of DOCA and renovascular hypertensive rats, suggesting that in these states as in the SHR, PGs may be released in a compensatory fashion to offset these prohypertensive stimuli. In adrenal regeneration hypertension, administration of PGE_2 resulted in a significant fall, whereas indomethacin produced a marked rise in blood pressure [230], results compatible with a role for renal PG deficiency in this condition.

Human Essential Hypertension

Measurements of PGA and PGE have been performed by radioimmunoassay in the plasma, urine, and kidney tissue of hypertensive man, utilizing age- and sex-matched normotensive man as controls, to determine whether aberrations in renal PG synthesis may underlie certain human hypertensive states.

NORMOTENSIVE HUMANS

Although many PGs are natriuretic, Lee [161], Zusman et al. [313], and Payakkapan et al. [232] reported that peripheral plasma immunoreactive PGA (iPGA) increases markedly in normal subjects on a low salt diet, and this effect is accompanied by a rise in PRA and aldosterone. These results suggested that circulating iPGA is not a natriuretic factor and in fact may act in normotensive man as an antinatriuretic agent, with possible important effects in mediating renin release and ultimately aldosterone generation. Indeed, Golub et al. [109] found that subdepressor doses of PGA_1 in normal man lead to a significant increase in PRA and aldosterone at a time when volume was maintained by saline infusion. Since sodium intake did not affect this renin-releasing activity, it would appear that PGA_1 may directly stimulate renin release independently of changes in sodium balance [260].

In addition to volume depletion initiated by sodium restriction, volume depletion induced by diuretics (furosemide, ethacrynic acid, chlorazanil) leads to an increase in urinary PG excretion that is inhibited by indomethacin [299,302]. Furthermore, furosemide-induced decrease in blood pressure and increase in PRA were almost completely inhibited by indomethacin in both normotensive and hypertensive man [69,228], suggesting that the ameliorative effects of furosemide on blood pressure may be mediated by PG release. This is substantiated by the finding of Abe et al. [2] that urinary iPGE rose from 26.6 ± 3.0 to 64.5 ± 11.3 ng/ hr following intravenous administration of furosemide in normotensive individuals. A third type of volume depletion, that following hemodialysis, has also been shown to result in a rise in plasma iPGA (but not iPGE) in both nephrectomized and nonnephrectomized individuals [136].

Evidence to date suggests therefore that plasma and urine prostaglandins rise during various maneuvers producing volume depletion. Volume depletion leads to a rise in the renin-angiotensin axis that is believed to be responsible at least in part for the increase in renal, circulating, or vascular PGs. It is possible that the beneficial effects of low sodium intake and diuretic therapy in hypertensive man may be the result of an increase in vasodilating PGs, which physiologically antagonize the prohypertensive renin-angiotensin axis and the sympathetic nervous system. Since a decreased vascular reactivity to angiotensin and norepinephrine is a hallmark of volume depletion, this property has been utilized extensively to explain the blood pressure lowering effect of the combination of low sodium intake with diuretic therapy. Since the decrease in vascular reactivity can be reversed by indomethacin, which increases pressor responsiveness to angiotensin and norepinephrine, a possibly critical role in maintaining normotension during volume depletion is suggested for PGs, which otherwise might be expected to result in blood pressure elevation because of the rise in the renin-angiotensin-aldosterone axis.

Although the schema whereby volume depletion leads to enhance-

ment of PG production is attractive, it must be remembered that renal
nerve stimulation and angiotensin infusion in turn stimulate renal PG
production [4,70,184], and that the hypotensive effect of β-adrenergic
blockade is inhibited by indomethacin [75]. Thus a complex servo-
regulatory mechanism exists between the prohypertensive and antihypertensive activities of the kidney.

HYPERTENSIVE PATIENTS

Since volume depletion (low sodium diet, diuretics, hemodialysis) in
normotensive and hypertensive man leads to normotension with an
increase in plasma and urinary PGs, and since indomethacin administration in normotensive man reproduces the syndrome of hyporeni-
nemic, hypoaldosteronism observed in patients with low renin hypertension [228], recent studies have explored the possibility that certain
states of human hypertension may be associated with a deficiency in
circulating or renal PGs as originally postulated following the discovery
of the renal PGs [159]. In human renovascular hypertension, the results
of renal or peripheral plasma levels of PGE and PGA have been conflicting, with reports of an increase in these compounds in certain studies
[126,128,129] and a decrease in others [277]. The role of renal PGs in
human renovascular hypertension remains unresolved.

In early investigations PGA-like material was reported to be lower in
the peripheral plasma of patients with essential hypertension as compared to controls [161], although peripheral plasma PGA_1-like material
has more recently been reported to be elevated in essential hypertension
[129]. More meaningful results have recently been obtained by measurement of urinary iPGE, which is believed to represent primarily PGE
synthesized by the renal medulla. Utilizing bioassay techniques, it has
been shown that urinary PGE-like material is low in essential hypertensives and decreases with age and severity of the hypertension [226].
With more specific immunoassay techniques, recent studies have revealed low urinary iPGE (11.9 $\pm$ 2.7 ng/hr) in hypertensive patients as
compared to normotensive subjects (26.2 $\pm$ 3.0 ng/hr) [2]. The normal
increase in response to furosemide was much less than in normal subjects, suggesting an impairment of the ability of the hypertensive kidney
to synthesize PGs during a volume-depleting stimulus. There was a
significant positive correlation between sodium excretion and urinary
iPGE in these patients [302], but not with the renin-aldosterone axis [57].
Interestingly, urinary kinin, like $iPGE_2$, was low in patients with essential
hypertension and increased to a significantly lesser extent than in normotensive subjects following furosemide administration [1]. Since urinary iPGE decreased in hypertensive patients on a normal (but not on
a low) sodium diet following the infusion of the angiotensin II antagonist
Sar^1-Ile^8-angiotensin II, Yasujima et al. [303] concluded that the synthesis
and release of renal PGs may be regulated by angiotensin II in patients
with essential hypertension. The significance of this finding remains to
be elucidated. Although a circadian rhythm exists for urinary iPGE in

normal subjects [48], no comparable data are available for hypertensive subjects.

Since indomethacin administration to normal subjects results in clinical and laboratory findings almost identical to those for patients with low renin hypertension [50], it is of interest that plasma iPGA and urinary iPGE have recently been reported to be markedly lower in patients with low renin hypertension as compared with normal renin hypertensives [50,269]. Furthermore, the normal rise in PRA and plasma iPGA following the administration of furosemide was significantly less than in normal renin hypertensives [50]. At present, it appears that a deficient synthesis of vasodilatory PGs or PG intermediates in the cascade from arachidonic acid may underlie certain states of human essential hypertension, particularly the low renin subgroup.

ACKNOWLEDGMENTS

This work was supported by grants 1453 and K016 from the New York State Health Research Council and grant 400965 from the Saudi Arabian Educational Mission. A. A. Attallah is supported by a fellowship from the Saudi Arabian Educational Mission, Houston, Texas. The authors thank Audrey Lee for preparation of the manuscript. The section on the renin–angiotensin axis has been reprinted in part with permission of Clin. Nephrol. 14:159–163, 1980.

REFERENCES

1. Abe, K., Seino, M., Yasujima, M., Chiba, S., Sakurai, Y., Irokawa, N., Miyazaki, S., Saito, K., Ito, T., Otsuka, Y., and Yoshinaga, K. (1977) Studies on renomedullary prostaglandin and renal kallikrein-kinin system in hypertension. Jpn. Circ. J. 41, 873–880.

2. Abe, K., Yasujima, M., Chiba, S., Irokawa, N., Ito, T., and Yoshinaga, K. (1977) Effect of furosemide on urinary excretion of prostaglandin E in normal volunteers and patients with essential hypertension. Prostaglandins, 14, 513–521.

3. Ahnfelt-Rønne, I., and Arrigoni-Martelli, E. (1977) Renal prostaglandin metabolism to spontaneously hypertensive rats. Biochem. Pharmacol. 26, 485–488.

4. Aiken, J. W., and Vane, J. R. (1973) Intrarenal prostaglandin release attenuates the renal vasoconstrictor activity of angiotensin. J. Pharmacol. Exp. Ther. 184, 678–687.

5. Altsheler, P., Klahr, S., Roschbaum, R., and Slatopolsky, E., (1978) Effects of inhibitors of prostaglandin synthesis on renal sodium excretion in normal dogs and dogs with decreased renal mass. Am. J. Physiol. 235, F338–F344.

6. Anderson, R. J., Berl, T., McDonald, K. M., and Schrier, R. W. (1975) Evidence for an in vivo antagonism between vasopressin and prostaglandin in the mammalian kidney. J. Clin. Invest. 56, 420–426.

7. Anderson, R. J., Taher, M. S., Cronin, R. E., McDonald, K. M., and Schrier, R. W. (1975) Effect of β-adrenergic blockade and inhibitors of angiotensin II and prostaglandin on renal autoregulation. Am. J. Physiol. 229, 731–736.

8. Änggård, E., Larsson, C., and Samuelsson, B. (1971) The distribution of 15-hydroxy-prostaglandin dehydrogenase and prostaglandin Δ-13-reductase in tissues of the swine. Acta Physiol. Scand. 81, 396–404.

9. Änggård, E., and Samuelsson, B. (1964) Prostaglandins and related factors. 28. Metabolism of prostaglandin E_1 in guinea pig lung. The structures of two metabolites. J. Biol. Chem. 239, 4097–4102.

10. Änggård, E., and Samuelsson, B. (1966) Metabolism of prostaglandins in the lung. Acta Physiol. Scand. 68 (Suppl. 277), 232.

11. Antonello, A., Tremolda, C., Baggio, B., Burn, F., Favaro, S., Piccoli, A., and Borsatti, A. (1978) In vivo activation of renal phospholipase activity by bradykinin in rat. Prostaglandins 16, 23–29.

12. Armstrong, J. M., Blackwell, G. J., Flower, R. J., McGiff, J. C., Mullane, K. M., and Vane, J. R. (1976) Genetic hypertension in rats is accompanied by a defect in renal prostaglandin catabolism. Nature (London) 260, 582–586.

13. Armstrong, J. M., Dusting, G. J., Moncada, S., and Vane, J. R. (1978) Cardiovascular actions of prostacyclin (PGI$_2$), a metabolite of arachidonic acid which is synthesized by blood vessels. Circ. Res. (Suppl. I), 43, I112–I119.

14. Armstrong, J. M., Lattimer, N., Moncada, S., and Vane, J. R. (1978) Comparison of the vasodepressor effects of prostacyclin and 6-oxoprostaglandin F$_{1\alpha}$ with those of prostaglandin E$_2$ in rats and rabbits. Br. J. Pharmacol. 62, 125–130.

15. Attallah, A. A., Duchesne, M. J., and Lee, J. B. (1975) Metabolism of prostaglandin A. II. Isolation, characterization and synthesis of PGA$_1$ renal metabolites. Life Sci. 16, 1743–1752.

16. Attallah, A. A., and Lee, J. B. (1973) Radioimmunoassay of prostaglandin A. Intrarenal PGA$_2$ as a factor mediating saline induced natriuresis. Circ. Res. 33, 696–703.

17. Attallah, A. A., and Lee, J. B. (1980) Indomethacin, salicylates and prostaglandin binding. Prostaglandins 19, 311–318.

18. Attallah, A. A., Stahl, R. A., Bloch, D. L., and Lee, J. B. (1979) Furosemide stimulates and saralasin inhibits renal prostaglandin E$_2$ biosynthesis. Clin. Res. 27, 599A.

19. Attallah, A. A., Stahl, R. A., Bloch, D. L., Ambrus, J. L., and Lee, J. B. (1980) Effect of Sar^1-Ile^8-angiotensin II and SQ 14225 on rabbit urinary PGE$_2$ excretion and renal tissue PGE$_2$ production. Physiologist 23, 180.

20. Attallah, A. A., Stahl, R. A., Bloch, D. L., Ambrus, J. L., and Lee, J. B. (1981) Inhibition of rabbit renal prostaglandin E$_2$ biosynthesis by chronic potassium deficiency. J. Lab. Clin. Med. 97, 205–212.

21. Attallah, A. A., Stahl, R. A., Lee, J. B., and Ambrus, J. L. (1981) Furosemide and indomethacin: Effects on rabbit renal PGE$_2$ biosynthesis and urinary salt and water excretion. J. Lab. Clin. Med. (submitted for publication).

22. Attallah, A. A., Stahl, R. A., Bloch, D. L., Ambrus, J. L., and Lee, J. B. (1981) Effect of Sar^1-Ile^8-angiotensin II and SQ 14225 on renal PGE$_2$ biosynthesis and excretion. Hypertension (submitted for publication).

23. Bailie, M. D., Barbour, J. A., and Hook, J. B. (1975) Effects of indomethacin on furosemide-induced changes in renal blood flow. Proc. Soc. Exp. Biol. Med. 148, 1173–1176.

24. Bailie, M. D., Crosslan, K., and Hook, J. B. (1976) Natriuretic effect of furosemide after inhibition of prostaglandin synthetase. J. Pharmacol. Exp. Ther. 199, 469–476.

25. Barry, E., and Hall, W. J. (1969) Stimulation of sodium movement across frog skin by prostaglandin E$_1$. J. Physiol. (London) 200, 83–84.

26. Bartter, F. C. (1977) Bartter's syndrome. Urol. Clin. North Am. 4, 253–261.

27. Bartter, F. C., Provone, P., Gill, J. R., MacCardle, R. C., and Diller, E. (1962) Hyperplasia of the juxtaglomerular complex with hyperaldosteronism and hypokalemic alkalosis. Am. J. Med. 33, 811–828.

28. Beck, N. P., Kaneko, T., Zor, U., Field, J. B., and Davis, B. B. (1971) Effects of vasopressin and prostaglandin E$_1$ on the adenyl cyclase–cyclic 3',5'-adenosine monophosphate system of the renal medulla of the rat. J. Clin. Invest. 50, 2461–2465.

29. Beck, N., and Shaw, J. O. (1979) Thromboxane and prostaglandin E in K$^+$-depleted rat kidney. Am. Soc. Nephrol. 78A.

30. Bell, C., and Mya, M. K. K. (1977) Release by vasopressin of E-type prostaglandins from the rat kidney. Clin. Sci. Mol. Med. 52, 103–106.

31. Berg, K. J. (1977) Acute effects of acetylsalicylic acid on renal function in normal man. Eur. J. Clin. Pharmacol. 11, 117–123.

32. Berg, K. J., and Loew, D. (1977) Inhibition of furosemide-induced natriuresis by acetylsalicylic acid in dogs. Scand. J. Clin. Lab. Invest. 37, 125.

33. Bergström, S., Carlson, L. A., Ekelund, L. G., and Orö, L. (1965) Cardiovascular and metabolic response to infusions of prostaglandin E_1 and to simultaneous infusions of noradrenaline and prostaglandin E_1 in man. Acta Physiol. Scand. 64, 332–339.

34. Bergström, S., Düner, H., von Euler, U. S., Pernow, B., and Sjövall, J. (1959) Observations on the effects of infusion of prostaglandin E in man. Acta Physiol. Scand. 45, 145–151.

35. Berl, T., Henrich, W. L., Erickson, A. L., and Schrier, R. W. (1979) Prostaglandins in the beta-adrenergic and baroreceptor-mediated secretion of renin. Am. J. Physiol. 236, F472–F477.

36. Berl, T., Raz, A., Wald, H., Horowitz, H., and Czaczkes, W. (1977) Prostaglandin synthesis inhibition and the action of vasopressin. Studies in man and rat. Am. J. Physiol. 232, F529–F537.

37. Bito, L. Z. (1976) Inhibition of renal prostaglandin metabolism and excretion by probenecid, bromcresol green and indomethacin. Prostaglandins 12, 639–646.

38. Blasingame, M. C., and Nasjletti, A. (1979) Contribution of renal prostaglandins to the natriuretic action of bradykinin in the dog. Am. J. Physiol. 237, F182–F187.

39. Bohman, S. O. (1977) Demonstration of prostaglandin synthesis in collecting duct cells and other cell types of the rabbit renal medulla. Prostaglandins 14, 729–744.

40. Bohman, S. O., and Larsson, C. (1975) Prostaglandin synthesis in membrane fractions from the rabbit renal medulla. Acta Physiol. 94, 244–258.

41. Bolger, P. M., Eisner, G. M., Ramwell, P. W., and Slotkoff, L. M. (1976) Effect of prostaglandin synthesis on renal function and renin in the dog. Nature (London) 259, 244–245.

42. Bolger, P. M., Eisner, G. M., Ramwell, P. W., Slotkoff, L. M., and Corey, E. J. (1978) Renal actions of prostacyclin. Nature (London) 271, 467–469.

43. Bolger, P. M., Eisner, G. M., Shea, P. T., Ramwell, P. W., and Slotkoff, L. M. (1977) Effects of PGD_2 on canine renal function. Nature (London) 267, 628–630.

44. Borgeat, P., and Samuelsson, B. (1979) Arachidonic acid metabolism in polymorphonuclear leukocytes: Effects of ionophore A23187. Proc. Natl. Acad. Sci. (US) 76, 2148–2152.

45. Borgeat, P., and Samuelsson, B. (1979) Arachidonic acid metabolism in polymorphonuclear leukocytes: Unstable intermediate in formation of dihydroxy acids. Proc. Natl. Acad. Sci. (US) 76, 3213–3217.

46. Bourland, W. A., Day, D. K., and Williamson, H. E. (1977) The role of the kidney in the early nondiuretic action of furosemide to reduce elevated left atrial pressure in the hypervolemic dog. J. Pharmacol. Exp. Ther. 202, 221–229.

47. Bowden, R. E., Gill, J. R., Radfar, N., Taylor, A. A., and Keiser, H. R. (1978) Effect of different prostaglandin synthetase inhibitors on immunoreactive prostaglandin E excretion in Bartter's syndrome. J. Am. Med. Assoc. 239, 117–121.

48. Bowden, R. E., Ware, J. H., Demets, D. L., and Keiser, H. R. (1977) Urinary excretion of immunoreactive prostaglandin E: A circadian rhythm and the effect of posture. Prostaglandins 14, 151–161.

49. Brennan, L. A., Bonjour, J. P., and Malvin, R. L. (1971) ADH levels during salt depletion in dogs. Eur. J. Clin. Invest. 2, 43–46.

50. Brooks, C. S., Talwalker, R. T., and Kotchen, T. A. (1977) Renin reactivity in plasma of patients with normal renin and low renin essential hypertension. J. Clin. Endocrinol. Metab. 44, 322–329.

51. Carlson, L. A., Ekelund, L. G., and Orö, L. (1970) Clinical metabolic and cardiovascular effects of different prostaglandins in man. Acta Med. Scand. 188, 553–559.

52. Carr, A. A. (1970) Hemodynamic and renal effects of a prostaglandin, PGA_1 in subjects with essential hypertension. Am. Med. Sci. 259, 21–26.

53. Carr, A. A. (1973) Effect of PGA_1 on renin and aldosterone in man. Prostaglandins 3, 621–628.

54. Carrière, A., Fribourg, J., and Guay, J. P. (1971) Vasodilators, intrarenal blood flow and natriuresis in the dog. Am. J. Physiol. 221, 92–98.

55. Chang, L. C. T., Spławiński, J. A., Oates, J. A., and Nies, A. S. (1975) Enhanced renal prostaglandin in the dog. 2. Effects on intrarenal hemodynamics. Circ. Res. 36, 204–207.

56. Chapnick, B. M., Paustian, P. W., Feigen, L. P., Joiner, P. D., Hyman, A. L., and Kadowitz, P. J. (1977) Influence of inhibitors of prostaglandin synthesis on renal vascular resistance and on renal vascular responses to vasopressor and vasodilator agents in the cat. Circ. Res. 40, 348–354.

57. Chiba, S., Abe, K., Yasujima, M., Irokawa, N., Seino, M., Sakurai, Y., Sato, M., Otsuka, Y., and Yoshinaga, K. (1978) Effect of spironolactone on urinary excretion of immunoreactive prostaglandin E in essential hypertension. Tohoku J. Exp. Med. 124, 297–305.

58. Damas, J., and Deby, C. (1974) Prostaglandin release by bradykinin in the rat. C. R. Soc. Biol. 168, 375–378.

59. Damas, J., and Deby, C. (1976) Correlation between inhibition by antiinflammatory substances, of arachidonic acid-induced hypotension, and of prostaglandin biosynthesis in vitro. Biochem. Pharmacol. 25, 983–985.

60. Daniels, E. G., Hinman, J. W., Johnson, B. A., Kupiecki, F. P., Nelson, J. W., and Pike, J. E. (1965) Identification of prostaglandin E_2 as the principal vasodepressor lipid of rabbit renal medulla. Nature (London) 215, 1298–1299.

61. Danon, A., Chang, L. C. T., Sweetman, B. J., Nies, A. S., and Oates, J. A. (1975) Synthesis of prostaglandins by the rat renal papilla in vitro. Mechanisms of stimulation by angiotensin II. Biochim. Biophys. Acta 388, 71–83.

62. Danon, A., Knapp, H. R., Oelt, O., and Oates, J. A. (1978) Stimulation of prostaglandin biosynthesis in the renal papilla by hypertonic medium. Am. J. Physiol. 234, F64–F67.

63. Data, J. L., Gerber, J. G., Crump, W. J., Frölich, J. C., Hollifield, J. W., and Nies, A. S. (1978) The prostaglandin system: A role in canine baroreceptor control of renin release. Circ. Res. 42, 454–458.

64. Data, J. L., Rane, A., Gerkens, J., Wilkinson, G. R., Nies, A. S., and Branch, R. A. (1978) The influence of indomethacin on the pharmacokinetics, diuretic response and hemodynamics of fuorsemide in the dog. J. Pharmacol. Exp. Ther. 206, 431–438.

65. Davila, D., Davila, E., Olin, E., and Änggård, E. (1978) The influence of dietary sodium on urinary prostaglandin excretion. Acta Physiol. Scand. 103, 100–106.

66. Davis, H., and Horton, E. W. (1972) Output of prostaglandins from the rabbit kidney: Its increase on renal nerve stimulation and its inhibition by indomethacin. Br. J. Pharmacol. 46, 658–675.

67. Desaulles, E., and Schwartz, J. (1979) A comparative study of the action of furosemide and methyclothiazide on renin release by rat kidney slices and the interaction with indomethacin. Br. J. Pharmacol. 65, 193–196.

68. Dew, M. E., and Michelakis, A. M. (1976) Effect of prostaglandins on renin release in vitro. Pharmacologist 16, 198.

69. Donker, A. J. M., Arisz, L., Brentjens, I. H., van der Hem, G. K., and Hollemans, H. J. G. (1976) The effect of indomethacin on kidney function and plasma renin activity in man. Nephron 17, 288–296.

70. Dunham, E. W., and Zimmerman, B. G. (1970) Release of prostaglandin-like material from the dog kidney during nerve stimulation. Am. J. Physiol. 219, 1279–1285.

71. Dunn, M. J. (1976) Renal prostaglandin synthesis in the spontaneously hypertensive rat. J. Clin. Invest. 58, 862–870.

72. Dunn, M. J., Greely, H. P., Valtin, H., Kinter, L. B., and Beeuwkes, R., III, (1978) Renal excretion of prostaglandins E_2 and $F_{2\alpha}$ in diabetes insipidus rats. Am. J. Physiol. 235, F624–F627.

73. Dunn, M. J., and Howe, D. (1977) Prostaglandins lack a direct inhibitory action on

electrolyte and water transport in the kidney and the erythrocyte. Prostaglandins 13, 417–429.

74. Dunn, M. J., Staley, R. S., and Harrison, M. (1976) Characterization of prostaglandin production in tissue culture of rat renal medullary cells. Prostaglandins 12, 38–49.

75. Durao, V., Prata, M. M., and Goncalves, L. M. P. (1977) Modification of antihypertensive effect of β-adrenoceptor-blocking agents by inhibition of endogenous prostaglandin synthesis. Lancet 2, 1005–1007.

76. Düsing, R., Attallah, A. A., Prezyna, A. P., and Lee, J. B. (1978) Renal biosynthesis of prostaglandin E_2 and $F_{2\alpha}$: Dependence on extracellular potassium. J. Lab. Clin. Med. 92, 669–677.

77. Düsing, R., Melder, B., and Kramer, H. J. (1976) Prostaglandins and renal function in acute extracellular volume expansion. Prostaglandins 12, 3–10.

78. Düsing, R., Melder, B., and Kramer, H. J. (1977) Effects of prostaglandin inhibition on intrarenal hemodynamics in acutely saline-loaded rats. Circ. Res. 41, 287–291.

79. Düsing, R., Opitz, W. D., and Kramer, H. J. (1977) The role of prostaglandins in the natriuresis of acutely salt-loaded rats. Nephron 18, 212–219.

80. Dusting, G. T., Moncada, S., and Vane, J. R. (1977) Prostacyclin (PGI_2) is a weak contractor of coronary arteries of the pig. Eur. J. Pharmacol. 45, 301–304.

81. Dusting, G. J., Moncada, S., and Vane, J. R. (1977) Prostacyclin (PGX) is the endogenous metabolite responsible for relaxation of coronary arteries induced by arachidonic acid. Prostaglandins 13, 3–15.

82. Dusting, G. J., Moncada, S., and Vane, J. R. (1978) Recirculation of prostacyclin (PGI_2) in the dog. Br. J. Pharmacol. 64, 315–320.

83. Feigen, L. P., Chapnick, B. M., Flemming, J. E., Flemming, J. M., and Kadowitz, P. J. (1977) Renal vascular effects of endoperoxide analogs, prostaglandins and arachidonic acid. Am. J. Physiol. 233, H573–H579.

84. Feigen, L. P., Chapnick, B. M., Gorman, R. R., Hyman, A. L., and Kadowitz, P. J. (1978) The effects of PGH_2 on blood flow in the canine renal and superior mesenteric vascular beds. Prostaglandins 16, 803–813.

85. Fejes-Tóth, G., Magyar, A., and Walter, J. (1977) Renal response to vasopressin after inhibition of prostaglandin synthesis. Am. J. Physiol. 232, F416–F423.

86. Feldman, D., Loose, D. S., and Tan, S. Y. (1978) Nonsteroidal antiinflammatory drugs cause sodium and water retention in the rat. Am. J. Physiol. 234, F490–F496.

87. Ferreira, S. H., and Vane, J. R. (1967) Prostaglandins: Their disappearance from and release into the circulation. Nature (London) 216, 868–873.

88. Ferris, T. F. (1978) Prostaglandins, potassium and Bartter's syndrome, J. Lab. Clin. Med. 92, 663–668.

89. Fichman, M. P., Telfer, N., Zia, P., Speckart, P., Golub, M., and Rude, R. (1976) Role of prostaglandins in the pathogenesis of Bartter's syndrome. Am. J. Med. 60, 185–797.

90. Fine, L. G., and Trizna, W. (1977) Influence of prostaglandins on sodium transport of isolated medullary nephron segments. Am. J. Physiol. 232, F383–F390.

91. Finn, W. F., and Arendshorst, W. J. (1976) Effect of prostaglandin synthetase inhibitors on renal blood flow in the rat. Am. J. Physiol. 321, 1541–1545.

92. Fitzpatrick, T. M., Alter, I., Corey, E. J., Ramwell, P. W., Rose, J. C., and Kot, P. A. (1978) Cardiovascular responses to PGI_2 (prostacyclin) in the dogs. Circ. Res. 22, 192–194.

93. Folkert, V. W., and Schlondorff, D. (1979) Prostaglandin synthesis in isolated glomeruli. Prostaglandins 17, 79–86.

94. Fram, M. H., and Hedqvist, P. (1975) Evidence for prostaglandin mediated prejunctional control of renal sympathetic transmitter release and vascular tone. Br. J. Pharmacol. 58, 189–196.

95. Friesinger, C., Oelz, O., Sweetman, B. J., Nies, A. S., and Data, J. L. (1978) Prostaglandin D_2, another renal prostaglandin? Prostaglandins 15, 969–981.

96. Frölich, J. C., Hollifield, J. W., Dormois, J. C., Frölich, B. L., Seyberth, H., Michelakis,

A. M., and Oates, J. A. (1976) Suppression of plasma renin activity by indomethacin in man. Circ. Res. 39, 447–452.

97. Frölich, J. C., Hollifield, J. W., Michelakis, A. M., Vesper, A. S., Wilson, J. P., Shand, D. G., Seyberth, H. J., Frölich, W. H., and Oates, J. A. (1979) Reduction of plasma renin activity by inhibition of the fatty acid cyclooxygenase in human subjects: Independence of sodium retention. Circ. Res. 44, 781–787.

98. Frölich, J. C., Wilson, T. W., Sweetman, B. J., Smigel, M., Nies, A. S., Carr, K., Watson, J. T., and Oates, J. A. (1975) Urinary prostaglandins. Identification and origin. J. Clin. Invest., 55, 763–770.

99. Fülgraf, G., Brandenbusch, G., and Heintze, K. (1974) Dose-response relation of the renal effects of PGA_1, PGE_2 and $PGF_{2\alpha}$ in dogs. Prostaglandins 8, 21–30.

100. Gafni, Y., Schwartzma, M., and Raz, A. (1978) Prostaglandin biosynthesis in rabbit kidney medulla: Inhibition in vitro vs. in vivo by aspirin, indomethacin and meclofenamic acid. Prostaglandins 15, 759–772.

101. Galvez, O. G., Roberts, B. W., Bay, W. H., and Ferris, T. F. (1976) Studies of the mechanism of polyuria with hypokalemia. Kidney Int. 10, 583.

102. Gerber, J. G., Branch, R. A., Nies, A. S., Gerkens, J. F., Shand, D. G., Hollifield, J., and Oates, J. A. (1978) Prostaglandins and renin secretion following infusion of PGI_2, E_2 and D_2 into the renal artery of anesthetized dogs. Prostaglandins 15, 81–88.

103. Gerber, J. G., Data, J. L., and Nies, A. S. (1978) Enhanced renal prostaglandin production in the dog kidney. The effect of sodium arachidonate in nonfiltering kidney. Circ. Res. 42, 43–45.

104. Gerber, J. G., Ellis, E., Hollifield, J., and Nies, A. S. (1979) Effect of prostaglandin endoperoxide analogue on canine renal function. Hemodynamics and renin release. Eur. J. Pharmacol. 53, 239–246.

105. Gerber, J. G., Hubbard, W. C., and Nies, A. S. (1979) The role of renal metabolism of PGE_2 in determining its activity as a renal vasodilator in the dog. Prostaglandins 17, 323–336.

106. Gill, J. R., and Bartter, F. C. (1978) Evidence for a prostaglandin-independent defect in chloride reabsorption in the loop of Henle as a proximal cause of Bartter's syndrome. Am. J. Med. 65, 776–772.

107. Gill, U. R., Jr., Frölich, J. C., Bowden, R. E., Taylor, A. A., Keiser, H. R., Seyberth, H. W., Oates, J. A., and Bartter, F. C. (1976) Bartter's syndrome: A disorder characterized by high urinary prostaglandins and a dependency of hyperrreninemia on prostaglandin synthesis. Am. J. Med. 61, 43–51.

108. Gimbrone, M. A., and Alexander, R. W. (1975) Angiotensin II stimulation of prostaglandin production in cultured human vascular endothelium. Science 189, 219–220.

109. Golub, M. S., Speckart, P. F., Zia, P. K., and Horton, R. (1976) The effect of prostaglandin A_1 on renin and aldosterone in man. Circ. Res. 39, 574–579.

110. Grantham, J. J., and Orloff, J. (1968) Effect of prostaglandin E_1 on the permeability response of the isolated collecting tubule to vasopressin, adenosine 3',5'-monophosphate and theophylline. J. Clin. Invest. 47, 1154–1161.

111. Greenberg, S. (1976) Evidence for enhanced venous smooth muscle turnover of prostaglandin-like substance in portal veins from spontaneously hypertensive rats. Prostaglandins 11, 163–193.

112. Grenier, F. C., and Smith, W. L. (1978) Formation of 6-keto-$PGF_{1\alpha}$ by collecting duct cells isolated from rabbit renal papilla. Prostaglandins 16, 759–772.

113. Gross, J. B., and Bartter, F. C. (1973) Effects of prostaglandins E_1, A_1 and $F_{2\alpha}$ on renal handling of salt and water. Am. J. Physiol. 225, 218–223.

114. Gryglewski, R., Korbut, R., and Ocetkiewicz, A. (1978) Generation of prostacyclin by lungs in vivo and its release into the arterial circulation. Nature (London) 273, 765–767.

115. Gryglewski, R. J., Korbut, R., Ocetkiewicz, A., Spławiński, J., Wojtaszek, B., and Swies, J. (1978) Lungs as a generator of prostacyclin—hypothesis on physiological significance. Naunyn-Schmiedebergs Arch. Pharmakol. 304, 45–50.

116. Halushka, P. V., Wohltmann, H., Privitera, P. J., Hurwitz, G., and Margolius, H. S. (1977) Bartter's syndrome: Urinary prostaglandin E-like material and kallikrein; Indomethacin effects. Ann. Intern. Med. 78, 281–286.

117. Hamberg, M. (1969) Biosynthesis of prostaglandins in the renal medulla of rabbit. FEBS Lett. 5, 127–130.

118. Hamberg, M., Hedqvist, P., Strandberg, K., Svensson, J., and Samuelsson, B. (1975) Prostaglandin endoperoxides: Effects on smooth muscle. Life Sci. 16, 541–561.

119. Hamberg, M., and Samuelsson, B. (1973) Detection and isolation of an endoperoxide intermediate in prostaglandin biosynthesis. Proc. Natl. Acad. Sci. (US) 70, 899–903.

120. Hamberg, M., Svensson, J., and Samuelsson, B. (1975) Thromboxanes: A new group of biologically active compounds derived from prostaglandin endoperoxides. Proc. Natl. Acad. Sci. (US) 72, 2994–2998.

121. Hassid, A., Konieczkowski, M., and Dunn, M. J. (1979) Prostaglandin synthesis in isolated rat kidney glomeruli. Proc. Natl. Acad. Sci. (US) 76, 1155–1159.

122. Henrich, W. L., Anderson, R. J., Berns, A. S., McDonald, K. M., Paulsen, P. J., Berl, T., and Schrier, R. W. (1978) The role of renal nerves and prostaglandins in control of renal hemodynamics and plasma renin activity during hypotensive hemorrhage in the dog. J. Clin. Invest. 61, 744–750.

123. Herman, C. A., Zenser, T. V., and Davis, B. B. (1977) Prostaglandin E_2 production by renal inner medullary tissue slices: Effect of metabolic inhibitors. Prostaglandins 14, 679–687.

124. Higashihara, E., Stokes, J. B., Kokko, J. P., Campbell, W. B., and Dubose, T. D., Jr. (1979) Cortical and papillary micropuncture examination of chloride transport in segments of the rat kidney during inhibition of prostaglandin production. Possible role for prostaglandins in the chloruresis of acute volume expansion. J. Clin. Invest. 64, 1277–1287.

125. Hood, V. L., and Dunn, M. J. (1978) Urinary excretion of prostaglandin E_2 and prostaglandin $F_{2\alpha}$ in potassium deficient rats. Prostaglandins 15, 273–280.

126. Hornych, A., Bedrossian, J., Bariety, J., Menard, J., Corvol, P., Safar, M., Fontaliran, F., and Milliez, P. (1975) Prostaglandins and hypertension in chronic renal disease. Clin. Nephrol. 4, 144–150.

127. Hornych, A., Safar, M., Papanicolaou, N., Meyer, P., and Milliez, P. (1973) Renal and cardiovascular effects of prostaglandin A_2 in hypertensive patients. Eur. J. Clin. Invest. 3, 391–398.

128. Hornych, A., Safar, M., Weiss, Y., Menard, J., Corvol, P., Bariety, J., and Milliez, P. (1976) Prostaglandins and essential hypertension. Eur. J. Clin. Invest. 6, 314.

129. Hornych, A., Weiss, Y., Safar, M., Menard, J., Corvol, P., Fontaliran, F., Bariety, J., and Milliez, P. (1976) Radioimmunoassay of prostaglandins, A and B in human blood. Prostaglandins 12, 383–397.

130. Hoult, J. R. S., and Moore, P. K. (1977) Pathways of prostaglandin $F_{2\alpha}$ metabolism in mammalian kidneys. Br. J. Pharmac. 61, 615–626.

131. Iino, Y., and Masoshi, I. (1978) Effects of prostaglandins on sodium transport in isolated collecting tubule. Pflügers Arch. 373, 125–132.

132. Itskovitz, H. D., Terragno, N. A., and McGiff, J. C. (1974) Effect of renal prostaglandin on distribution of blood flow in the isolated canine kidney. Circ. Res. 34, 770–776.

133. Jaffe, B. M., Parker, C. W., Marshall, G. R., and Needleman, P. (1972) Renal concentration of PGE in acute and chronic renal ischemia. Biochem. Biophys. Res. Commun. 49, 799–805.

134. Johns, E. J., Murdock, R., and Singer, B. (1977) The effect of angiotensin I converting enzyme inhibitor (SQ 20881) on the release of prostaglandins by rabbit kidney, in vivo. Br. J. Pharmacol. 60, 573–581.

135. Juan, H. (1977) Mechanism of action of bradykinin-induced release of prostaglandin E. Naunyn-Schmiedebergs Arch. Pharmakol. 300, 77–85.

136. Juncos, L. I., Fuller, T. J., and Cade, J. R. (1977) Effects of ultrafiltration on peripheral

plasma renin activity and prostaglandin concentration in hemodialysis patients with and without bilateral nephrectomy. J. Lab. Clin. Med. 90, 904–913.

137. Kalisker, A., and Dyer, D. C. (1972) In vitro release of prostaglandins from the renal medulla. Eur. J. Pharmacol. 19, 305–309.

138. Katzen, D. R., Pong, S. S., and Levine, L. (1975) Distribution of prostaglandin E 9-ketoreductase and NAD$^+$-dependent and NADP$^+$-dependent 15-hydroxyprostaglandin dehydrogenase in the renal cortex and medulla of various species. Res. Commun. Chem. Pathol. Pharmacol. 12, 781–787.

139. Kauker, M. L. (1977) Prostaglandin E$_2$ effect from the luminal side on renal tubular ^{22}Na efflux: Tracer microinjection studies. Proc. Soc. Exp. Biol. 154, 274–277.

140. Keiser, H. R., Andrews, M. J., Guyton, R. A., Margolius, H. S., and Pisano, J. J. (1976) Urinary kallikrein in dogs with constriction of one renal artery. Proc. Soc. Exp. Biol. Med. 151, 53–56.

141. Keiser, H. R., Geller, R. G., Margolius, H. S., and Pisano, J. J. (1976) Urinary kallikrein in hypertensive animal models. Fed. Proc. 35, 199–202.

142. Keiser, H. R., Seyberth, H. W., Oates, J. A., and Bartter, F. C. (1976) Bartter's syndrome: A disorder characterized by high urinary prostaglandin and a dependence of hyperreninemia on prostaglandin synthesis. Am. J. Med. 61, 43–51.

143. Kimberly, R. P., Gill, J. R., Bowden, R. E., Keiser, H. R., and Plotz, P. H. (1978) Elevated urinary prostaglandins and the effects of aspirin on renal function in lupus erythematosus. Ann. Intern. Med., 83, 336–341.

144. Kirschenbaum, M. A. (1977) The effect of prostaglandin inhibition on the natriuresis of drug-induced renal vasodilation. Prostaglandins 13, 1103–1112.

145. Kirschenbaum, M. A., and Stein, J. H. (1976) The effect of inhibition of prostaglandin synthesis on urinary sodium excretion in the conscious dog. J. Clin. Invest. 57, 517–521.

146. Kirschenbaum, M. A., and Stein, J. H. (1977) The effect of prostaglandin inhibition on sodium excretion during expansion of the extracellular fluid volume. J. Lab. Clin. Med. 90, 46–56.

147. Kirschenbaum, M. A., White, N., and Stein, J. H. (1974) Redistribution of renal cortical blood flow during inhibition of prostaglandin synthesis. Am. J. Physiol. 227, 801–805.

148. Köver, S., and Tost, H. (1977) The effect of indomethacin on kidney function: Indomethacin and furosemide antagonism. Pflügers Arch. 372, 215–220.

149. Krakoff, L. R., De Guia, D., Vlachakis, N., Stricker, J., and Goldstein, M. (1973) Effect of sodium balance on arterial blood pressure and renal responses to prostaglandin A$_1$ in man. Circ. Res. 33, 539–546.

150. Krakoff, L. R., Vlachakis, N. D., and De Guia, D. (1977) Effect of prostaglandin A$_1$ infusion in hypertensive patients with renal artery stenosis. Prostaglandins 14, 1153–1164.

151. Kulkarni, P. S., Roberts, R., and Needleman, P. (1976) Paradoxical endogenous synthesis of a coronary dilating substance from arachidonate. Prostaglandins 12, 337–353.

152. Kunze, H., and Vogt, W. (1971) Significance of phospholipase A for prostaglandin formation. Ann. NY Acad. Sci. 180, 123–125.

153. Larsson, C., and Änggård, E. (1973) Arachidonic acid lowers and indomethacin increases the blood pressure of the rabbit. J. Pharm. Pharmacol. 25, 653–655.

154. Larsson, C., and Änggård, E. (1973) Regional differences in the formation and metabolism of prostaglandins in the rabbit kidney. Eur. J. Pharmacol. 21, 30–36.

155. Larsson, C., and Änggård, E. (1974) Increased juxtamedullary blood flow on stimulation of intrarenal prostaglandin biosynthesis. Eur. J. Pharmacol. 25, 326–334.

156. Larsson, C., Weber, P., and Änggård, E. (1976) Arachidonic acid increases and indomethacin decreases plasma renin activity in the rabbit. Eur. J. Pharmacol. 28, 391–394.

157. Larsson, C., Weber, P., and Änggård, E. (1976) Stimulation and inhibition of renal

PG biosynthesis: Effects on renal blood flow and on plasma renin activity. Acta Biol. Med. Ger. 35, 1195–1200.

158. Leary, W. P., Asmal, A. C., and Botha, J. (1977) Pulmonary inactivation of prostaglandin by hypertensive rats. Prostaglandins 13, 679–700.

159. Lee, J. B. (1967) Antihypertensive activity of the kidney. The renomedullary prostaglandins. New Engl. J. Med. 277, 1073–1079.

160. Lee, J. B. (1967) Chemical and physiological properties of renal prostaglandins: The antihypertensive effects of medullin in essential human hypertension. In: S. Bergström and B. Samuelsson (eds.), Nobel Symposium 2: Prostaglandins, Almqvist and Wiksell, Stockholm, pp. 197–210.

161. Lee, J. B. (1973) Hypertension, natriuresis and the renomedullary prostaglandins: An overview, Prostaglandins 3, 511–579.

162. Lee, J. B., Covino, B. G., Takman, B. H., and Smith, E. R. (1965) Renal medullary vasodepressor substance medullin: Isolation, chemical characterization and physiological properties. Circ. Res. 17, 57–77.

163. Lee, J. B., Crowshaw, K., Takman, B. H., Attrep, K. A., and Gougoutas, J. Z. (1967) The identification of prostaglandins E_2, $F_{2\alpha}$ and A_2 from rabbit kidney medulla. Biochem. J. 105, 1251–1260.

164. Lee, J. B., McGiff, J. C., Kannegiesser, H., Aykent, Y. Y., Mudd, J. G., and Frawley, T. F. (1971) Prostaglandin A_1: Antihypertensive and renal effects. Ann. Intern. Med. 74, 703–710.

165. Lee, S. C., and Levine, L. (1975) Prostaglandin metabolism. II. Identification of two 15-hydroxyprostaglandin dehydrogenase types. J. Biol. Chem. 250, 548–552.

166. Lee, S. C., Pong, S. S., Katzen, D., Wu, K. Y., and Levine, L. (1975) Distribution of prostaglandin E 9-ketoreductase and types I and II 15-hydroxy-prostaglandin dehydrogenase in swine kidney medulla and cortex. Biochemistry 14, 142–145.

167. Levy, J. V. (1977) Changes in systolic arterial blood pressure in normal and spontaneously hypertensive rats produced by acute administration of inhibitors of prostaglandin biosynthesis. Prostaglandins 13, 153–160.

168. Lifschitz, M. D., Patak, R. V., Padem, S. Z., and Stein, J. H. (1978) Urinary prostaglandin E excretion: Effect of chronic alterations in sodium intake and inhibition of prostaglandin synthesis in the rabbit. Prostaglandins 16, 607–619.

169. Limas, C. J., and Limas, C. (1977) Vascular prostaglandin synthesis in the spontaneously hypertensive rat. Am. J. Physiol. 233, H493–H499.

170. Lipson, L. C., and Sharp, G. W. G. (1971) Effect of prostaglandin E_1 on sodium transport and osmotic water flow in the toad bladder. Am. J. Physiol. 220, 1046–1052.

171. Littlewood, J. M., Lee, M. R., and Meadow, S. R. (1976) Treatment of childhood Bartter's syndrome with indomethacin. Lancet 2, 795.

172. Lonigro, A. J., Itskovitz, H. D., Crowshaw, K., and McGiff, J. C. (1973) Dependency of renal blood flow on prostaglandin synthesis in the dog. Circ. Res. 32, 712–717.

173. Lonigro, A. J., Terragno, N. A., Malik, K. U., and McGiff, J. C. (1973) Differential inhibition by prostaglandins of the renal actions of pressor stimuli. Prostaglandins 3, 595–606.

174. Lopez-Ovejero, J. A., Weber, M. A., Drayer, J. I. M., Sealey, J. E., and Laragh, J. H. (1978) Effects of indomethacin alone and during diuretic or β-adrenoreceptor-blockade therapy on blood pressure and the renin system in essential hypertension. Clin. Sci. Mol. Med. 55, 203s–205s.

175. Lum, G. M., Aisenberry, G. A., Dunn, M. J., Berl, T., Schrier, R. W., and McDonald, K. M. (1977) In vivo effect of indomethacin to potentiate the renal medullary cyclic AMP response to vasopressin. J. Clin. Invest. 59, 8–13.

176. Malik, K. U. (1978) Prostaglandins—Modulation of adrenergic nervous system. Fed. Proc. 37, 203–207.

177. Malik, K. U., and McGiff, J. C. (1975) Modulation by prostaglandins of adrenergic transmission in the isolated perfused rabbit and rat kidney. Circ. Res. 36, 599–609.

178. Malik, K. U., and Nasjletti, A. (1979) Attenuation by bradykinin of adrenergically

induced vasoconstriction in the isolated perfused kidney on the rabbit: Relationship to prostaglandin synthesis. Br. J. Pharmacol. 57, 269–275.

179. Margolius, H. S., Horwitz, D., Geller, R. G., Alexander, R. W., Gill, J. R., Pisano, J. J., and Keiser, H. R. (1971) Urinary kallikrein excretion in normal man. Relationship to sodium intake and sodium retaining steroids. Circ. Res. 35, 812–819.

180. Margolius, H. S., Horwitz, D., Pisano, J. J., and Keiser, H. R. (1976) Relationships among urinary kallikrein mineralocorticoids and human hypertensive disease. Fed. Proc. 35, 203–206.

181. Martinez-Maldonaldo, M., Tsaparas, N., Eknoyan, G., and Suki, W. N. (1972) Renal actions of prostaglandins: Comparison with acetylcholine and volume expansion. Am. J. Physiol. 222, 1147–1152.

182. Marumo, F., and Edelman, I. S. (1971) Effects of Ca^{++} and prostaglandin E_1 on vasopressin activation of renal adenyl cyclase. J. Clin. Invest. 50, 1613–1620.

183. Mauk, R. H., Patak, R. V., Padem, S. Z., Lifschitz, M. D., and Stein, J. H. (1977) Effect of prostaglandin E administration in a nephrotoxic and a vasoconstrictor model of acute renal failure. Kidney Int. 12, 122–130.

184. McGiff, J. C., Crowshaw, K., Terragno, N. A., and Lonigro, A. J. (1970) Release of prostaglandin-like substance into renal venous blood in response to angiotension II. Circ. Res. (Suppl. I) 26, I121–I130.

185. McGiff, J. C., Itskovitz, H. D., and Terragno, N. A. (1975) The actions of bradykinin and eledoisine in the isolated kidney. Relationship to prostaglandins. Clin. Sci. Mol. Med. 49, 125–131.

186. McGiff, J. C., Terragno, N. A., Malik, K. U., and Lonigro, A. J. (1972) Release of a prostaglandin E-like substance from canine kidney by bradykinin. Circ. Res. 31, 36–43.

187. McQueen, D., and Bell, K. (1976) The effect of prostaglandin E_1 and sodium meclofenamate on blood pressure in renal hypertensive rats. Eur. J. Pharmacol. 37, 223–235.

188. Mills, J. H., and Obika, L. (1977) Increased urinary kallikrein excretion during prostaglandin E_1 infusion in anesthetized dogs and its relation to natriuresis and diuresis. J. Physiol. 273, 459–474.

189. Mimran, A., Casellas, D., Dupont, M., and Baron, P. (1975) Effect of a competitive antagonist on the renal hemodynamic changes induced by inhibition of prostaglandin synthesis in rats. Clin. Sci. Mol. Med. 48, 299s–302s.

190. Moncada, S., Gryglewski, R., Bunting, S., and Vane, J. R. (1976) An enzyme isolated from arteries transforms prostaglandin endoperoxides to an unstable substance that inhibits platelet aggregation. Nature (London) 263, 663–665.

191. Moncada, S., Higgs, E. A., and Vane, J. R. (1977) Human arterial and venous tissues generate prostacyclin (prostaglandin X), a potent inhibitor of platelet aggregation. Lancet 1 (801), 18–20.

192. Montgomery, R. G., Patel, N. C., and Lee, J. G. (1973) A comparison of the diuretic effects of prostaglandin A_1, sodium ethacrynate, and placebo. Prostaglandins 4, 381–394.

193. Morrison, A. R., Nishikawa, K., and Needleman, P. (1977) Unmasking of thromboxane A_2 synthesis by ureteral obstruction in the rabbit kidney. Nature (London) 267, 259–269.

194. Morrison, A. R., and Needleman, P. (1979) Biochemistry and pharmacology of renal prostaglandins. In: B. Brenner and J. Stein (eds.), Hormonal Functions of the Kidney, Churchill Livingstone, New York, pp. 68–88.

195. Muirhead, E. E., Brooks, B., and Brosius, W. L. (1976) Indomethacin and blood pressure control. J. Lab. Clin. Med. 88, 578–583.

196. Muirhead, E. E., Rightsel, W. A., Leach, B. E., Byers, L. W., Pitcock, J. A., and Brooks, B. (1977) Reversal of hypertension by transplants and lipid extracts of cultured renomedullary interstitial cells. Lab. Invest. 35, 162–172.

197. Nasjletti, A., and Colina-Chovrio, J. (1976) Interaction of mineralocorticoids, renal prostaglandins and the renal kallikrein-kinin system. Fed. Proc. 35, 189–193.

198. Needleman, P., Bronson, S. D., Wyche, A., and Sivokoff, M. (1978) Cardiac and renal PGI₂ biosynthesis and biological effects in isolated perfused rabbit tissues. J. Clin. Invest. 61, 839–849.

199. Needleman, P., Kauffman, A. H., Douglas, J. R., Jr., Johnson, E. M., and Marshall, G. R. (1973) Specific stimulation and inhibition of renal prostaglandin release by angiotensin analogs. Am. J. Physiol. 224, 1415–1419.

200. Needleman, P., Marshall, G. R., and Sobel, B. E. (1975) Hormone interactions in the isolated rabbit heart: Synthesis and coronary vasomotor effects of prostaglandins, angiotensin and bradykinin. Circ. Res. 37, 802–808.

201. Needleman, P., Minke, M., and Raz, A. (1976) Thromboxanes: Selective biosynthesis and distinct biological properties. Science 193, 163–165.

202. Negus, P., Tannen, R. L., and Dunn, M. J. (1976) Indomethacin potentiates the vasoconstrictor actions of angiotensin II in normal man. Prostaglandins 12, 175–180.

203. Norbiato, G., Raggi, U., Fasoli, A., Bevilacqua, M., and Micossi, P. (1976) Inhibition of prostaglandin synthesis and Bartter's syndrome. Lancet 2, 1144.

204. Norby, L., Framenbaum, W., Lehtz, R., and Ramwell, P. W. (1976) Prostaglandins and aspirin therapy in Bartter's syndrome, Lancet 2, 604–606.

205. Nugteren, D. H., and Hazelhof, E. (1973) Isolation and properties of intermediates in prostaglandin biosynthesis. Biochim. Biophys. Acta 326, 448–461.

206. Okada, F., Nukada, T., Yamauchi, Y., and Abe, K. (1974) The hypotensive effect of prostaglandin E₁ on hypertensive cases of various types. Prostaglandins 7, 99–106.

207. Oliw, E. (1978) Acute unilateral ureteral occlusion increases plasma renin activity and contralateral urinary prostaglandin excretion in rabbits. Eur. J. Pharmacol. 53, 95–102.

208. Oliw, E., Köver, S., Larsson, C., and Änggård, E. (1976) Reduction by indomethacin of furosemide effects in the rabbit. Eur. J. Pharmacol. 38, 95–110.

209. Oliw, E., Lundén, I., and Änggård, E. (1978) In vivo inhibition of prostaglandin synthesis in rabbit kidney by nonsteroidal anti-inflammatory drugs. Acta Pharmacol. Toxicol. 42, 179–184.

210. Olsen, U. B. (1976) Clonidine-induced increase of renal prostaglandin activity and water diuresis in conscious dogs. Eur. J. Pharmacol. 36, 95–101.

211. Olsen, U. B. (1977) Prostaglandin/kinin activity related to changed renal compliance after bumetanide in dogs. Acta Pharmacol. Toxicol. 40, 430–438.

212. Olsen, U. B. (1978) Kidney volume expansion and prostaglandin release by bradykinin. The effect of indomethacin pretreatment. Acta Physiol. Scand. 102, 129–136.

213. Olsen, U. B., and Ahnfelt-Rønne, I. (1976) Bumetanide-induced increase of renal blood flow in conscious dogs and its relation to local renal hormones. Acta Pharmacol. Toxicol. 38, 219–228.

214. Olsen, U. B., and Ahnfelt-Rønne, I. (1978) Enhancement of urine prostaglandin excretion by chlorazanil in dogs. Acta Pharmacol. Toxicol. 43, 233–239.

215. Olsen, U. B., and Arrigoni-Martelli, E. (1979) The effects of kinase II inhibition by SQ14225 on kidney kallikrein-kinin and prostaglandin systems in conscious dogs. Eur. J. Pharmacol. 54, 229–234.

216. Omini, C., Moncada, S., and Vane, J. R. (1977) The effects of prostacyclin (PGI₂) on tissues which detect prostaglandins (PGs). Prostaglandins 14, 625–632.

217. Orloff, J., Handler, J. S., and Bergström, S. (1965) Effect of prostaglandin (PGE₁) on the permeability response of toad bladder to vasopressin, Theophylline and adenosine 3',5'-monophosphate. Nature (London) 205, 397–398.

218. Owen, T. L., Ehrhart, I. C., Weidner, J. W., Scott, J. B., and Haddy, F. J. (1975) Effects of indomethacin on local blood flow regulation in canine heart and kidney. Proc. Soc. Exp. Biol. Med. 149, 871–876.

219. Pace-Asciak, C. R. (1976) Biosynthesis and catabolism of prostaglandins during animal development. In: B. Samuelsson and R. Paoletti (eds.) Advances in Prostaglandin and Thromboxane Research Vol. 1, Raven Press, New York, pp. 35–46.

220. Pace-Asciak, C. R. (1976) Isolation, structure and biosynthesis of 6-keto-prostaglandin $F_{1\alpha}$ in the rat stomach. J. Am. Chem. Soc. 98, 2348–2349.

221. Pace-Asciak, C. R. (1976) Decreased renal prostaglandin catabolism precedes onset of hypertension in the developing spontaneously hypertensive rat. Nature (London) 263, 510–512.

222. Pace-Asciak, C. R., Carrara, M. C., and Comazet, Z. (1977) Identification of the major urinary metabolites of 6-keto-prostaglandin $F_{1\alpha}$ (6K-PKF$_{1\alpha}$) in the rat. Biochem. Biophys. Res. Commun. 78, 115–121.

223. Pace-Asciak, C. R., Carrara, M. C., and Nicolaou, K. C. (1978) Prostaglandin I_2 has more potent properties than prostaglandin E_2 in the normal and spontaneously hypertensive rat. Prostaglandins 15, 999–1003.

224. Pace-Asciak, C. R., Carrara, M. C., Rangaraj, G., and Nicolaou, K. C. (1978) Enhanced formation of PGI$_2$, a potent hypotensive substance by aortic rings and homogenates of the spontaneously hypertensive rat. Prostaglandins 15, 1005–1012.

225. Pace-Asciak, C. R., and Nashat, M. (1975) Catabolism of an isolated, purified intermediate of prostaglandin biosynthesis by regions of the adult rat kidney. Biochim. Biophys. Acta 388, 243–253.

226. Papanicolaou, N., Mountokalasis, T. H., Safar, M., Bariety, J., and Milliez, P. (1976) Deficiency in renomedullary prostaglandin synthesis related to the evolution of essential hypertension. Experientia 32, 1015–1017.

227. Papanicolaou, N., Safar, M., Hornych, A., Fontaliran, F., Weiss, Y., Bariety, J., and Milliez, P. (1975) The release of renal prostaglandins during saline infusion in normal and hypertensive subjects. Clin. Sci. Mol. Med. 49, 459–463.

228. Patak, R. V., Mookerjee, B. K., Bentzel, C. J., Hysert, P. E., Babej, M., and Lee, J. B. (1975) Antagonism of the effects of furosemide by indomethacin in normal and hypertensive man. Prostaglandins 10, 649–659.

229. Patak, R. V., Fadem, S. Z., Rosenblatt, S. G., Lifschitz, M. D., and Stein, J. H. (1979) Diuretic-induced changes in renal blood flow and PGE$_2$ excretion in dog. Am. J. Physiol. 236, F494–F504.

230. Paulson, D. J., and Eversole, J. (1977) Effects of prostaglandin E_2 and prostaglandin inhibitors on adrenal regeneration hypertension. Am. J. Physiol. 232, E95–E99.

231. Paulsrud, J. R., and Miller, O. N. (1974) Inhibition of 15-OH-prostaglandin dehydrogenase by several diuretic drugs. Fed. Proc. 33, 590a.

232. Payakkapan, W., Attallah, A. A., Lee, J. B., and Carr, A. A. (1975) Effect of sodium intake on prostaglandin A, renin and aldosterone in normotensive humans. Kidney Int. (Suppl) 8, 283–290.

233. Pong, S. S., and Levine, L. (1976) Biosynthesis of prostaglandins in rabbit renal cortex. Res. Commun. Chem. Pathol. Pharmacol. 13, 115–123.

234. Pugsley, D. J., Berlen, L. J., and Petro, R. (1975) Renal prostaglandin synthesis in the Goldblatt hypertensive rat. Circ. Res. (Suppl. I) 36, 37, 181–188.

235. Radfar, N., Gill, J. R., Jr., Bartter, F. C., Bravo, E., Taylor, A. A., and Bowden, R. E. (1978) Hypokalemia, in Bartter's syndrome and other disorders, produces resistance to vasopressors via prostaglandin overproduction. Proc. Soc. Exp. Biol. Med. 158, 502–507.

236. Raz, A. (1972) Interaction of prostaglandins with blood plasma proteins: Comparative binding of prostaglandins A_2, $F_{2\alpha}$ and E_2 to human plasma proteins. Biochem. J. 130, 631–636.

237. Raz, A., Isakson, P. C., Minkes, M. S., and Needleman, P. (1977) Characterization of a novel metabolic pathway of arachidonate in coronary arteries which generates a potent endogenous coronary vasodilator. J. Biol. Chem. 252, 1123–1126.

238. Rennick, B. R. (1977) Renal tubular transport of prostaglandins: Inhibition by probenecid and indomethacin. Am. J. Physiol. 233, F133–F137.

239. Rioux, F., Quirion, R., and Regoli, D. (1977) The role of prostaglandins in hypertension. I. The release of prostaglandins by aorta strips of renal DOCA-salt and spontaneously hypertensive rats. Can. J. Pharmacol. 55, 1330–1338.

240. Rioux, F., and Regoli, D. (1975) In vitro production of prostaglandins by isolated aorta strips of normotensive and hypertensive rats. Can. J. Physiol. Pharmacol. 53, 673–677.

241. Romero, J. C., and Strong, C. G. (1977) The effect of indomethacin blockade of prostaglandin synthesis on blood pressure of normal rabbits and rabbits with renovascular hypertension. Circ. Res. 40, 35–41.

242. Romero, J. C., and Strong, C. G. (1977) Hypertension and the interrelated renal circulatory effects of prostaglandins and the renin-angiotension system. Mayo Clin. Proc. 52, 462–464.

243. Romero, J. C., Strong, C. G., Ott, C. E., Walker, R., Schryver, S., and Manahan, D. (1975) The effect of indomethacin on the renin-angiotensin system. Clin. Res. 23, 372A.

244. Rose, J. C., Kot, P. A., Ramwell, P. W., Doykos, M., and O'Neill, W. P. (1976) Cardiovascular responses to three prostaglandin endoperoxide analogs in the dog. Proc. Soc. Exp. Biol. Med. 153, 209–212.

245. Rosenblatt, S. G., Patak, R. V., and Lifschitz, M. D. (1978) Organic acid secretory pathway and urinary excretion of prostaglandin E in the dog. Am. J. Physiol. 234, F473–F479.

246. Rosenthal, J., Simone, P. G., and Silbergleit, A. (1974) Effects of prostaglandin deficiency on natriuresis, diuresis and blood pressure. Prostaglandins 5, 435–440.

247. Rumpf, K. W., Frenzel, S., Lowetz, H. D., and Scheler, F. (1975) The effect of indomethacin on plasma renin activity in man under normal conditions and after stimulation of tbe renin-angiotensin system. Prostaglandins 10, 641–648.

248. Rumpf, K. W., Frenzel, S., Lowetz, H. D., and Scheler, F. (1976) Die Wirkung von Indomethacin auf die vasale und stimumierte Plasmareninaktivitat beim Menschen. Klin. Wochenschr. 54, 255–259.

249. Samuelsson, B. (1977) The role of prostaglandin endoperoxides and thromboxanes as bioregulators. In: N. Kharasch and J. Fried (eds.) Biochemical Aspects of Prostaglandins and Thromboxanes: Proceedings of the 1976 Intra-science Foundation Symposium, Academic Press, New York, pp. 133–154.

250. Samuelsson, B. (1978) Prostaglandins and thromboxanes. Rec. Prog. Hormone Res. 34, 239–258.

251. Scherer, B., Siess, W., and Weber, P. C. (1977) Radioimmunological and biological measurement of prostaglandin in rabbit urine: Decrease of PGE_2 excretion at high NaCl intake. Prostaglandins 13, 1127–1139.

252. Scherer, B., and Weber, P. C. (1979) Time dependent changes in prostaglandin excretion in response to furosemide in man. Clin. Sci. 56, 77–81.

253. Schölkens, B. A., and Steinbach, R. (1975) Increase of experimental hypertension following inhibition of prostaglandin biosynthesis. Arch. Int. Pharmacodyn. 214, 328–334.

254. Schwartz, W. B., and Relman, A. S. (1967) Effects of electrolyte disorders on renal structure and function. New Engl. J. Med. 276, 383–389.

255. Seymour, A. A., Davis, J. O., Freeman, R. H., DeForrest, J. M., Rowe, B. P., and Williams, G. M. (1979) Renin release from filtering and nonfiltering kidneys stimulated by PGI_2 and PGD_2. Am. J. Physiol. 237, F285–F290.

256. Seymour, A. A., and Zehr, J. E. (1979) Influence of renal prostaglandin synthesis on renin control mechanisms in the dog. Circ. Res. 45, 13–25.

257. Share, L., Claybaugh, J. R., Hatch, F. E., Jr., Johnson, J. G., Lee, S., Muirhead, E. E., and Shaw, P. (1972) Effects of change of posture and of sodium depletion on plasma levels of vasopressin and renin in normal human subjects. J. Lab. Clin. Med. 35, 171–174.

258. Smith, W. L., and Bell, T. G. (1978) Immunohistochemical localization of the prostaglandin-forming cyclo-oxygenase in renal cortex. Am. J. Physiol. 235, F451–F457.

259. Smith, W. L., Bell, T. G., and Needleman, P. (1979) Increased renal tubular synthesis

of prostaglandins in the rabbit kidney in response to ureteral obstruction. Prostaglandins 18, 269–277.

260. Speckart, P., Zia, P., Zipser, R., and Horton, R. (1977) The effect of sodium restriction and prostaglandin inhibition on the renin-angiotensin system in man. J. Clin. Endocrinol. Metab. 44, 832–837.

261. Stahl. R., Dienemann, H., Kneissler, U., Christ, H., and Helmchen, U. (1979) Indomethacin-induced hypotension in sodium and volume depleted rats. Klin. Wochenschr. 57, 143–145.

262. Stahl, R. A. K., Attallah, A. A., Bloch, D. L., and Lee, J. B. (1979) Stimulation of rabbit renal PGE_2 biosynthesis by dietary sodium restriction. Am. J. Physiol. 237, F344–F349.

263. Stone, K. J., and Hart, M. (1976) Inhibition of renal PGE_2-9-keto-reductase by diuretics. Prostaglandins 12, 197–208.

264. Strandboy, J. W., Ott, C. E., Schneider, E. G., Willis, L. R., Beck, N. P., Davis, B. B., and Knox, F. G. (1974) Effects of prostaglandins E_1 and E_2 on renal sodium reabsorption and starling forces. Am. J. Physiol. 226, 1015–1021.

265. Sugawara, S., and Zimmerman, B. G. (1978) Influence of angiotensin antagonists on renal vascular resistance and prostaglandin E release. Clin. Exp. Hypertension 1, 11–24.

266. Sun, F. F., and Taylor, B. M. (1978) Metabolism of prostacyclin in rat. Biochemistry 17, 4096–4101.

267. Svensson, J., and Hamberg, M. (1976) Thromboxane A_2 and prostaglandin H_2: Potent stimulators of the swine coronary artery. Prostaglandins 12, 943–950.

268. Swain, J. A., Hendricks, G. R., Boettcher, D. H., and Vatner, S. F. (1975) Prostaglandin control of renal circulation in the unanesthetized dog and baboon. Am. J. Physiol. 229, 826–830.

269. Tan, S. Y., Sweet, P., and Mulrow, P. J. (1978) Impaired renal production of prostaglandin E_2: A newly identified lesion in human essential hypertension. Prostaglandins 15, 139–150.

270. Tannenbaum, J., Spławiński, J. A., Oates, J. A., and Nies, A. S. (1975) Enhanced renal prostaglandin production in the dog. I. Effects on renal function. Circ. Res. 36, 197–203.

271. Terashima, R., Anderson, F. L., and Jubiz, W. (1976) Prostaglandin E release in the dog: Effect of sodium. Am. J. Physiol. 321, 1429–1432.

272. Terragno, D. A., Crowshaw, K., Terragno, N. A., and McGiff, J. C. (1975) Prostaglandin synthesis by bovine mesenteric arteries and veins. Circ. Res. (Suppl. I) 36, I176–I180.

273. Terragno, N. A., McGiff, J. C., Smigel, M., and Terragno, D. A. (1978) Patterns of prostaglandin production in the bovine fetal and maternal vasculature. Prostaglandins 16, 847–855.

274. Terragno, N. A., Terragno, D. A., and McGiff, J. C. (1977) Contribution of prostaglandin to the renal circulation in conscious, anesthetized and laparotomized dogs. Circ. Res. 40, 590–595.

275. Tobian, L., and O'Donnell, M. (1976) Renal prostaglandins in relation to sodium regulation and hypertension. Fed. Proc. 35, 2388–2392.

276. Tuveno, T., and Wide, L. (1973) Prostaglandin release from the human umbilical artery in vitro. Prostaglandins 4, 689–694.

277. Vance, V. K., Attallah, A., Prezyna, A., and Lee, J. B. (1973) Human renal prostaglandins. Prostaglandins 3, 647–667.

278. Vander, A. J. (1968) Direct effects of prostaglandin on renal function and renin release in anesthetized dog. Am. J. Physiol. 214, 218–221.

279. Vargaftig, B. B. (1966) Effet des analgésiques non narcotiques sur l'hypotension due à la bradykinine. Experientia 22, 182–183.

280. Vargaftig, B. B. and Dao Hai, N. (1972) Selective inhibition by mepacrine of the

release of "rabbit aorta contracting substance" evoked by the administration of bradykinin. J. Pharm. Pharmacol. 24, 159–161.

281. Venuto, R. C., O'Dorisio, T., Ferris, T. F., and Stein, J. H. (1975) Prostaglandin and renal function, II. The effect of prostaglandin inhibition on autoregulation of blood flow in the intact kidney of the dog. Prostaglandins 9, 817–828.

282. Verberckmoes, R., van Damme, B., Clemen, J., Amery, A., and Michielsen, P. (1976) Bartter's syndrome with hyperplasia of renomedullary cells: Successful treatment with indomethacin. Kidney Int. 9, 302–307.

283. Villa, S., and de Gaetano, G. (1977) Prostacyclin-like activity in rat vascular tissues. Fast, long-lasting inhibition by treatment with lysine acetylsalicylate. Prostaglandins 14, 1117–1124.

284. Vinci, J. M., Gill, J. R., Bowden, R. E., Pisano, J. J., Izzo, J. L., Radfar, N., Taylor, A. A., Zusman, R. M., Bartter, F. C., and Keiser, H. H. (1978) The kallikrein-kinin system in Bartter's syndrome and its response to prostaglandin synthetase inhibition. J. Clin. Invest. 61, 1671–1682.

285. Walker, L. A., Whorton, A. R., Smigel, M., France, R., and Frölich, J. C. (1978b) Antidiuretic hormone increases renal prostaglandin synthesis in vivo. Am. J. Physiol. 235, F180–F185.

286. Weber, P. C., Holzgreve, H., Stephan, R., and Herbst, R. (1975) PRA and sodium and water excretion following infusion of arachidonic acid in rats. Eur. J. Pharmacol. 34, 299–304.

287. Weber, P. C., Larsson, C., Änggård, E., Hamberg, M., Corey, E. J., Nicolaou, K. C., and Samuelsson, B. (1976) Stimulation of renin release from rabbit renal cortex by arachidonic acid and prostaglandin endoperoxide. Circ. Res. 39, 868–873.

288. Weber, P. C., Larsson, C., and Scherer, B. (1977) Prostaglandin E_2-9-ketoreductase as a mediator of salt intake-related prostaglandin-renin interaction. Nature (London) 266, 65–66.

289. Weber, P. C., Scherer, B., Lange, H. H., Held, E., and Schnermann, J. (1978) Renal prostaglandins and renin release relationship to regulation of electrolyte excretion and blood pressure. Proceedings of the Seventh International Congress on Nephrology, Montreal, pp. 99–106.

290. Weber, P. C., Scherer, B., and Larsson, C. (1977) Increase in free arachidonic acid by furosemide in man as the cause of prostaglandin and renin release. Eur. J. Pharmacol. 41, 329–332.

291. Weksler, B. B., Marcus, A. J., and Jaffe, E. A. (1977) Synthesis of prostaglandin I_2 (prostacyclin) by cultured human and bovine endothelial cells. Proc. Natl. Acad. Sci. (US) 74, 3922–3926.

292. Wennmalm, Å. (1974) Hypertensive effect of prostaglandin synthesis inhibitor indomethacin. Res. Clin. Pharmacol. Ther. 2, 1099.

293. Wennmalm, Å. (1977) Vasodilatory action of arachidonic acid in humans following indomethacin treatment. Prostaglandins 13, 809–810.

294. Werning, C., Vetter, W., Weidmann, P., Schweikert, H. U., Stiel, D., and Siegenthaler, W. (1971) Effect of prostaglandin E_1 on renin in the dog. Am. J. Physiol. 220, 852–856.

295. Westura, E. E., Kannegiesser, H., O'Tool, J. B., and Lee, J. B. (1970) Antihypertensive effects of prostaglandin A_1 in essential hypertensive. Circ. Res. 27 (Suppl. I) I131–I140.

296. Whorton, A. R., Misano, K., Hollifield, J., Frölich, J. C., Inagami, T., and Oates, J. A. (1977) Prostaglandin and renin release. I. Stimulation of renin release from rabbit renal cortical slices by PGI_2. Prostaglandins 14, 1095–1104.

297. Whorton, A. R., Smigel, M., Oates, J. A., and Frölich, J. C. (1978) Regional differences in prostacyclin formation by the kidney. Prostacyclin is a major prostaglandin of renal cortex. Biochim. Biophys. Acta 529, 176–180.

298. Williams, W. M., Frölich, J. C., Nies, A. S., and Oates, J. A. (1976) Urinary prostaglandins: Site of entry into renal tubular fluid. Kidney Int. 11, 256–260.

299. Williamson, H. E., Bourland, W. A., and Marchand, G. R. (1975) Inhibition of furosemide-induced increase in renal blood flow by indomethacin. Proc. Soc. Exp. Biol. Med. 148, 164–165.

300. Williamson, H. E., Bourland, W. A., Marchand, G. R., Farley, D. B., and van Orden, D. E. (1975) Furosemide-induced release of prostaglandin E to increase renal blood flow. Proc. Soc. Exp. Med. 150, 104–106.

301. Williamson, H. E., Marchand, G. R., Bourland, W. A., Farley, D. B., and van Orden, D. E. (1976) Ethacrynic acid induced release of prostaglandin E to increase blood flow. Prostaglandins 11, 519–522.

302. Yasujima, Y., Abe, K., Irokawa, N., Chiba, S., Sato, M., Seino, M., Sakurai, Y., Saito, K., Ito, T., Ritsu, K., and Yoshinaga, K. (1978) Urinary prostaglandin and sodium metabolism in patients with essential hypertension. Tohoku J. Exp. Med. 124, 277–283.

303. Yasujima, M., Abe, K., Otsuka, Y., Chiba, S., Ritsu, K., Irokawa, N., Seino, M., Sakurai, Y., Saito, K., Ito, T., and Yoshinaga, K. (1977) Effects of Sar[1]-Ile[8]-angiotensin II on urinary prostaglandin excretion in patients with essential hypertension. Tohoku J. Exp. Med. 123, 271–278.

304. Yun, J., Kelly, G., Bartter, F. C., and Smith, Jr., H. (1977) Role of prostaglandins in the control of renin secretion in the dog. Circ. Res. 40, 459–464.

305. Yun, J., Kelly, C. H., Bartter, F. C., and Smith H., Jr. (1978) Role of prostaglandins in the control of renin secretion in the dog. Life Sci. 23, 945–952.

306. Zenser, T. V., and Davis, B. B. (1978) Antioxidant inhibition of prostaglandin production by rat renal medulla, Metabolism 27, 227–233.

307. Zenser, T. V., Levitt, M. J., and Davis, B. B. (1977) Possible modulation of rat renal prostaglandin production by oxygen. Am. J. Physiol. 233, F539–F543.

308. Zenser, T. V., Levitt, M. J., and Davis, B. B. (1977) Effect of oxygen and solute on PGE and PGF production by the rat kidney slices. Prostaglandins 13, 143–151.

309. Zimmerman, B. G. (1978) Effect of meclofenamate on renal vascular resistance in early Goldblatt hypertension in conscious and anesthetized dog. Prostaglandins 15, 1027–1034.

310. Zimmerman, B. G., Mommsen, C., and Kraft, E. (1980) Interrelationship between renal prostaglandin E, renin and renal vascular tone in conscious dogs. In: B. Samuelsson, P. W. Ramwell, and R. Paoletti (eds.), Advances in Prostaglandin and Thromboxane Research, Vol. 7, Raven Press, New York, pp. 1153–1157.

311. Zins, G. (1975) Renal prostaglandins. Am. J. Med. 58, 14–24.

312. Zipser, R. D., Hoefs, J. C., Speckart, P. F., Zia, P. K., and Horton, R. (1979) Prostaglandins: Modulators of renal function and pressor resistance in chronic liver disease. J. Clin. Endocrinol. Metab. 48, 895–900.

313. Zusman, R. M., Caldwell, B. V., Mulrow, P. J., and Speroff, L. (1973) The role of prostaglandin A in the control of sodium homeostasis and blood pressure. Prostaglandins 3, 679–690.

314. Zusman, R. M., and Keiser, H. R. (1977) Prostaglandin E$_2$ biosynthesis by rabbit renomedullary interstitial cells in tissue culture. Mechanism of stimulation by angiotensin II, bradykinin and arginine vasopressin. J. Biol. Chem. 252, 2069–2071.

315. Zusman, R. M., and Keiser, H. R. (1977) Prostaglandin biosynthesis by rabbit renomedullary interstitial cells in tissue culture. Stimulation by angiotensin II, bradykinin and arginine vasopressin. J. Clin. Invest. 60, 215–223.

316. Zusman, R. M., Keiser, H. R., and Handler, J. S. (1977) Vasopressin-stimulated prostaglandin E biosynthesis in the toad urinary bladder. Effect on water flow. J. Clin. Invest. 60, 1339–1347.

317. Zusman, R. M., Keiser, H. R., and Handler, J. S. (1977) Inhibition of vasopressin-stimulated prostaglandin E biosynthesis by chlorpropamide in the toad urinary bladder. J. Clin. Invest. 60, 1348–1353.

318. Zusman, R. M., Keiser, H. R., and Handler, J. S. (1978) Effect of adrenal steroids on vasopressin-stimulated PGE synthesis and water flow. Am. J. Physiol. 234, F532–F540.
319. Zusman, R. M., Spector, D., Caldwell, B. V., Speroff, L., Schneider, G., and Mulrow, P. J. (1973) The effect of chronic sodium loading and sodium restriction of plasma prostaglandin A, E and F. Concentrations in human beings. J. Clin. Invest. 52, 1093–1098.

RYSZARD J. GRYGLEWSKI, M.D.

PROSTACYCLIN, PROSTAGLANDINS, THROMBOXANES, AND PLATELET FUNCTION

POLYUNSATURATED FATTY ACIDS (PUFA)

Polyunsaturated fatty acids (PUFAs) are closely associated with platelet function. PUFAs are the constituents of membrane phospholipids, and some of them are the substrates for the generation of biologically active lipids such as prostaglandin endoperoxides, primary prostaglandins, prostacyclin, thromboxanes, leukotriens hydroperoxy fatty acids, and phosphatidic acid [164,178,262] (Fig. 1).

PUFAs of Biological Interest

PUFAs are olefins. Their chain contains 18 to 24 carbon atoms and one to six nonconjugated double bonds, ending with a carboxylic group. Biologically essential PUFAs are of the "all-cis" configuration. The most important group of PUFAs derives from linoleic acid ($18:2\omega6$). This family contains dihomo-γ-linolenic ($20:3\omega6$, DHLA) and arachidonic ($20:4\omega6$, AA) acids—the direct precursors for monoenoic and dienoic prostaglandin endoperoxides (PGG_1 and PGG_2). By elongation and desaturation of α-linolenic acid ($18:3\omega3$), there arises 5,8,11,13,17-eicosapentaenoic

From the Department of Pharmacology, Copernicus Academy of Medicine in Cracow, Cracow, Poland.

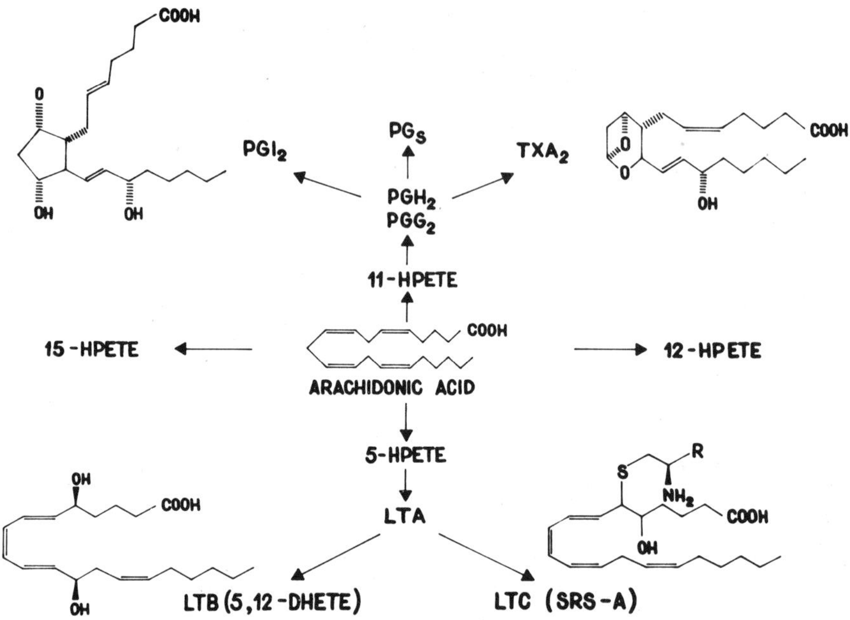

FIGURE 1. Oxidative metabolism of arachidonic acid: HPETE, hydroperoxy eicosate-tranoic acids: PGG$_2$ and PGH$_2$, prostaglandin endoperoxides: PGs, primary prostaglandins: PGI$_2$, prostacyclin; TXA$_2$, thromboxane A$_2$, LTA, leukotrien A: LTB, leukotrien B (5,12-dixydroxy eicosatetranoic acid): LTC, leukotrien C (a slow reacting substance).

acid (20:5ω3, EPA), the precursor for a trienoic prostaglandin endope-roxide (PGG$_3$). The third family of PUFAs is headed by oleic acid (18:1ω9). The family members have no appreciable biological activity. The molar ratio of linoleic, oleic, and arachidonic acids in the phospholipids of freshly isolated platelet membranes is approximately 1:3.5:7 [58]; eico-sapentaenoic acid is practically absent in the plasma phospholipids of Europeans [66].

Arachidonic Acid and Platelets

In platelet-rich plasma (PRP) AA promotes platelet aggregation [271, 311], most likely via its cyclooxygenation to prostaglandin endoperoxides [117,220,341] and/or because of the isomerization of these substances to thromboxane A$_2$ [120]. The participation of the products of AA lipoxy-genation in the aggregatory response to AA cannot be excluded [178, 313]. In an artificial medium AA causes lysis of human platelets [305], and therefore washed platelets should be protected by the addition of albumin when aggregated with AA. The susceptibility of PRP to the proaggregatory action of AA is species dependent. The threshold effec-tive concentrations of AA are as follows: in human, PRP 200–600 μM

[292,293], in cat and rabbit, PRP 40–100 μM [177], dog PRP seems to be resistant to the proaggregatory action of AA [44], at least in the majority of animals [146]. In diabetic and atherosclerotic [293] patients, the sensitivity of platelets to the proaggregatory action of AA is increased.

In vivo AA has also a prothrombotic action. An intravenous injection of AA (1.4 mg/kg) in rabbits causes sudden death, as the result of obturation of their pulmonary circulation with platelet clumps [272]. Aspirin but not heparin offers the protection against AA-induced thrombosis in rabbits. Four healthy, brave volunteers ingested ethyl arachidonate at a dose of 6 g daily for a period of 2–3 weeks. They survived, but the aggregability of their platelets was essentially increased [263].

PUFAs and Platelets

The remaining PUFAs at millimolar concentrations have weak antiaggregatory properties in vitro (Fig. 2). This action is the most evident when prostaglandin endoperoxides or their synthetic analogues are used as proaggregatory agents. DHLA [342] and EPA [65,66,115] (Fig. 2) have a stronger antiaggregatory activity in vitro than other PUFAs. Since both are substrates for cyclooxygenase, it may be suspected that antiaggregatory metabolites (e.g. PGE_1 or PGD_3) are generated in PRP [271]. In the case of EPA this possibility was excluded [115] (Fig. 2). Either EPA prevents platelet aggregation by competing with AA for cyclooxygenase,

FIGURE 2. Inhibition by unsaturated fatty acid (FAs) of aggregation of human PRP induced by U46619 (11,9-epoxymethano analogue of PGH_2): γ-linolenic acid (18:3 ω 3), linoleic acid (18:2 ω 6). α-linolenic acid (18:3 ω 6), oleic acid (18:1 ω 9), eicosapentaenoic acid (20:5 ω 3), and arachidonic acid (20:4 ω 6). When 20:4 ω 6 was used, PRP was pretreated with aspirin (0.5 mM) for 5 minutes, to prevent the proaggregating action of 20:4 ω 6. FAs were preincubated with PRP at 37°C for 10 minutes before U46619 was added. [After Gryglewski et al. [115].]

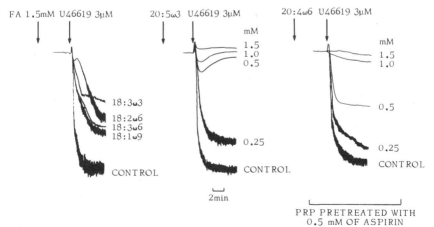

thus hindering PGG$_2$ formation [212], or EPA acts directly to inhibit platelet aggregation by blocking receptors for proaggregatory metabolites of AA [115]. There is also a third possibility. Labeled AA or EPA is readily and similarly incorporated in vitro into platelet phospholipids and can be released again by activation of phospholipase A$_2$ with stimuli such as thrombin. The slow replacement of AA by EPA in platelet phospholipids could contribute to its antiaggregatory effect in vitro.

The past few decades have seen innumerable studies of the in vivo effects of vegetable oils (Table 1) on atherogenesis and thrombogenesis in humans and in experimental animals, but the results have been inconclusive. A relationship between a diet high in saturated fatty acids and atherosclerosis has been demonstrated, whereas PUFAs are thought to have antiatherosclerotic and antithrombotic effects [137,217]. However, peanut oil produces atherosclerosis when fed to monkeys.

The atherogenic effect of peanut oil is similar to that of coconut oil, and both are considerably more harmful for arteries than corn oil or peanut oil from which arachidonic and behenic acids have been removed [158,346]. On the other hand, thrombosis and myocardial infarction occur in dogs fed coconut oil but not cottonseed oil [172]. Platelets of rabbits fed a butter diet are activated and generate more thromboxanes than do platelets prepared from rabbits fed corn oil [3]. The results of human epidemiological studies are difficult to assess. For example, a large multicenter study in Norway [207] aiming at a comparison of the effects of dietary vegetable oils on the incidence of coronary heart disease failed to reach a hard conclusion. Large amounts of margarine given to a healthy volunteers at a single meal [222] or in a course of 2–4 weeks [144] decreased platelet activity. These reports are of clinical importance; however pure PUFAs rather than vegetable oils should be used for a detailed study of the effects of PUFAs on platelet function in vivo. There is a considerable amount of experimental and clinical evidence that linoleic acid (18:2ω6) and DHLA (20:3ω6) may have antithrombotic properties [137,153,223,273,286,315], although the mechanism of their ben-

TABLE 1. The Fatty Acid Composition of Vegetable Oils

Vegetable oil	Fatty acids (g/100 g fat)			
	18:1 ω 9	18:2 ω 6	18:3 ω 3	Saturated
Soybean	22.8	50.8	6.8	15.1
Cottonseed	18.1	50.3	0.4	26.1
Corn	24.6	57.3	0.8	12.7
Safflower	11.9	73.3	0.5	9.5
Peanut	45.6	31.0	—	17.3
Coconut	5.7	1.8	—	86.3
Palm	37.9	9.0	0.3	47.9
Sunflower seed	21.7	66.4	0.3	10.3

Extracted from data of Weihrauch et al. [325].

eficial action is not fully elucidated. Also, more experiments are needed to prove or to disprove the antiaggregatory action of EPA (20:5ω3) in vivo [65,66,115].

In summary, linoleic acid, γ-linolenic acid, DHLA, or EPA may be found to be clinically useful in the prevention and treatment of thrombosis and atherosclerosis; however more knowledge about their mechanism of action must be accumulated. AA, and saturated and monounsaturated fatty acids, are thrombogenic in vivo [217]. Peroxidized PUFAs are inhibitors of prostacyclin synthetase [104,255] and therefore they may activate platelet aggregability in vivo. The concepts of the significance of deficiency of DHLA metabolites for development of atherosclerosis [153,286] and schizophrenia [138] remain to be tested.

PRIMARY PROSTAGLANDINS

Aggregating platelets release primary prostaglandins E_2, F_{2a} [278,279], and D_2 [281]. Monoenoic and trienoic prostaglandins are hardly detected in platelets, since DHLA constitutes only a small portion (0.6%) of fatty acids in platelet phospholipids hydrolyzates [48] and EPA is practically absent [66]. When thromboxane synthetase [120] and lipoxygenase [119,218] were discovered, it became obvious that AA metabolites formed by these two enzymatic routes dominate in platelets, and the formation of primary PGs constitutes only a narrow stream of the overall AA metabolism in platelets. Nonetheless, PGE_1, PGD_2, and PGD_3 have a potent antiaggregatory effect by stimulating platelet receptors, which are closely associated with adenylate cyclase [191]. PGE_2 has inhibitory effects on primary aggregation, and stimulatory effect on secondary aggregation, but only at high concentration [268]. $PGF_{1\alpha}$ and $PGF_{2\alpha}$ are inactive [40]. 16,16-Dimethyl PGE_2 has a strong proaggregatory action [88]. Recently, it has been proposed that PGE_1 may also induce formation of an antiaggregatory macromolecule in plasma [274].

Antiaggregating Effect of PGE_1

Kloetze [155], in 1967, first showed that PGE_1 inhibited ADP-induced aggregation of rat, pig, and human platelets. It has subsequently been found that PGE_1 inhibits aggregation by most of known proaggregatory agents [279], and this biological activity of PGE_1 is mediated through stimulation of platelet adenylate cyclase [17,91,189,299], and thus, by inhibition, platelet contractility [161] as well as inhibition of the release of arachidonic acid from phospholipids [82]. In platelets the receptor site for adenylate cyclase that is activated by PGE_1 is similar to or identical with that which is sensitive to prostacyclin (PGI_2) but distinct from that which is activated by PGD_2 [330,337]. SQ 22536 (9-tetrahydro-2-furyl)adenine), an inhibitor of adenylate cyclase in platelets, prevents the inhibitory effect of PGE_1 on platelet function [258].

PGE_2 antagonizes weakly the antiaggregatory action of PGE_1 [155].

PGE_1 inhibits ADP-induced platelet aggregation in human, dog, rat, rabbit, sheep, and horse PRP and its antiaggregatory potency (IC_{50}) in these species is in the range of 25–125 nM [337].

The physiologic relevance of the antiaggregating activity of PGE_1 is difficult to assess. Low concentrations of PGE_1 have been detected by radioimmunoassay in unextracted plasma [183]. Such amounts of PGE_1 may be higher in subjects fed a DHLA-rich diet, especially during concomitant vitamin C therapy [176]. Basal level of PGE_1 in human platelets is claimed to be higher than that of PGE_2; however during platelet activation, no change in PGE_1 concentration occurs [162]. The pitfalls of radioimmunoassay should be kept in mind.

PGE_1 was shown to stimulate de novo synthesis of phospholipids in human platelets [285] and to increase the sensitivity of adenylate cyclase to the action of adenosine [143]. Because of its vasodilator and antiaggregatory properties, PGE_1 was used for the treatment of obstructive vascular diseases [225] as well as for preservation of platelets during in vitro simulation of cardiopulmonary bypass [2].

Antiaggregating Effects of PGD_2 and PGD_3

The antiaggregatory property of PGD_2 was discovered by three independent research groups [190,216,280]. This biologic activity of PGD_2 is related to its stimulatory effect on platelet adenylate cyclase through a receptor [191] that is different from that activated by PGE_1. Compound N-0164 [sodium-p-benzyl-4-(1-oxo-2-(4-chlorobenzyl)-3-phenyl-propyl)phenyl phosphate], which is a prostaglandin antagonist [67] and a thromboxane A_2 synthetase inhibitor [68], selectively antagonizes the antiaggregatory action of PGD_2 but fails to affect the antiaggregatory action of PGE_1 [170] or PGI_2 [337]. Adenine derivatives that are adenylate cyclase inhibitors are equally effective against PGE_1, PGD_2, and PGI_2, and thus lack this kind of selectivity [258]. The distribution of the platelet "PGD_2 receptor" varies among species. Human, sheep, and horse platelets are equally sensitive to the antiaggregatory action of PGD_2. In these species PGD_2 is twice as potent as PGE_1. On the other hand, rabbit and dog platelets, respectively, are 25 and 100 times less sensitive to the antiaggregatory action of PGD_2 as compared to that of PGE_1, whereas rat platelets, being highly sensitive to PGE_1 (IC_{50} = 25 nM), are completely resistant to the antiaggregatory action of PGD_2 [337]. The occurrence of a species-specific and separate site for PGD_2 on platelets raises the question of its biologic significance. It may well be that the cyclic AMP content in platelets is controlled by two independent mechanisms. The first, a universal one, is designed for prostacyclin (PGI_2), and additionally it can be set in motion by PGE_1. The second mechanism operates in only a few species (including man), and it is triggered by PGD_2.

PGD_2 can be formed nonenzymatically from prostaglandin endoperoxides (PGG_2 and PGH_2), and this conversion is greatly enhanced by silica gel [276] and by the presence of plasma proteins [121]. Whittle et al. [337] demonstrated that in species in which PGD_2 had little antiaggregatory activity, the conversion by plasma protein of PGH_2 to PGD_2 was low; however, a high conversion rate of an endoperoxide to PGD_2 occurred in plasma of species in which platelet receptors were highly susceptible to stimulation by PGD_2. In some species, the authors speculate, PGD_2 deriving from endoperoxides released by platelets into the plasma may play a role as an endogenous antiaggregatory factor along with prostacyclin (PGI_2), which is generated by the vascular walls [104,193].

Indeed, PGD_2 has been detected in human PRP aggregated by thrombin, collagen, epinephrine [224], and PGH_2 [276,281]. The amounts of PGD_2 generated are small but sufficient to oppose, at least partially, the action of proaggregatory agents. We observed [115] that PRP from several human donors was resistant to the proaggregatory action of PGH_2. An explanation could be that in these particular specimens of PRP an endoperoxide was more avidly converted by plasma to PGD_2 than by platelets to thromboxane A_2. It has been also reported [5] that frozenthawed platelets synthesize PGD_2 at a rate equal to that for synthesis of thromboxane B_2. The existence of platelet intracellular PGH_2/PGD_2 isomerase was postulated, similar to that shown in other cells and tissues [1,220].

As mentioned above, not all samples of human PRP are irreversibly aggregated by PGH_2, but in those that are, PGH_3 induces an immediate and always fully reversible aggregation [115]. After a 4-minute incubation of nonaggregating doses of PGH_2 or PGH_3 (100–300 nM) with PRP, stable antiaggregatory compounds are generated. The amount of this antiaggregatory activity obtained from PGH_3 is 10 times higher than that obtained from PGH_2. The antiaggregating compounds were identified by mass spectrometry as PGD_2 and PGD_3, respectively [115]. It may well be that the antiaggregatory potency of PGD_3 is higher than that of PGD_2 [212]. If, however, the antiaggregating potency of PGD_3 is equal to that of PGD_2 (Udo Axen, personal communication), an alternative explanation could be offered [115,276]. We attribute the apparent difference in antiaggregatory potency between PGD_2 and PGD_3 generated in PRP from PGH_2 and PGH_3 to the concurrent production of PGE_2 and PGE_3. PGE_2 prevents the antiaggregatory action of PGD_2, whereas PGE_3 does not affect the activity of PGD_3 [115].

PGD_2 was considered for many years to be a curiosity in the prostaglandin family, a less important isomer of PGE_2, with little biological activity. However the studies of past 5 years have shown that PGD_2 is the most active primary prostaglandin in the circulatory system. Its potent antiaggregatory activity is mediated through platelet receptors different from those activated by PGE_1 and PGI_2. This peculiarity may be of clinical importance. Cooper et al. [49] have shown that activation of platelet adenylate cyclase by PGD_2 in patients with myeloproliferative disorders was less effective than in normal controls, whereas the responsiveness of platelets of those patients to PGE_1 and PGI_2 was not disturbed. The authors conclude that the observed platelet abnormal response to PGD_2 represents an intrinsic membrane abnormality characteristic of all the myeloproliferative disorders in man.

THROMBOXANES AND PROSTAGLANDIN ENDOPEROXIDES

The mechanisms that govern shape change, aggregation, and the release reaction of platelets are not fully understood and frequently are the subject of controversy. It appears that the natural inducers of aggregation, such as thrombin or collagen, release from platelets either ADP or prostaglandin endoperoxides or both, or some still unknown factors that change the function of platelets. Although the effects of ADP and prostaglandin endoperoxides on platelets are interrelated exogenous ADP will aggregate platelets after pretreatment of PRP with aspirin, therefore in absence of prostaglandin endoperoxides, whereas AA will cause aggregation in the absence of releasable ADP [124]. On the other hand, thrombin-induced aggregation will proceed in the absence of either endogenous ADP or prostaglandin endoperoxides. This fact lead Smith et al. [284], Vargaftig [313], and Chinard et al. [45] to postulate the existence of the "third intraplatelet route," which may be used during thrombin-induced aggregation.

At the time of the first demonstration that AA is a proaggregating agent in PRP [278,311,341], it was obvious that none of primary prostaglandin could be responsible for platelet aggregation. It was claimed from the very beginning that highly unstable metabolites of AA are the true inducers of platelet aggregation [311,341]. Because these metabolites were characterized by their contractile action on a strip of rabbit aorta, they used to be known as "rabbit aorta contracting substances" (RCSs) or "labile aggregation-stimulating substances" (LASSs) [341]. Presently we know that these acronyms denominated a mixture composed of thromboxane A_2 and prostaglandin endoperoxides.

Discovery of Rabbit Aorta Contracting Substances, Prostaglandin Endoperoxides, and Thromboxane A_2

Using the bioassay cascade of superfused detector-organs invented by Vane [308], in 1969 Piper and Vane [236] detected the release from immunologically triggered perfused lungs of sensitized guinea pigs of a substance that was highly unstable and contracted a strip of rabbit aorta. The authors called this substance RCS. The release of RCS from lungs was blocked by prostaglandin biosynthesis inhibitors (e.g. aspirin). RCS may be released from lungs by a number of stimuli, including AA, and it is also generated by slices of spleen [101] and by blood platelets [311].

In 1972 Gryglewski and Vane [102] suggested that RCS generated by splenic microsomes could be an unstable intermediate in the biosynthesis of prostaglandins, the existence of which had been postulated by Samuelsson [259] and by Nugteren et al. [219].

In 1973 the forecast existence of an unstable metabolite between AA and primary prostaglandins was successfully demonstrated by Hamberg and Samuelsson [117] and by Nugteren and Hazelhof [220]. It turned out that there are two unstable metabolites named (because of their chemical structure) prostaglandin endoperoxides. 15-Hydroperoxy (PGG_2) and 15-hydroxy (PGH_2) endoperoxides have been isolated as the immediate products of the cyclooxygenation of AA by microsomal preparations. The corresponding endoperoxides from the enzymatic conversion of DHLA (PGG_1 and PGH_1) and of EPA (PGH_3) [208,212,276] have also been isolated.

All the prostaglandin endoperoxides contract rabbit aortic strip, therefore Nugteren and Hazelhof [220] equated the endoperoxides (PGG_2 and PGH_2) with the RCS of Piper and Vane [236]. However, more detailed studies revealed differences between the RCS from lungs and the endoperoxides from seminal vesicle microsomes [118]. The former has a half-life of less than 2 minutes whereas the half-lives of endoperoxides are about 5 minutes. This and other discrepancies induced Samuelsson's group to look among the arachidonic acid metabolites for an additional unstable substance that would match more closely the properties of RCS from lungs [236], from spleen [101], or from platelets [311]. This research led to the discovery of thromboxane A_2.

When prostaglandin endoperoxides (PGG_2 or PGH_2) are allowed to decompose spontaneously in a buffer, PGD_2, PGE_2, $PGF_{2\alpha}$, malondialdehyde (MDA), and the C17 hydroxy acid (HHT, 12-L-hydroxy-5,8,10-heptadecatrienoic acid) are formed. When prostaglandin endoperoxides are incubated with washed platelets, however, along with the products above a new unstable product with nonprostaglandin structure is formed. This product was named by the discoverers [120,122] thromboxane A_2 (TXA_2). TXA_2 has a half-life of 30 seconds at 37°C and is spontaneously decomposed to a stable and biologically inactive thromboxane B_2 (TXB_2), which is metabolized to a number of products that are excreted in urine [141].

TXA_2 is more than 50 times more potent in contracting rabbit aortic strip than is PGG_2 [209]. Thus the activity of RCS from lungs, platelet, or spleen is mainly due to TXA_2 and only partially due to PGG_2 or PGH_2, although RCS from other biological sources may be entirely composed of the prostaglandin endoperoxides [102]. TXA_2 synthetase (an enzyme that converts PGH_2 to TXA_2) has been found in horse and human platelet microsomes [209,288] and has been separated from the cyclooxygenase component [296,297].

TXA_2, although highly unstable, seems to be an important mediator in the interaction between blood platelets and the vascular wall. Its powerful vasoconstrictor action is combined with proaggregatory properties [120,209].

Release of Arachidonic Acid During Platelet Aggregation

Platelets aggregate in the presence of free AA [278,311,341]; however the concentration of free AA in PRP is usually too low [179] to initiate spontaneous aggregation. Delayed spontaneous aggregation of PRP occurs only in some atherosclerotic patients and at the same time thresholds proaggregatory concentrations of AA in PRP of those patients are very low [292,293]. Bills et al. [21–23] and Schoene and Lacono [265] showed that aggregating agents trigger the release of AA from the platelet phosphatide fraction. Blackwell et al. [24] demonstrated that only trace amounts of free AA are found in platelets, and that the amounts present as neutral lipid esters are also extremely low. Although 16–23 ng of AA is found per 10^6 platelets, 97% of this is bound in the platelet phosphatide fraction. Similar patterns of AA distribution in platelets were reported earlier by other authors [22,179]. Following aggregation of platelets with collagen or thrombin, there is a consistent fall (up to 80%) in the phospholipid AA content, mainly from phosphatidylethanolamine in rabbit platelets [24], and from phosphatidylcholine [23,248] and phosphatidylinositol in human platelets [22]. Interestingly, AA is not liberated by aggregating agents from platelet phosphatidylserine [24]. Simultaneously there appear the products of cycloxygenation (TXB$_2$ and PGs) and lipoxygenation (HETE) of AA [24]. Clearly, the released AA is partially used for the generation of proaggregatory endoperoxides and TXA$_2$. This "mobilization" of the substrate, which occurs during contact of platelets with collagen or thrombin, is blocked by a phospholipase A$_2$ inhibitor, mepacrine, but not by a cyclooxygenase inhibitor, indomethacin. On the other hand, indomethacin and mepacrine block the generation of proaggregatory products of AA cyclooxygenation [24]. The authors conclude that aggregating agents, by activating phospholipase A$_2$, release free AA and thus initiate its enzymic transformation to proaggregatory endoperoxides and TXA$_2$. In this process the two rate-limiting enzymatic steps, phospholipase A$_2$ and cyclooxygenase, have been shown to be targets for different types of antiaggregatory drug.

This clear picture of AA transformation in aggregating platelets is not the complete one. It has been shown that when washed platelets prelabled with [1-^{14}C] AA are aggregated with thrombin, the radioactivity deriving from the released AA is partially incorporated into neutral lipids and phosphatidic acid [164,165] or into the portion of phosphatidylethanolamine that is in plasmalogen form [246,254]. At present it is difficult to evaluate the significance of the "other route" of metabolism of AA for platelet aggregability. Vargaftig [313] has suggested that nonprostaglandin, nonthromboxane lipids mediate the carrageenan-induced and thrombin-induced aggregation of rabbit platelets. It may well be that these products are members of the recently discovered family of leukotriens [262] or phosphatidic acid [84,164], or simply lipoperoxides or yet unknown metabolites of AA [313].

Platelet phospholipase A$_2$ has an absolute requirement for Ca^{2+}, has optimum activity at pH 9.5, and is possible located on the inner layer of the platelet membrane [58]. Thrombin stimulates more release of AA in intact platelets than in membrane preparations. This might indicate the participation of intracellular stores of Ca^{2+} in activation of phospholipase A_2 by thrombin [233,247,248]. Indeed, platelet phospholipase A_2 activity is initiated by ionophore A23187 even in the absence of external calcium, indicating that the Ca^{2+} requirement for phospholipase A_2 activation can be satisfied by mobilization of Ca^{2+} from the intracellular stores [234,247]. The ionophore-induced activation of phospholipase A_2 requires neither cofactors nor intact platelet energy metabolism. It is also independent of the release reaction. In contrast to ionophore, thrombin activation of the enzyme requires metabolic ATP [247]. Nonetheless, in both instances the availability of intracellular Ca^{2+} through activation of phospholipase A_2 governs the generation of prostaglandin endoperoxides, TXA_2, and other AA-derived products with proaggregatory properties. One of those is a platelet-activating factor (PAF) recently described by Chignard et al. [45]. The thrombin- or collagen-activated protease has been also proposed to be involved in the activation of platelet phospholipase A_2 [13,70].

Endoperoxides and Platelet Aggregation

Blood platelets contain a fatty acid cyclooxygenase that transforms AA into PGG_2 [117,119,220].

DHLA is a somewhat worse substrate for platelet cyclooxygenase than AA [333], and EPA is hardly converted to PGH_3 at all [276]. Little is known about enzymatic reduction of PGG_2 to PGH_2 in platelets, but this conversion has been claimed to be crucial in an inflammatory processes [159]. When added to PRP, PGH_2 forms a stable 12-L-hydroxy-5,8,10-heptadecatrienoic acid (HHT) with a release of malondialdehyde (MDA) and a labile thromboxane A_2 [242]. In addition, platelets appear to possess a PGH_2/PGE_2 isomerase activity that is manifested when TXA_2 synthetase is inhibited [241]. A role for 15-hydroxy-PG dehydrogenase in regulation of platelet aggregability has been also proposed [322]. Another route of biochemical transformation of AA in platelets leads to 12-L-hydroperoxy-5,8,10,14-eicosatetranoic acid (HPETE) followed by reduction to HETE [119,218]. Among these products of AA metabolism, only PGH_2 PGG_2, and TXA_2 were shown to aggregate platelets, although the importance of a lipoxygenase pathway for irreversible aggregation induced by PGH_2 was claimed.

When PGH_2 (1–2 μM) is added to human PRP, aggregation occurs and TXA_2 is formed [72]. However, some specimens of human PRP do not aggregate to PGH_2 at a concentration as high as 16 μM [115]. The most plausible explanation for this occasional failure of PGH_2 to aggregate PRP is that in some of PRP specimens PGH_2 is converted more avidly to PGD_2 than to TXA_2. The stimulatory effect of plasma proteins on the conversion of an endoperoxide to an antiaggregatory prostaglandin is even better seen in the case of PGH_3. PGH_3 is a weak inducer of platelet aggregation owing to its rapid conversion into PGD_3 in human PRP, although TXA_3 is proaggregatory [115] and a vasoconstrictor [209]. On the other hand, PGH_1 neither induces aggregation nor forms vasoactive TXA_1 [240].

The proaggregating properties of PGH_2 are mimicked by a number of synthetic stable analogues of PGH_2 that possess 9,11-epoxymethano or azo bridges and therefore cannot be isomerized to prostaglandins or thromboxanes [50,174]. Some synthetic analogues of PGE_2 or $PGF_{2\alpha}$ can induce aggregation of human blood platelets [88], although PGE_2 and $PGF_{2\alpha}$ themselves are inactive [40]. All these prostaglandins trigger platelet aggregation at the same receptor site and release 5-hydroxytryptamine from platelet-dense bodies but do not release lysosomal hydrolases from platelet α-granules [171]. Holmsen [133] considers the generation and action of prostaglandin endoperoxides in platelets to be a part of a positive feedback loop in the propagation of platelet response during the "basic platelet reaction." It has been claimed also that PGH_2 (or TXA_2) directly triggers dense-body granule secretion and that the released ADP subsequently causes shape change and platelet aggregation [260,261] or that PGH_2 and PGG_2 release calcium ions from the membrane vesicles to the cytoplasm [83]. A part of the proaggregatory activity of endoperoxides also might be due to the release of endogenous AA by exogenous PGG_2 [256]. This fraction of proaggregatory activity of endoperoxides is sensitive to inhibition by indomethacin. PGG_2 may produce reversible platelet aggregation without secretion or irreversible platelet aggregation with secretion of platelet constituents, depending on the concentration of an endoperoxide used for aggregation [256,282]. The cAMP-lowering effect of PGH_2 in PRP is independent of the platelet release reaction [94]. The action of endoperoxides on platelets is complex, and agreement has not been reached on the most important issue: namely, is the proaggregatory action of endoperoxides mediated by TXA_2?

Thromboxane A_2 and Platelet Aggregation

There is no doubt that platelets possess a very efficient enzymatic system—thromboxane synthetase—that converts prostaglandin endoperoxides into thromboxane A_2 [209]. Apart from platelets, leukocytes [35], macrophages [201,324], and lung fibroblasts [135] also generate TXA_2. The enzyme is located in the microsomal fraction of platelet homogenates, and unlike cyclooxygenase it does not require heme or phenolic cofactors for optimal activity [296]. Thromboxane synthetase is insensitive to typical cyclooxygenase inhibitors, but it is effectively inhibited by the synthetic substrate analogues [33,73,90,92,288]. When human or animal PRP is aggregated by AA, considerable amounts of vasoconstrictor material are generated [177,293,311,341]. Its half-life, its biologic properties, and its ability to cause spontaneous conversion to TXB_2 clearly indicate that this material is identical to the substance that was named TXA_2 [120,260,261]. The peak concentration of TXA_2 in cat PRP aggregated with AA may reach a value as high as 3000 ng/ml [177].

Collagen-induced aggregation is associated with the generation of TXA_2 in PRP at a maximal concentration of 200–400 ng/ml. Even during ADP-induced aggregation, a sharp peak of TXA_2 (up to 100 ng/ml) appears at the beginning of the second wave of aggregation [177]. Also the second wave of serotonin-induced aggregation is associated with the production of TXB_2 [187]. Thrombin-induced aggregation is accompanied by generation of thromboxanes; however there exist distinct species differences. Human and dog platelets produce large amounts, horse platelets medium amounts, mink, pig, and cow platelets low amounts, and cat platelets hardly a trace of thromboxanes in response to thrombin [177,186]. In humans, the plasma level of TXB_2 is 0.08–0.32 ng/ml, as estimated by radioimmunoassay, but during cardiopulmonary bypass it rises to 0.5–2.0 ng/ml [53]. These last levels imply sufficient in vivo TXA_2 production to cause platelet activation and myocardial ischemia from coronary artery occlusion. In patients who survive myocardial infarction, platelets generate excessive amounts of TXA_2 [292].

There is common agreement that the products of AA cyclooxygenation in platelets play a role in their aggregatory response to AA as well as to other proaggregatory agents [133]. However, the functional role of TXA_2 versus PGG_2 and PGH_2 in platelet aggregation is a subject of controversy. According to Needleman et al. [208,211] and Raz et al. [240, 242], the conversion of PGG_2 or PGH_2 to TXA_2 is not a necessary step for AA-induced aggregation. Endoperoxides themselves are considered to possess intrinsic proaggregatory properties, whereas their transformation into TXA_2 seems to be important only for the amplification of their vasoconstrictor activity. This concept designates TXA_2 to a platelet-derived vasoconstrictor that may be responsible for acute ischemia during intravascular platelet aggregation [55,69,202,264]. The foregoing conclusions are based mainly on the comparative study of proaggregatory and vasoconstrictor properties of endoperoxides and thromboxanes deriving from DHLA, AA, and EPA, as well as the finding that in AA-induced platelet aggregation, imidazole inhibits TXA_2 formation with no apparent effect on aggregation. The release of Ca^{2+} from platelet membrane vesicles by PGH_2 or PGG_2 is also not influenced by imidazole [83]. In contrast, Gorman et al. [89,90,92] and Fitzpatrick and Gorman [72] have found that PRP transforms exogenous PGH_2 into TXA_2 immediately before the initiation of irreversible aggregation. The thromboxane synthetase inhibitor, 9,11-azaprosta-5,13-dienoic acid, blocks platelet aggregation induced by PGH_2, as well as the cAMP-lowering activity of PGH_2. These data indicate to the authors cited that to induce platelet aggregation or to lower cAMP in platelets, PGH_2 must be converted into TXA_2.

Thromboxane A_2, Endoperoxides, Calcium Ions, and Cyclic-AMP in Platelets

Evidence from many laboratories seems to indicate that an important intracellular messenger in the regulation of platelet function is the calcium ion (Ca^{2+}) [124]. PGG_2 and PGH_2 release Ca^{2+} from the platelet membrane vesicles [83]. An increase in its concentration in the cytosol evokes shape change, aggregation, and the release reaction: conversely, lowering of Ca^{2+} in the cytosol preserves the integrity of the platelets. This effect of Ca^{2+} on the platelet function is accomplished in two ways— directly via activation of the contractile machinery of the platelets [124], and by indirect influence on AA metabolism in platelets [82,164,192]. In turn, prostaglandin endoperoxides and cAMP may regulate intracellular compartmentization of Ca^{2+} [334]. As already mentioned, PGI_2, PGD_2, and PGE_1 increase levels of cAMP in platelets and inhibit aggregation. A similar antiaggregatory effect has been reported for inhibitors of di-butyryl -cAMP and cAMP phosphodiesterase [312]. On the other hand, a pharmacologic inhibition of platelet adenylate cyclase is followed by enhancement of platelet activity [257]. The first concept was that cAMP inhibits selectively the formation of RCS but not the formation of pros-tagladins in platelets [312]. The next concept was that cAMP inhibits cyclooxygenase and therefore prevents formation of endoperoxides and TXA_2 in platelets [175]. It is now assumed that cAMP inhibits membrane phospholipase in platelets and therefore diminishes the availability of AA for cyclooxygenase [82,164,192]. It should be reminded that phos-pholipase A_2 is activated by Ca^{2+} [58], and cAMP sequestrates Ca^{2+} the internal compartments of platelets [334].

The most interesting hypothesis on the mechanism of proaggregatory action of the endoperoxides and TXA_2 was recently presented by Gorman et al. [89,93,94]. As already mentioned, these authors are convinced that the endoperoxides must be converted to TXA_2 to induce aggregation or to lower cAMP in platelets. The proposed mechanism of the aggregating section of TXA_2 is as follows. TXA_2 mobilizes Ca^{2+} within the platelet, possibly from the dense tubular system [85,334]. Indeed, TXA_2 has been proposed to act as an ionophore and selectively transport Ca^{2+} [335]. Mobilized Ca^{2+} inhibits adenylate cyclase and brings about a fall in cAMP. Since cAMP enhances Ca^{2+} sequestration and therefore inhibits phospholipase A_2 activity [82,164,165,192], the TXA_2-induced fall in the cytoplasmic concentration of this nucleotide will cause a further rise in Ca^{2+} and AA inside the platelet, thus making it prone to aggregatory response. TXA_2-induced aggregation may occur in the absence of the platelet release reaction [43,94]. However, at a high level of stimulation, the TXA_2 generated via Ca^{2+} may initiate ADP release from dense-body granules. As noted before, the cAMP-lowering activity of TXA_2 can be divorced from the platelet release reaction. If this phenomenon occurs, however, released ADP may perturb the platelet membrane, enhance Ca^{2+} mobilization, and finally amplify the initial aggregatory stimulus. Gorman et al. [94] have presented only indirect evidence that Ca^{2+} ac-tually mediates the cAMP-lowering activity of TXA_2. From their exper-iments, however, it is clear that ADP is not a primary inhibitor of aden-ylate cyclase in human platelets aggregated by TXA_2 and that the direct inhibition of adenylate cyclase by TXA_2 is independent of the release of ADP by TXA_2 from platelets. In our concern with the mechanism of proaggregatory action of the PGH_2 -TXA_2 system, we should not over-look the alternative routes that lead to a rise in cytoplasmic Ca^{2+}. One of those routes may start at the moment of formation of phosphatidic acid [165].

By an interaction with platelet membrane, thrombin collagen or ADP may initiate the breakdown of d-phosphatidyl-inositol to 1.2-diacylglycerol, which is then converted to phosphatidic acid. This is a releaser of Ca^{2+} from platelet intracellular stores [84]. Phosphatidic acid is also the substrate phospholipase A_2, and the released AA may be converted to PGH_2 and TXA_2.

PROSTACYCLIN

Among the metabolites of arachidonic acid, PGG_2, PGH_2, and TXA_2 have been established as the endogenous stimulators of platelet aggregation, and their action seems to be mediated by the release of Ca^{2+} from the dense tubular system and by the lowering of cAMP in platelets. Although PGE_1 and PGD_2 inhibit platelet aggregation, sequestrate Ca^{2+}, and increase cAMP in platelets (see above, "Primary Prostaglandins") the physiologic significance of these findings is not clear, since these antiaggregatory prostaglandins are not generated in sufficient quantities in vivo to counterbalance the effects of TXA_2. Prostacyclin (PGI_2) is a much more potent antiaggregatory agent than either PGE_1 or PGD_2, and it is generated in the right place and in the right amounts to be important in maintaining homeostasis in the circulation.

Biosynthesis, Metabolism, and Distribution of Prostacyclin

In 1976, in collaboration with Bunting, Moncada, and Vane [34,104, 193,194], we discovered that the endoperoxides PGG_2 and PGH_2 are transformed by aortic microsomes to an unstable substance with antiaggregatory and vasodilator properties. This factor was called PGX and later, when it was synthesized, its name was changed to prostacyclin (PGI_2) [148]. Prostacyclin is spontaneously broken down to 6-keto-prostaglandin $F_{1\alpha}$ (6-keto-$PGF_{1\alpha}$). The velocity of this decomposition is pH and temperature dependent. In the extravasated blood at 37°C the half-life of prostacyclin is 3 minutes [63]. It has been reported that in whole blood prostacyclin is trapped by erythrocytes and platelets, while in plasma prostacyclin activity is relatively stable (half-life > 30 minutes) [339]. In a buffer of pH 7.4 at 37°C, prostacyclin decomposes in a couple of minutes, but in a buffer of 10.5 at 4°C prostacyclin does not lose biologic activity for a least 3 days. The stable metabolite of prostacyclin (6-keto-$PGF_{1\alpha}$) was originally isolated and characterized by Pace-Asciak [226,229].

In most biologic systems 6-keto-$PGF_{1\alpha}$ is relatively inactive. Although chemically stable, 6-keto-$PGF_{1\alpha}$ is metabolized in vivo. It has been claimed [227] that the main pathway of metabolism of 6-keto-$PGF_{1\alpha}$ in rats is via β- and ω-oxidation, not via the prostaglandin 15-hydroxy dehydrogenase. This assumption has recently been questioned [291]. Partially purified rhesus monkey lung prostaglandin 15-hydroxy dehydrogenase catalyzes oxidation of 6-keto-PGF$_{1\alpha}$ and prostacyclin to 6,15-diketo-PGF$_{1\alpha}$. Prostacyclin is oxidized four to six times faster than 6-keto-PGF$_{1\alpha}$, suggesting that the metabolism of prostacyclin probably proceeds through a bicyclic 15-keto intermediate before chemically decomposing to the final stable product, 6,15-diketo-PGF$_{1\alpha}$ [185]. Prostacyclin is extensively metabolized when infused or injected into rats, and at least seven metabolites of PGI$_2$ appear in the urine. These include the products of β- and ω-oxidation as well as the products of dehydrogenation at the 15 position and reduction at 13,14 double bond [289,290].

The data above indicate that the metabolism of prostacyclin in vivo may be different from that of 6-keto-PGF$_{1\alpha}$ [291]. Species differences in metabolizing prostacyclin are highly probable. In dogs about 50% of prostacyclin infused into the aorta is inactivated in one complete circulation [63]. Prostacyclin is mainly removed by liver and in peripheral circulation. In vitro rat liver endothelial cells have been reported to synthesize prostacyclin, and this synthesis is inhibited by PGE$_2$ [304]. Prostacyclin escapes inactivation by the lungs. On the contrary, the lungs seem to secrete prostacyclin continuously into the arterial blood [107,110,111,199] (Fig. 3), although the physiologic concentration of PGI$_2$ in blood (100–200 pg/ml) [111] is probably too low to affect platelet cAMP and platelet aggregability [125] or to lower blood pressure [283]. This subthreshold concentration of circulating prostacyclin may, however, amplify the antiaggregating action of endothelial prostacyclin in the arteries. The generation of prostacyclin by the lung is enhanced by hyperventilation [107], pulmonary emboli, and angiotensin II [116].

Another organ that may be a source of circulating prostacyclin is the kidney. Prostacyclin is the major metabolite of AA or PGG$_2$ in renal cortex [338], and it may be also metabolized there [228]. A more recent

FIGURE 3. Differences in concentration of an antiaggregating substance between aortic (A) and mixed venous (V) blood of an anesthetized cat. Heparinized A and V blood superfused in two parallel collagen strips [112]. Note the slower rise in weight of the strip bathed in A blood as compared to that bathed in V blood. Also a disaggregating potency of exogenous prostacyclin (PGI$_2$, 5 ng/ml) was higher on the aortic site. This is evidence [107,110,111] in favor of the concept that prostacyclin is a circulating hormone released by the lungs.

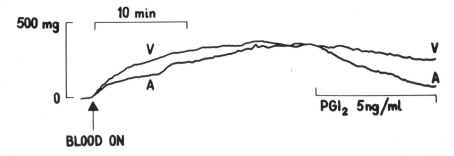

study revealed that renal medulla also is capable of synthesizing prostacyclin, and this synthesis is stimulated by angiotensin II [270]. In vivo
both angiotensin II [267] and bradykinin [203] stimulate dog kidneys to
release substantial amounts of prostacyclin into circulation. The stimulated release of prostacyclin either from the lungs [107,116] or from the
kidneys [267] is of so great an order of magnitude that the aggregability
of the circulating platelets is severely depressed.

There is no doubt that prostacyclin is the major metabolite of AA in
most of the vascular tissues that have been investigated [27,104,197,
238,302,317] and that the intensity of its biosynthesis is highest in the
endothelial layer [36,128,197], although subendothelial layers also generate substantial amounts of prostacyclin [19,136,306]. Interestingly, in
cultured endothelial cells [169,193,328,329] and in aortic slices [154] the
generation of prostacyclin is stimulated by the same factors that enhance
the release of TXA_2 from platelets, namely, by thrombin, trypsin, and
the ionophore A23187, but it is inhibited by β-thromboglobulin [134].
Another product of the platelet release reaction, factor 4, does not influence the generation of prostacyclin by arterial endothelial cells. In
arteries, prostacyclin synthetase (the enzyme that converts PGH_2 to PGI_2)
seems to be far more efficient than cyclooxygenase. We originally suggested that platelets can "feed" arterial walls with the endoperoxides
and thus accelerate the intramural formation of prostacyclin [104,194].
This mechanism of in vitro platelet-endothelium interaction was confirmed in one laboratory [298], and denied in another [136].

In addition, there have been reports of the in vitro generation of
prostacyclin by perfused rabbit heart [54,56,62,140], rabbit pericardium,
pleura, and peritoneum [129], rat, guinea pig, and sheep myometrium,
decidua, and placenta [149,205,340], bovine corpora lutea [321], rat stomach microsomes [104,226,229] and gastric mucosa [336], bovine [321] and
ram [41,51] seminal vesicle microsomes, and murine Lewis lung carcinoma cells [237].

In their elegant study Salmon et al. [255] confirmed that porcine aorta
microsomes contain the enzyme that converts PGH_2 to prostacyclin.
Prostacyclin synthetase displays a broad pH spectrum (pH 6.5–8.0) and
catalyzes a rapid conversion of 80% of PGH_2 to prostacyclin when incubated at 37°C. Prostacyclin is never formed spontaneously from the
endoperoxides; thus, unlike the cases of PGE_2, $PGF_{2\alpha}$, and PGD_2 there
is an absolute requirement for an enzymic reaction to take place. The
isomerases that convert the endoperoxides to PGE_2 and PGD_2 are not
detected in the arterial wall. An exception to this rule consists of isolated
cerebral microvessels that seem to convert considerable amounts of PGH_2
to PGE_2, their biosynthetic capacity is stimulated by glutathione [86].

Prostacyclin synthetase from porcine aortic microsomes is selectively
inhibited by low concentrations (IC_{50} = 1.5 μM) of 15-hydroxyarachi-
donic acid [104] Salmon et al. [25] confirmed this observation and found
that hydroperoxides of several unsaturated fatty acids as well as of their
methyl esters are potent inhibitors of the enzyme and act in a time-
dependent manner. Otherwise prostacyclin synthetase is resistant to a

vast number of enzymatic inhibitors [104], and only few drugs can influence its activity.

Vascular Action of Prostacyclin

Prostacyclin relaxes superfused strips of rabbit mesenteric and coeliac arteries [34], human or baboon basilar, middle cerebral, vertebral, and common carotid arteries [27], and bovine coronary artery [62]. Aortic strips and vein strips are resistant to this action of prostacyclin. In rats and rabbits intravenous prostacyclin causes systemic hypotension and is two to eight times more potent as a vasodepressor agent that PGE_2 and 125–250 times more potent than 6-keto-$PGF_{1\alpha}$ [14]. In rats and rabbits vasodepressor responses induced by prostacyclin are similar in magnitude after either intravenous or intraaortic administration, indicating that prostacyclin does not lose its biologic activity on passage through the lungs. In dogs prostacyclin causes a dose-dependent decrease in systemic and pulmonary arterial blood pressure. Since left ventricular end-diastolic, left atrial, and right atrial pressures as well as cardiac output are not essentially affected by prostacyclin, it may be concluded that prostacyclin decreases vascular resistance both in the pulmonary and in the systemic circulations [150]. Prostacyclin is the only known metabolite of arachidonic acid that dilatates pulmonary circulation.

When prostacyclin is infused intravenously in man at doses of 5–20 ng/kg/min, there is a moderate fall in diastolic blood pressure, erythema appears in the regions of the face, palms, and feet, and the skin temperature of these regions rises by 0.5–1.5°C [114,294]. An intraarterial infusion of prostacyclin (5–10 ng/kg/min) into the femoral artery results in profound redness of the infused limb, but no edema appears [295]. These vascular effects of prostacyclin, in addition to its antiaggregatory properties and cytoprotective action, might be of value for preserving myocardial tissue in acute myocardial ischemia [166].

Prostacyclin and Platelet Aggregation

The first biological activity of prostacyclin to be discovered was inhibition of platelet aggregation [104,193]. Platelets from humans and several animal species have uniformly high sensitivity to the antiaggregatory action of prostacyclin against ADP-induced aggregation (IC_{50} = 0.5–3.7 ng/ml) [337]. Prostacyclin also inhibits aggregation induced by AA, PGH_2, PGG_2, TXA_2, synthetic analogues of PGH_2, collagen, thrombin, and a-drenaline. In human PRP antiaggregatory activity of prostacyclin is 20 times greater than that of PGD_2, 40 times greater than that of PGE_2 [337], and 1000 greater than that of adenosine [26]. Therefore, prostacyclin is the most potent and the most universal endogenous inhibitor of platelet aggregation so far discovered. Prostacyclin has also a disaggregatory action; that is, it disperses platelet clumps in circulating blood of animals [108,109] and humans [114,294]. The disaggregatory action of prostacyclin is at least 30,000 times more potent than that of adenosine (Fig.

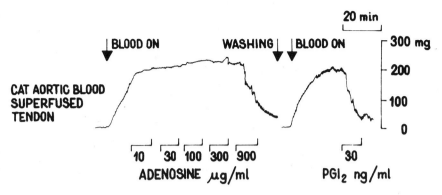

FIGURE 4. Disaggregatory action of adenosine and prostacyclin (PGI$_2$) on platelet clumps that were formed on the surface of blood-superfused collagen tendon [112]. Prostacyclin is at least 30,000 times more potent than adenosine.

4). Prostacyclin prevents thrombus formation in several animal models [4,108,109,130,307] and is successfully used in the treatment of arteriosclerosis obliterans in humans [295].

In humans intravenous prostacyclin (5–10 ng/kg/min) doubles template bleeding time [114,294]. Also in rabbits infusion of prostacyclin elongates bleeding time [307]. On the other hand, the formation of endogenous prostacyclin has little influence on template bleeding time, since in rabbits immunized against a 6-keto-PGF$_{1\alpha}$–albumin conjugate, bleeding time does not differ from that of control animals, whereas PRP from immunized animals is highly resistant to the antiaggregatory action of exogenous prostacyclin [284]. Immune injury to human platelets by drugs, bacteria, and viruses is mediated by the IgG Fc receptor. Prostacyclin prevents binding of IgG-covered cells to human platelets and protects platelets from the IgG Fc-mediated injury, being the most active protective substance so far known. Indeed, it is hoped that prostacyclin will exhibit the same action in vivo against allergic thrombocytopenia [126].

Arterial rings [34], aortic microsomes [132], and vascular endothelial cells [328], when incubated with PRP, either inhibit or reverse platelet aggregation induced by a wide variety of aggregating agents. This is due to the generation of prostacyclin by the vascular preparations in PRP. The antiaggregatory effect of natural or synthetic prostacyclin is not mediated by an interaction with "TXA$_2$ receptors" [132], rather, it is due to the stimulation of platelet adenylate cyclase by prostacyclin [91,299], followed by an accumulation of cAMP in platelets. Phosphodiesterase inhibitors enhance the antiaggregatory action of prostacyclin [108]. When added to human PRP prostacyclin is 10 times more active than PGD$_2$, 30 times more active than PGE$_1$, and 1000 times more active than 6-oxo-PGF$_{1\alpha}$ in raising cAMP [299]. An additional feature of prostacyclin-induced elevation of cAMP in platelets is its persistence for almost 3 minutes, in contrast to the effects of PGE_1 and PGD_2, which start to disappear after 30 seconds [91].

Prostacyclin is also a potent stimulator of platelet adenylate cyclase in isolated membrane preparations [89]. The molecular mechanisms by which an elevated cAMP level inhibits platelet aggregation still need to be investigated. At present, the most convincing concept is that cAMP, by sequestration of Ca^{2+} in intracellular compartments [8,89,334], inhibits phospholipase A_2 [164,192] and subsequently hinders the generation of proaggregatory metabolites of AA. Indeed, prostacyclin abolishes the oxygen burst and aggregation response induced by collagen in washed platelet suspensions [30]. However, in human PRP aggregated with AA, prostacyclin also suppresses the generation of TXA_2 by 50–80%, whereas in platelet homogenates prostacyclin does not influence the conversion of AA to TXA_2 [95]. Therefore, it may be concluded that the prostacyclin-cAMP system in platelets inhibits indirectly the oxygenative metabolism of both endogenous and exogenous AA. This last inhibition takes place only in intact platelets. Therefore the prostacyclin-cAMP system may prevent the penetration of exogenous AA inside the platelet or, alternatively, exogenous AA may make platelets aggregate by activation of phospholipase and release of the endogenous substrate.

It should be also mentioned that aspirinized prostacyclin-treated PRP is resistant to the proaggregatory action of exogenous TXA_2 [95]. The data above point to the possibility that inhibition of platelet aggregation by the prostacyclin-cAMP system also occurs by mechanisms other than inhibition of phospholipase A_2 activity. Another mechanism of antiaggregatory action of prostacyclin may involve the suppression of the ADP-induced increase in the number of available binding sites for fibrinogen on platelets [127].

Gorman [89] has proposed that the balance between cAMP-lowering activity of the PGH_2-TXA_2 system in the platelet, and the cAMP-stimulating properties of prostacyclin, not only controls platelet aggregation but also may be of importance in the regulation of cellular function in other tissues.

Prostacyclin and Atherosclerosis

In one of the pioneering papers on the discovery of prostacyclin [104] we described how 15-hydroperoxyarachidonic acid ($IC_{50} = 1.5\ \mu M$) and tranylcypromine ($IC_{50} = 600\ \mu M$) inhibit prostacyclin synthetase in procine aortic microsomes. 15-Hydroperoxyarachidonic acid also inhibits generation of prostacyclin in arterial slices [194] and in cultured endothelial cells [180]. Later a powerful inhibition of prostacyclin synthetase by other lipid peroxides was reported.

We put forward the hypothesis that an increase in lipid peroxidation promotes the development of atherosclerosis by decreasing of the ratio of PGI_2 to TXA_2 in the circulatory system [56,106,350] and that prostacyclin is a natural antiatherosclerotic hormone [100]. Indeed, an atherogenic diet in rabbits causes a dramatic suppression of prostacyclin generation by arteries, heart, kidney, and lungs [56,57,106]. This suppression may be observed as early as one week after feeding the animals an atherogenic diet [181]. An increase in the biosynthesis of PGE_2 during experimental atherosclerosis [20] may be considered to represent a diversion of PGH_2 metabolism from prostacyclin to primary prostaglandins owing to the blockade of prostacyclin synthetase. Only at a later stage of development of atherosclerosis does there occur an overproduction of TXA_2 by rabbit [350] and human [292,293] platelets.

We have no direct evidence that during experimental atherosclerosis the formation of lipid peroxides is increased. However, lipoperoxides have been found in human atheromatic arteries [79,87] in retina during ocular siderosis [131], and in ceroid atheromatous plaques from human arteries [123]. In human atheromatous plaques hardly any prostacyclin is generated [11], although experimental venous thrombosis is not associated with a decrease in prostacyclin-generating capacity of damaged rat veins [206]. Interestingly, feeding rabbits a diet enriched with safflower oil decreases the formation of prostacyclin in the vascular endothelium [345]. Safflower oil (Table 1) is the richest plant source of PUFAs, which are prone to oxidation. Swines kept on a corn-soybean diet, free of cholesterol and saturated fat, develop atherosclerosis identical to that seen in humans [300]. On the other hand, antioxidants protect rats against the vascular damage of acute choline deficiency, which by itself increases lipid peroxidation in the body [344]. Species differences should be taken into the consideration. In minipigs fed an atherogenic diet, the generation of prostacyclin by vascular tissue is increased [275]. Our evidence for the involvement of prostacyclin in the pathogenesis of atherosclerosis in humans is the evidence ex iuvantibus. Prostacyclin alleviates the symptoms of advanced peripheral arteriosclerosis [295] in patients who are resistant to other pharmacological treatment [47].

To summarize, we postulate that atherosclerosis is a disease resulting from a deficiency of prostacyclin. This hormonal defect is due to intoxication of prostacyclin synthetase with lipid peroxides or with corresponding free radicals. Cells and tissues are protected against oxidizing free radicals by several complex antioxidant mechanisms [61]. In disease these mechanisms may fail. A special case is atherosclerotic hyperlipidemia with a surplus of circulating lipids to be peroxidized. Deficiency of prostacyclin leads to a decrease in cAMP levels both in platelets and in arterial walls, thus increasing platelet aggregability [89] and endothelial permeability [221]. When deprived of its capacity to synthesize prostacyclin, the arterial endothelium becomes a surface prone to platelet adhesion and aggregation.

The decisive role of platelets in the initiation of atherosclerosis is evidenced by the resistance to atherosclerosis of pigs with von Willebrand's disease [80]. Aggregating platelets are activated not only by a lack of "prostacyclin barrier" at the endothelial surface, but also by low concentrations of circulating prostacyclin and by a diversion of AA metabolism from prostacyclin to the proaggregatory metabolites. Activated platelets aggregate and adhere to the defenseless endothelial cells. At this stage no arterial thrombosis occurs, but mural microthrombi are formed. The focal microaggregates release enzymes and mediators that cause endothelial damage and mural inflammatory response. Vascular wall, when denuded from endothelium, is prone to a more intensive platelet aggregation. Platelet-derived growth factor (PDGF) is released [12,250] triggering the proliferation of fibroblasts and the migration of myocytes, and finally an atheromatic plaque is formed [251]. The secondary ulceration of atheromatic plaques may lead to a massive intraarterial thrombosis.

Clinical Perspectives on Prostacyclin Therapy

The only published clinical use of prostacyclin is in the treatment of atherosclerosis. Prostacyclin was administered intraarterially (5–10 ng/kg/min for 72 hours) into five patients suffering from advanced arteriosclerosis obliterans of the lower extremities [295]. All patients had chronic ischemic ulcers and focal necrosis was present in three. The lesions were painful and had resisted healing from 3 months to 3 years. Conservative treatment had been tried in the past, and no further treatment except for amputation could be offered. In all patients, pain was extinguished 2 days after prostacyclin infusion, and in three of them regression of necrosis and healing of ischemic ulcers occurred 4–8 weeks later. The striking clinical improvement after prostacyclin therapy was accompanied by a persistent increase in capillary blood flow, but the anatomical obstruction to the major arteries remained unchanged, as evidenced by angiography.

We believe that the powerful antiaggregating and disaggregating properties of prostacyclin caused the nonobstructed small arteries and capillaries to be cleared of platelet microaggregates. Thus atherogenesis was arrested, peripheral blood flow increased, and possibly the vascular endothelium, which had been deprived of prostacyclin synthetase, had a chance to rebuild the lacking enzyme. A transient vasodilatation produced by prostacyclin during the infusion period is an unlikely cause of clinical improvement, since increased capillary blood flow was observed 6 weeks after termination of prostacyclin infusion and the curative effects of prostacyclin persisted for at least 3 months of the observation period. Prostacyclin might, however, act directly on blood vessels by stimulating proliferation of new capillaries into the ischemic area. Prostacyclin increases cAMP in vascular walls, [57] and cAMP stimulates the proliferation of vascular tissues [221].

The effectiveness of prostacyclin in advanced arteriosclerosis obliterans created a sound basis for further clinical trials of prostacyclin therapy in atherosclerosis of the coronary and cerebral arteries. Diabetic angiopathy might be another indication for administration of prostacyclin, especially since in patients with juvenile-onset diabetes the generation of PGI_2 by vascular tissues is diminished [269]. On the other hand, in patients with renal failure increased amounts of prostacyclin are produced by vascular tissue [245]. Plasma of uremic patients as well as those with advanced hepatic dysfunction stimulates prostacyclin release from arterial slices [310]. It has been proposed that the overproduction of prostacyclin in such patients may contribute to the prolonged bleeding time experienced by those individuals. The purified active plasma fraction of patients with renal or hepatic failure might be tried, as well as angiotensin analogues [100,116], to stimulate prostacyclin generation in patients with intraarterial thrombosis. The drug that seems to exert an antithrombotic effect through the stimulation of prostacyclin release from blood vessels is 1-(2-(β-naphthyloxy)ethyl)-3-methyl-2-pyrazolin-5-one (BAY g 6575) [39,266]. Dipyridamole [182] was claimed to have a similar effect. The development of this kind of drug will constitute a new therapeutic approach to the treatment of thrombosis and atherosclerosis.

The final goal that emerges from the discovery of prostacyclin is to obtain new antithrombotic and, hopefully, antiatherosclerotic drugs. This may be done by administration of prostacyclin itself into patients [114,294,295], or by stimulation of its endogenous release [100,116, 266,310], or by replacement of prostacyclin with its synthetic analogues. The synthetic analogues of prostacyclin [52,78,81,113,213,326] should be more stable but not necessarily more potent than the natural hormone. They should be active orally. Perhaps prostacyclin analogues may be used in hormone substitution therapy in diseases that are resistant to heparin and K antivitamin treatment, such as a number of peripheral artery diseases, acute myocardial infarction, "crescendo angina," acute cerebral ischemia, and disseminated intravascular thrombosis.

The use of prostacyclin in extracorporeal circulation systems such as cardiopulmonary bypass or artificial kidney has been also suggested [200]. Indeed, strong experimental evidence was recently presented that prostacyclin can replace heparin during hemodialysis [347,348] and can prevent a fall of platelet count and fibrinogen levels in blood during charcoal hemoperfusion [349]. Prostacyclin offers not only a simple replacement for heparin but also a safer one.

Heparin is a potent anticoagulant; however it exerts a paradoxical platelet-aggregating activity and therefore causes thrombocytopenia, disseminated intravascular thrombosis, and formation of microaggregates, which constitute serious complications in heparin therapy. This proaggregating action of heparin is probably accomplished by the inhibition of platelet adenylate cyclase that is sensitive to PGE_1 [243] and PGI_2 [170]. Heparin also potentiates the synthesis of TXA_2 in platelets [10]. Platelets defend themselves against heparin by generating several antiheparin proteins (e.g. PF4) [253]. Prostacyclin and PF4 antagonize heparin at different molecular levels, and it is possible that prostacyclin acts at the regulatory subunit of platelet adenylate cyclase. The inhibition of the secretory platelet response by prostacyclin is sufficient not only to preserve platelet integrity but also to prevent the release of platelet factors, which initiate blood coagulation in a dialysis machine. During charcoal hemoperfusion prostacyclin alone cannot prevent blood from clotting, and the cooperation of heparin and prostacyclin is necessary.

INTERFERENCE IN ARACHIDONIC ACID CASCADE IN PLATELETS AND IN VASCULAR WALLS

Pharmacologic interference in the metabolism of arachidonic acid [239] both in platelets and in vascular endothelium may change the function of the circulating platelets. This section deals with the drugs that influence the generation of either TXA_2 in platelets or prostacyclin in blood vessels.

Phospholipase A_2 Inhibitors

In 1975 Gryglewski et al. [103] discovered that glucocorticosteroids inhibit the liberation of AA from its phospholipid stores. This action of glucocorticosteroids is mediated through the induction of the intracellular biosynthesis of a phospholipase A_2 inhibitor [77]. These findings explain the inability of glucocorticosteroids to inhibit the liberation of AA (thus its cyclooxygenation) in tissue homogenates as well as in platelets [96,231]. Platelets have no nuclei; therefore the transcription and transformational nuclear actions that are necessary for the generation of a phospholipase A_2 inhibitor cannot be performed by glucocorticosteroids in platelets. There are, however, direct inhibitors of phospholipase A_2, such as mepacrine and bromophenacetyl bromide [313]. These drugs inhibit collagen-, thrombin-, and carrageenan-induced platelet aggregation [24,313], but are ineffective against AA-induced aggregation [24].

The data above clearly indicate that several proaggregating agents release endogenous AA from platelets by activation of phospholipase A_2, although it is less clear whether the subsequent cyclooxygenation of free AA is an indispensable step in the aggregatory response [313]. Mepacrine and bromophenacetyl bromide are used only as chemical tools for studying metabolism of AA in platelets.

Cyclooxygenase Inhibitors

In 1971 Vane [309], Smith and Willis [277], and Ferreira et al. [71] discovered that aspirin and indomethacin inhibit prostaglandin biosynthesis in lung homogenates, in platelets, and in perfused spleen. Nonsteroidal antiinflammatory drugs inhibit the first step of AA transformation by the microsomal multienzymic system (fatty acid cyclooxygenase) [75,76], which eventually leads to formation of prostaglandins, TXA_2, or prostacyclin. Thus aspirinlike drugs are cyclooxygenase inhibitors: that is, they inhibit the conversion of AA to PGG_2.

The effects of cyclooxygenase inhibitors on platelet function have been reviewed many times [75,97–99,204], and their clinical efficacy in thrombosis has also been investigated [25,145,316]. Eicosatetraynoic acid

(ETY), an antimetabolite of AA, acts like aspirin on platelets [343]. Aspirin inhibits the release reaction induced in human PRP by ADP, adrenaline, and thrombin, and this inhibitory effect of aspirin is prevented by incubation of PRP with a nonaggregating concentration of AA [167]. Aspirinlike drugs effectively inhibit AA-induced platelet aggregation, shift dose-response curves for collagen and thrombin-induced aggregation to the right, prevent the "second wave" of aggregation induced by low concentrations of ADP and adrenaline, and partially antagonize the proaggregatory action of low concentrations of endoperoxides and of their synthetic analogues. Cyclooxygenase inhibitors do not influence platelet aggregation induced by supramaximal concentrations of ADP, adrenaline, endoperoxides, and their analogues. The clinical effectiveness of cyclooxygenase inhibitors in the prevention of the secondary myocardial infarction [29,303] and other thrombotic diseases [145] is still under investigation, and in spite of several favorable reports [29,303], no conclusion has been reached [16,25,145,316].

Acetylsalicylic acid (aspirin), frequently combined with dipyridamole (persantin), and sulfinpyrazone (anturan) have gained the keen attention of clinicians. In theory, cyclooxygenase inhibitors can hinder the formation of both products of AA cyclooxygenation in the circulatory system, that is, formation of TXA_2 in platelets and prostacyclin in vascular endothelium. When treating intraarterial thrombosis, we would prefer to see a selective inhibition of AA cyclooxygenation in platelets, rather than the complete elimination of AA metabolites. Therefore numerous laboratory and clinical studies focused on the problem of the site of action of aspirin in the circulatory system.

In vitro aspirin selectively and irreversibly acetylates active sites of platelet cyclooxygenase [252] and inhibits the spontaneous generation of AA metabolites from superfused platelets [231]. Also in vivo this enzymatic inactivation is irreversible, and platelets from aspirin-treated volunteers (a single oral dose of 600 mg) do not convert AA to PGE_2, MDA, or TXA_2 for at least 2 days [142,156,287,292]. The gradual reappearance of the capability of PRP to generate TXA_2 is a manifestation of the expulsion of new platelets by the bone marrow into the peripheral blood, and therefore this simple technique may be used for determination of platelet life span [287,292]. The presence of an acetyl group in the molecule of aspirin is an absolute requirement for its activity, since unlike aspirin, salicylic, gentisic, and salicyluric acids [314] fail to inhibit the generation of TXA_2 in platelets after in vivo administration to the rat. Aspirin does not inhibit platelet adherence to collagen or to the subendothelium at a normal hematocrit [38]. Cyclooxygenase inhibitors are not effective inhibitors of the platelet release of PDGF [139]. In consequence, pretreatment with aspirin does not inhibit myointimal thickening of rat arterial walls denuded of endothelium [46], although when applied topically, aspirin inhibits electrically induced white platelet thrombus formation in a mesenteric artery of the rat [28]. In fact, aspirin at high doses (200 mg/kg) is thrombogenic in rabbits, presumably because it inhibits the biosynthesis of prostacyclin in arterial walls [152].

The basal production of prostacyclin by arterial segments from rats is strongly inhibited for 2 days after a single oral administration of aspirin at a dose of 300 mg/kg [15]. In rabbits, aspirin (100 mg/kg, intravenously) inhibits prostacyclin generation in arterial and venous tissues, both by endothelial and nonendothelial cells [31]. After 20 hours only a half the control amount of prostacyclin is generated by arteries. This suppression of prostacyclin biosynthesis by aspirin is associated with an increase in platelet adhesion in mechanically induced injury sites in carotid arteries [32].

There have been repeated reports of platelets having a high susceptibility to the inhibitory action of aspirin, compared to arterial cyclooxygenase. Korbut and Moncada [157] and Amezcua et al. [9] have proposed that by lowering the dose of aspirin, it is possible to produce selective inhibition of platelet aggregability without damage to the prostacyclin-generating system. Indeed, the authors have shown that aspirin at low doses not only abolishes the prothrombotic effect of AA but also unmasks the antiaggregatory effect of AA in vivo. In rats aspirin at a dose of 3.6 mg/kg inhibits by half the formation of MDA in platelets, whereas ID_{50} for inhibition of prostacyclin generation in arteries is 25 mg/kg [168]. Also the inhibitory effect of aspirin in platelets lasts longer (96–120 hours) than in arterial tissues (< 24 hours) [168]. Aspirin inhibits AA-stimulated generation of TXB_2 in human platelets at IC_{50} (3.2 μg/ml) [332], whereas the inhibitory effect of aspirin on the generation of prostacyclin in rabbit aortic slices is much weaker (IC_{50} 140 μg/ml) [331]. AA (1.4 mg/kg) infused intravenously into rabbits causes a rise in plasma TXB_2 and 6-keto-$PGF_{1\alpha}$ levels up to 156 and 5.8 ng/ml, respectively. The animals die from pulmonary thrombosis and hypotension. Treatment of the animals with aspirin (25 mg/kg) before an infusion of AA keeps plasma TXB_2 level down to 2.5 ng/ml and does not influence AA-induced increases in 6-keto-$PGF_{1\alpha}$; however this dose of aspirin protects only 50% of the animals against AA-induced death [184]. On the other hand, in man aspirin at a single oral dose as low as 0.3 g completely abolishes generation of TXB_2 by platelets as well as production of prostacyclin by vein specimens obtained at biopsy [230]. The data from our laboratory [18] indicate that in rabbits there exists only a narrow range of doses of aspirin (10–15 mg/kg) that selectively suppress the generation of TXA_2 in platelets without affecting prostacyclin synthesis in arteries. In rabbits aspirin at a single oral dose of 15 mg/kg does not influence the capacity of arterial walls to synthesize prostacyclin. If, however, this dose of aspirin is administered daily during three consecutive days, there occurs a 40% inhibition of prostacyclin formation in arteries (Gryglewski, unpublished data). Therefore, we feel that aspirin is not a good antithrombotic drug, and if used it should be administered at a low dose every second or third day.

The influence of aspirin on bleeding has been investigated by a number of authors [9,64,145,232,319,323]. The concept that low doses prolong and high doses shorten bleeding time [9] has been criticized [64]. At most, aspirin doubles template bleeding time in man, although Mielke et al. [188] suggest that the effect of aspirin on hemostasis is minimal.

Another controversial issue is the appreciation of the effects of dipyridamole (persantin) on platelet function and its interaction with aspirin [57,60,182,198,214,232,319]. Dipyridamole has a multidirectional biochemical action on platelets and on blood vessels. The vascular and platelet effects of dipyridamole have been attributed to its inhibitory effects on cAMP phosphodiesterase [198], inhibition of intracellular uptake of adenosine [57], inhibition of TXA_2 formation [7,214], or stimulation of prostacyclin release [182]. Dipyridamole has been claimed to potentiate [198] or to attenuate [60] the antiaggregating action of prostacyclin. A more detailed discussion on the mode of action of dipyridamole is beyond the scope of this chapter.

Recently reports have appeared on new drugs with antiaggregating activity, that potentiate prostacyclin generation by arteries rather than inhibiting it. These drugs are BAY g 6575 [39,266], suloctidil [163,318], and ticlopidine [147,244].

Thromboxane Synthetase Inhibitors

By definition, thromboxane synthetase inhibitors invalidate the conversion of endoperoxides to TXA_2. A selective thromboxane synthetase inhibitor is expected not to influence the activities of cyclooxygenase and prostacyclin synthetase. The superiority of thromboxane synthetase inhibitors over cyclooxygenase inhibitors is based on the failure of the former to inhibit the generation of prostacyclin by vascular walls. Depending on whether one chooses Needleman's [208] or Gorman's [89] point of view (see "Thromboxane A_2 and Platelet Aggregation," under the section "Thromboxanes and Prostaglandin Endoperoxides," above), a search for selective thromboxane synthetase inhibitors may be considered to be a search for drugs that will alleviate acute ischemia occurring during intravascular platelet aggregation [66,202,264] or a search for potential antithrombotic agents that may replace heparin, K antivitamins, aspirin, sulfinpyrazone, dipyridamole, and clofibrate in the prevention of myocardial reinfarction, as well as a supplement for prostacyclin in the treatment of atherosclerosis [295].

The known thromboxane synthetase inhibitors do not constitute a homogeneous group, either chemically or pharmacologically [59,210, 296]. Two nonacidic antiinflammatory drugs, first known as cyclooxygenase inhibitors—benzydamine [195] and nictindole (L-8027) [105]—were reported to inhibit TXA_2 synthetase at IC_{50} of 300 and 1 μM, respectively. Both drugs at the concentrations given do not influence cyclooxygenase activity from ram seminal vesicle microsomes. The inhibition of thromboxane synthetase by benzydamine was denied [59]. It was confirmed for nictindole [59]; however in vivo it is practically impossible a separate inhibition of thromboxane synthetase from inhibition of cyclooxygenase by nictindole [112].

Imidazole, a compound first known as a stimulator of cAMP phosphodiesterase [37], has been found to inhibit thromboxane synthetase [59,196,210,215,296]. Imidazole is a weak (IC_{50} 375 µM) but selective thromboxane synthetase inhibitor [196]. Therefore, imidazole derivatives [196,297], histamine, and antagonists of H_2 histamine receptors such as burimamide, metiamide, and cimetidine [6] have been studied as potential thromboxane synthetase inhibitors. Among histamine antagonists, only burimamide inhibits TXA_2 synthetase (IC_{50} 25 µM) [6]. Monosubstituted alkyl and arylalkyl derivatives of imidazole such as 1-butylimidazole or 1-(2-isopropylphenyl)imidazole [297] are much better inhibitors of the enzyme than the parent compound.

Unexpectedly, the influence of imidazole on platelet aggregation is rather erratic. Imidazole causes a delay in platelet aggregation in PRP but is without any effect in washed platelet suspensions aggregated with AA or with PGH_2 [208,210,211]. At high concentrations, imidazole may in fact enhance platelet aggregability through a mechanism that is independent of thromboxane synthesis [73]. Perhaps a direct stimulatory effect of imidazole on phosphodiesterase activity [37] or on Ca^{2+} transport through biomembranes [151] may offer an explanation for the proaggregatory action of this compound. Imidazole is an irritant to mammalian tissues. Thus for different reasons both nictindole and imidazole are useless for the in vivo inhibition of thromboxane synthetase.

Eakins et al. [67] have demonstrated that p-benzyl-4-(1-oxo-(4-chlorobenzyl)-3-phenyl propyl) phenyl phosphate (N-0164) at concentrations of 1–10 µM antagonizes the contractile action of prostaglandins at their "receptor sites" in gastrointestinal smooth muscle. Later it was shown that N-0164 selectively blocks "receptor sites" for PGD_2 and fails to antagonize the action of PGE_1 and PGI_2 on platelet membranes [170,171, 336]. In addition, high concentrations of N-0164 (20–100 µM) inhibit TXA_2 synthetase in human platelets [68,160]. Again, the inhibition of platelet aggregation by N-0164 cannot be considered to be a result of the selective inhibition of thromboxane synthetase in platelets; rather, it may be attributed to the extracellular action of N-0164.

Thromboxane synthetase was also claimed to be inhibited by nicotinic acid [320], extracts from onion (*Allium cepa*) and garlic (*Allium sativum*) [173], and microsomes from the bovine heart [42].

A new approach to the selective inhibition of thromboxane synthetase was initiated by the synthesis of the substrate analogues for this enzyme. The chemical group composed of the synthetic endoperoxide analogues and related prostanoic structures is of great biologic interest. A replacement of the 9,11 oxygen-oxygen bridge in a molecule of PGH_2 by an azo [50] or an epoxymethano [288] bridge yields prostanoids that mimic biologic activity of the parent structure; that is, they induce platelet aggregation and contract aortic strips [174,177], although in platelet microsomes they may inhibit thromboxane synthetase [288]. Synthetic analogues of PGH_2 cannot be converted to TXA_2-like material by platelet microsomes; possibly therfore there still exist differences between their proaggregating and prosecretory actions and those of original PGH_2 [43].

If in the azo or epoxyimino analogues of PGH_2 the 15-hydroxy group is replaced by a hydrogen atom, there arises a series of potent and markedly selective thromboxane synthetase inhibitors [33,73,90,92,235]. The most thoroughly investigated was 9,11-azaprosta-5,13-dienoic acid (U-81606) [73,89,90,92], which inhibits TXA_2 generation and PGH_2-induced platelet aggregation both in washed platelet suspension and in PRP [211]. Another analogue, U-51605, also inhibits the activity of cyclooxygenase in ram seminal vesicle microsomal preparation and prostacyclin synthetase from sheep aorta and rabbit lungs. It is, however, in this respect 10–40 times weaker than a thromboxane synthetase inhibitor in human platelet microsomes [235]. An even more interesting inhibitor of PGH_2-induced aggregation of human platelets is 9,11-epoxyiminoprosta-5,13-dienoic acid [33,74]. This analogue seems to antagonize directly the "receptor sites" for TXA_2 in platelets [74]. It has been rightly pointed out by the authors that: "Just as experiments with dichloroisoproterenol advanced the understanding of the β-adrenergic receptor, we believe that experiments with 9,11-epoxyiminoprosta-5,13-dienoic acid will advance the understanding of TXA_2 receptors in platelets."

Prostacyclin Synthetase Inhibitors

It was mentioned earlier that prostacyclin synthetase from porcine aortic microsomes is effectively inhibited by 15-hydroperoxyarachidonic acid [104] and by a number of other lipid peroxides [255]. A much weaker inhibitor of the enzyme is tranylcypromine [104]. Tranylcypromine (10 mg/kg, intraperitoneally) enhances platelet aggregation in murine cerebral microvessels, whereas another monoaminoxidase inhibitor (iproniazed), which is devoided of inhibitory action on prostacyclin synthetase, inhibits platelet aggregation [249]. In the same experimental model imidazole failed to influence platelet aggregation. These data support our concept [104] that prostacyclin is an important physiologic inhibitor of platelet aggregation, whereas the in vivo role of TXA_2 for the platelet aggregability is of a smaller importance.

In perfused rabbit heart, nicotine inhibits the transformation of AA to 6-keto-$PGF_{1\alpha}$ and diverts AA metabolism to PGE_2 [327] much as in perfused guinea pig lungs, imidazole diverts AA metabolism from TXA_2 to $PGF_{2\alpha}$ [215]. Nicotine also inhibits the release of prostacyclin from pulsating rat aorta [301].

CONCLUSIONS

The role of the metabolites of arachidonic acid in platelet function is not fully understood. Several proaggregating agents liberate arachidonic acid from platelet phosphatides and thus promote its enzymatic transformation or incorporation into other chemical units. The first enzymatic step is lipoxygenation of arachidonic acid to the corresponding hydroperoxy eicosatetraenoic acid (HPETE). The significance of various

HPETEs for platelet function remains unknown. Are they the substrates for the generation of leukotriens in platelets? Do they stabilize the irreversible phase of the endoperoxide-induced aggregation? Do they participate in the initiation of the release reaction?

At least the fate of 11-HPETE in platelets is known. It is cyclooxygenized to an endoperoxide, PGG_2, which in turn is the substrate for a peroxidase that transforms PGG_2 to PGH_2. Prostaglandin endoperoxides (PGG_2 and PGH_2) aggregate platelets and induce the release reaction, although the phenomena can be separated. Endoperoxide-induced aggregation is essentially resistant to the inhibitory action of cyclooxygenase inhibitors (e.g. aspirin), whereas the effects of thromboxane synthetase inhibitors on the endoperoxide-induced aggregation are not unequivocal. Imidazole does not inhibit the PGH_2-induced aggregation in a suspension of washed platelets, but 9,11-azaprosta-5,13-dienoic acid blocks the cAMP-lowering activity of PGH_2 and the PGH_2-induced aggregation in platelet-rich plasma. Is then thromboxane A_2 or PGH_2 a primary proaggregating metabolite of arachidonic acid?

The next uncertainty is the mode of proaggregatory action of the PGH_2-TXA_2 system. It seems that TXA_2 acts as an ionophore: thus by increasing the concentration of Ca^{2+} in cytosol it promotes the contractile events in platelets, activates phospholipase A_2, and inhibits adenylate cyclase. What is the relative importance of this PGH_2-TXA_2-mediated route in comparison to the ADP-mediated, phosphatidic acid–mediated, or thrombin-mediated independent routes to platelet activation? The answer to this question is crucial for the relevance of the therapeutic and preventive treatment of thrombosis with aspirin, sulfinpyrazone, and thromboxane synthetase inhibitors.

On the other hand, two metabolites of arachidonic acid, prostacyclin (PGI_2) and prostaglandin D_2 (PGD_2), are potent inhibitors of platelet aggregation and of the release reaction. The antiaggregating properties of prostacyclin and PGD_2 are mediated by the activation of two different receptors that are closely associated with the platelet adenylate cyclase. Prostacyclin receptor is identical to that for prostaglandin E_1 (PGE_1). In contrast to the effects produced by PGD_2 and PGE_1, a prostacyclin-induced rise in platelet cAMP is long-lasting. Phosphodiesterase inhibitors potentiate the antiaggregating effects of prostacyclin.

Prostacyclin is generated enzymatically from prostaglandin endoperoxides by vascular walls, lungs, and kidneys. The in vivo release of prostacyclin into the circulation is stimulated by angiotensin II, bradykinin, hyperventilation, and pulmonary embolism. Prostacyclin synthetase is selectively inhibited by linear lipid peroxides, which are likely to accumulate in the body during atherosclerotic hyperlipidemia. There is no conclusive evidence that PGE_1 and PGD_2 are generated in vivo in sufficient amounts to influence platelet aggregability, nor that the generation of PGE_1 and PGD_2 is an enzymatic process. At least there are no known specific inhibitors of the corresponding isomerases.

On the contrary, PGH_2 is easily converted to PGD_2 in the presence of silica gel or albumin, and in the absence of any enzymic protein. In my opinion prostacyclin is the only physiologically important substance that prevents platelets from aggressive behavior and shields arteries against mural thrombosis, and therefore against atherosclerosis. Just as insulin is the only powerful hypoglycemic hormone, the action of which is opposed by multiple hyperglycemic mechanisms, prostacyclin alone fights against a variety of endogenous thrombogenic factors. Continuing this analogy, atherosclerosis may be considered to be a disease resulting from a deficiency of prostacyclin, just as juvenile diabetes is the disease resulting from a deficiency of insulin. Indeed, an intraarterial infusion of prostacyclin has been shown to alleviate the signs and symptoms of advance arteriosclerosis obliterans.

REFERENCES

1. Abdel-Halim, M. S., Hamberg, M., Sjöquist, B., and Änggård E. (1977) Identification of prostaglandin D_2 as a major prostaglandin in homogenates of rat brain. Prostaglandins 14, 633–643.

2. Addonizio, V. P., Macarak, E.J., Niewiarowski, S., Colman, R.W., and Edmunds, L. H. (1979) Preservation of human platelets with prostaglandin E_1 during in vitro simulation of cardiopulmonary bypass. Circ. Res. 44, 350–357.

3. Agradi, E., Tremoli, E., Petroni, A., Colombo, C., and Galli, C. (1979) Effects of dietary fatty acids on platelet aggregation and platelet thromboxane B_2 production in the rabbit. Thromb. Haemostasis 42, 405 (Abstr.).

4. Aiken, J. W., Gorman, R. R., and Shebuski, J. J. (1979) Prevention of blockade of partially obstructed coronary arteries with prostacyclin correlates with inhibition of platelet aggregation. Prostaglandins 17, 483–494.

5. Ali, M., Cerskus, A. L. Zamecnik, J., and McDonald, J. W. D. (1977) Synthesis of prostaglandin D_2 and thromboxane B_2 in human platelets. Thromb. Res. 11, 485–496.

6. Allan, G., and Eakins, K. (1978) Burimamide is a selective inhibitor of thromboxane A_2 biosynthesis in human platelet microsomes. Prostaglandins 15, 659–661.

7. Ally, A. I., Manku, M. S., Horrobin, D. F., Morgan, R. O., Karmazin, M., and Karmali, R. A. (1977) Dipyridamole a possible potent inhibitor of thromboxane A_2 synthetase in vascular smooth muscle. Prostaglandins 14, 607–609.

8. Ally, A. I., Barrete, W. E., Cunnane, S., Horrobin, D. F., Karmali, R. A., Karmazyn, M., Manku, M. S., Morgan, R. O., and Nicolaou, K. C. (1978) Prostaglandin I_2 (prostacyclin) inhibits intracellular calcium release. J. Physiol. 276, 40P.

9. Amezcua, J. L., Parsons, M., and Moncada, S. (1978) Unstable metabolites of arachidonic acid, aspirin and the formation of the haemostatic plug. Thromb. Res. 13, 477–488.

10. Anderson, W. H., Mohammad, S. F., Chuang, H. Y. K., and Mason, R. G. (1979) Heparin potentiates synthesis of thromboxane A_2 in human platelets. Abstracts of the Fourth International Prostaglandin Conference, Washington, D.C., May 27–31, 1979, p. 5.

11. Angelo, V., Myśliwiec, M., Donati, M. B., and Gaetano, G. (1978) Defective fibrinolytic and prostacyclin-like activity in human atheromateous plaques. Thromb. Haemostasis 39, 535–536.

12. Antoniades, H. N., Scher, C. D., and Stiles, C. D. (1979) Purification of human platelet-derived growth factor. Proc. Natl. Acad. Sci. (USA) 76, 1809–1813.

13. Aoki, N., Naito, K., and Yoshida, N. (1978) Inhibition of platelet aggregation by protease inhibitors. Possible involvement of proteases in platelet aggregation. Blood 52, 1–12.

14. Armstrong, J. M., Lattimer, N., Moncada, S., and Vane, J. R. (1978) Comparison of

the vasodepressor effects of prostacyclin and 6-oxo-prostaglandin $F_{1\alpha}$ with those of prostaglandin E_2 in rats and rabbits. Br. J. Pharmacol. 62, 125–130.

15. Ashida, S., and Abiko, Y. (1978) Effect of ticlopidine and acetylsalicylic acid on generation of prostaglandin I_2-like substance in rat arterial tissue. Thromb. Res. 13, 901–908.

16. Avellone, G., Davi, G., and Novo, S. (1978) Platelet anti-aggregants and ischemic heart disease. In: L. A. Carlson, R. Paoletti, C. R. Sirtori, and G. Weber (eds), International Conference on Atherosclerosis, Raven Press, New York, pp. 623–629.

17. Ball, G., Brereton, G. G., Fulwood, M., Ireland, D. M., and Yates, P. (1970) Effect of prostaglandin E_1 alone and in combination with theophylline or aspirin on collagen-induced platelet aggregation and on platelet nucleotides including adenosine 3′: 5′-cyclic monophosphate. Biochem. J. 120, 709–718.

18. Basista, M., Dobranowski, J., and Gryglewski, R. J. (1978) Prostacyclin and thromboxane generating systems in rabbits pretreated with aspirin. Pharmacol. Res. Commun. 10, 759–763.

19. Baumgartner, H. R., and Tschopp, T. B. (1979) Platelet interaction with aortic subendothelium (SE) in vitro: Locally produced PGI_2 inhibits adhesion and formation of mural thrombi in flowing blood. Thromb. Haemostasis 42, 6 (Abstr.).

20. Berberian, P. A., Ziboh, V. A., and Hsia, S. L. (1976) Prostaglandin E_2 biosynthesis: Changes in rabbit aorta and skin during experimental atherosclerosis. J. Lipid Res. 17, 46–52.

21. Bills, T. K., and Silver, M. J. (1975) Phosphatidylcholine is the primary source of arachidonic acid utilized by platelet prostaglandin synthetase. Fed. Proc. 34, 790.

22. Bills, T. K., Smith, J. B., and Silver, M. J. (1976) Metabolism of $[1-^{14}C]$-arachidonic acid by human platelets. Biochim. Biophys. Acta 241, 303–314.

23. Bills, T. K., Smith, J. B., and Silver, M. J. (1977) Selective release of arachidonic acid from phospholipids of human platelets in response to thrombin. J. Clin. Invest. 60, 1–6.

24. Blackwell, G. J., Duncombe, W. G., Flower, R. J., Parsons, M. F., and Vane, J. R. (1977) The distribution and metabolism of arachidonic acid in rabbit platelets during aggregation and its modification by drugs. Br. J. Pharmacol. 59, 353–366.

25. Blakely, J. A. (1978) Platelet suppressing drugs in arterial disease. Thromb. Haemostasis 39, 294–303.

26. Born, G. V. R. (1962) Aggregation of blood platelets by adenosine diphosphate and its reversal. Nature (London) 194, 927–929.

27. Boullin, D. J., Bunting, S., Blaso, W. P., Hunt, T. M., and Moncada, S. (1979) Responses of human and baboon arteries to prostaglandin endoperoxides and biologically generated and synthetic prostacyclin: Their relevance to cerebral arterial spasm in man. Br. J. Clin. Pharmacol. 7, 139–147.

28. Bourgain, R. H. (1978) The effect of indomethacin and ASA on in vivo induced white platelet arterial thrombus formation. Thromb. Res. 12, 1079–1086.

29. Breddin, K., Uberla, K., and Walter, E. (1977) German-Austrian multicenter two-year prospective studies on the prevention of the secondary myocardial infarction by ASA in comparison to phencumaron and placebo. Thromb. Haemostasis 38, 168 (Abstr.).

30. Bressler, N. M., Broekman, M. J., and Marcus, A. J. (1977) Simultaneous studies of oxygen consumption and aggregation collagen-stimulated human platelets. Blood 50 (Suppl. 1), 235 (Abstr.).

31. Buchanan, M. R., Dejana, E., Cazenave, J. P., Mustard, J. F., and Hirsh, J. (1979) PGI_2 production and effect of aspirin on endothelial cells and non-endothelial cells of the vessel wall. Thromb. Haemostasis 42, 156 (Abstr.).

32. Buchanan, M. R., Dejana, E., Mustard, J. F., and Hirsh, J. (1979) Prolonged inhibition of PGI_2 production and associated increased thrombogenic effect in arteries after aspirin administration. Thromb. Haemostasis 42, 61 (Abstr.).

33. Bundy, G. L., and Peterson, D. C. (1978) The synthesis of 15-deoxy-9,11-epoxyimino prostaglandins, potent thromboxane synthetase inhibitors, Tetrahedron Lett. 1, 41–44.

34. Bunting, S., Gryglewski, R. J., Moncada, S., and Vane, J. R. (1976) Arterial walls generate from prostaglandin endoperoxides a substance (prostaglandin X) which relaxes strips of mesenteric and coeliac arteries and inhibits platelet aggregation. Prostaglandins 12, 897–913.

35. Bunting, S., Higgs, G. A., Moncada, S., and Vane, J. R. (1976) Generation of thromboxane A_2-like activity from prostaglandin endoperoxides by polymorphonuclear leukocyte homogenates. Proc. Br. Pharmacol. Soc. 296P.

36. Bunting, S., Moncada, S., and Vane, J. R. (1977) Antithrombotic properties of vascular endothelium. Lancet 2, 1075–1076.

37. Butcher, R. W., and Sutherland, E. W. (1962) Adenosine 3',5'-phosphate in biological materials. I. Purification and properties of cyclic-3',5'-nucleotide phosphodiesterase and use of this enzyme to characterize adenosine 3',5'-phosphate in human urine. J. Biol. Chem. 237, 1244–1252.

38. Cazenave, J. R., Kinlough-Rathbone, R. L., Packham, M. A., and Mustard, J. F. (1978) The effect of acetylsalicylic acid and indomethacin on rabbit platelet adherence to collagen and the subendothelium in the presence of a low or high hematocrit. Thromb. Res. 13, 971–981.

39. Chamone, D. A. F., Vermylen, J., and Verstraete, M. (1979) Bay g 6575, an antithrombotic compound that stimulates prostacyclin release from the vessel wall. Thromb. Haemostasis 42, 369 (Abstr.).

40. Chandra Sekhar, N. (1970) Effect of eight prostaglandins on platelet aggregation. J. Med. Chem. 13, 39–44.

41. Chang, W. C., and Murota, S. I. (1977) Identification of 6-keto-prostaglandin $F_{1\alpha}$ formed from arachidonic acid in bovine seminal vesicles. Biochim. Biophys. Acta 486, 136–141.

42. Chanh, P. H., Sokan, I., Chanh, A. P. H., and Clavel, P. (1979) A comparative study of anti-thromboxane synthetase activity of the microsomes from different parts of the bovine heart. Abstracts of the Fourth International Prostaglandin Conference, Washington, D.C. May 27–31, 1979, p. 19.

43. Charo, J. F., Feinman, R. D., Detwills, T. C., Smith, J. B., Ingerman, C. M., and Silver, M. J. (1977) Prostaglandin endoperoxides and thromboxane A_2 can induce platelet aggregation in the absence of secretion. Nature (London) 269, 66–69.

44. Chignard, M., Lefort, J., and Vargaftig, B. B. (1977) Platelet effects of arachidonic acid in dog blood. I. Lack of involvement of cyclo-oxygenase in the in vivo situation. Prostaglandins 14, 909.

45. Chignard, M., Le Couedic, J. O., Tnacè, M., Benveniste, J., and Vargaftig, B. B. (1979) Platelet release new mediator, platelet-activating factor, which accounts for ADP and thromboxane-independent aggregation. Thromb. Haemostasis 42, 246 (Abstr.).

46. Clowes, A. W., and Karnovsky, M. J. (1977) Failure of certain antiplatelet drugs to affect myointimal thickening following arterial endothelial injury in the rat. Lab. Invest. 36, 452–464.

47. Coffman, J. D. (1979) Drug therapy: Vasodilator drugs in peripheral vascular disease. New Engl. J. Med. 300, 713–721.

48. Cohen, P., and Derksen, A. (1969) Comparison of phospholipids and fatty acid composition of human erythrocytes and platelets. Br. J. Haematol. 17, 359–371.

49. Cooper, B., Schafer, A. I., Puchalsky, D., and Handin, R. (1978) Platelet resistance to prostaglandin D_2 in patients with myeloproliferative disorders. Blood 52, 618–626.

50. Corey, E. J., Nicolaou, K. C., Machida, Y., Malmsten, C. L., and Samuelsson, B. (1975) Synthesis and biological properties of a 9,11-aza-prostanoid; Highly active biochemical mimic of prostaglandin endoperoxides. Proc. Natl. Acad. Sci. (USA) 72, 335–338.

51. Cottee, F., Flower, R. J., Salmon, J. A., and Vane, J. R. (1977) Synthesis of 6-keto-$PGF_{1\alpha}$ by ram seminal vesicle microsomes. Prostaglandins 14, 413–423.

52. Crane, B. H., Maish, T. L., Maddox, Y. T., Corey, E. J., Szekely, I., and Ramwell, P. W. (1978) Effect of prostaglandin I_2 and analogs on platelet aggregation and smooth muscle contraction. J. Pharmacol. 206, 132–138.

53. Davies, G. C., Sobel, M., and Salzman, E. W. (1979) Plasma thromboxane B₂ (TxB₂) and fibrinopeptide A (FpA) in patients with thrombosis and during contact of blood with artificial surfaces. Thromb. Haemostasis 42, 72 (Abstr.).

54. De Deckere, E. A. M., Nugteren, D. H., and Ten Hoor, F. (1977) Prostacyclin is the major prostaglandin released from the isolated perfused rabbit and rat heart. Nature (London) 268, 160–163.

55. Dejana, E., Castelli, M. G., de Gaetano, G., and Bonaccorsi, A. (1978) Contribution of platelets to the cardiovascular effects of ADP in the rat. Thromb. Haemostasis 39, 135–145.

56. Dembińska-Kieć, A., Gryglewska, T., Żmuda, A., and Gryglewski, R. J. (1977) The generation of prostacyclin by arteries and by the coronary vascular bed is reduced in experimental atherosclerosis in rabbits. Prostaglandins 14, 1025–1035.

57. Dembińska-Kieć, A., Rücker, W., and Schönhöfer, P. (1979) Effects of dipyridamole in vivo on ATP and cAMP content in platelets and arterial wall and atherosclerotic plaque formation. Naunyn-Schmiedebergs Arch. Pharmakol. 309, 59–64.

58. Derksen, A., and Cohen, P. (1975) Patterns of fatty acid release from endogenous substrates by human platelet homogenates and membranes. J. Biol. Chem. 250, 9342–9347.

59. Diczfalusy, W., and Hammarström, S. (1977) Inhibitors of thromboxane synthase in human platelets. FEBS. Lett. 82, 107–110.

60. Di Minno, G., de Gaetano, G., and Silver, M. J. (1979) Dipyridamole reduced the effectiveness of prostaglandin (PG) I₂, PGD₂ and PGE₁ as inhibitors of platelet aggregation in human platelet rich plasma (PRP). Thromb. Haemostasis 41, 198 (Abstr.).

61. Dormandy, T. L. (1978) Free-radical oxidation and antioxidants. Lancet 1, 647–650.

62. Dusting, G. J., Moncada, S., and Vane, J. R. (1977) Prostacyclin (PGX) is the endogenous metabolite responsible for relaxation of coronary arteries induced by arachidonic acid. Prostaglandins 13, 3–15.

63. Dusting, G. J., Moncada, S., and Vane, J. R. (1978) Recirculation of prostacyclin (PGI₂) in the dog. Br. J. Pharmacol. 64, 315–320.

64. Dybdahl, J. H., Eika, C., Daae, L., Dodal, H. C., Frislid, K., Wiik, I., and Larsen, S. (1979) Similar prolongation of bleeding time after low and high doses of acetylsalicylic acid. Thromb. Haemostasis 42, 241 (Abstr.).

65. Dyeberg, J., and Bang, H. O. (1978) Dietary fat and thrombosis. Lancet 1, 152.

66. Dyeberg, J., and Bang, H. O., Stoffersen, E., Moncada, S., and Vane, J. R. (1978) Eicosapentanoic acid and prevention of thrombosis and atherosclerosis? Lancet 2, 117–119.

67. Eakins, K. E., Rajadhyaksha, V., and Schroer, R. (1976) Prostaglandin antagonism by sodium p-benzyl-4-(1-oxo-2-(-4-chlorobenzyl)-3-phenyl propyl) phenyl phosphonate (N-0164). Br. J. Pharmacol. 58, 333.

68. Eakins, E. K., and Kulkarni, P. S. (1977) Selective inhibitory actions of sodium p-benzyl-4-(1-oxo-2-(4-chlorobenzyl)-3-phenyl propyl) phenyl phosphonate (N-0164) and indomethacin on the biosynthesis of prostaglandins and thromboxanes from arachidonic acid. Br. J. Pharmacol. 60, 135–140.

69. Ellis, E. F., Oelz, O., Roberts, L. J., Payne, N. A., Sweetman, B. J., Nies, A.S., and Oates, J. A. (1976) Coronary arterial smooth muscle contraction by a substance released from platelets: Evidence that it is thromboxane A₂. Science 193, 1135–1137.

70. Feinstein, M. B., Becker, E. L., and Fraser, C. (1977) Thrombin, collagen and A23187 stimulated endogenous platelet arachidonate metabolism: Differential inhibition by PGE₁, local anaesthetics and a serine-protease inhibitor. Prostaglandins 14, 1075–1093.

71. Ferreira, S. H., Moncada, S., and Vane, J. R. (1971) Indomethacin and aspirin abolish protaglandin release from the spleen. Nature (London) New Biol. 231, 237–239.

72. Fitzpatrick, F. A., and Gorman, R. R. (1977) Platelet rich plasma transforms exogenous prostaglandin endoperoxide H₂ into thromboxane A₂. Prostaglandins 14, 881–889.

73. Fitzpatrick, F. A., and Gorman, R. R. (1978) A comparison of imidazole and 9,11-

azaprosta-5,13-dienoic acid—Two selective thromboxane synthetase inhibitors. Biochim. Biophys. Acta 539, 162–172.

74. Fitzpatrick. F. A., Bundy, G. L., Gorman, R. R., and Honohan, T. (1978) 9,11-Epoxyiminoprosta-5,13-dienoic acid is thromboxane A_2 antagonist in human platelets. Nature (London) 275, 4230–4231.

75. Flower, R. J. (1974) Drugs which inhibit prostaglandin biosynthesis. Pharmacol. Rev. 26, 33–67.

76. Flower, R. J., Gryglewski, R. J., Herbaczyńska-Cedro, K., and Vane, J. R. (1972) The effect of anti-inflammatory drugs on prostaglandin biosynthesis. Nature (London) New Biol. 238, 104–106.

77. Flower, R. J., and Blackwell, G. J. (1979) Anti-inflammatory steroids induce the biosynthesis of a phospholipase A_2 inhibitor which prevents prostaglandin generation. Nature (London) 278, 456–459.

78. Fried, J., and Barton, J. (1977) Synthesis of 13,14-dehydroprostacyclin methyl ester: A potent inhibitor of platelet aggregation. Proc. Natl. Acad. Sci. (USA) 74, 2199–2203.

79. Fukuzumi, K. (1969) Lipids of atherosclerotic artery. The cause of atherosclerosis from the view point of fact chemistry. Fette Seifen Anstrichm. 11, 953–960.

80. Fuster, V., Bowie, E. J. W., Lewis, J. C., Fass, D. N., Owen, C. A., and Brown, A. L. (1978) Resistance to arteriosclerosis in pigs with von Willebrand's disease. J. Clin. Invest. 61, 722–730.

81. Gandolfi, C. A., and Gryglewski, R. J. (1978) 20-Methylprostacyclin analogs—A two-stage screening procedure for biological properties. Pharmacol. Res. Commun. 10, 885–896.

82. Gerrard, J. M., Peller, J. D., Krick, T. P., and White, J. G. (1977) Cyclic AMP and platelet prostaglandin synthesis. Prostaglandins 14, 39–50.

83. Gerrard, J. M., Butler, A. M., Graff, G., Stoddard, S. F., and White, J. G. (1978) Prostaglandin endoperoxides promote calcium release from a platelet membrane fraction in vitro. Prostaglandins Med. 1, 373–385.

84. Gerrard, J. M., Butler, A. M., Peterson, D. A., and White, J. G. (1978) Phosphatidic acid release calcium from a platelet membrane fraction in vitro. Prostaglandins Med. 1, 387–396.

85. Gerrard, J. M., Butler, A. M., and White, J. G. (1978) Calcium release from a platelet-sequestrating membrane fraction by arachidonic acid and its prevention by aspirin. Prostaglandins 15, 703 (Abstr.).

86. Gerritsen, M. E. (1979) Prostaglandin endoperoxide metabolism in isolated microvessels. Presented during Conference on Prostaglandins and Microvasculatory Function, New York Medical College, Valhalla, July 19–20, 1979.

87. Glavind, J., Hartman, S., Clemensen, J., Jessen, K. E., and Dam, H. (1952) Studies on the role of lipid peroxides in human pathology. II. The presence of peroxidized lipids in the atherosclerotic aortas. Acta Pathol. Microbiol. Scand. 30, 1–6.

88. Gordon, J. L., and MacIntyre, D. E. (1976) Stimulation of platelets by bisenoic prostaglandins. Br. J. Pharmacol. 58, 298P–299P.

89. Gorman, R. R. (1979) Modulation of human platelet function by prostacyclin and thromboxane A_2. Fed. Proc. 38, 83–88.

90. Gorman, R. R., Bundy, G. L., Peterson, D. C. Sun, F. F., Miller, O. V., and Fitzpatrick, F. A. (1977) Inhibition of human platelet thromboxane synthetase by 9,11-azaprosta-5,13-dienoic acid. Proc. Natl. Acad. Sci. (USA) 74, 4007–4011.

91. Gorman, R. R., Bunting, S., and Miller, O. V. (1977) Modulation of human platelet adenylate cyclase by prostacyclin (PGX). Prostaglandins 13, 377–388.

92. Gorman, R. R., Fitzpatrick, F. A., and Miller, O. V. (1977) A selective thromboxane synthetase inhibitor blocks the cAMP lowering activity of PGH_2. Biochem. Biophys. Res. Commun. 79, 305–313.

93. Gorman, R. R., Fitzpatrick, F. A., and Miller, O. V. (1978) Reciprocal regulation of human platelet cAMP levels by thromboxane A_2 and prostacyclin. In: W. J. George

and L. J. Ignarro (eds.), Advances in Cyclic Nucleotide Research, Vol. 9, Raven Press, New York, pp. 597–609.

94. Gorman, R. R., Wierenga, W., and Miller, O. F. (1979) Independence of the cyclic AMP-lowering activity of thromboxane A_2 from the platelet release reaction. Biochim. Biophys. Acta 572, 95–104.

95. Grodzińska, L., and Marcinkiewicz, E. (1979) The generation of TXA_2 in human platelet rich plasma and its inhibition by nictindole and prostacyclin. Pharmacol. Res. Commun. 11, 133–146.

96. Gryglewski, R. J. (1976) Steroid hormones, anti-inflammatory steroids and prostaglandins. Pharmacol. Res. Commun. 8, 337–351.

97. Gryglewski, R. J. (1977) Screening for inhibitors of prostaglandin and thromboxane biosynthesis. In: F. Berti, B. Samuelsson, and G. P. Velo (eds.) Prostaglandin and Thromboxanes, Plenum Press, New York and London, pp. 85–109.

98. Gryglewski, R. J. (1978) Screening and assessment of potency of anti-inflammatory drugs in vitro. In: J. R. Vane and S. H. Ferreira (eds.), Handbook of Experimental Pharmacology, Vol. 50, Part 2, Springer-Verlag, Berlin, Heidelberg and New York, pp. 1–43.

99. Gryglewski, R. J. (1978) Pharmacological interference in biotransformation of arachidonic acid. In: B. B. Vargaftig (ed.), Advances in Pharmacology and Therapeutics, Vol. 4, Pergamon Press, Oxford and New York, pp. 53–62.

100. Gryglewski, R. J. (1979) Prostacyclin as a circulatory hormone. Biochem. Pharmacol. 28, 3161–3166.

101. Gryglewski, R. J., and Vane, J. R. (1972) The release of prostaglandins and rabbit aorta contracting substance (RCS) from rabbit spleen and its antagonism by antiinflammatory drugs. Br. J. Pharmacol. 45, 37–47.

102. Gryglewski, R. J., and Vane, J. R. (1972) The generation from arachidonic acid of rabbit aorta contracting substance (RCS) by microsomal enzyme preparation which also generates prostaglandins. Br. J. Pharmacol. 46, 449–457.

103. Gryglewski, R. J., Panczenko, B., Kerbut, R., Grodzińska, L., and Ocetkiewicz, A. (1975) Corticosteroids inhibit prostaglandin release from perfused lungs of sensitized guinea pigs. Prostaglandins 10, 343–355.

104. Gryglewski, R. J., Bunting, S., Moncada, S., Flower, R. J., and Vane, J. R. (1976) Arterial walls are protected against deposition of platelet thrombi by a substance (prostaglandin X) which they make from prostaglandin endoperoxides. Prostaglandins 12, 685–713.

105. Gryglewski, R. J., Żmuda, A., Korbut, R., Kręcioch, E., and Bieroń, K. (1977) Selective inhibition of thromboxane A_2 biosynthesis in blood platelets. Nature (London) 267, 627–628.

106. Gryglewski, R. J., Dembińska-Kieć, A., Chytkowski, A., and Gryglewska, T. (1978) Prostacyclin and thromboxane A_2 biosynthesis capacities of heart, arteries and platelets at various stages of experimental atherosclerosis in rabbits. Atherosclerosis 31, 385–394.

107. Gryglewski, R. J., Korbut, R., and Ocetkiewicz, A. (1978) Generation of prostacyclin by lungs in vivo and its release into the arterial circulation. Nature (London) 273, 765–767.

108. Gryglewski, R. J., Korbut, R., and Ocetkiewicz, A. (1978) De-aggregatory action of prostacyclin in vivo and its enhancement by theophylline. Prostaglandins 15, 637–644.

109. Gryglewski, R. J., Korbut, R., and Ocetkiewicz, A. (1978) Reversal of platelet aggregation by prostacyclin. Pharmacol. Res. Commun. 10, 185–189.

110. Gryglewski, R. J., Korbut, R., Ocetkiewicz, A., Spławiński, J., Wojtaszek, B., and Swiens, J. (1978) Lungs, a generator of prostacyclin–Hypothesis on physiological significance. Naunyn-Schmiedebergs Arch. Pharmacol. 304, 45–50.

111. Gryglewski, R. J., Korbut, R., and Spławiński, J. (1978) A new endocrine-like function of lungs: Generation of prostacyclin. Mater. Med. Pol. 10, 247–253.

112. Gryglewski, R. J., Korbut, R., Ocetkiewicz, A., and Stachura, J. (1978) In vivo method for quantitation of antiplatelet potency of drugs. Naunyn-Schmiedebergs Arch. Pharmac. 302, 25–30.

113. Gryglewski, R. J., and Nicolaou, K. C. (1978) A triple test for screening biological activity of prostacyclin analogues. Experientia 34, 1336–1337.

114. Gryglewski, R. J., Szczeklik, A., and Niżankowski, R. (1978) Anti-platelet action of intravenous infusion of prostacyclin in man. Thromb. Res. 13, 153–163.

115. Gryglewski, R. J., Salmon, J. A., Ubatuba, F. B., Weathery, B. C., Moncada, S., and Vane, J. R. (1979) Effects of all cis-5,8,11,14,17-eicosapentaenoic acid and PGH_3 on platelet aggregation. Prostaglandins 18, 453–478.

116. Gryglewski, R. J., Korbut, R., and Spławiński, J. (1979) Endogenous mechanisms which regulate prostacyclin release. Haemostasis 8, 294–299.

117. Hamberg, M., and Samuelsson, B. (1973) Detection and isolation of an endoperoxide intermediate in prostaglandin biosynthesis. Proc. Natl. Acad. Sci. (USA) 70, 899–903.

118. Hamberg, M., and Samuelsson, B. (1974) Prostaglandin endoperoxides. VII. Novel tranformation of arachidonic acid in guinea pig lung. Biochem. Biophys. Res. Commun. 61, 942–949.

119. Hamberg, M., and Samuelsson, B. (1974) Prostaglandin endoperoxides. Novel transformations of arachidonic acid in human platelets. Proc. Natl. Acad. Sci. (USA) 71, 3400–3404.

120. Hamberg, M., Svensson, J., and Samuelsson, B. (1975) Thromboxanes: A new group of biologically active compounds derived from prostaglandin endoperoxides. Proc. Natl. Acad. Sci. (USA) 72, 2994–2998.

121. Hamberg, M., and Fredholm, B. B. (1976) Isomerization of prostaglandin H_2 into prostaglandin D_2 in the presence of serum albumin. Biochim. Biophys. Acta 431, 189–193.

122. Hamberg, M., Svensson, J., and Samuelsson, B. (1976) Novel transformations of prostaglandin endoperoxides and formation of thromboxanes. In: B. Samuelsson and R. Paoletti (eds.), Advances in Prostaglandin and Thromboxane Research, Vol. 1, Raven Press, New York, pp. 19–27.

123. Hartroft, W. S., and Prta, E. A. (1965) Ceroid. Am. J. Med. Sci. 250, 324–344.

124. Haslam, R. J., Davidson, M. M. L., Davies, T., Lynham, J. A., and McClenaghan, M. D. (1978) Regulation of blood platelet function by cyclic nucleotides. In: W. J. George and L. J. Ignarro (eds.), Advances in Cyclic Nucleotide Research, Vol. 9, Raven Press, New York, pp. 533–552.

125. Haslam, R. J., and McClenaghan, M. D. (1979) An assay for activators of platelet adenylate cyclase present in rabbit blood: Evidence that prostacyclin (PGI_2) is not a circulating hormone. Thromb. Haemostasis 42, 117 (Abstr.).

126. Hawiger, J., Parkinson, S. K., Timmons, S., and Glick, A. D. (1979) Immune injury to human platelets mediated by IgG Fc receptor is prevented by prostacyclin. Thromb. Haemostasis 42, 256 (Abstr.).

127. Hawiger, J., Parkinson, S., and Timmons, S. (1979) Mobilization of fibrinogen receptor sites on human platelets stimulated with ADP is prevented by prostacyclin. Thromb. Haemostasis 42, 359 (Abstr.).

128. Herman, A. G., Moncada, S., and Vane, J. R. (1977) Formation of prostacyclin (PGI_2) by different layers of the arterial wall. Arch. Int. Pharmacodyn. 227, 162–163.

129. Herman, A. G., Claeys, M., Moncada, S., and Vane, J. R. (1978) Prostacyclin production by rabbit aorta, pericardium, pleura, peritoneum and dura mater. Arch. Int. Pharmacodyn. 236, 303–304.

130. Higgs, E. A., Higgs, G. A., Moncada, S., and Vane, J. R. (1978) Prostacyclin (PGI_2) inhibits the formation of platelet thrombi in arterioles and venules of the hamster cheek pouch. Br. J. Pharmacol. 63, 535–539.

131. Hiramitsu, T., Majima, T., Hasegava, Y., Hirata, K., and Yaki, K. (1976) Lipidperoxide formation in the retina in ocular siderosis. Experientia 32, 1324–1327.

132. Ho, P. P. K., Herrmann, R. G., Towner, R. D., and Walters, C. P. (1977) Reversal of platelet aggregation by aortic microsomes. Biochem. Biophys. Res. Commun. 74, 514–519.

133. Holmsen, H. (1977) Prostaglandin endoperoxide–thromboxane synthesis and dense granule secretion as positive feedback loops in the propagation of platelet responses during "the basic platelet reaction." Thromb. Haemostasis 38, 1030–1041.

134. Hope, W., Chesterman, C. N., Dusting, G. J., Smith, I., Morgan, F. J., and Martin, T. J. (1979) Inhibition by β-thromboglobulin PGI$_2$ formation in arterial endothelial cells. Thrombos. Haemostasis 42, 8 (Abstr.).

135. Hopkins, N. K., Sun, F. F., and Gorman, R. R. (1978) Thromboxane A$_2$ biosynthesis in human lung fibroblasts WI-38. Biochem. Biophys. Res. Commun. 85, 827–836.

136. Hornstra, G., Haddeman, E., and Don, J. A. (1978) Some investigations into the role of prostacyclin in thromboregulation. Thromb. Res. 12, 367–374.

137. Hornstra, G., and Vles, R. (1978) Effects of dietary fats on atherosclerosis and thrombosis. In: International Conference on Atherosclerosis, Milan, 1977, L. A. Carlson, R. Paoletti, C. R. Sirtori, and G. Weber (eds), Raven Press, New York, pp. 471–476.

138. Horrobin, D. F. (1979) Schizophrenia: Reconciliation of the dopamine, prostaglandin and opioid concepts and the role of the pineal. Lancet 1, 529–532.

139. Ihnatowycz, I. O., Cazenave, J. P., Mustard, J. F., and Moore, S. (1979) Effect of indomethacin, sulfinpyrazone and dipyridamole on the release of the platelet-derived growth factor. Thromb. Res. 14, 311–321.

140. Isakson, R. C., Raz, A., Denny, S. E., Pure, E., and Needleman, P. (1977) A novel prostaglandin is the major product of arachidonic acid metabolism in rabbit heart. Proc. Natl. Acad. Sci. (USA) 74, 101–110.

141. Jackson-Roberts, L., II, Sweetman, B. J., and Oates, J. A. (1978) Metabolism of thromboxane B$_2$ in the monkey. J. Biol. Chem. 253, 5305–5318.

142. Jafari, E., Saleem, A., Shaikh, B. S., and Demers, L. M. (1976) Effect of aspirin on prostaglandin synthesis by human platelets. Prostaglandins 12, 829–835.

143. Jakobs, K. H., Saur, W., and Johnson, R. A. (1979) Regulation of platelet adenylate cyclase by adenosine. Biochim. Biophys. Acta 583, 409–421.

144. Jakubowski, J. A., and Ardlie, N. G. (1978) Modification of human platelet function by a diet enriched in saturated or polyunsaturated fat. Atherosclerosis 31, 335–344.

145. Jobin, F. (1978) Acetylsalicylic acid, hemostasis and human thromboembolism, Semin. Thromb. Hemostasis 4, 199–240.

146. Johnson, G. J., Leis, L. A., Rao, G. H. R., and White, J. G. (1979) Arachidonate-induced platelet aggregation in the dog. Thromb. Res. 14, 147–154.

147. Johnson, M., and Heywood, J. B. (1979) Possible mode of action of ticlopidine: A novel inhibitor of platelet aggregation. Thromb. Haemostasis 42, 367.

148. Johnson, R. A., Morton, D. R., Konner, J. H., Gorman, R. R., McGuire, J. C., Sun, F. F., Whittaker, N., Bunting, S., Salmon, J., Moncada, S., and Vane, J. R. (1976) The chemical structure of prostaglandin X (prostacyclin). Prostaglandins 12, 915–928.

149. Jones, R. L., Poyser, N. L., and Wilson, N. H. (1977) Production of 6-oxo-prostaglandin F$_{1\alpha}$ by rat, guinea pig, and sheep uteri in vitro. Proc. Br. Pharmacol. Soc. 5–7 January, 1977, p. 40.

150. Kadowitz, P. J., Chapnick, B. M., Feigen, L. P., Hyman, A. L., Nelson, P. K., and Spannhake, E. W. (1978) Pulmonary and systemic vasodilator effects of the newly discovered prostaglandin, PGI$_2$. J. Appl. Physiol. 45, 408–413.

151. Kazic, T. (1977) Action of methylxanthines and imidazole on the contractility of the terminal ileum of guinea pig. Eur. J. Pharmacol. 41, 103–109.

152. Kelton, J. G., Hirsh, J., Carter, C. J., and Buchanan, M. R. (1978) Thrombogenic effect of high-dose aspirin in rabbits. Relationship to inhibition of vessel wall synthesis of prostaglandin I$_2$-like activity. J. Clin. Invest. 62, 892–895.

153. Kernoff, P. B. A., Willis, A. L., Stone, K. J., Davies, J. A., and McNicol, G. P. (1977) Antithrombotic potential of dihomo-γ-linolenic acid in man. Br. Med. J. 2. 1441–1444.

154. Kitani, T., Kawamura, T., Okuda, S., Watada, M., Nakagawa, M., and Ijichi, H. (1979) Acceleration of prostacyclin release from aorta by thrombin and collagen. Thromb. Haemostasis 42, 233 (Abstr.).

155. Kloetze, J. (1967) Influence of prostaglandins on platelet adhesiveness and platelet aggregation. In: S. Börgstrom and B. Samuelsson (eds.) Prostaglandins, Proceedings of the Second Nobel Symposium, Almqvist and Wiksell, Stockholm, p. 241.

156. Kocsis, J. J., Hernandovich, J., Silver, M. J., Smith, J. B., and Ingerman, C. (1973) Duration of inhibition of platelet prostaglandin formation and aggregation by ingested aspirin or indomethacin. Prostaglandins 3, 141–154.

157. Korbut, R., and Moncada, S. (1978) Prostacyclin (PGI$_2$) and thromboxane A$_2$ interaction in vivo. Regulation by aspirin and relationship with anti-thrombotic therapy. Thromb. Res. 13, 489–500.

158. Kritchevsky, D., Tepper, S. A., Vesselinovitch, D., and Wissler, R. W. (1971) Cholesterol vehicle in experimental atherosclerosis. Part 11. Peanut oil. Atherosclerosis 14, 53–59.

159. Kuehl, F. A., Humes, J. L., Egan, W. R., Ham, E. A., Beveridge, G. C., and Van Arman, C. G. (1977) Role of prostaglandin endoperoxide PGG$_2$ in inflammatory processes. Nature (London) 265, 170–173.

160. Kulkarni, P. S., and Eakins, K. E. (1976) N-0164 inhibition generation of thromboxane A$_2$-like activity from prostaglandin endoperoxides by human platelet microsomes. Prostaglandins 12, 465–469.

161. Kuntamukkula, M. S., McIntire, L. V., Moake, J. L., Peterson, D. M., and Thompson, W. J. (1978) Rheological studies on the contractile force within platelet-fibrin clots: Effects of prostaglandin E$_1$, dibutyryl-cAMP and dibutyryl-cGMP. Throb. Res. 13, 957–969.

162. Lagarde, M., and Dechavanne, M. (1979) Basal level of human platelet prostaglandins: PGE$_1$ is more elevated than PGE$_2$. Prostaglandins 17, 685–705.

163. Lansen, J., Biagi, G., Niebes, P., Gordon, J., and Roncucci, R. (1979) Effect of suloctidil on PGI$_2$ production and inhibition of platelet aggregation. Thromb. Haemostasis 42, 368 (Abstr.).

164. Lapetina, E. G., Schmitges, C. J., Chandrabose, K., and Cuatrecasas, P. (1977) Cyclic adenosine 3′,5′-monophosphate and prostacyclin inhibit phospholipase activity in platelets. Biochem. Biophys. Res. Commun. 76, 828–835.

165. Lapetina, E. G., Chandrabose, K. A., and Cuatrecasas, P. (1978) Ionophore A 23187 and thrombin-induced platelet aggregation: independence from cyclo-oxygenase products. Proc. Natl. Acad. Sci. (USA) 75, 818–821.

166. Lefer, A. M., Ogletree, M. L., Smith, J. B., Silver, M. J., Nicolaou, K. C., Barnette, W. E., and Gasic, G. P. (1978) Prostacyclin: A potentially valuable agent for preserving myocardial ischemia. Science 200, 52–54.

167. Leonardi, R. G., Alexander, B., White, F., and Parts, A. (1978) Effects of arachidonic acid on some inhibitors of the human platelet release reaction. Biochem. Pharmacol. 27, 2131–2138.

168. Livio, M., Villa, S., and de Gaetano, G. (1979) Aspirin as a potential antithrombotic drug: An experimental approach for more rational clinical use. Thromb. Haemostasis 42, 156 (Abstr.).

169. Lollar, P., and Owen, W. G. (1979) Thrombin-induced release of prostaglandins from cultured endothelium. Thromb. Haemostasis 42, 232 (Abstr.).

170. MacIntyre, D. E. (1977) Selective inhibition of platelet responses to bisenoic prostaglandins. Br. J. Pharmacol. 60, 293P–294P.

171. MacIntyre, D. E., Salzman, E. W., and Gordon, J. L. (1978) Prostaglandin receptors on human platelets, Structure-activity relationship of stimulatory prostaglandins. Biochem. J. 174, 921–929.

172. Mahley, R. W., Nelson, A. W., Ferrans, V. J., and Fry, D. L. (1976) Thrombosis in association with atherosclerosis induced by dietary perturbations in dogs. Science 192, 1139–1141.

173. Makheja, A. N., Vanderhoek, J. Y., and Bailey, J. M. (1979) Properties of inhibitor of platelet aggregation and thromboxane synthesis isolated from onion and garlic. Thromb. Haemostasis 42, 74 (Abstr.).

174. Malmsten, C. (1976) Some biological effects of prostaglandin endoperoxide analogs. Life Sci. 18, 169–174.

175. Malmsten, C., Granström, E., and Samuelsson, B. (1976) Cyclic AMP inhibits synthesis of prostaglandin endoperoxide (PGG_2) in human platelets. Biochem. Biophys. Res. Commun. 68, 569–576.

176. Manku, M. S., Oka, M., and Horrobin, D. F. (1979) Differential regulation of the formation of prostaglandins and related substances from arachidonic acid and from dihomogammalinolenic acid. II. Effects of vitamin C. Prostaglandins Med. 3, 129–137.

177. Marcinkiewicz, E., Grodzińska, L., and Gryglewski, R. J. (1978) Platelet aggregation and thromboxane A_2 formation in cat platelet rich plasma. Pharmacol. Res. Commun. 10, 1–12.

178. Marcus, A. J. (1978) The role of lipids in platelet function: With particular reference to arachidonic acid pathway. J. Lipid Res. 19, 793–826.

179. Marcus, A. J., Ullman, H. L., and Safier, L. B. (1969) Lipid composition of subcellular particles of human blood platelets. J. Lipid Res. 10, 108–114.

180. Marcus, A. J., Weksler, B. B., and Jaffe, E. A. (1978) Enzymatic conversion of prostaglandin endoperoxide H_2 and arachidonic acid to prostacyclin by cultured human endothelial cells. J. Biol. Chem. 253, 7138–7141.

181. Masotti, G., Galanti, G., Poggesi, L., Curcio, A., and Neri Serneri, G. G. (1979) Early changes of the endothelial antithrombotic properties in cholesterol fed rabbits. Decreased PGI_2 production by aortic wall. Thromb. Haemostasis 42, 423 (Abstr.).

182. Masotti, G., Poggesi, L., Galanti, G., and Neri Serneri, G. G. (1979) Increase of circulating PGI_2 and PGI_2 released by vessel wall after dipyridamole. Thromb. Haemostasis 42, 197 (Abstr.).

183. McCosh, E. J., Meyer, D. L., and Dupont, J. (1976) Radioimmunoassay of prostaglandins E_1, E_2 and F_2 in unextracted plasma, serum and myocardium. Prostaglandins 12, 471–486.

184. McDonald, J. W. D., Cerskus, A. L., and Ali, M. (1979) Effects of aspirin and sulfinpyrazone on thromboxane and prostacyclin synthesis in rabbits. Thromb. Haemostasis 42, 100 (Abstr.).

185. McGuire, J. C., and Sun, F. F. (1978) Metabolism of prostacyclin: Oxidation by rhesus monkey lung 15-hydroxyl prostaglandin dehydrogenase. Arch. Biochem. Biophys. 189, 92–96.

186. Meyers, K. M., Holmsen, H., Seachord, C. I., and Smith, J. B. (1979) Platelet activation pathways of domestic animals. Thromb. Haemostasis 42, 247 (Abstr.).

187. Meyers, K. M., Seachord, C. I., Prieur, D., and Holmsen, H. (1979) A serotonin induced biphasic aggregation by platelets from cats with Chediak-Higashi syndrome. Thromb. Haemostasis 42, 195 (Abstr.).

188. Mielke, C. H., Jr., Ramos, J., and Rodvien, R. (1979) Template bleeding time (TBT): Influence of venostasis and direction of incision upon the influence of aspirin (ASA). Thromb. Haemostasis 42, 241 (Abstr.).

189. Mills, D. C., and Smith, J. B. (1971) The influence on platelet aggregation of drugs that affect the accumulation of adenosine 3': 5'-cyclic monophosphate in platelets. Biochem. J. 121, 185–196.

190. Mills, D. C. B., and Macfarlane, D. E. (1974) Stimulation of human platelet adenylate cyclase by prostaglandin D_2. Thromb. Res. 5, 401–403.

191. Mills, D. C. B., and Macfarlane, D. E. (1977) Platelet receptors. In: J. L. Gordon (ed.), Platelets in Biology and Pathology, Elsevier–North Holland Biomedical Press, Amsterdam, pp. 159–201.

192. Minkes, M., Stanford, N., Chi, M. M.-Y., Roth, G. J., Raz, A., Needleman, P., and Majerus, P. W. (1977) Cyclic adenosine 3',5'-monophosphate inhibits the availability

of arachidonate to prostaglandin synthetase in human platelet suspensions. J. Clin. Invest. 59, 449–454.

193. Moncada, S., Gryglewski, R. J., Bunting, S., and Vane, J. R. (1976) An enzyme isolated from arteries transforms prostaglandin endoperoxides to an unstable substance that inhibits platelet aggregation. Nature (London) 263, 663–665.

194. Moncada, S., Gryglewski, R. J., Bunting, S., and Vane, J. R. (1976) A lipid peroxide inhibits the enzyme in blood vessel microsomes that generates from prostaglandin endoperoxides the substance (prostaglandin X) which prevents platelet aggregation. Prostaglandins 12, 715–733.

195. Moncada, S., Needleman, P., Bunting, S., and Vane, J. R. (1976) Prostaglandin endoperoxide and thromboxane generating systems and their selective inhibition. Prostaglandins 12, 323–335.

196. Moncada, S., Bunting, S., Mullane, K., Thorogood, P., and Vane, J. R. (1977) Imidazole: A selective inhibitor of thromboxane synthetase. Prostaglandins 13, 611–618.

197. Moncada, S., Herman, A. G., Higgs, E. A., and Vane, J. R. (1977) Differential formation of prostacyclin (PGX or PGI$_2$) by layers of the arterial wall. An explanation for the anti-thrombotic properties of vascular endothelium. Thromb. Res. 11, 323–344.

198. Moncada, S., and Korbut, R. (1978) Dipyridamole and other phosphodiesterase inhibitors act as antithrombotic agents by potentiating endogenous prostacyclin. Lancet 1, 1286–1289.

199. Moncada, S., Korbut, R., Bunting, S., and Vane, J. R. (1978) Prostacyclin is a circulating hormone. Nature (London) 273, 767–768.

200. Moncada, S., and Vane, J. R. (1978) Prostacyclin (PGI$_2$) the vascular wall hormone and vasodilator, In: P. M. Vanhoutte and J. Leusen (eds.), Mechanisms of Vasodilatation, Karger, Basel, pp. 107–121.

201. Morley, J., Bray, M. A., Jones, R. W., Nugteren, D. H., and van Dorp, D. A. (1979) Prostaglandin and thromboxane production by human and guinea-pig macrophages and leucocytes. Prostaglandins 17, 730–736.

202. Morooka, S., Kobayashi, M., and Shimamoto, T. (1977) Experimental ischemic heart disease induced by thromboxane A$_2$ in rabbits. Jpn. Circ. J. 41, 1373–1379.

203. Mullane, K. M., Moncada, S., and Vane, J. R. (1979) Prostacyclin release induced by bradykinin may contribute to the anti-hypertensive action of angiotensin converting enzyme inhibitors. Abstracts of the Fourth International Prostaglandin Conference, Washington, D.C. 27–31 May 1979, p. 84.

204. Mustard, J. F., and Packham, M. A. (1975) Platelets, thrombosis and drugs. Drugs 9, 19–76.

205. Myatt, L., and Elder, M. C. (1977) Inhibition of platelet aggregation by placental substance with prostacyclin-like activity. Nature (London) 268, 159–162.

206. Myśliwiec, M., Villa, S., de Gaetano, G., and Donati, M. B. (1979) Decreased plasminogen activator (PA) but normal prostacyclin (PGI$_2$) activity in veins with experimental thrombosis. Thromb. Haemostasis 42, 7 (Abstr.).

207. Natvig, H., Borchgrevink, C. F., Dedichen, J., Orwen, A., Schiotz, F. H., and Wesilund, K. (1968) A controlled trial of the effect of linolenic acid on incidence of coronary heart disease. The Norwegian vegetable oil experiment of 1965–66. Scand. J. Clin. Lab. Invest. 22 (Suppl.), 1–20.

208. Needleman, P., Minkes, M., and Raz, A. (1976) Thromboxanes: Selective biosynthesis and distinct biological properties. Science 193, 163–165.

209. Needleman, P., Moncada, S., Bunting, S., Vane, J. R., Hamberg, M., and Samuelsson, B. (1976) Identification of an enzyme in platelet microsomes which generates thromboxane A$_2$ from prostaglandin endoperoxides. Nature (London) 261, 558–560.

210. Needleman, P., Bryan, B., Wyche, A., Bronson, S. D., Eakins, K., Ferendelli, J. A., and Minkes, M. (1977) Thromboxane synthetase inhibitors as pharmacological tools: Differential biochemical and biological effects on platelet suspensions. Prostaglandins 14, 897–907.

211. Needleman, P., Raz, A., Ferrendelli, A. J., and Minkes, M. (1977) Application of imidazole as a selective inhibitor of thromboxane synthetase in human platelets. Proc. Natl. Acad. Sci. (USA) 74, 1716–1720.

212. Needleman, P., Raz, A., Minkes, M. S., Ferrendelli, J. A., and Sprecher, H. (1979) Triene prostaglandins: Prostacyclin and thromboxane biosynthesis and unique biological properties. Proc. Natl. Acad. Sci. (USA) 76, 944–949.

213. Nemesánszly, E., Blaskó, G. Stadler, I., Sas, G., and Pálos, L. A. (1979) Effects of PGI_2 and its more stable forms on the aggregation and on the cAMP content of human platelets. Thromb. Haemostasis 42, 118 (Abstr.).

214. Neri-Serneri, G. G., Gensini, G. F., Abbate, R., Favilla, S., and Laureano, R. (1979) Modulation by dipyridamole of the arachidonic acid metabolic pathway in platelets. An in vivo and in vitro study. Thromb. Haemostasis 42, 197 (Abstr.).

215. Nijkamp, F. P., Moncada, S., White, H. L., and Vane, J. R. (1977) Diversion of prostaglandin endoperoxide metabolism by selective inhibition of thromboxane A_2 biosynthesis in lung, spleen or platelets. Eur. J. Pharmacol. 44, 179–186.

216. Nishizawa, E. E., Miller, W. L., Gorman, R. R., and Bundy, G. L. (1975) Prostaglandin D_2 as a potential antithrombotic agent. Prostaglandins 9, 109–121.

217. Nordøy, A. (1974) Platelets and fatty acids. Editorial items. Biochem. Exp. Biol. 1, 295–305.

218. Nugteren, D. H. (1975) Arachidonate lipoxygenase in blood platelets. Biochim. Biophys. Acta 380, 299–307.

219. Nugteren, D. H., Beerthius, R. K., and van Dorp, D. A. (1966) The enzymic conversion of all-cis-8,11,14-eicosatrienoic acid into prostaglandin E_1. Rec. Trav. Chim. Pays-Bas 85, 405–419.

220. Nugteren, D. H., and Hazelhof, E. (1973) Isolation and properties of intermediates in prostaglandin biosynthesis. Biochim. Biophys. Acta 326, 448–461.

221. Numano, F. (1977) Progression and regression of atherosclerosis. Asian Med. J. 20, 625–644.

222. O'Brien, J. R., Etherington, M. D., and Jamieson, S. (1976) Acute platelet changes after large meals of saturated and unsaturated fats. Lancet 1, 878–880.

223. Oelz, O., Seberth, H. W., Knapp, H. R., Sweetman, B. J., and Oates, J. A. (1976) Effects of feeding ethyl-dihomo-γ-linolenate on prostaglandin biosynthesis and platelet aggregation in the rabbit. Biochim. Biophys. Acta 431, 268–277.

224. Oelz, O., Oelz, R., Knapp, H. R., Sweetman, B. J., and Oates, J. A. (1977) Biosynthesis of prostaglandin D_2. I. Formation of prostaglandin D_2 by human platelets. Prostaglandins 13, 225–234.

225. Olsson, A. G., and Jogestrand, T. (1978) Effects of prostaglandin E_1 in peripheral vascular disease. In: L. A. Carlson, R. Paoletti, C. R. Siroti, and G. Weber (eds.), International Conference on Atherosclerosis, Milan, 1977, Raven Press, New York, pp. 403–407.

226. Pace-Asciak, C. (1976) Isolation, structure and biosynthesis of 6-keto-prostaglandin $F_{1\alpha}$ in the rat stomach. J. Am. Chem. Soc. 98, 2348–2349.

227. Pace-Asciak, C. R., Carrara, M. C., and Domazet, Z. (1977) Identification of the major urinary metabolite of 6-keto-prostaglandin $F_{1\alpha}$ (6K-$PGF_{1\alpha}$) in the rat. Biochem. Biophys. Res. Commun. 78, 115–121.

228. Pace-Asciak, C. R., Domazet, Z., and Carrara, M. (1977) Catabolism of 6-ketoprostaglandin $F_{1\alpha}$ by the rat kidney cortex. Biochim. Biophys. Acta 487, 400–404.

229. Pace-Asciak, C., and Rangaraj, G. (1977) Distribution of prostaglandin biosynthetic pathways in several rat tissues. Formation of 6-keto prostaglandin $F_{1\alpha}$. Biochim. Biophys. Acta 486, 579–582.

230. Pareti, F. I., Smith, J. B., D'Angelo, A., and Mannucci, P. M. (1979) Aspirin (ASA) inhibits both prostacyclin and thromboxane formation in man. Thromb. Haemostasis 42, 156 (Abstr.).

231. Patrono, C., Ciabattoni, G., and Grossi-Belloni, D. (1975) Release of prostaglandin

$F_{1\alpha}$ and $F_{2\alpha}$ from superfused platelets: Quantitative evaluation of the inhibitory effect of some aspirin-like drugs. Prostaglandins 9, 557–568.

232. Penny, A. F., Crow, M. J., Rajah, S. M., and Kester, R. C. (1979) The combined effect of dipyridamole and acetyl salicylic acid on platelet function and bleeding time: Evaluation of dose for prophylaxis of thrombosis. Thromb. Haemostasis 42, 242 (Abstr.).

233. Pickett, W. C., Jesse, R. L., and Cohen, P. (1976) Trypsin-induced phospholipase activity in human platelets. Biochem. J. 160, 405–408.

234. Pickett, W. C., Jesse, R. L., and Cohen, P. (1977) Initiation of phospholipase A_2 activity in human platelets by the calcium ion ionophore A23187. Biochim. Biophys. Acta 486, 209–213.

235. Pike, J. E. (1978) The synthesis and biological activities of analogs of prostaglandins and other arachidonic acid cascade metabolites. Abstracts of the First Soviet Union Conference on Prostaglandins, Moscow, 18–20 April 1978, p. 18.

236. Piper, P. J., and Vane, J. R. (1969) Release of additional factors in anaphylaxis and its antagonism by antiinflammatory drugs. Nature (London) 233, 29–35.

237. Poggi, A., Dall'Olio, A., Balconi, G., Delaini, F., de Gaetano, G., and Donati, M. B. (1979) Generation of prostacyclin (PGI_2) activity by Lewis lung carcinoma (3LL) cells. Thromb. Haemostasis 42, 339 (Abstr.).

238. Powell, W. S., and Solomon, S. (1977) Formation of 6-oxoprostaglandin $F_{1\alpha}$ by arteries of the fetal calf, Biochem. Biophys. Res. Commun. 75, 815–818.

239. Ramwell, P. W., Leovey, E. M. K., and Sintetos, A. L. (1977) Regulation of arachidonic acid cascade. Biol. Reprod. 16, 70–84.

240. Raz, A., Minkes, M. S., and Needleman, P. (1977) Endoperoxides and thromboxanes. Structural determinants for platelet aggregation and vasoconstriction. Biochim. Biophys. Acta 488, 305–311.

241. Raz, A., and Aharony, D. (1978) Prostaglandin biosynthesis in platelets: Demonstration and role of prostaglandin $H_2 \rightarrow E_2$ isomerase. Res. Commun. Chem. Pathol. Pharmacol. 21, 507–515.

242. Raz, A., Aharony, D., and Kenig-Wakshal, R. (1978) Biosynthesis of thromboxane B_2 and 12-L-hydroxy-5,8,10-heptadecatrienoic acid in human platelets. Evidence for a common enzymatic pathway. Eur. J. Biochem. 86, 447–454.

243. Reches, A., Eldor, A., and Salomon, Y. (1979) Heparin inhibits PGE_1-sensitive adenylate cyclase and antagonizes PGE_1 antiaggregating effect in human platelets. J. Lab. Clin. Med. 93, 638–644.

244. Reece, A. H., and Walton, P. L. (1979) Inhibition of intimal proliferation of rabbit aorta by ticlopidine. Thromb. Haemostasis 42, 367 (Abstr.).

245. Remuzzi, G., Cavenaghi, A. E., Mecca, G., Donati, M. B., and de Gaetano, G. (1977) Prostacyclin (PGI_2) and bleeding time in uremic patients. Thromb. Res. 11, 919–920.

246. Rittenhouse-Simmons, S., Russell, F. A., and Deykin, D. (1976) Transfer of arachidonic acid to human platelet plasmogen in response to thrombin. Biochem. Biophys. Res. Commun. 70, 295–301.

247. Rittenhouse-Simmons, S., and Deykin, D. (1977) The mobilization of arachidonic acid in platelets exposed to thrombin or ionophore A23187. J. Clin. Invest. 60, 495–498.

248. Rittenhouse-Simmons, S., and Deykin, D. (1978) The activation by Ca^{2+} of platelet phospholipase A_2. Effects of dibutyryl cyclic adenosine monophosphate and 8-(N,N-diethylamino)-octyl-3,4,5-trimethoxybenzoate. Biochim. Biophys. Acta 543, 409–422.

249. Rosenblum, W. I., and El-Sabban, F. (1978) Enhancement of platelet aggregation by tranylcypromine in mouse cerebral microvessels. Circ. Res. 43, 238–241.

250. Ross, R., Glomset, J., Kariya, R., and Harker, L. (1974) A platelet-dependent serum factor that stimulates the proliferation of arterial smooth muscle cells in vitro. Proc. Natl. Acad. Sci. (USA) 71, 1207–1210.

251. Ross, R., and Harker, L. (1976) Hyperlipidemia and atherosclerosis. Science 193, 1094–1100.

252. Roth, G. J., Stanford, N., and Majerus, P. (1975) Acetylation of prostaglandin synthetase by aspirin. Proc. Natl. Acad. Sci. (USA) 72, 3073–3076.

253. Rucinski, B., Niewiarowski, S., James, P., Walz, D. A., and Budzynski, A. Z. (1979) Antiheparin proteins secreted by human platelets. Purification, characterization and radioimmunoassay. Blood 53, 47–62.

254. Russell, F. A., and Deykin, B. (1976) The effect of thrombin on the uptake and transformation of arachidonic acid by human platelets. Am. J. Hematol. 1, 59–70.

255. Salmon, J. A., Smith, D. R., Flower, R. J., Moncada, S., and Vane, J. R. (1978) Further studies on the enzymatic conversion of prostaglandin endoperoxide into prostacyclin by porcine aorta microsomes. Biochim. Biophys. Acta 523, 250–262.

256. Salzman, E. W. (1977) Interrelation of prostaglandin endoperoxide (prostaglandin G_2) and cyclic 3',5'-adenosine monophosphate in human blood platelets. Biochim. Biophys. Acta 499, 48–60.

257. Salzman, E. W., MacIntyre, D. E., Gordon, J. L., and Steer, M. (1977) Enhancement of platelet activity by inhibition of adenylate cyclase. Thromb. Haemostasis 38, 6 (Abstr.).

258. Salzman, E. W., MacIntyre, D. E., Steer, M. L., and Gordon, J. L. (1978) Effect on platelet activity of inhibition of adenylate cyclase. Thromb. Res. 13, 1089–1101.

259. Samuelsson,B. (1965) On the incorporation of oxygen in the conversion of 8,11,14-eicosatrienoic acid to prostaglandin E_1. J. Am. Chem. Soc. 87, 3011–3013.

260. Samuelsson, B., Hamberg, M., Malmsten, C., and Svensson, J. (1976) The role of prostaglandin endoperoxide and thromboxanes in platelet aggregation. In: B. Samuelsson and R. Paoletti (eds.), Advances in Prostaglandin and Thromboxane Research, Vol, 2, Raven Press, New York, pp. 737–746.

261. Samuelsson, B., Folco, G., Granström, E., Kindahl, H., and Malmsten, C. (1978) Prostaglandins and thromboxanes: Biochemical and physiological considerations. In: F. Coceani and P. M. Olley (eds.), Advances in Prostaglandin and Thromboxanes Research, Vol. 4, Raven Press, New York, pp. 1–25.

262. Samuelsson, B., Borgeat, P., Hammarström, S., and Murphy, R. C.(1979) Introduction of a nomenclature: Leukotriens. In: Abstracts of International Conference on Prostaglandins, Washington, D.C., 28 May 1979, pp. 1–3.

263. Sayberth, H. W., Oelt, O., Kennedy, T., Sweetman, B. J., Danon, A., Frölich, J. C., Heimberg, M., and Oates, J. A. (1975) Increase arachidonate in lipids after administration to man: Effects on prostaglandin biosynthesis. Clin. Pharmacol. Ther. 18, 521.

264. Schneider, M. D., and Kelman, B. J. (1979) A proposed mechanism(s) of transistory ischemic injury to myocardium. Am. J. Vet. Res. 40, 170–182.

265. Schoene, N. W., and Lacono, J. M. (1975) Stimulation of phospholipase activity by aggregating agents. Fed. Proc. 34, 257 (Abstr.).

266. Seuter, F., Busse, W. D., Meng, K., Hoffmeister, F., Möller, E., and Horstmann, H. (1979) The antithrombotic activity of BAY g 6575. Arzneim.-Forsch. 29, 54–59.

267. Shebuski, R. J., and Aiken, J. W. (1979) Angiotensin II induced renal prostacyclin release suppresses platelet aggregation in the anesthetized dog. Abstracts of the Fourth International Prostaglandin Conference, Washington, D.C., May 27–31, 1979, p. 106.

268. Shio, H., and Ramwell, P. (1972) Effect of prostaglandin E_2 and aspirin on the secondary aggregation of human platelets. Nature (London) New Biol. 236, 45–46.

269. Silberbauer, K., Schernthaner, G., Sinzinger, H., Clopath, P., Piza-Katzer, H., and Winter, M. (1979) Diminished prostacyclin generation in human and experimentally induced (streptozotocin, alloxan) diabetes mellitus. Thromb. Haemostasis 42, 334 (Abstr.).

270. Silberbauer, K., Sinzinger, H., and Winter, M. (1979) Prostacyclin activity in rat kidney stimulated by angiotensin II. Br. J. Exp. Pathol. 60, 38–44.

271. Silver, M. J., Smith, J. B., Ingerman, C., and Kocsis, J. J. (1973) Arachidonic acid

induced human platelet aggregation and prostaglandin formation. Prostaglandins 4, 863.

272. Silver, M. J., Hoch, W., Kocsis, J. J., Ingerman, C. M., and Smith, J. B. (1974) Arachidonic acid causes sudden death in rabbits. Science 183, 1085–1087.

273. Sim, A. K., and McCraw, A. P. (1977) The activity of γ-linolenate and dihomo-γ-linolenate methyl esters in vitro and in vivo on blood platelet function in non-human primates and in man. Thromb. Res. 10, 385–397.

274. Sinha, A. K., and Colman, R. W. (1978) Prostaglandin E_1 inhibits platelet aggregation by a pathway independent of adenosine, 3',5'-monophosphate. Science 200, 202–203.

275. Sinzinger, H., Clopath, P., and Silberbauer, K. (1979) Increased prostacyclin generation in minipig vascular tissue after atherogenic diet. Thromb. Haemostasis 42, 424 (Abstr.).

276. Smith, D. R., Weatherly, B. C., Salmon, J. A., Ubatuba, F. B., Gryglewski, R. J., and Moncada, S. (1979) Preparation and biochemical properties of PGH_3. Prostaglandins 18, 423–438.

277. Smith, J. B., and Willis, A. L. (1971) Aspirin selectively inhibits prostaglandin production in human platelets. Nature (London) New Biol. 231, 235–237.

278. Smith, J. B., Ingerman, C., Kocsis, J. J., and Silver, M. J. (1973) Formation of prostaglandins during the aggregation of human blood platelets. J. Clin. Invest. 52, 965–969.

279. Smith, J. B., and Macfarlane, D. E. (1974) Platelets. In: P. W. Ramwell (ed.), The Prostaglandins, Vol. 2, Plenum Press, New York and London, pp. 293–343.

280. Smith, J. B., Silver, M. J., Ingerman, C. M., and Kocsis, J. J. (1974) Prostaglandin D_2 inhibits the aggregation of human platelets. Thromb. Res. 5, 291–299.

281. Smith, J. B., Ingerman, C. M., and Silver, M. J. (1976) Formation of prostaglandin D_2 during endoperoxide-induced platelet aggregation. Thromb. Res. 9, 413–418.

282. Smith, J. B., Sedar, A. W., Ingerman, C. M., and Silver, M. J. (1977) Prostaglandin endoperoxides: Platelet shape change, aggregation and the release reaction. In: D. C. B. Mills and J. F. Pareti (eds.), Platelets and Thrombosis, Academic Press, London, New York, San Francisco, pp. 83–95.

283. Smith, J. B., Ogletree, M. L., Lefer, A. M., and Nicolaou, K. C. (1978) Antibodies which antagonize the effects of prostacyclin. Nature (London) 274, 64–65.

284. Smith, J. B., Ingerman, C. M., and Silver, M. J. (1979) Normal bleeding times in rabbits containing antibodies that bind prostacyclin (PGI_2). Thromb. Haemostasis 42, 7 (Abstr.).

285. Srivastava, K. C., and Rastogi, S. C. (1977) Effects of prostaglandins E_1 and E_2 on the de novo synthesis of lipids in human platelets and whole boood. Indian J. Biochem. Biophys. 14, 98–99.

286. Stone, K. J., Willes, A. L., Hart, M., Kirtland, S. J., Kernoff, P. B. A., and McNicol, G. P. (1979) The metabolism of dihomo-γ-linolenic acid in man. Lipids 14, 174–180.

287. Stuart, M. J., Murphy, S., and Oski, F. A. (1975) A simple non-radioisotope technique for the determination of platelet life-span, New Engl. J. Med. 1, 1310–1316.

288. Sun, F. F. (1977) Biosynthesis of thromboxanes in human platelets. I. Characterization and assay of thromboxane synthetase. Biochem. Biophys. Res. Commun. 74, 1432–1440.

289. Sun, F. F., McGuire, J. C., and Taylor, B. (1978) Metabolism of prostacyclin (PGI_2). Prostaglandins 15, 724 (Abstr.).

290. Sun, F. F., and Taylor, B. M. (1978) Metabolism of prostacyclin in rat. Biochemistry 17, 4096–4112.

291. Sun, F. F., Taylor, B. M., Sutter, D. M., and Weeks, J. R. (1979) Metabolism of prostacyclin. III. Urinary metabolite profile of 6-keto-$PGF_{1\alpha}$ in rat. Protaglandins 17, 753–759.

292. Szczeklik, A., and Gryglewski, R. J. (1978) Thromboxane A_2 synthesis in platelets of

patients with coronary heart disease. In: L. A. Carlson, R. Paoletti, C. R. Siroti, and G. Weber (eds.), International Conference of Atherosclerosis, Milan 1977, Raven Press, New York, pp. 597–606.

293. Szczeklik, A., Gryglewski, R. J., Musiał, J., Grodzińska, L., Serwońska, M., and Marcinkiewicz, E. (1978) Thromboxane generation and platelet aggregation in survivals of myocardial infarction. Thromb. Haemostasis 40, 66–74.

294. Szczeklik, A., Gryglewski, R. J., Niżankowski, R., Musiał, J., Piętoń, R., and Mruk, J. (1978) Circulatory and anti-platelet effects of intravenous prostacyclin in healthy men. Pharmacol. Res. Commun. 10, 545–556.

295. Szczeklik, A., Niżankowski, R., Skawiński, S., Szczeklik, J., Głuszko, P., and Gryglewski, R. J. (1979) Successful therapy of advanced arteriosclerosis obliterans with prostacyclin. Lancet, 1, 1111–1114.

296. Tai, H.-H., and Yuan, B. (1978) Studies on the thromboxane synthesizing system in human platelet microsomes. Biochim. Biophys. Acta. 531, 286–294.

297. Tai, H.-H., and Yuan, B. (1978) On the inhibitory potency of imidazole and its derivatives on thromboxane synthetase. Biochem. Biophys. Res. Commun. 80, 236–242.

298. Tansik, R. L., Namm, D. H., and White, H. L. (1978) Synthesis of prostaglandin 6-keto $PGF_{1\alpha}$ by cultured aortic smooth muscle cells and stimulation of its formation in a coupled system with platelet lysates. Prostaglandins 15, 399–408.

299. Tateson, J. E., Moncada, S., and Vane, J. R. (1977) Effects of prostacyclin (PBX) on cyclic AMP concentrations in human platelets. Prostaglandins 13, 389–397.

300. Taura, S., Taura, M., and Kummerow, F. A. (1978) Human arterio- and atherosclerosis: Identical to that in 6 and 36 months old swine fed a corn soy diet free of cholesterol and saturated fat. Artery 4, 100–106.

301. Ten Hoor, F., and Quadt, J. F. A. (1979) Effect of nicotine on prostacyclin production by the isolated pulsatingly perfused rat aorta. Abstracts of the Fourth International Prostaglandin Conference in Washington, D. C., May 28–31, 1979, p. 52.

302. Terragno, N. A., Terragno, A., McGiff, J. C., and Rodriguez, D. J. (1977) Synthesis of prostaglandins by the ductus arteriosus of the bovine fetus. Prostaglandins 14, 721–727.

303. The Anturan Reinfarction Trial Research Group (1978) Sulfinpyrazone in the prevention of cardiac death after myocardial infarction. New Engl. J. Med. 298, 289–298.

304. Tomasi, V., Meringolo, C., Bartolini, G., and Orlandi, M. (1978) Biosynthesis of prostacyclin in rat liver endothelial cells and its control by prostaglandin E_2. Nature (London) 273, 670–671.

305. Tsao, C., and Holly, C. M. (1979) Arachidonic acid causes lysis of human platelets in an artificial medium: Protection by plasma. Prostaglandins 17, 775–784.

306. Tschopp, T. B., and Baumgartner, H. R. (1979) Platelet adhesion and aggregation in arteries of rats, rabbits and guinea pigs in vivo correlate negatively with their prostacyclin (PGI_2) production. Thromb. Haemostasis 42, 174 (Abstr.).

307. Ubatuba, F. B., Moncada, S., and Vane, J. R. (1979) The effect of prostacyclin (PGI_2) on platelet behaviour, thrombus formation in vivo and bleeding time. Thromb. Haemostasis 41, 425–435.

308. Vane, J. R. (1964) The use of isolated organs for detecting active substances in the circulating blood. Br. J. Pharmacol. 23, 360–373.

309. Vane, J. R. (1971) Inhibition of prostaglandin synthesis as a mechanism of action of aspirin-like drugs. Nature (London) New Biol. 231, 232–235.

310. Van Hoff. A., Chamone, D. A. F., and Vermylen, J. (1979) Plasma from patients with hepatic or renal failure stimulates prostacyclin release from "exhausted" rat aorta slices. Thromb. Haemostasis 42, 43 (Abstr.).

311. Vargaftig, B. B., and Zirinis, R. B. (1973) Platelet aggregation induced by arachidonic acid is accompanied by release of potential inflammatory mediators distinct from PGE_2 and $PGF_{2\alpha}$. Nature (London) New Biol. 244, 114–116.

312. Vargaftig. B. B., and Chignard, M. (1975) Substances that increase the cyclic AMP

content prevent platelet aggregation and the concurrent release of pharmacologically active substances evoked by arachidonic acid. Agents Actions 5 (2), 137–144.

313. Vargaftig, B. B. (1977) Carrageenan and thrombin trigger prostaglandin synthetase-independent aggregation of rabbit platelets: Inhibition by phospholipase A_2 inhibitors. J. Pharm. Pharmacol. 29, 222–228.

314. Vargaftig, B. B. (1978) Salicylic acid fails to inhibit generation of thromboxane A_2 activity in platelets after in vivo administration to the rat. J. Pharm. Pharmacol. 30, 101–104.

315. Vergroesen, A. J. (1978) The biology of linolenic acid. In: Z. M. Bacq (ed.), Colloque Consacré aux Acides Gras Polyinsaturés du 14 Octobre 1978, Palais des Academies, Bruxelles, pp. 47–61.

316. Verstraete, M. (1978) Antiplatelet agents in coronary disease: Are they of prophylactic value? Drugs 15, 464–471.

317. Villa, S., and de Gaetano, G. (1977) Prostacyclin-like activity in rat vascular tissues. Fast, long-lasting inhibition by treatment with lysine acetylsalicylate. Prostaglandins 14, 1117–1124.

318. Villa, S., Cavenaghi, A. E., and de Gaetano, G. (1979) Suloctidil does not inhibit vascular prostacyclin activity in rats. Thromb. Haemostasis 42, 368 (Abstr.).

319. Villa, S., and de Gaetano, G. (1979) Aspirin, dipyridamole, prostacyclin (PGI_2) and bleeding time in rats. Thromb. Haemostasis 42, 242 (Abstr.).

320. Vincent, J. E., and Zijlstra, F. J. (1978) Nicotinic acid inhibits thromboxane synthesis and platelets. Prostaglandins 15, 629–636. (Abstr.).

321. Wallach, D. (1978) Biosynthesis of 6-keto $PGF_{1\alpha}$ by microsomal acetone-pentane powder preparations from hog aorta, ram seminal vesicles and bovine corpora lutea: Properties of same. Prostaglandins 15, 671–684.

322. Wallis, R. B. (1978) The role of prostaglandins in the ADP-induced aggregation of rabbit platelets shown by the use of 15-hydroxyprostaglandin dehydrogenase. Thromb. Haemostasis 39, 725–732.

323. Walter, E., Siess, R., Zimmermann, R., and Weber, E. (1979) Also high dose of aspirin prolongs bleeding time, but later after ingestion. Thromb. Haemostasis 42, 242 (Abstr.).

324. Weidemann, M. J., Peskar, B. A., Wrogemann, K., Rietschel, E. T., Staudinger, H., and Fischer, H. (1978) Prostaglandin and thromboxane synthesis in a pure macrophage population and the inhibition by E-type prostaglandins of chemiluminescence. FEBS Let. 89, 136–139.

325. Weihrauch, J. L., Brignoli, C. A., Reeves, J. N., and Iverson, L. (1977) Fatty acid composition of margarines, processed fats and oils. Food Technol. 1, 80–85.

326. Weithmann, K. U., Bartmann, W., Beck, G., Lerch, U., Konz, E., and Schölkens, B. A. (1979) Comparisons of biochemical and pharmacological properties of prostacyclins with modified ω-side chain. Thromb. Haemostasis 42, 119 (Abstr.).

327. Wennmalm, A. (1978) Effects of nicotine on cardiac prostaglandin and platelet thromboxane synthesis. Br. J. Pharmacol. 64, 559–563.

328. Weksler, B. B., Marcus, A. J., and Jaffe, E. A. (1977) Synthesis of prostaglandin I_2 (prostacyclin) by cultured human and bovine endothelial cells. Proc. Natl. Acad. Sci. (USA) 74, 3922–3926.

329. Weksler, B. B., Ley, C. W., and Jaffe, E. A. (1978) Stimulation of endothelial cell prostacyclin production by thrombin, trypsin and the ionophore A23187. J. Clin. Invest. 923–930.

330. Westwick, J., and Webb, H. (1978) Selective antagonism of prostaglandin (PG) E_1, PGD_2 and prostacyclin (PGI_2) on human and rabbit platelets by di-4-phloretin phosphate (DPP). Thromb. Res. 12, 973–978.

331. Westwick, J., Webb, J., and Lewis, G. P. (1979) The effect of sulfinpyrazone, aspirin, and their metabolites on prostacyclin production by rabbit aortic rings. Thromb. Haemostasis 42, 99 (Abstr.).

332. Westwick, J., Webb, H., and Lewis, G. P. (1979) Comparison of sulfinpyrazone and

its metabolites on TxB$_2$ and PGE$_2$ generation by human platelets. Thromb. Haemostasis 42, 402 (Abstr.).

333. White, H. L., and Glassman, A. T. (1976) Biochemical properties of the prostaglandin/thromboxane synthetase of human blood platelets and comparison with the synthetase of bovine seminal vesicles. Prostaglandins 12, 811–828.

334. White, J. G., and Gerrard, J. M. (1976) Ultrastructural features of abnormal blood platelets. Am. J. Pathol. 83, 589–632.

335. White, J. G., and Gerrard, J. M. (1978) Platelet morphology and the ultrastructure of regulatory mechanisms involved in platelet activation. In: G. de Gaetano and S. Garatini (eds.), Platelets: A Multidisciplinary Approach, Raven Press, New York, pp. 17–34.

336. Whittle, B. J. R., Moncada, S., and Vane, J. R. (1978) Formation of prostacyclin by the gastric mucosa and its actions on gastric function. Prostaglandins 15, 704 (Abstr.).

337. Whittle, B. J. R., Moncada, S., and Vane, J. R. (1978) Comparison of the effects of prostacyclin (PGI$_2$). prostaglandin E$_1$ and D$_2$ on platelet aggregation in different species. Prostaglandins 16, 373–388.

338. Whorton, A. R., Smigiel, M., Oates, J. A., and Fröhlich, J. C. (1978) Regional differences in prostacyclin formation by the kidney. Prostacyclin is a major metabolite of renal cortex. Biochim. Biophys. Acta 529, 176–180.

339. Willems, C., van Aken, W. G., Peuscher-Prakke, E. M., and van Mourik, J. A. (1979) Synthesis of PGI$_2$ by cultured human vascular endothelial cells and stabilization of PGI$_2$ by blood components. Thromb. Haemostasis 42, 6 (Abstr.).

340. Williams, K. I., Dembińska-Kieć, A., Zmuda, A., and Gryglewski, R. J. (1978) Prostacyclin formation by myometrial and decidual fractions of pregnant rat uterus. Prostaglandins 15, 343–350.

341. Willis, A. L. (1974) Isolation of a chemical trigger for thrombosis. Prostaglandins 5, 1–25.

342. Willis, A. L., Comai, K., Kuhn, D. C., and Paulsrud, J. (1974) Dihomo-γ-linolenate suppresses platelet aggregation when administered in vitro and in vivo. Prostaglandins 8, 509–519.

343. Willis, A. L., Kuhn, D. C., and Weiss, H. J. (1974) Acetylenic analog of arachidonate that acts like aspirin on platelets. Science 183, 327–329.

344. Wilson, R. B., Kula, N. S., Newberne, P. M., and Conner, M. W. (1973) Vascular damage and lipid peroxidation in choline-deficient rats. Exp. Mol. Pathol. 18, 357–368.

345. Winocour, P. D., Groves, H. M., Dejana, E., Kinlough-Rathbone, R. L., and Mustard, F. J. (1979) The effects of dietary fats in rabbits on platelet survival, platelet turnover, platelet density, PGI$_2$ production and thrombus formation in response to an aortic indwelling cannula. Thromb. Haemostasis 42, 423 (Abstr.).

346. Wissler, R. W., Vesselinowitch, D., Goetz, G. S., and Hughes, R. H. (1967) Aortic lesions and blood lipids in rhesus monkeys fed three different food fats. Fed. Proc. 26, 371–382.

347. Woods, H. F., Ash, G., Weston, M. J., Stuart, S., Moncada, S., and Vane, J. R. (1978) Prostacyclin can replace heparin in haemodialysis in dogs. Lancet 2, 1075–1077.

348. Woods, H. F., and Weston, M. J. (1979) Prostacyclin can replace heparin for haemodialysis in dogs, Thromb. Haemostasis 42, 131 (Abstr.).

349. Woods, H. F., and Weston, M. J. (1979) The use of prostacyclin (PGI$_2$) during charcoal haemoperfusion. Thromb. Haemostasis 42, 131 (Abstr.).

350. Zmuda, A., Dembińska-Kieć, A., Chytkowski, A., and Gryglewski, R. J. (1977) Experimental atherosclerosis in rabbits: Platelet aggregability, thromboxane A$_2$ generation and anti-aggregatory potency of prostacyclin. Prostaglandins 14, 1035–1042.

LAWRENCE G. RAISZ, M.D.

PROSTAGLANDINS
AND SKELETAL METABOLISM

INTRODUCTION

The role of prostaglandins and related compounds in skeletal metabolism is not as well established as that for the cardiovascular and reproductive systems. Nevertheless, there is substantial evidence that prostaglandins may mediate pathologic changes in bone, cartilage, and associated connective tissues. There is less evidence for a physiologic role for this class of compounds in skeletal growth and remodeling, but such a role seems likely on the basis of the potency of their skeletal action and the known sites of production. This chapter summarizes available data on the effects of prostaglandins on bone and cartilage, the production of prostaglandins by these tissues, and the role of prostaglandins in the pathologic destruction of skeletal tissue in malignancy and inflammatory disease.

Since there is a detailed discussion of bone metabolism at the cell and organ level and its regulation by hormones in another volume of this series, only a few general points concerning skeletal structure and function are made here, to indicate the sites at which prostaglandins might have an effect. Cartilage and bone are closely linked in skeletal growth. Developmentally, cartilage provides the template for initial bone for-

From the Section of Endocrinology and Metabolism, Department of Medicine, University of Connecticut Health Center, Farmington, Connecticut.

mation, which begins as a thin periosteal collar around the cartilage core in much of the skeleton; later trabecular bone is formed on the template of calcified cartilage in the primary spongiosa. Some membranous bones particularly in the skull may arise without a cartilage anlage. Hence, cartilage growth is most important for initial development and subsequent linear growth. This process is regulated by the growth hormone–dependent somatomedins, by the steroid hormones, including sex hormones, and probably also by calcium-regulating hormones. Prostaglandins are present at those sites and may have regulatory functions as well. As skeletal development is completed, more and more of the activity of bone cells is devoted to remodeling rather than to initial bone formation. Many humoral mechanisms can affect remodeling, and it is likely that prostaglandins are involved in this process. Calcium-regulating hormones affect the remodeling process through their influence on osteoclastic bone resorption and on matrix formation and mineral deposition. These hormones are largely controlled by body needs for calcium and phosphate. Parathyroid hormone (PTH) and the active metabolite of vitamin D (1,25-dihydroxyvitamin D or calcitriol) increase skeletal breakdown and may decrease skeletal growth when calcium and phosphate are in short supply. However, when mineral supplies are adequate the increases in bone resorption and intestinal absorption produced by these hormones may be associated with increased bone formation. One reason for this association is that the formation of new bone in the adult skeleton is largely at sites of previous resorption. This occurs in Haversian remodeling when resorption cavities formed by osteoclasts are refilled by concentric layers of osteoblasts, and in trabecular remodeling when scalloped resorption surfaces (Howship's lacunae) are the sites of new bone deposition. This coupling presumably is determined locally and the humoral factors involved are unknown, but a role for prostaglandins has been suggested.

Metabolic bone diseases that impair skeletal structure and function usually disrupt orderly coupling. In age-related bone loss there are many local areas of intense resorption where formation does not keep pace, producing loss of trabecular bone and increased cortical porosity. Disorderly coupling may occur in Paget's disease, in which bone formation is accelerated in response to the abnormal proliferation of osteoclasts, which is the primary lesion. The trabecular structure becomes distorted and the skeleton is structurally impaired, with resulting deformities. Irregular bone formation can also occur in malignancy, where osteolysis by tumor cells or their products is the primary lesion.

These basic principles of skeletal function in health and disease should be kept in mind in considering the implications of a particular effect of a prostaglandin on bone metabolism. Unfortunately, we have few data concerning the physiologic effects of prostaglandins in vivo. Most of the data have been obtained in vitro, or under unusual pathologic circumstances. Nevertheless, the effects of prostaglandins on skeletal tissue are striking and the amounts involved relatively small; thus it seems likely that many examples of prostaglandin-mediated alterations in bone and cartilage metabolism will be encountered in the future.

EFFECTS OF PROSTAGLANDINS

Effects on Bone Resorption

The first indication that there might be a role for prostaglandins in skeletal metabolism came from the finding that PGE_1 and PGE_2 could increase cyclic adenosine 3',5'-monophosphate (cAMP) content in fetal rat calvaria [20] and stimulate resorption of fetal rat long bone shafts [62]. It has been widely assumed that these two phenomena are related, and, as discussed below, structure-activity relations for stimulation of bone resorption and increases in adenyl cyclase activity or tissue cAMP content in bone cells are generally parallel. However, the bone cell populations that have been shown to respond to prostaglandins do not consist of resorptive cells or their precursors alone. In fact, extensive studies on cAMP have been done on an osteosarcoma cell line, which is more closely related to osteoblastic than to osteoclastic cells [2,3,71]. Because of this, and because the effects on osteoclastic cells are believed to be of the greatest importance for the pathologic effects of prostaglandins, these are discussed first and the cAMP studies considered separately.

Most of the data show that prostaglandins of the E series are the most potent stimulators of bone resorption (Table 1). The number of double bonds in the side chain has some effect on potency, PGE_1 is less potent than PGE_2, whereas both 13,14-dihydro-PGE_2 and PGE_1 are less potent than the most unsaturated compounds. The 15-hydroxyl group seems to be of considerable importance, since 15-keto compounds are relatively

TABLE 1. Relative Potencies of Various Prostaglandins in Stimulation of Bone Resorption in Vitro and Cyclic AMP Production in Osteosarcoma Cells

Agent	Bone resorption	Cyclic AMP production
PGE_2	100	100
PGE_1	50	100
PGI_2	10–100*	10
$PGF_{2\alpha}$	5–10†	5
PGA_2	5–10	5
PGB_2	1	1
PGD_2	1	1
Thromboxane B_2	1	1
6-K to $PGF_{1\alpha}$	1	1
13,14-Dihydro-PGE_2	10–50	50
15-Keto-13,14-dihydro-PGE_2	1	1

Note: Approximate potencies relative to PGE_2 are based on a compilation of published data [2,3,23, 26,28,116]. Values of 1 indicate that only mineral resorption or cyclic AMP production was found, or high concentrations, usually 10^{-5} M.

*Potency estimated from multiple injections or continuous infusion.

†In one study $PGF_{2\alpha}$ was more potent than PGE_2 (28).

inactive. The configuration of oxygen groups on the pentane ring also has an important effect. Prostaglandins of the F series are generally less potent than those of the E series in long bone cultures, and similar results have been obtained in mouse calvaria, although in one report $PGF_{2\alpha}$ was found to be more effective than PGE_2 [28]. The reason for the latter discrepancy is not clear, but the binding or stability of the compound in the culture media used may be implicated [26]. Among the other prostaglandins, PGA and PGB and PGD show decreasing activity, in the order given. Since PGD_2, the enantiomer of PGE_2, was almost inactive, it was tested as a possible antagonist, but it did not block the response to PGE_2 (L. G. Raisz and H. A. Simmons, unpublished observations). The other stable products of the arachidonate pathway, thromboxane B_2 and 6-keto-$PGF_{1\alpha}$, which are the degradation products of the short-lived compounds thromboxane A_2 and prostacyclin (PGI_2), are also relatively inactive [88,116]. The dose-response curves for prostaglandin stimulation of bone resorption differ in different culture systems. A steep dose-response curve is obtained using mouse calvaria [28,116]. Using rat long bone shafts the dose-response curve is relatively flat, extending from 10^{-7} to 10^{-5} M with inhibition at higher concentrations, which may indicate toxicity (Fig. 1). In contrast, PTH has a more rapid effect and a steeper dose-response curve, with a response that remains constant at supramaximal doses [83].

Qualitatively, there seems to be little difference in the resorptive response to prostaglandins and to other stimulators, despite the differences in time course and slope of the dose-response curve. Resorption is by osteoclasts, large multinucleated cells with an active pinocytotic ruffled border and a surrounding clear zone that may facilitate attachment of the cell to bone [50,51]. Increases in osteoclast size and disproportionate increases in ruffled border and clear zone area have been found using quantitative electron microscopy, similar to the effects of PTH (Table 2). Increased numbers of osteoclasts are found in mouse calvaria cultured with PGE_2 [101a]. Prostaglandins also produce an early release of lysosomal enzymes similar to that produced by PTH [32]. Collagenase activity may also be increased, but this is a late effect [99a]. Calcitonin and colchicine can block PGE_2-stimulated bone resorption and lysosomal enzyme release. Glucocorticoids can also inhibit PGE-stimulated resorption, although the effect is somewhat variable [85].

TABLE 2. Areas of Total Cell, Ruffled Border, and Clear Zone in Osteoclasts of Fetal Rat Bones Cultured with PGE_2 (10^{-6} M) for 24 Hours

Treatment	Cell	Ruffled border	Clear zone
Control	250	3	6
PGE_2	490*	24*	19*
PTH	430*	21*	18*

Note: Values are means (μ^2) for 35–110 osteoclast profiles, modified from Holtrop and Raisz [52].
*Significantly different from control, $p < 0.01$.

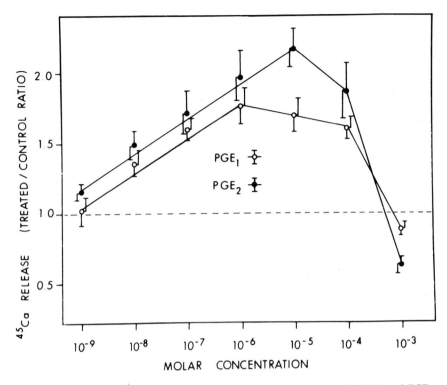

FIGURE 1. Dose-response curve for stimulation of bone resorption by PGE_2 and PGE_1. Resorption is measured as the ratio of the release of previously incorporated ^{45}Ca from prostaglandin-treated bones to the paired, untreated controls. Points represent the mean and vertical lines, standard error for 4–16 pairs. (From Dietrich et al. [26].)

The effects of the short-lived intermediates of prostaglandin synthesis have not been studied extensively. Multiple doses of the endoperoxides PGG_2 and PGH_2 caused a transient release of calcium from cultured fetal rat long bones at 6 hours, but no prolonged resorption at 48 hours [88]. In contrast, multiple injections of PGI_2, as well as PGE_2, for 6 hours, produced a prolonged resorptive response at 48 hours, when the bones were transferred to medium without added prostaglandin [90]. Prostacyclin and the endoperoxides were administered in this fashion because of their short half-life. An infusion of prostacyclin has also produced a resorptive response [9]. These effects correlate well with the effects on cAMP production [23]. In preliminary studies thromboxane A_2 produced by adding platelets and arachidonate to bone cultures did not stimulate resorption (W. A. Soskolne and L. G. Raisz, unpublished observations), and addition to osteosarcoma cells had little effect on cAMP levels (T. J. Martin, personal communication). Stable analogues of these short-lived compounds have also been studied. Endoperoxide analogues in which the oxygen bridge was replaced by methoxy or diazo groups were inactive in stimulating bone resorption [116]. In contrast, among the stable sulfur analogues of prostacyclin, the unoxidized thiaprostacyclin did stimulate bone resorption, but the oxidized sulfona and sulfoxo analogues were ineffective [90].

The induction of prolonged resorption after brief application of PGE_2 and PGI_2 may represent an important mechanism for stimulation of bone resorption, although prostaglandins appear to be less effective than PTH, osteoclast-activating factor (OAF), or vitamin D metabolites in this regard [83]. If pulsatile prostaglandin release can activate the osteoclast for long periods, intermittent production may produce a resorptive response that does not correlate with prostaglandin levels in the tissues at the same time resorption is most active.

There are a few studies of the interactions between prostaglandins and other bone-resorbing agents. Recently, we found that the stimulation of bone resorption by endotoxin and PGE_2 may be synergistic, in that concentrations of either agent that are minimally effective in stimulating bone resorption can produce a large increase when added together (C. B. Alander, W. A. Soskolne, and L. G. Raisz, unpublished observations) (Table 3). Another more complex form of interaction was recently described by Yoneda and Mundy [127], who showed that PGE secretion from macrophages was essential for production of OAF by lymphocytes. It had been shown earlier that lymphocytes that had been stimulated by mitogens could not produce OAF in the absence of macrophages. The finding that this lymphocyte-macrophate synergy could

TABLE 3. Interaction Between *S. Typhimurium* Endotoxin (Endo) and Prostaglandin (PGE_2) in Stimulation of Resorption in 5-Day Cultures of Fetal Rat Long Bones

Treatment	^{45}Ca released (%)	Ratio of treated cultures to controls
Control	36 ± 1	
Endo		
0.25 µg/ml	46 ± 4	1.27 ± 0.12*
0.06 µg/ml	36 ± 6	1.01 ± 0.16
PGE_2		
10^{-7} M	47 ± 6	1.32 ± 0.17*
10^{-8} M	38 ± 3	1.04 ± 0.10
PGE_2 10^{-8} + endo 0.25 µg/ml	72 ± 5	2.01 ± 0.13†
PGE_2 10^{-8} + endo 0.06 µg/ml	64 ± 6	1.79 ± 0.16†

Note: Values are means ± standard error for six cultures (unpublished data of C. B. Alander and L. G. Raisz).
*Significantly greater than 1.0; $p < .05$.
†Significantly greater than 1.0; $p < .01$.

be replaced by the addition of low concentration of prostaglandin to the medium, coupled with the observation that macrophages produce prostaglandins, indicates another indirect role for prostaglandins in mediating bone resorption under pathologic circumstances. PGE production by macrophages may also be important in facilitating collagenase release from these cells [123], which in turn can resorb bone directly [77].

Bone cells can produce prostaglandins under a wide variety of conditions, and this can result in increased resorption. Prostaglandin production in organ cultures, sufficient to stimulate a resorptive response, was first demonstrated after the addition of complement-sufficient serum and antibodies to cell surface antigens [87,90,100]. The response was dependent on late components and was absent in C_6-deficient serum but was independent of whether activation of complement was by the classical or the alternative pathway. The resorptive response and prostaglandin production can be greatly enhanced by the addition of high concentrations of arachidonic acid to the culture medium. Prostaglandin synthesis in bone has also been produced by treatment with a crude bacterial collagenase [27] and with phorbol esters or mellitin [120], which would share with activated complement the ability to produce cell membrane damage. It seems likely that these agents could activate membrane phospholipase and release arachidonate [10]. There may be an additional effect to increase prostaglandin synthetase activity or access to this enzyme complex, since the effect of exogenous arachidonate is seen only in the presence of complement. Recently, Tashjian and Levine [119] reported that prostaglandins mediate the stimulation of bone resorption produced by low concentrations of epidermal and fibroblastic growth factors (EGF and FGF), peptides that bind to cell membranes but certainly have not been implicated as lytic agents. This mechanism, which was observed in calvaria from neonatal mice, was not found in fetal rat long bone cultures. In the latter FGF had no effect on resorption and EGF stimulated resorption by a mechanism independent of prostaglandin synthesis [106].

Other resorptive effects may involve prostaglandin synthesis, by bone itself. Goldhaber et al. described an effect of gingival extracts on mouse calvaria that could be blocked by indomethacin [40]. Stern et al. [110] found that the bone-resorbing activity in bovine serum albumin is partially inhibited by indomethacin. Similarly, we found bone-resorbing activity of fetal calf serum that could be partially inhibited by indomethacin [67]. Since these proteins were inactivated by heat, the effect could not be ascribed to complement. Recently, Goodson et al. [43] reported that indomethacin treatment of pregnant rats resulted in an increase in sensitivity of the fetal bones to exogenous prostaglandins. This suggested that the endogenous prostaglandin synthesis was normally present and that removal of this source might cause increased sensitivity. Goodson also reported that the bone-resorbing activity of endotoxin could be inhibited by indomethacin [43], but this finding has not been confirmed by other investigators [48]. Finally, in isolated bone cells it has been possible to show that prostaglandin production can be stimulated by pressure or stretch on the dish to which the cells were attached [45].

Effects on Bone Formation

Studies on effects of prostaglandins on skeletal growth in vitro have shown that PGE_2 or PGE_1 inhibits collagen synthesis in fetal rat calvaria at concentrations of 10^{-6} and 10^{-5} M [84]. These concentrations do not inhibit the synthesis of noncollagen protein. Some other prostaglandins have a more general inhibitory effect on protein synthesis; for example, in an action similar to its effect on cartilage, PGA_2 at 10^{-5} and 10^{-4} M inhibits both collagen and noncollagen protein synthesis. PGE_1 has also been found to inhibit collagen synthesis in isolated bone cells [46]. There is one report of increased incorporation of proline into collagen with prostaglandin treatment of chick bone rudiments, but effects on amino acid uptake or precursor pools were not ruled out [11].

The role of endogenous prostaglandins in regulating bone formation is unknown. In organ cultures of fetal rat calvaria, complement increases prostaglandin release and produces a marked inhibition of protein synthesis with some selective reduction of osteoblastic activity, but this effect cannot be reversed by inhibitors of prostaglandin cyclooxygenase, although a small increase in collagen labeling is observed (Table 4). In contrast, cultured bone cells that increase prostaglandin synthesis in response to mechanical stress show an increase in cell replication [107a]. Thus, it is possible that prostaglandins have different effects on differentiated osteoblasts and on their precursors.

TABLE 4. Effect of Complement (Unheated Rabbit Serum) and Drugs That Block Prostaglandin Cyclooxygenase on the Incorporation of [³H] Proline into Collagenase-Digestible Protein (CDP) and Noncollagen Protein (NCP) in Fetal Rat Calvaria

	Effect (dpm/μg dry weight) on		Collagen synthesis (%)
	CDP	NCP	
Heat-inactivated rabbit serum	43 ± 3*	55 ± 2*	12.6 ± 0.7*
Unheated rabbit serum	12 ± 1	34 ± 2	6.0 ± 0.4
Unheated rabbit serum + indomethacin, 10^{-5} M	19 ± 1*	36 ± 2	8.7 ± 0.5*
Unheated rabbit serum + flufenamic acid, 10^{-5} M	17 ± 2*	35 ± 3	8.1 ± 0.5*

Note: Values are means ± standard error for eight bone cultures 24 hours in 5% serum, and pulsed for the last 2 hours with [³H]proline (unpublished data of B. E. Kream and L. G. Raisz).
*Significantly different from unheated rabbit serum; $p < .02$.

Effects on Cartilage

High concentrations of prostaglandins have been shown to inhibit cartilage proteoglycan synthesis [33,34,61,63,65,68]. Protein and nucleic acid synthesis are also inhibited, but the effect does not appear to be ascribable to nonspecific cell damage [33]. Prostaglandin A_2 appears to be the most potent of the prostaglandins in producing this effect, though high concentrations are still required (10^{-5} to 10^{-4} M). Data on the effects of lower concentrations of prostaglandins are relatively few. Small stimulatory effects have been described [19,63], but there are no studies of specificity or structure-activity relations. Decreased incorporation of labeled sulfate into cartilage has been reported in animals on diets deficient in essential fatty acids [80], but it has not been possible to reverse this defect with specific prostaglandins. There is a report that high concentrations of prostaglandins can produce cartilage degradation directly, with release of proteoglycan aggregates [121]. Thus it is possible that prostaglandin production is important in the pathogenesis of articular damage in various forms of arthritis. On the other hand in vivo studies show that prostaglandin therapy can actually result in improvement in experimental arthritis. This beneficial effect may be due to suppression of the cell-mediated immune response [13,130]. Prostaglandins can also inhibit the release of degradative enzymes from polymorphonuclear leukocytes, which could be involved in cartilage breakdown in inflammation [57].

Cartilage contains the enzymes for both synthesis and degradation of prostaglandins [79,125,126]. Synthetic activity appears to be greatest in the early hypertrophic zone, whereas degradative activity appears to be greatest in calcified cartilage. These results could indicate that prostaglandins play a role in the differentiation and mineralization of cartilage. Perhaps such a role might explain the observation that treatment with the prostaglandin synthesis inhibitor, indomethacin, can delay healing of experimental fractures [93,112]. Indomethacin treatment not only causes prolongation of the early phases during which cartilaginous transformation and remodeling predominate, but also results in a larger hematoma, perhaps related to an effect on platelets or blood vessels. Prostaglandins have also been reported both to stimulate and to inhibit fibroblast, collagen, and proteoglycan synthesis [13,19,24,80].

Effects on Cyclic Nucleotides

The original demonstration that prostaglandins can stimulate bone resorption was stimulated by the finding that these compounds increase cyclic AMP content of fetal rat calvaria in a manner similar to PTH. A number of subsequent studies have confirmed that prostaglandins activate adenyl cyclase in bone or bone cells and produce a rapid increase in cyclic AMP content [49,59,69,91,128,129]. This initial marked increase is transient, lasting less than an hour, although values may remain slightly above the initial control level for up to 24 hours. The time course is usually similar to that for PTH, but prolonged subcultivation of bone cells can produce populations that respond more slowly to PGE than to PTH [91]. Malignant cell lines from a rat osteosarcoma also show a response to both hormones, although dissociation can occur upon subculture [2,3].

The initial exposure to PGE produces desensitization to its subsequent administration. This desensitization has been observed in isolated bone cells [49] and in osteosarcoma cells [72], as well as in organ cultures of fetal rat and mouse calvaria [49]. In organ culture desensitization is generally hormone specific; that is, the initial exposure to PGE reduces the response to a second dose of PGE but not to a second dose of PTH, and vice versa. However, in cell cultures PGE pretreatment can decrease the subsequent response to PTH [59].

It is not yet possible to determine whether increases in cyclic AMP are more closely related to the effects of prostaglandins on osteoclastic bone resorption or osteoblastic bone formation or are equally important for both responses. Most of the studies have been carried out in cell preparations in which osteoblasts predominate or in osteosarcoma cells, which are derived from osteoblasts. On the other hand, PGE can increase cAMP concentrations in cells derived from giant cell tumors of bone, which may be related to osteoclasts [40a]. Moreover, the structure-activity relations for increasing cAMP with different prostaglandins in osteosarcoma cells closely parallel their relative potencies for stimulation of bone resorption (Table 1). In cartilage the inhibitory effects on proteoglycan synthesis that are produced by PGA are clearly dissociated from cAMP, which is most affected by PGE [34]. Of course, prostaglandins can increase cAMP concentration in other cell types including lymphocytes and fibroblasts [14,40,123].

Effects on Calcium

Studies on the mechanism of action of PTH have suggested that not only cyclic nucleotides, but also calcium ions may act as messengers in transmitting the hormone effect from the cell membrane to the cytosol and nucleus. Evidence that prostaglandins have a similar effect on calcium transport in skeletal tissue was reported recently [70]. The effects of prostaglandins on calcium transport and binding in other tissues are complex [54,92]. An initial increase and a subsequent decrease have been described, and these effects are consistent with the biphasic dose-response curves observed for prostaglandin stimulation of many processes, including bone resorption. Prostaglandins can also complex with calcium [1], and since they are lipid soluble, they may exhibit some of the properties of a calcium ionophore [60].

Effects on Calcium Regulation and Bone Metabolism In Vivo

All the other known potent stimulators of bone resorption can produce hypercalcemia. Hence there have been numerous attempts to produce hypercalcemia by administration of prostaglandins in vivo. Most of these have been unsuccessful [6,62], but in two studies small increases in serum calcium concentration were observed after short-term intravenous or intraarterial infusion [37,94]. In another study when 16-dimethyl PGE_2, which is resistant to inactivation by prostaglandin 15-dehydrogenase, was administered for prolonged periods, osteoclast number increased, but serum calcium concentration decreased [101]. Local injection of prostaglandins on the surface of rat calvaria produced a bone lesion in which there was evidence of resorption [42a]. The most striking evidence for the importance of prostaglandin stimulation of bone resorption in vivo is from animals bearing prostaglandin-producing tumors, which develop hypercalcemia and show increases in osteoclast number (see below).

It is possible that some of the effects of prostaglandins on serum calcium concentration in vivo are indirect, resulting from changes in the synthesis or secretion of calcium-regulating hormones. Stimulation has been reported of both calcitonin and PTH secretion [16,99], so that either hyper- or hypocalcemia might result.

PROSTAGLANDINS AS MEDIATORS

Hypercalcemia and Osteolysis in Malignancy

In 1972 Tashjian et al. [114] reported that the bone-resorbing factor secreted by cultures of the mouse HSDM 1 fibrosarcoma, was prostaglandin, mainly PGE_2. Moreover, mice bearing this tumor showed hypercalcemia that responded to treatment with indomethacin [115]. They postulated that the hypercalcemia of malignancy in this animal model was mediated by the synthesis and secretion of PGE_2 [64]. Even more striking results were obtained with another animal model, the Walker VX_2 carcinoma in the rabbit [122]. Animals bearing this tumor developed severe hypercalcemia, which could be prevented or reversed by treatment with indomethacin, and the tumor produced large amounts of PGE_2 in vitro. In vivo, however, in both the mouse and rabbit models, the concentration of PGE_2 in the serum was not high. It is likely that PGE_2 was being produced but rapidly metabolized, since the major metabolite, 13,14-dihydro-15-keto-PGE_2, was found in relatively high concentrations [104,117,118]. As noted above, this compound is not a potent bone resorber and therefore either PGE_2 itself, the 13,14-dihydro metabolite, which is biologically active, or some other prostaglandin may have been responsible for production of hypercalcemia. Animals bearing this tumor show morphologic evidence of osteoclastic bone destruction at sites distant from the primary lesion but also show inhibited bone formation [55,124]. It is possible that local skeletal production is involved rather than production by the tumor, for example, by one of the immune mechanisms described above. The hypercalcemic effect of the tumor apparently depends to some extent on its location. Hypercalcemia is striking when the VX_2 tumor is implanted subcutaneously, but not when the tumor is growing in the peritoneal cavity [127]. Other hypercalcemic animal tumors have been found to respond to indomethacin in vivo or

in vitro [81,111]. Prostaglandin production by the Walker 256 rat carcinosarcoma has been reported [108], but others have found that this
tumor secretes immunoreactive PTH [75]. It is possible that different cell
lines derived from the same tumor may show different behavior.

A number of studies have been carried out to determine the importance of prostaglandin synthesis in human hypercalcemia of malignancy,
and these have been critically analyzed in many reviews and editorials
[5,30,38,39,44,76,78,86,89,102,105,113]. Many human tumors have been
shown to produce prostaglandins in vitro. Among these renal cell carcinoma [4] is of particular interest, since this lesion frequently produces
hypercalcemia without metastasizing to bone. A number of patients
reported to have indomethacin-responsive hypercalcemia had renal cell
carcinoma [15,95,96]. However the most common tumor associated with
hypercalcemia is breast cancer with bone metastases. In vitro, breast
cancer tissue has been found to synthesize and release prostaglandin
[7,8,28]. A correlation between the amount of prostaglandin produced
and the frequency of hypercalcemia or osteolytic bone metastases has
been reported in human breast cancer [8,28,30], but this observation has
not been made consistently [12,18]. Moreover the ability to make prostaglandins is not limited to malignant tissue. Nonmalignant breast tissue
may produce prostaglandins [29,73], but preformed prostaglandin levels
are reported to be higher in malignancy [109]. Since so many tissues can
produce prostaglandins in vitro, this finding is not sufficient to implicate
these agents as the pathogenetic factor in hypercalcemia or osteolysis,
particularly since attempts to reduce hypercalcemia with inhibitors of
prostaglandin synthesis in breast cancer patients have been generally
unsuccessful [21,22].

The most convincing evidence that prostaglandins play a role in hypercalcemia in human malignancy was the report in 1974 by Seyberth
and associates [103], namely, that changes in serum calcium concentration and urine calcium excretion were correlated with the urinary excretion of a metabolite of PGE_2, termed PGE-M. The majority of the
patients were males with carcinoma of the lung. In patients without
evidence of bone metastases, hypercalcemia, hypercalciuria, and increased PGE-M excretion were all reversed by treatment with aspirin or
indomethacin. The changes in all three parameters in response to treatment were strikingly parallel (Fig. 2). Patients with bone metastases also
showed high PGE-M excretion that was decreased by inhibitors of prostaglandin synthesis, but unfortunately their hypercalcemia persisted.

The experience of physicians who treat a large number of patients
with hypercalcemia has been that treatment with indomethacin and
aspirin is only occasionally effective. There are many possible explanations for the disappointing results of inhibitor therapy. The most
obvious is that the tumor produces bone-resorbing factors other than
prostaglandins. There is evidence that breast cancer produces a
nonprostaglandin stimulator of bone resorption [30]. In hematologic
neoplasms, particularly multiple myeloma, another potent bone resorber
has been isolated, which appears to be the bone-resorbing lymphokine,

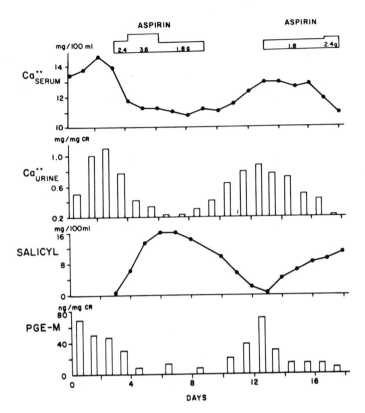

FIGURE 2. The effects of aspirin on serum calcium concentration, urine calcium excretion, and urinary excretion of 7α-hydroxy-5,11-diketo-tetranorprostane-1,16-dioic acid (PGE-M) in a 50-year-old patient with hypercalcemia due to squamous cell carcinoma of the pancreas with no evidence of bone metastases. (From Seyberth et al. [103].)

osteoclast-activating factor [76,86]. OAF is also secreted by antigen- or mitogen-stimulated normal lymphocytes and may play a role in bone loss associated with chronic inflammation. Although OAF has not been fully characterized chemically, it is clearly not a prostaglandin but a peptide. Some tumors may also produce PTH ectopically, though this is probably relatively rare [82,107]. Finally metastatic tumors may produce osteolysis directly without the intervention of osteoclasts [36,38,39]. This phenomenon has been observed in vitro with breast cancer cells [31].

Another possibility is that prostaglandins are important mediators in hypercalcemia but that the inhibitors are ineffective. One reason for this might be that the important source of prostaglandins in malignancy is not production by the tumor itself, but local production in bone. This might be much harder to inhibit with a circulating drug. Activated macrophages can produce prostaglandins [14,123], and these cells can accumulate around metastatic deposits in bone. Antigens from the tumor might become bound to cell surfaces, and antibodies to these antigens might then initiate complement-mediated prostaglandin production by the bone [87]. Alternatively, antibodies to the tumor could cross-react with bone cell surface antigens. Finally, low concentrations of prostaglandins might stimulate OAF production, as described above [126]. It is also possible that other oxygenated fatty acid products that are not produced by prostaglandin cyclooxygenase are involved, such as the unsaturated hydroperoxy fatty acids. Much further work needs to be done to clarify the precise mechanisms; however the fundamental observation that prostaglandins can play a role in hypercalcemia of malignancy seems reasonably well established.

Bone Destruction and Inflammation

Localized bone loss is regularly observed adjacent to sites of chronic inflammations. Bone loss around inflamed joints is an important factor in the osteopenia associated with rheumatoid arthritis, although other factors such as immobilization and the use of glucocorticoid therapy also contribute. In 1975 Robinson et al. [98] showed that the medium from cultured rheumatoid synovium contains bone-resorbing activity that could be essentially completely accounted for by the amount of PGE produced by that synovial culture. Synthesis of PGE by rheumatoid synovium could be blocked with indomethacin and enhanced with colchicine, with parallel changes in bone-resorbing activity [97]. Moreover prostaglandins have been identified in rheumatoid synovium in vivo [56].

Localized bone loss is also a major clinical problem in patients with periodontal disease when the loss of alveolar bone is the principal cause of loss of teeth [40]. In 1973 Harris and associates [47] showed that dental cysts that produce local alveolar bone loss contain substantial amounts of prostaglandin. Subsequently, Goodson et al. [42] demonstrated prostaglandins in inflamed gingiva. Bone-resorbing activity has also been found in the media of cultured gingival tissue [35,41], but this activity may not be entirely attributed to preformed prostaglandins. Goldhaber et al. [40] suggested that there was a macromolecular material released from gingiva that could stimulate bone resorption in culture. This effect was blocked by adding indomethacin to the bone cultures, suggesting that the gingival factor stimulated prostaglandin production by bone tissue. No measurements of prostaglandin production were reported. Gomes et al. [41] found bone-resorbing activity in monkey gingiva, which they attributed to PGE production; but in their studies there was no difference between inflamed and normal gingival tissue. Nevertheless prostaglandin can produce changes in gingival tissue [58].

A major problem in interpretation of all these studies, as with those on cultured breast tissue, has been the possibility that prostaglandin production in culture may not reflect production in vivo. It is difficult to prevent prostaglandin production during the handling of freshly isolated tissue. Recently, Hopps and associates [53] studied gingival tissue that was rapidly placed in liquid nitrogen and maintained at low temperature while it was dried and powdered. When this material was incubated in culture medium it released substantial amounts of bone-resorbing activity. This release was not inhibited by the addition of indomethacin and could not be accounted for by preformed PGE, which was present only at low concentrations. Moreover, the material did not increase prostaglandin synthesis in bone. Subsequent studies showed that this bone-resorbing activity was correlated with the presence of gingival inflammation (W. A. Soskoline, K. Nuki, and L. G. Raisz, unpublished observation). The effect might be attributable to bacterial endotoxins present on the surface of inflamed gingival tissue. Endotoxin effects might be enhanced by the small amount of prostaglandin present since, as noted above, these two agents can produce synergistic stimulation of resorption.

Prostaglandins may also be involved in other skeletal lesions. High concentrations of PGE were found in the calcium deposits in a patient with calcinosis circumscripta [17] and in another with myositis ossificans [74]. The potent bone-resorbing capacity of PGI_2, which is produced by vascular endothelium, suggests another pathogenetic mechanism. Vascular invasion is regularly associated with local bone resorption in chronic inflammation or in such lesions as hemangiomatosis (Gorham's disease), as well as in normal bone remodeling.

CONCLUSIONS

Prostaglandins clearly have important effects on skeletal metabolism and are potent stimulators of bone resorption. Pathologically, an effect on bone resorption is likely to be of importance in some patients with hypercalcemia and osteolysis due to malignancy and in localized bone loss associated with inflammation. It is also possible that prostaglandins mediate cartilage destruction in some forms of arthritis and bone loss associated with vascular invasion. These pathologic states may be characterized by complex interactions between one or more prostaglandins and other mediators of bone resorption, which make it difficult to assess the role of one particular agent. There is no proof that prostaglandins are physiologic modulators of bone or cartilage metabolism, but this is an attractive possibility. Particularly worthy of further study is the suggestion that prostacyclin released by vascular endothelium may mediate Haversian and metaphyseal remodeling in which osteoclastic activity is closely associated with vascular invasion. Another attractive hypothesis is that mechanical stress on bone cells results in prostaglandin production, which then mediates local changes in bone resorption or formation.

Further research will clarify these issues and generate new questions concerning the role of prostaglandins. However it seems inevitable that prostaglandins will receive increasing attention as physiologic and pathologic regulators of skeletal structure and function, and that the skeleton as an organ system will be as important in prostaglandin research as the cardiovascular and reproductive systems, which have received so much attention in the past.

REFERENCES

1. Advani, A. T., and Pettit, L. D. (1973) The formation constants of the proton and calcium complexes of prostaglandins PGE_1 and PGF_1. Chem. Biol. Interactions 7, 181–184.

2. Atkins, D., and Martin, T. J. (1977) Rat osteogenic sarcoma cells: Effects of some prostaglandins, their metabolites and analogues on cyclic AMP production. Prostaglandins 13, 861–871.

3. Atkins, D., Hunt, N. H., Ingleton, P. M., and Martin, T. J. (1977) Rat osteogenic sarcoma cells. Isolation and effects of hormones on the production of cyclic AMP and cyclic GMP. Endocrinology 101, 555–561.

4. Atkins, D., Ibbotson, K. J., Hillier, K., Hunt, N. H., Hammonds, J. C., and Martin, T. J. (1977) Secretion of prostaglandins as bone resorbing agents by renal cortical carcinoma in culture. Br. J. Cancer 36, 601–607.

5. Atkins, D., Greaves, M., Ibbotson, K. J., and Martin, T. J. (1979) Role of prostaglandins in bone metabolism: A review. J. R. Soc. Med. 72, 27.

6. Beliel, O. M., Singer, F. R., and Coburn, J. W. (1973) Prostaglandins: Effect on plasma calcium concentration. Prostaglandins 3, 237–241.

7. Bennett, A., Simpson, J. S., McDonald, A. M., and Stamford, I. F. (1975) Breast cancer, prostaglandins and bone metastases. Lancet 1, 1218–1220.

8. Bennett, A., Charlier, E. M., McDonald, A. M., Simpson, J. S., Stamford, I. F., and Zebro, T. (1977) Prostaglandins and breast cancer. Lancet 2, 624–626.

9. Bennett, A., Edwards, D. A., Ali, N. N., Auger, D. W., and Harris, M. (1979) Prostacyclin potently resorbs bone in vitro. Paper presented at the Fourth International Prostaglandin Conference, Washington, D. C., May 27–31.

10. Blackwell, G. J., Flower, R. J., Nijkamp, F. P., and Vane, J. R. (1977) Phospholipase A_2 activity of guinea-pig perfused lungs: Stimulation and inhibition by anti-inflammatory steroids. Proc. Br. J. Pharmacol. 59, 441P.

11. Blumenkrantz, N., and Sondergaard, J. (1972) Effect of prostaglandins E_1 and $F_{1\alpha}$ on biosynthesis of collagen. Nature (London) New Biol. 239, 246.

12. Bockman, R. S., Myers, W. P. L., Kempin, S., and Bajorunas, D. (1977) Prostaglandin E in cancer patients. Clin. Res. 25, 387A.

13. Bonta, I. L., and Parnham, M. J. (1978) Prostaglandins and chronic inflammation Biochem. Pharmacol. 26, 1611–1623.

14. Bray, M., Gordon, D., Morley, J., and Myatt, L. (1975) Macrophages on intrauterine contraceptive devices produce prostaglandins. Nature (London) 257, 227–228.

15. Breeton, H. D., Halushka, P. V., Alexander, R. W., Mason, D. M., Keiser, H. R., and De Vita, V. T., Jr. (1974) Indomethacin responsive hypercalcemia in a patient with renal-cell adenocarcinoma. New Engl. J. Med. 291, 83–85.

16. Brown, E. M., Gardner, D. G., Windeck, R. A., Hurwitz, S., Brennan, M. F., and Aurbach, G. D. (1979) β-Adrenergically stimulated adenosine 3',5'-monophosphate accumulation in and parathyroid hormone release from dispersed human parathyroid cells. J. Clin. Endocrinol. Metab. 48, 618–626.

17. Caniggia, A., Gennari, C., Vattimo, A., Runci, F., and Bombardieri, S. (1978) Prostaglandin PGE_2: A possible mechanism for bone destruction in calcinosis circumscripta. Calcif. Tissue Res. 25, 53–57.

18. Caro, J. F., Besarab, A., and Flynn, J. T. (1979) Prostaglandin E and hypercalcemia in breast carcinoma: Only a tumor marker? A need for perspective. Am. J. Med. 66, 337–341.

19. Chang, W. C., Abe, M., and Murota, S. I. (1977) Stimulation by prostaglandin $F_{2\alpha}$ of acidic glycosaminoglycan production in cultured fibroblasts. Prostaglandins 13, 55–63.

20. Chase, L. R., and Aurbach, G. D. (1970) The effect of parathyroid hormone on the concentration of adenosine $3',5'$-monophosphate in skeletal tissue in vitro. J. Biol. Chem. 245, 1520–1526.

21. Coombes, R. C., Neville, A. M., Bondy, P. K., and Powles, T. J. (1976) Failure of indomethacin to reduce hydroxyproline excretion or hypercalcemia in patients with breast cancer. Prostaglandins 12, 1027.

22. Coombes, R. C., Powles, T. J., and Joplin, G. F. (1977) Calcium metabolism in breast cancer. Proc. R. Soc. Med. 70, 195–199.

23. Crawford, A., Atkins, D., and Martin, T. J. (1978) Rat osteogenic sarcoma cells: Comparison of the effects of prostaglandins E_1, E_2, I_2 (prostacyclin), 6-keto $F_{1\alpha}$ and thromboxane B_2 on cyclic AMP production and adenylate cyclase activity. Biochem. Biophys. Res. Commun. 82, 1195–1201.

24. Denko, C. W., and Petricevic, M. (1977) Prostaglandin A_2 and ^{35}S uptake in connective tissue. Prostaglandins 14, 701–707.

25. Dietrich, J. W., and Raisz, L. G. (1975) Prostaglandin in calcium and bone metabolism. Clin. Orthop. 111, 228–237.

26. Dietrich, J. W., Goodson, J. M., and Raisz, L. G. (1975) Stimulation of bone resorption by various prostaglandins in organ culture. Prostaglandins 10, 231.

27. Dowsett, M., Eastman, A. R., Easty, D. M., Easty, G. C., Powles, T. J., and Neville, A. M. (1976) Prostaglandin mediation of collagenase induced bone resorption. Nature (London) 263, 72–74.

28. Dowsett, M., Easty, G. C., Powles, T. J., Easty, D. M., and Neville, A. M. (1976) Human breast tumor-induced osteolysis and prostaglandins. Prostaglandins 11, 447–455.

29. Dowsett, M., Gazet, J. C., Powles, T. J., Easty, G. C., and Neville, A. M. (1976) Benign breast lesions and osteolysis. Lancet 1, 970–971.

30. Easty, G. C., Dowsett, M., Powles, T. J., Easty, D. M., Gazet, J. C., and Neville, A. M. (1977) Hypercalcemia in malignant disease. Proc. R. Soc. Med. 70, 191–201.

31. Eilon, G., and Mundy, G. R. (1978) Direct resorption of bone by human breast cancer cells in vitro. Nature (London) 276, 726–728.

32. Eilon, G., and Raisz, L. G. (1978) Comparison of the effects of stimulators and inhibitors of resorption on the release of lysosomal enzymes and radioactive calcium from fetal bone in organ culture. Endocrinology 103, 1969–1975.

33. Eisenbarth, G. S., Beuttel, S. C., and Lebovitz, H. E. (1974) Inhibition of cartilage macromolecular synthesis by prostaglandin A_1. J. Pharmacol. Exp. Ther. 189, 213–220.

34. Eisenbarth, G. S., and Lebovitz, H. E. (1974) Prostaglandin inhibition of cartilage chondromucoprotein synthesis; Concept of "intrinsic activity." Prostaglandins 7, 11–20.

35. Elattar, T. M. A. (1976) Prostaglandin E_2 in human gingiva in health and disease and its stimulation by female sex steroids. Prostaglandins 11, 311.

36. Faccini, J. M. (1974) The mode of growth of experimental metastases in rabbit femora. Virchows Arch. Pathol. Anat. 364, 249–263.

37. Franklin, R. B., and Tashjian, A. H., Jr. (1975) Intravenous infusion of prostaglandin E_2 raises plasma calcium concentration in the rat. Endocrinology 97, 240–243.

38. Galasko, C. S. B. (1976) Mechanisms of bone destruction in the development of skeletal metastases. Nature 263, 507–508.

39. Galasko, C. S. B., and Bennett, A. (1976) Relationship of bone destruction in skeletal metastases to osteoclast activation and prostaglandins. Nature (London) 263, 508–510.

40. Goldhaber, P., Rabadjija, L., Beyer, W. R., and Kornhauser, A. (1973) Bone resorption in tissue culture and its relevance to periodontal disease. J. Am. Dent. Assoc. 87, 1027–1032.

40a. Goldring, S. R., Dayer, J. M., and Krane, S. M. (1979) Regulation of hormone-induced cyclic AMP response to parathyroid hormone and prostaglandin E_2 in cells cultured from human giant cell tumors of bone. Calcif. Tiss. Int. 29, 193.

41. Gomes, B. C., Hausmann, E., Weinfeld, N., and De Luca, C. (1976) Prostaglandins: Bone resorption stimulating factors released from monkey gingiva. Calcif. Tissue Res. 19, 285–293.

42. Goodson, J. M. Dewhirst, F. E., and Brunetti, A. (1974) Prostaglandin E_2 levels and human periodontal disease. Prostaglandins 6, 81–85.

42a. Goodson, J. M., McClatchy, K., and Revell, C. (1974) Prostaglandin-induced resorption of the adult rat calvarium. J. Dent. Res. 53, 670–677.

43. Goodson, J. M., Offenbacher, S., and Bloomfield, R. B. (1979) Effects of indomethacin pretreatment on prostaglandin and lipopolysaccharide stimulated bone resorption, J. Dent. Res. 58, 120.

44. Greaves, M., Ibbotson, K. J., Atkins, D., and Martin, T. J. (1979) Prostaglandins extracted from tumors and produced by cultures of renal cortical carcinoma and benign and malignant breast tumors: Relation to bone resorption. Clin. Sci. 58, 201–210.

45. Harell, A., Dekel, S., and Binderman, I. (1977) Biochemical effect of mechanical stress on cultured bone cells. Calcif. Tissue Res. 22, 202–207.

46. Harper, R., Heersche, J. N. M., and Sodek, J. (1979) Effects of parathyroid hormone and prostaglandin E_1 on collagen metabolism and cAMP response in isolated bone cells. J. Dent. Res. 58, 155, 251.

47. Harris, M., Jenkins, M. V., Bennett, A., and Wills, M. R. (1973) Dental cysts, prostaglandins and bone resorption. Nature (London) 245, 213–215.

48. Hausmann, E., Luderitz, O., Knox, K., and Weinfeld, N. (1975) Structural requirements for bone resorption by endotoxin and lipoteichoic acid. J. Dent. Res. Special Issue B54, B94–B99.

49. Heersche, J. N. M., Heyboer, M. P. M., and Ng, B. (1978) Hormone specific suppression of adenosine $3',5'$-monophosphate responses in bone in vitro during prolonged incubation with parathyroid hormone, prostaglandin E_1 and calcitonin. Endocrinology 103, 333–340.

50. Holtrop, M. E. (1975) The ultrastructure of bone. Ann. Clin. Lab. Sci. 5, 264–271.

51. Holtrop, M. E., and King, G. J. (1977) The ultrastructure of the osteoclast and its functional implications. Clin. Orthop. 123, 177–196.

52. Holtrop, M. E., and Raisz, L. G. (1979) Comparison of the effects of 1,25-dihydroxycholecalciferol prostaglandin E_2 and osteoclast activating factor with parathyroid hormone on the ultrastructure of osteoclasts in cultured long bones of fetal rats. Calc. Tissue Int. 29, 201.

53. Hopps, R. M., Nuki, K., and Raisz, L. G. (1979) Demonstration of bone resorptive activity in freeze-dried gingiva. J. Dent. Res. 58, 99.

54. Horrobin, D. F. (1977) Interactions between prostaglandins and calcium—Importance of bell-shaped dose response curves. Prostaglandins 14, 667–677.

55. Hough, A., Seyberth, H., Oates, J., and Hartmann, W. (1977) Changes in bone and bone marrow of rabbits bearing the VX_2 carcinoma. Am. J. Pathol. 87, 537–547.

56. Husby, G., Bankhurst, A. D., and Williams, R. C., Jr. (1977) Immunohistochemical localization of prostaglandin E in rheumatoid synovium tissue. Arthritis Rheum. 20, 784–791.

57. Ignarro, L. J., and Cech, S. Y. (1975) Inhibition of human neutrophil-mediated cartilage degradation by prostaglandins and glucocorticoids. Arthritis Rheum. 18, 406.

58. Kafrawy, A. H., and Mitchell, D. F. (1977) Effects of prostaglandin E_1 on periodontium of rats. J. Dent. Res. 56, 1132–1133.

59. Kent, G. R., and Cohn, D. V. (1979) Interaction of bone active agents on cAMP production in isolated bone cells. Programs and Abstracts, 61st Annual Meeting, Endocrine Society, p. 84.

60. Kirtland, S. J., and Baum, H. (1972) Prostaglandin E₁ may act as a calcium ionophore. Nature (London) New Biol. 236, 47–49.
61. Kirkpatrick, J. C., and Gardner, D. L. (1976) Chondrocyte growth inhibition by prostaglandin A₁. J. Cell Biol. 70, 168a.
62. Klein, D. C., and Raisz, L. G. (1970) Prostaglandins: Stimulation of bone resorption in tissue culture. Endocrinology 86, 1436–1440.
63. Kleine, T. O., and Jungmann, U. (1977) Inhibitory and stimulating effects of prostaglandins A, E, F on the in vitro biosynthesis and glycosaminoglycans and protein from calf rib cartilage. Pharmacol. Res. Commun. 9, 823–831.
64. Levine, L., Hinkle, P. M., Voelkel, E. F., and Tashjian, A. H., Jr. (1972) Prostaglandin production by mouse fibrosarcoma cells in culture: By indomethacin and aspirin. Biochem. Biophys. Res. Commun. 47, 888–896.
65. Lippiello, L., Yamamoto, K., Robinson, D. R., and Makin, H. J. (1978) Involvement of prostaglandins from rheumatoid synovium in inhibition of articular cartilage net. Arthritis Rheum. 21, 909–917.
67. Lorenzo, J. L., and Raisz, L. G. (1979) Bone-resorbing activity in fetal calf serum. First Annual Meeting of the American Society for Bone Mineral Research, June 11–12, Anaheim, Calif., p. 3A.
68. Malemud, C. J., and Sokoloff, L. (1977) Effect of prostaglandins on cultured lapine articular chondrocytes. Prostaglandins 13, 845–860.
69. Marcus, R., and Orner, F. B. (1977) Cyclic AMP production in rat calvaria in vitro—Interactions of prostaglandins with parathyroid hormone. Endocrinology 101, 1570–1578.
70. Marcus, R., Orner, F., and Keutman, H. (1979) Effects of parathyroid hormone (PTH) and prostaglandins (PG) on calcium uptake in bone cells. First Annual Meeting of the American Society for Bone Mineral Research, June 11–12, Anaheim, Calif., p. 3A.
71. Martin, T. J., Ingleton, P. M., Underwood, J. C. E., Michelangeli, V. P., Hunt, N. H., and Melick, R. A. (1976) Parathyroid hormone-responsive adenylate cyclase in induced transplantable osteogenic rat sarcoma. Nature (London) 260, 436–437.
72. Martin, T. J., Partridge, N. C., Greaves, M., Atkins, D., and Ibbotson, K. J. (1980) Prostaglandin effects on bone and role in cancer hypercalcemia. Endocrinology, in press.
73. Marx, S. J., Zusman, R. M., and Umiker, W. O. (1977) Benign breast dysplasia causing hypercalcemia. J. Clin. Endocrinol. Metab. 45, 1049–1052.
74. Maxwell, W. A., Halushka, P. V., Miller, R. L., Spicer, S. S., Westphal, M. C., and Penny, L. D. (1978) Elevated prostaglandin production in cultured cells from a patient with fibrodysplasia ossificans progressiva. Prostaglandins 15, 123–129.
75. Minne, H., Ziegler, R., and Arnaud, C. D. (1977) Paraneoplastic parathyroid hormone production by the hypercalcemic Walker carcinosarcoma 256 of the rat. In: D. H. Copp and R. V. Talmage (eds.), Endocrinology of Calcium Metabolism, Proceedings of the Sixth Parathyroid Conference, Vancouver, B. C., Canada, June 12–17, Excerpta Medica, Amsterdam.
76. Mundy, G. R. (1978) Calcium and cancer. Life Sci. 23, 1735–1744.
77. Mundy, G. R., Altman, A. J., Gondek, M. D., and Bandelin, J. G. (1977) Direct resorption of bone by human monocytes. Science 196, 1109–1111.
78. Murray, T. M., Josse, R. G., and Heersche, J. N. M. (1978) Review article: Hypercalcemia and cancer: An update. Can. Med. Assoc. J. 119, 915–920.
79. Northington, F. K., Oglesby, T. D., Ishikawa, Y., and Wuthier, R. E. (1978) Localization of prostaglandin synthetase in chicken epiphyseal cartilage. Calcif. Tissue Res. 26, 227–336.
80. Parnham, M. J., Shoshan, S., Bonta, I. L., and Neimanwollner, S. (1977) Increased collagen metabolism in granulomata induced in rats deficient in endogenous prostaglandin precursors. Prostaglandins 14, 709–714.

81. Powles, T. J., Clark, S. A., Easty, D. M., Easty, G. C., and Neville, A. M. (1973) The inhibition by aspirin and indomethacin of osteolytic tumor deposits and hypercalcemia in rats with Walker tumor and its possible application to human breast cancer. Br. J. Cancer 28, 316–321.

82. Powell, D., Singer, F. R., Murray, T. M., Minkin, C., and Potts, J. T., Jr. (1973) Non-parathyroid humoral hypercalcemia in patients with neoplastic diseases. New Engl. J. Med. 289, 176–181.

83. Raisz, L. G. (1972) Mechanisms in bone resorption. In: E. E. Astwood and R. Greep (eds.), Handbook of Physiology, section on Endocrinology, Vol. 7, Williams and Wilkins, Baltimore, pp. 117–136.

84. Raisz, L. G., and Koolemans-Beynen, A. R. (1974) Inhibition of collagen synthesis by prostaglandin E_2 in organ culture. Prostaglandins 8, 377–385.

85. Raisz, L. G., Trummel, C. L., Wener, J. A., and Simmons, H. A. (1972) Effect of glucocorticoids on bone resorption in tissue culture. Endocrinology 90, 961–967.

86. Raisz, L. G., Mundy, G. R., and Luben, R. A. (1974) Skeletal reactions to neoplasms. Ann. NY Acad. Sci. 230, 473–475.

87. Raisz, L. G., Sandberg, A., Goodson, J. M., Simmons, H. A. and Mergenhagen, S. E. (1974) Complement-dependent stimulation of prostaglandin synthesis and bone resorption. Science 185, 789–791.

88. Raisz, L. G., Dietrich, J. W., Simmons, H. A., Seyberth, H. W., Hubbard, W., and Oates, J. A. (1977) Effect of prostaglandin endoperoxides and metabolites on bone resorption in vitro. Nature (London) 267, 532–534, 1977.

89. Raisz, L. G., Mundy, G. R., and Eilon, G. (1977) Hypercalcemia of neoplastic diseases. In "Endocrinology of Calcium Metabolism," D. H. Copp and R. V. Talmage (eds.), Proceedings of the Sixth Parathyroid Conference, Vancouver, B. C., Canada, June 12–17, Excerpta Medica, Amsterdam, pp. 64–70.

90. Raisz, L. G., Vanderhoek, J. Y., Simmons, H. A., Kream, B. E., and Nicolaou, K. C. (1979) Prostaglandin synthesis by fetal rat bone in vitro: Evidence for a role of prostacyclin. Prostaglandins 7, 905–914.

91. Rao, L. G., Ng, B., Brunette, D. M., and Heersche, J. N. M. (1977) Parathyroid hormone and prostaglandin E_1-response in a selected population of bone cells after repeated subculture and storage at $-80°C$. Endocrinology 100, 1233–1241.

92. Reed, P. W., and Knapp, H. R. (1978) Prostaglandins and calcium. Ann. NY Acad. Sci. 307, 445–447.

93. Ro, J., Sudmann, E., and Marton, P. F. (1976) Effect of indomethacin on fracture healing in rats. Acta Orthop. Scand. 47, 588–599.

94. Robertson, R. P., and Baylink, D. J. (1977) Hypercalcemia induced by prostaglandin E_2 in thyroparathyroidectomized but not intact rats. Prostaglandins 13, 1141–1145.

95. Robertson, R. P., Baylink, D. J., Marini, J. J., and Adkison, H. W. (1975) Elevated prostaglandins and suppressed parathyroid hormone associated with hypercalcemia and renal cell carcinoma. J. Clin. Endocrinol. Metab. 41, 164–167.

96. Robertson, R. P., Baylink, D. J., Metz, S. A., and Cummings, K. B. (1976) Plasma prostaglandin E in patients with cancer with and without hypercalcemia. J. Clin. Endocrinol. Metab. 43, 1330–1335.

97. Robinson, D. R., Smith, H., McGuire, M. B., and Levine, L. (1975) Prostaglandin synthesis by rheumatoid synovium and its stimulation by colchicine. Prostaglandins 10, 67–85.

98. Robinson, D. R., Tashjian, A. H., Jr., and Levine, L. (1975) Prostaglandin stimulated bone resorption by rheumatoid synovia. Possible mechanisms for bone destruction in rheumatoid arthritis. J. Clin. Invest. 56, 1181.

99. Roos, B. A., Bundy, L. L., Miller, E. A., and Deftos, L. J. (1975) Calcitonin secretion by monolayer cultures of human C-cells derived from medullary thyroid carcinoma. Endocrinology 97, 39–45.

99a. Sakamoto, S. M., Sakamoto, P., Goldhaber, M. J., and Glimcher, M. J. (1979) Col-

lagenase activity and morphological and chemical bone resorption induced by prostaglandin E_2 in tissue culture. Proc. Soc. Exp. Biol. Med. 161, 99.

100. Sandberg, A. L., Raisz, L. G., Goodson, J. M., Simmons, H. A., and Mergenhagen S. E. (1977) Initiation of bone resorption by the classical and alternative C pathways and its mediation by prostaglandins. J. Immunol. 119, 1378–1381.

101. Santoro, M. G., Jaffe, B. M., and Simmons, D. J. (1977) Bone resorption in vitro and in vivo in PGE treated mice. Proc. Soc. Exp. Biol. Med. 156, 373–377.

101a. Schelling, S. H., Wolfe, H. J., and Tashjian, A. H. (1980) Role of the osteoclast in prostaglandin E_2 stimulated bone resorption; a correlative morphometric and bio-chemical analysis. Lab. Invest. 42, 290–299.

102. Seyberth, H. W. (1978) Prostaglandin mediated hypercalcemia: A paraneoplastic syn-drome. Klin. Wochenschr. 56, 373–378 (in English).

103. Seyberth, H. W., Segre, G. V., Morgan, J. L., Sweetman, B. J., Potts, J. T., Jr., and Oates, J. A. (1975) Prostaglandins as mediators of hypercalcemia associated with cancer. New Engl. J. Med. 293, 1278–1283.

104. Seyberth, H. W., Hubbard, W. C., Oelz, O., Sweetman, B. J., Watson, J. T., and Oates, J. A. (1977) Prostaglandin-mediated hypercalcemia in the VX_2 carcinoma bear-ing rabbit. Prostaglandins 14, 319–331.

105. Seyberth, H. W., Raisz, L. G., and Oates, J. A. (1978) Prostaglandins and hypercal-cemic states. Annu. Rev. Med. 29, 23–29.

106. Simmons, H. A., Canalis, E., and Raisz, L. G. (1979) Effect of epidermal growth factor on resorption of fetal rat long bone in vitro. First Annual Meeting of the American Society for Bone Mineral Research, June 11–12, Anaheim, Calif., p. 5A.

107. Singer, F. R., Sharp, C. F., and Rude, R. K. (1979) Pathogenesis of hypercalcemia in malignancy. Miner. Electrol. Metab. 2, 161.

107a. Somjen, D., Binderman, I., Berger, E., and Harell, A. (1980) Bone remodelling induced by physical stress is prostaglandin (PGE_2) mediated. Biochim. Biophys. Acta. 627, 91–100.

108. Spiro, T., and Mundy, G. R. (1979) Prostaglandins mediate in vitro bone resorption caused by cultured Walker rat 256 carcinoma cells. First Annual Meeting of the American Society for Bone Mineral Research, June 11–12, Anaheim, Calif. p. 22A.

109. Stamford, I. F., Wright, J. E., Bennett, A., Rowe, D. J. F., and Harris, M. (1979) Benign breast tumors: PG yield low with homogenisation but high with incubation. Fourth International Prostaglandin Conference May 27–31, p. 111.

110. Stern, P. H., Miller, J. C., Chen, S. F., and Kahn, D. J. (1978) A bone resorbing substance from bovine serum albumin. Calcif. Tissue Res. 25, 233–240.

111. Strausser, H. R., and Humes, J. L. (1975) Prostaglandin synthesis inhibition: Effect on bone changes and sarcoma tumor induction on BALB/c mice. Int. J. Cancer 15, 724–730.

112. Sudman, E., and Bang, G. (1979) Indomethacin-induced inhibition of Haversian remodeling in rabbits. Acta Orthop. Scand. 50, 621.

113. Tashjian, A. H., Jr. (1975) Prostaglandins, hypercalcemia and cancer. New Engl. J. Med. 293, 1317–1318.

114. Tashjian, A. H., Jr., Voelkel, E. F., Levine, L., and Goldhaber, P. (1972) Evidence that the bone resorption stimulating factor produced by mouse fibrosarcoma cells is prostaglandin E_2. A new model for the hypercalcemia of cancer. J. Exp. Med. 136, 1329–1343.

115. Tashjian, A. H., Jr., Voelkel, E. F., Goldhaber, P., and Levine, L. (1973) Successful treatment of hypercalcemia by indomethacin in mice bearing a prostaglandin-pro-ducing fibrosarcoma. Prostaglandins 3, 515–524.

116. Tashjian, A. H., Jr., Tice, J. E., and Sides, K. (1977) Biological activities of prosta-glandin analogues and metabolites on bone in organ culture. Nature (London) 266, 645–666.

117. Tashjian, A. H., Jr., Voelkel, E. F., and Levine, L. (1977) Effects of hydrocortisone

on the hypercalcemia and plasma levels of 13,14-dihydro-15-keto-prostaglandin E_2 in mice bearing the HSDMI fibrosarcoma. Biochem. Biophys. Res. Commun. 74, 199–207.

118. Tashjian, A. H., Jr., Voelkel, E. F., and Levine, L. (1977) Plasma concentrations of 13,14-dihydro-15-keto-prostaglandin E_2 in rabbits bearing VX_2 carcinoma effects of hydrocortisone and indomethacin. Prostaglandins 14, 309–317.

119. Tashjian, A. H., Jr., and Levine, L. (1978) Epidermal growth factor stimulates prostaglandin production and bone resorption in cultured mouse calvaria. Biochem. Biophys. Res. Commun. 85, 966–975.

120. Tashjian, A. H., Jr., Ivey, J. L., Delclos, B., and Levine, L. (1978) Stimulation of prostaglandin production in bone by phorbol diesters and mellitin. Prostaglandins 16, 221–232.

121. Teitz, C. C., and Chrisman, O. D. (1975) The effect of salicylate and chloroquinine on prostaglandin-induced articular damage in the rabbit knee. Clin. Orthop. 108, 264–274.

122. Voelkel, E. F., Tashjian, A. H., Jr., Franklin, E., Wasserman, E., and Levine, L. (1975) Hypercalcemia and tumor—Prostaglandins: The VX_2 carcinoma model in the rabbit. Metabolism 24, 973–986.

123. Wahl, L. M., Olsen, C. E., Sandberg, A. O., and Mergenhagen, S. E. (1977) Prostaglandin regulation of macrophage collagenase production. Proc. Natl. Acad. Sci. (US) 74, 4955–4958.

124. Wolfe, H. J., Bitman, W. R., Voelkel, E. F., Griffiths, H. J., and Tashjian, A. H., Jr. (1978) Systemic effects of the VX_2 carcinoma on the osseous skeleton: A quantitative study of trabecular bone. Lab. Invest. 38, 208–215.

125. Wong, P. Y. K., and Wuthier, R. (1974) Isolation and identification of prostaglandin PGB_1 in growth cartilage. Prostaglandins 8, 125–129.

126. Wong, P. Y. K., Majeska, R. J., and Wuthier, R. E. (1977) Biosynthesis and metabolism of prostaglandins in chick epiphyseal cartilage. Prostaglandins 14, 839–851.

127. Yoneda, T., and Mundy, G. R. (1979) Prostaglandins are necessary for osteoclast activating factor production by activated peripheral blood leukocytes. J. Exp. Med. 149, 279–283.

128. Young, D. M., Ward, J. M., and Prieur, D. J. (1978) Animal model of human disease. Am. J. Pathol. 93, 619–722.

129. Yu, J. H., Wells, H., Ryan, W. J., and Lloyd, W. S. (1976) Effects of prostaglandins and other drugs on cyclic AMP content of cultured bone cells. Prostaglandins 12, 501–513.

130. Yu, J. H., Wells, H., Moghadam, B., Ryan, W. J., Jr. (1979) Cyclic AMP formation and release by cultured bone cells stimulated with prostaglandin E_2. Prostaglandins 17, 61–70.

131. Zurier, R. B., and Quagliata, F. (1971) Effect of prostaglandin E on adjuvant arthritis. Nature (London) 234, 304–305.

INDEX

373

Secretion
  biliary, 119–120
  gastric, 115–118, 124–126
  intestinal, 118–119
  pancreatic, 120–124
  of saliva, 114–115
Serotonin, 4
Skin inflammations, 101–102
Small intestinal contractility, 137–143
Small intestinal motile function, 143–145
Sodium excretion, 259–269
Sodium homeostasis, 259–269
Sodium iodide, antiinflammatory effects of, 99
Splanchnic circulation
  and arachidonic acid, 185–186
  and prostacyclin, 203–204
Sponge-induced granuloma formation, 102–103
SRS, 72–77
Suppressor cells, 55–56
Suprofen, inhibition of PG biosynthesis by, 5

T
T cells, 54–57
Thromboxane(s)
  agents inhibiting formation of, 9–10; see also specific agent
  biosynthesis of, 7–10
  receptors, 18
Thromboxane A_2, 197–199
  and blood pressure, 198
  and cerebral circulation, 199
  and coronary circulation, 198–199
  discovery of, 311
  and platelet aggregation, 314–315, 316
  and renal circulation, 199

Thromboxane B_2
  and blood pressure, 200
  cardiac actions of, 200
  and pulmonary circulation, 200
Thromboxane synthetase inhibitors, 329–331
Tranylcypromine, inhibition of prostaglandin synthetase by, 331
L-Tryptophan, 4

U
Ulcer formation, 124–126
Umbilical circulation, PG levels in, 232
Uterine bleeding, 228–229
Uterine contractility, 219, 224, 226–227
  nonpregnant, 224–227
  pregnant, 224, 229
Uteroplacental circulation, and PGD_2, 197
Uterus, 232–233
  nonpregnant, 224–229
  pregnant, 229–233

V
Vasoactive compounds, 258
Vasodepressor effects, of prostacyclin, 320
Vasopressin, 269–270
Vinblastine, 24
Vitamin E, 4

W
Water excretion, 269–272

Z
Zn^{2+}, inhibition of thromboxane B_2 synthesis by, 10